Person Centered Psychiatry

Juan E. Mezzich · Michel Botbol
George N. Christodoulou
C. Robert Cloninger · Ihsan M. Salloum
Editors

Person Centered Psychiatry

Springer

Editors
Juan E. Mezzich
Professor of Psychiatry, Icahn School of Medicine at Mount Sinai
New York, NY
USA

Michel Botbol
Professor of Child and Adolescent Psychiatry
University of Western Brittany
Brest
France

George N. Christodoulou
Emeritus Professor of Psychiatry
University of Athens
Athens
Greece

C. Robert Cloninger
Wallace Renard Professor of Psychiatry, Genetics and Psychology
Washington University School of Medicine
Saint Louis, MO
USA

Ihsan M. Salloum
Professor of Psychiatry, Miller School of Medicine
University of Miami
Coral Gables, FL
USA

ISBN 978-3-319-39722-1   ISBN 978-3-319-39724-5 (eBook)
DOI 10.1007/978-3-319-39724-5

Library of Congress Control Number: 2016941285

Printed on acid-free paper

This Springer imprint is published by Springer Nature
The registered company is Springer International Publishing AG Switzerland

Contents

Contributors

Mohammed T. Abou-Saleh, MD, PhD Professor of Psychiatry, St George's Medical School, University of London, London, UK

Michaela Amering, MD Univ. Prof., Department of Psychiatry and Psychotherapy, Medical University of Vienna, Vienna, Austria

Maria Ammon, PhD Psychotherapist and Psychoanalyst, President of the German Academy for Psychoanalysis (DAP) and Secretary General of the World Association for Dynamic Psychiatry (WADP), Berlin, Germany

Dimitris Anagnostopoulos, MD, PhD Associate Professor of Child and Adolescent Psychiatry, Department of Child and Adolescent Psychiatry, University of Athens, General Pediatric Hospital of Athens "Agia Sofia", Athens, Greece

William Anthony, PhD Professor Emeritus, Center for Psychiatric Rehabilitation, Boston University, Boston, USA

James Appleyard, MA, MD, FRCPCH Former Consultant Pediatrician, Kent and Canterbury Hospital, Canterbury, UK; President, International College of Person Centered Medicine, London, UK

Said A. Azim, MD, PhD Professor Emeritus of Psychiatry, Cairo University, Giza, Egypt

Claudio E.M. Banzato, MD, PhD Associate Professor, Department of Psychiatry, Medical School, University of Campinas-UNICAMP, Campinas, Brazil

Rachid Bennegadi, MD Research and Teaching Pole, Centre Minkowska, Paris, France; University Diploma on Health, Disease, Care and Cultural Competence, University of Paris, Descartes, Paris, France

Moty Benyakar, MD, PhD Professor of Psychiatry, El Salvador Univ, Capital Federal, Buenos Aires, Argentina; President, Iberoamerican Ecobioethics Network for Education Science and Technology, Unesco Chair in Bioethics, Paris, France; Honorary Member, World Psychiatric Association, Geneva, Switzerland

Marco O. Bertelli, MD, PhD Research and Clinical Centre, San Sebastiano Foundation, Florence, Italy

Michel Botbol, MD Chief, Department of Child Psychiatry, Brest University Hospital, University of Western Brittany, Brest, France; Professor, Service Universitaire de Psychiatrie Infanto Juvénile, CHU de Brest, Hôpital de Bohars, Bohars, France

Lovorka Brajkovic, PhD Professor and Clinical Psychologist, Department of Psychiatry, University Hospital Centre Zagreb, Zagreb, Croatia

Marijana Braš, MD, PhD Associate Professor, Department of Psychological Medicine, Clinical Hospital Centre Zagreb, School of Medicine University of Zagreb, Zagreb, Croatia

Dawn J. Brooker, PhD Professor, Association for Dementia Studies, University of Worcester, Worcester, UK

Ilse Burbiel, PhD Psychotherapist and Psychoanalyst, Governor of the German Branch of WADP and Member of the World Psychiatric Association Psychoanalysis Section, Geneva, Switzerland

Megan M. Campbell, PhD Department of Psychiatry and Mental Health, University of Cape Town, Cape Town, South Africa

Eric Cassell, MD Emeritus Professor of Public Health, Weill Medical College of Cornell University, New York, USA; Adjunct Professor of Medicine, McGill University, Montréal, Canada; Attending Physician, New York Presbyterian Hospital, New York, USA

Angeliki Christodoulou, BSc, MA Psychologist, Scientific Collaborator, Child and Adolescent Mental Health Unit, Department of Psychiatry, Medical School, University of Athens, Athens, Greece

George N. Christodoulou, MD, PhD Emeritus Professor of Psychiatry, University of Athens, Athens, Greece

Nikos G. Christodoulou, MBBS, PhD, MRCPsych Honorary Assistant Professor in Psychiatry, University of Nottingham and Consultant Liaison Psychiatrist, Nottingham, UK; Department of Psychological Medicine, Queen's Medical Centre, Nottingham, UK

C. Robert Cloninger, MD, PhD Wallace Renard Professor of Psychiatry, Genetics, and Psychology, Director, Center for Wellbeing, Washington University School of Medicine, St Louis, MO, USA

Kevin M. Cloninger, PhD President, Anthropedia Foundation, St. Louis, MO, USA

Carlos Collazo, MD Professor of Psychiatry, El Salvador Univ, Capital Federal, Buenos Aires, Argentina; Honorary Chair, WPA Section on Disaster Psychiatry, Geneva, Switzerland; International Fellow, American Psychiatric Association, Arlington County, VA, USA

John Cox, MD Professor Emeritus, Keele University, Keele, Staffordshire, UK

Myriam Deveugele, MA, PhD Professor of Communication in Health Science, Department of Family Medicine and Primary Health Care, Faculty of Medicine, Ghent University, Ghent, Belgium

Veljko Djordjevic, MD, PhD Professor, Department of Psychological Medicine, Clinical Hospital Centre Zagreb and School of Medicine, University of Zagreb, Zagreb, Croatia

Athanassios Douzenis, MD, MMSc Associate Professor of Psychiatry, Forensic Psychiatry, 2nd Psychiatry Department, Attikon Hospital, National and Kapodistrian University of Athens Medical School, Athens, Greece

Marianne Farkas, ScD Professor, Center for Psychiatric Rehabilitation, Boston University, Boston, MA, USA

Arnstein Finset, PhD Professor, Department of Behavioral Sciences in Medicine, Institute of Basic Medical Sciences, Faculty of Medicine, University of Oslo, Oslo, Norway

Wolfgang Gaebel, MD Professor, Department of Psychiatry and Psychotherapy, Heinrich Heine University, Düsseldorf, Germany

Elena Gayvoronskaya, MD, PhD Assistant Professor of Psychiatry, N. N. Burdenko State Medical University, Voronezh, Russia

Tesfamicael Ghebrehiwet, PhD Former Consultant, Nursing and Health Policy, International Council of Nurses, Board Director, International College of Person-Centered Medicine, Calgary, Canada

Paul Glare, MD Palliative Medicine Service, Division of Supportive Care and Survivorship, Department of Medicine, Memorial Sloan Kettering Cancer Center, New York, NY, USA; Department of Medicine, Weill Cornell Medical College, New York, NY, USA

Fragiskos Gonidakis, MD, PhD Eating Disorders Unit, 1st Psychiatric Department, Medical School, National and Kapodistrian University of Athens, Athens, Greece

Luigi Grassi, MD Professor and Chair of Psychiatry, Program on Psycho-Oncology, University of Ferrara, Ferrara, Italy

Alison Gray, MD Cadbury Centre, Birmingham University, Birmingham, UK

Joanna Groves, BSc, MSc Board member, International College of Person Centered Medicine, Former Chief Executive Officer, International Alliance of Patients' Organizations, London, UK

Jeanine M. Hayes, RN, MSL Psychiatric Nurse and Master of Science in Health Law, Pittsburgh, PA, USA

Helen Herrman, MD Professor of Psychiatry, The National Center of Excellence in Youth Mental Health and the University of Melbourne, Geneva, Switzerland; President-Elect, World Psychiatric Association, Geneva, Switzerland

Ruben Hernandez, MD Professor of Forensic Psychiatry and Medico Legal Sexology, Universidad Central, Caracas, Venezuela

Miro Jakovljević, MD Professor of Psychiatry, Department of Psychiatry, University Hospital Centre Zagreb, School of Medicine, University of Zagreb, Zagreb, Croatia

D. Jousset MD, PhD University Lecturer, Director of Research, Program on Ethics, Professionalism, and Health, Department of Philosophy, University of Brest, Brest, France

Roy Abraham Kallivayalil MD, DPM, MAMS Vice-Principal, Professor and Head, Dept of Psychiatry, Pushpagiri Institute of Medical Sciences, Tiruvalla, Kerala, India; Secretary General, World Psychiatric Association, Geneva, Switzerland

Marianne C. Kastrup, MD, PhD Specialist in Psychiatry, Frederiksberg, Denmark

Levent Kirisci, PhD Professor, Department of Pharmaceutical Sciences, University of Pittsburgh School of Pharmacy, Pittsburgh, PA, USA

Laurence J. Kirmayer, MD, FRCP(C), FCAHS James McGill Professor and Director, Division of Social and Transcultural Psychiatry, McGill University, Montreal, Canada; Director, Culture and Mental Health Research Unit, Institute of Community and Family Psychiatry, Jewish General Hospital, Montreal, QC, Canada

Nestor Koldobsky, MD Professor of Psychiatry, Universidad de La Plata, La Plata, Argentina

Anne-Sophie Lancien, MD Department of Child and Adolescent Psychiatry, Brest University Hospital, University of Western Brittany, Brest, France

Dusica Lecic-Tosevski, MD, PhD Professor of Psychiatry and Director, Institute of Mental Health, University of Belgrade, Belgrade, Serbia

Nigel C. Lester, MD Clinical Researcher and Instructor of Psychiatry, Washington University School of Medicine, St. Louis, MO, USA

Igor Marinić, MD, PhD Associate Professor, Forensic Psychiatry Sub-Specialist, Department of Psychiatry, University Hospital Dubrava, Zagreb, Croatia

Juan E. Mezzich, MD, MA, MS, PhD Professor of Psychiatry, Icahn School of Medicine at Mount Sinai, New York, USA; Secretary General, International College of Person Centered Medicine, New York, USA; Editor in Chief, International Journal of Person Centered Medicine, New York, USA; Former President, World Psychiatric Association, Geneva, Switzerland

Helen L. Millar, MBChB, MRCPsych Consultant Psychiatrist, University of Dundee, Dundee, Scotland, UK; Carseview Centre, Dundee, UK

A. Mishara, PhD, PsyD Full Professor, Department of Clinical Psychology, Chicago School of Professional Psychology, Los Angeles, CA, USA

Roger Montenegro, MD President, Fundacion Contener, Buenos Aires, Argentina; Former Secretary of Education, World Psychiatric Association, Geneva, Switzerland; Former Director, Institute of Post Graduate Education, Association of Argentinean Psychiatrists, Buenos Aires, Argentina

Alexander Moreira-Almeida, MD Associate Professor of Psychiatry, School of Medicine, Federal University of Juiz de Fora, Minas Gerais, Brazil

Lana Mužinić, MD, PhD Associate Professor, Forensic Psychiatry Sub-Specialist, Department of Psychiatry, University Hospital Dubrava, Zagreb, Croatia

Felipe Navarro-Cremades PhD, MD Associate Professor, Faculty of Medicine, UMH, San Juan University, Alicante, Spain

Angel Otero, MD Professor of Psychiatry, University of La Habana, Havana, Cuba; Former Chair, Section on Classification, Diagnostic Assessment and Nomenclature, World Psychiatric Association, Geneva, Switzerland

Antonio Pacheco Palha, MD Professor of Psychiatry, Faculty of Medicine, Porto University, Porto, Portugal

Alberto Perales-Cabrera, MD, DMedSc Professor, Department of Psychiatry and Institute of Ethics in Health, Faculty of Medicine, Universidad Nacional Mayor de San Marcos, Lima, Peru; Honorary Member, Academia Nacional de Medicina, Lima, Peru

Sam Pfeifer, MD Professor of Psychotherapy and Psychiatry, Psychiatric Clinic Sonnenhalde, Riehen/Basel, Switzerland

Barbara Probst, PhD, LCSW Smith College, School for Social Work, Northampton, MA, USA

Varghese P. Punnoose, MD Professor of Psychiatry, Government Medical College Kottayam, Kottayam, Kerala, India

Peter Pype, MD, PhD Professor of Communication in Health Science, Department of Family Medicine and Primary Health Care, Faculty of Medicine, Ghent University, Ghent, Belgium

Rodrigo Ramalho, MD, PhD Department of Social and Community Health, School of Population Health, Centre for Addiction Research (CFAR), The University of Auckland, Auckland, New Zealand

Michelle Riba, MD Professor, Integrated Medical and Psychiatric Services, Department of Psychiatry, University of Michigan, Ann Arbor, MI, USA; Director, Psycho-Oncology Program, University of Michigan Comprehensive Cancer Center, Ann Arbor, MI, USA

Roger Ruiz, MD, PhD Professor of Medicine, Clinical Communication Skills Unit, School of Medicine, University Francisco de Vitoria, Madrid, Spain

Wolfgang Rutz, MD, PhD Professor of Social Psychiatry, University of Coburg, Coburg, Germany; Senior Consultant, International and Public Mental Health, Stockholm, Sweden

Javier E. Saavedra, MD, DrMedSc Executive Director of the Specialized Research and Teaching Office, Instituto Nacional de Salud Mental "Honorio Delgado—Hideyo Noguchi" and Professor of Psychiatry, Universidad Peruana Cayetano Heredia, Lima, Peru; Chair, Section on Diagnosis and Classification, Latin American Psychiatric Association, Lima, Peru

Ihsan M. Salloum, MD, MPH Professor of Psychiatry, University of Miami School of Medicine, Miami, FL, USA; Chair, Section on Classification, Diagnostic Assessment and Nomenclature, World Psychiatric Association, Geneva, Switzerland

Luis Salvador-Carulla, MD, PhD Professor, Centre for Disability Research and Policy, Faculty of Health Sciences, University of Sydney, Sydney, Australia

Margit Schmolke, PhD Psychologist, Psychoanalyst and Director of the Munich Training and Research Institute of the German Academy of Psychoanalysis, Munich, Germany

M. Schwartz, MD Clinical Professor of Psychiatry, Texas A & M Health Science Center, College of Medicine, Round Rock, TX, USA

Jon Snaedal, MD Professor of Geriatric Medicine, Landspitali University Hospital, Reykjavik, Iceland

Drozdstoj S. Stoyanov, MD, PhD Professor, Department of Psychiatry and Medical Psychology, Faculty of Medicine, Medical University of Plovdiv, Plovdiv, Bulgaria

Alessandro Svettini, MD Psychiatrist, Psychotherapist—Department of Psychiatry, Health Trust of Bolzano, Bolzano, Italy; European Federation of Associations of Families of People with Mental Illness (EUFAMI), Bolzano, Italy

Dragan M. Svrakic, MD, PhD Professor of Psychiatry, Washington University School of Medicine, St. Louis, MO, USA

Sigrid Steffen Past President, European Federation of Associations of Families of People with Mental Illness (EUFAMI), Salzburg, Austria

Dan J. Stein, MD Professor, Department of Psychiatry and Mental Health, University of Cape Town, and MRC Unit on Anxiety and Stress Disorders, Cape Town, South Africa

Ralph E. Tarter, PhD Professor, Center for Education and Drug Abuse Research, School of Pharmacy, University of Pittsburgh, Pittsburgh, PA, USA

C.W. Van Staden, MBChB, MMed (Psych), MD Nelson Mandela Professor of Philosophy and Psychiatry, University of Pretoria, Pretoria, South Africa

Eugenio Villar-Montesinos, MD, MSc Medical Scholar, Geneva, Switzerland

Juergen Zielasek, MD Department of Psychiatry and Psychotherapy, Heinrich Heine University, Düsseldorf, Germany

Spyros Zorbas Economist and Mental Health Advocate, Member, European Federation of Associations of Families of People with Mental Illness (EUFAMI), Athens, Greece

Introduction to Person-Centered Psychiatry

1

Juan E. Mezzich, MD, MA, MS, PhD, Michel Botbol, MD,
George N. Christodoulou, MD, PhD,
C. Robert Cloninger, MD, PhD
and Ihsan M. Salloum, MD, MPH

1.1 Conceptual Development of Person-Centered Psychiatry and Medicine

Person-Centered Psychiatry and Medicine are fundamentally aimed at promoting the health and well-being of the totality of the person [44, 49]. Here, the *person* is the key concept as the center and goal of health care [12].

J.E. Mezzich, MD, MA, MS, PhD (✉)
Professor of Psychiatry, Icahn School of Medicine at Mount Sinai, Fifth Avenue and 100th Street, Box 1093, New York, NY 10029, USA; Editor in Chief, International Journal of Person Centered Medicine, New York, USA; Secretary General, International College of Person Centered Medicine, New York, USA; Former President, World Psychiatric Association, Geneva, Switzerland
e-mail: juanmezzich@aol.com

M. Botbol, MD
Board Director, International College of Person Centered Medicine, Brest, France; Chair, World Psychiatric Association Section on Psychoanalysis in Psychiatry, Brest, France; Professor of Child and Adolescent Psychiatry, University of Western Brittany, Brest, France

G.N. Christodoulou, MD, PhD
Honorary Fellow, World Psychiatric Association, Athens, Greece; Former President, World Federation for Mental Health, Athens, Greece; Emeritus Professor of Psychiatry, University of Athens, Athens, Greece

C.R. Cloninger, MD, PhD
Wallace Renard Professor of Psychiatry, Genetics, and Psychology, and Director, Center for the Science of Wellbeing, Washington University in St. Louis, MO, USA

I.M. Salloum, MD, MPH
Professor of Psychiatry, University of Miami School of Medicine, Miami, FL, USA; Chair, Section on Classification, Diagnostic Assessment and Nomenclature, World Psychiatric Association, Geneva, Switzerland

J.E. Mezzich et al. (eds.), *Person Centered Psychiatry*,
DOI 10.1007/978-3-319-39724-5_1

Historical roots for person-centered care can be found in major Eastern civilizations, particularly Chinese and Ayurvedic, which are still alive and practiced today as traditional medicine. Both of them articulate a comprehensive and harmonious framework of health and life and promote a highly personalized approach for the treatment of specific diseases and the enhancement of quality of life [53]. In the West, the need for holism in medicine has been strongly advocated by ancient Greek philosophers and physicians. Socrates and Plato taught that "if the whole is not well it is impossible for the part to be well" [14]. This position was enriched by Aristotle, the philosopher and naturalist *par excellence* [34] and by Hippocrates, who brought theory, emotion, and individuality into the practice of medicine and delineated its ethical and person-centered foundations [36]. Prehispanic American medicine vision was holistic and integrative in context and in beliefs [40] and was consistent with concepts of medicine and health in the earliest Asian and Hellenic civilizations. Such broad and enlightened concept of health (full well-being and not only the absence of disease) has been incorporated into WHO's [70] definition of health. This notion has maintained its vitality throughout the vicissitudes of contemporary health care.

Modern medicine has brought a number of important advances in the scientific understanding of diseases and the development of valuable technologies for diagnosis and treatment. At the same time, it has led to a hyperbolic, impersonal, and dehumanizing focus on disease and organs, over-specialization of medical disciplines, fragmentation of health services, weakening of the clinician–patient relationship, and commoditization of medicine [30].

In response, proposals for re-prioritizing psychiatry, general medicine, and health care as person-centered are emerging, which cover a wide range of concepts, tasks, technologies, and practices that aim to put the whole person in context as a center of clinical practice and public health. Among contemporary antecedents of person-centered medicine, particularly prominent is the seminal work of Tournier [66], who wrote *Medicine de la Personne* in Switzerland. Also important are the contributions of Rogers' [55] person-centered approach in education and counseling focused on open communication and empowerment in the United States, McWhinney's [41] family medicine movement in the UK and Canada, and Alanen's [1] need-adaptive assessment and treatment approach in Finland.

An important implication is that the focus of contemporary medicine should be shifted from disease and patient to person [48, 51]. In the clinical arena, Heath [30] has spoken critically of "promotion of disease and distortion of medicine" and concerning public health, the World Health Organization's [70] broad definition of health focused on well-being is compelling. Concerning theoretical and practical purposes and vis-a-vis narrower approaches such as evidence-based medicine, person-centered medicine is promoting a view of evidence-, experience- and values-informed medicine oriented to the fulfillment of the whole person [67].

1.2 Mental Health Perspectives in Person-Centered Medicine

Complementing the broad Hellenic perspectives relevant to person-centered medicine mentioned earlier, Socrates stated that "everything comes from the psyche, bad things and good things for the body and the whole person" [24]. These considerations illustrate the ancient roots of holism and integrity of the person in medicine, as well as of the particular role of the psyche, i.e., mentation, emotions, and behavior, for health and well-being.

A brief discussion of the place and role of mental health in person-centered medicine should start with the various activities and manners through which mental health has contributed to the conceptualization and experience of person-centered medicine.

At the 54th World Health Assembly, Brundtland [11], former Prime Minister of Norway and then WHO Director General proclaimed "There is no development without health, and no health without mental health." This summarizes the growing perception of the crucial importance of mental health to achieving general health and well-being. The following sections illustrate why this is so, from various angles, particularly with attention to person-centered health and person-centered medicine.

1.2.1 The Importance of Behavioral Factors for Addressing Chronic Diseases

Chronic non-communicable diseases such as diabetes, cancer, and cardiovascular and respiratory illnesses are responsible for over 70 % of morbidity and mortality across the world. Their prominence as a global epidemic has attracted the urgent attention of the United Nations and the World Health Organization [72].

Addressing chronic disease is particularly pertinent for the International College of Person-Centered Medicine given that effective care for such conditions requires indispensably the engagement of persons and their sense of responsibility to adjust their life style actively and creatively [17, 28]. Consequently, the International College dedicated its 5th Geneva Conference to *Person Centered Care for Chronic Diseases* and issued its first Geneva Declaration, which was dedicated to this topic [35]. Among its recommendations are to monitor risk and protective factors (intrinsic and extrinsic; biological, psychological, and social), as well as outcomes for positive health (vitality and resilience despite exposure and adversity).

The World Health Alliance (World Medical Association, International Council of Nurses, International Dental Federation, and International Pharmaceutical Federation) has recently identified through a Health Improvement Card [61] a number of factors to prevent chronic diseases. The majority of such factors have to do with behavior and life style. Among these are: diet, exercise, avoidance of alcohol and other hazardous drugs, stress-control, adequate rest and sleep, and participation in social and creative activities.

1.2.2 Psychological Elements in Adaptive Systems for the Promotion of Well-Being

Keyes et al. [37] have shown the overlap of physical, mental and social well-being, as well as the inadequacy of focusing only on the presence of physical and mental disorders in assessing health. Flourishing involves dynamic interactions between healthy functioning, contributions to health and the experience of health. As argued by Herrman et al. [32], in order to develop well-being, people must be aware of the causes of both their distress and disability as well as of the paths open to them to develop in health and happiness with community support as well as personal effort.

Cloninger et al. [19] have endeavored to explain the dynamic origins of well-being. The causes of well-being and ill-being appear to involve a complex adaptive network of components and processes that are being gradually specified, measured and treated according to the principles of person-centered medicine. Some of the key factors promoting well-being involve the development of self-awareness, leading to greater self-directedness, cooperation, and self-transcendence, and in turn health [16].

1.2.3 The Importance of Subjectivity and Inter-subjectivity in Person-Centered Care

As noted by Botbol [8], person-centered medicine should not be reduced to individualization of care or respect for patients' rights, as it has wider aspirations. These include the recognition of the individual subjectivity of the whole person of the patient beyond what characterizes his or her illness or the status or role of patient. What is of interest here is dealing with the inner world of a patient in his particular situation of suffering and dependence caused by illness, as proposed in Aristotle's Nicomachean Ethics: "Cure of a unique person (not of a generalized nosological case), in a specific situation, within a specific, unrepeatable period of one's life" [69]. What becomes crucial here is the commitment of the mental health professional to approach the patient's subjectivity in such singular vital situation.

In addition to the attention paid to the medico-biological aspects of the person's health status, a person-centered assessment needs to give enough consideration to the patient's subjective feelings [10]. Whether or not one suspects a psychic or psychosomatic causality to the disorder that a patient brings to the clinic, it is essential to keep in perspective the factors involved in the patient's health situation. Beyond reasserting this principle, one needs to utterly enhance the methodology for accessing these subjective dimensions among different partners involved in the diagnostic process and the therapeutic relationship. For health professionals, the only way to access these subjective dimensions is through what the patient (and or his/her carers) says in words or shows in acting, as long as these words or acts can trigger in the professionals enough empathy to approach the patient's subjective feelings to which these expressions are related.

Working on a person-centered diagnostic approach has become an important element to meet this methodological goal. This diagnostic model includes, besides the objective elements about the patient and his or her context, the subjective elements reported by the idiographic formulations of the person who is being cared for, their carers and assisting professionals.

This approach appears to lead to a closer examination of the role of the professional's empathy as a way to access the subjectivity of the patient, trying to go beyond general assertions about the importance of this concept in therapeutic relationships and care activities [10].

At first seen as the professional's ability to listen sympathetically to the comments of the patient and to consider his wishes and needs, the notion of empathy has gradually widened to include representations that the physician (or other health professional) makes of the clinical situation in which the person in need of care is involved. In short, these are representations that the professional makes of the health situation of the person suffering through the professional's own empathy, triggered by the words and the acts of the patients and of their carers. This mechanism is well described by the concept of "metaphorizing-empathy" proposed by Lebovici [39] from his work with babies and their mothers. It is also close to the notion of "narrative empathy" proposed by Hochmann [33] based on his work with autistic children and on the philosophical ideas brought by Ricoeur [54] in his book "Time and Narrative." It is also consistent with Kleinman's [38] assumptions about illness narratives. This important development in person-centered medicine marks the full recognition of the role of the physician's subjectivity as a diagnostic and treatment tool within the framework of the physician–patient relationship. This recognition of the role of empathy corresponds to the concept of "resonance" in traditional medicine because both allow harmony to develop from the evocation of images, emotions, concepts that facilitate communication and understanding. Well-being involves a harmonious balance of physical, mental, and social processes that occur within each person, between persons, and in the collective whole of life.

1.2.4 Recovery Orientation in Mental Health and Its Relations to Medicine

Recovery-oriented concepts emerged from a coalescence of efforts from both service users and professional groups in the mental health field. On one hand, individuals who suffered and recovered from mental illnesses formed a recovery movement and a national and international community of activists. For example, Chamberlin [13] and Deegan [22] expressed their criticism against negatively experienced psychiatric treatment and demanded to be considered active protagonists and partners rather than passive recipients of care. On the other hand, well-known experts in the field of psychosocial rehabilitation, such as Anthony [2] welcomed the statements of service users and recognized the need to attend to their subjective experiences, speaking against improving just functioning and adaptation and not cultivating the flourishing of the individual human being. At least since the beginning of the 1990s, many professionals in rehabilitation and other fields and various service user groups have started substantial collaboration through joint publications and conferences. Recently, reflecting progress in this regard, Barber [6] has considered recovery as "the new medical model for psychiatry."

Recovery Orientation engages multidisciplinary cooperation, where professionals aim at helping not only to reduce symptoms, disease and disability but also to assist individuals to have a home again, to return to work, and to have friends. Key here is to cultivate a partnership attitude in which the individual can contribute actively based on his/her former illness experience and include family members and friends who know well the patient's needs. Furthermore, peer-support (a recovery-oriented development) is becoming frequently complementary to standard treatment in the United States, United Kingdom, and Australia [21].

Patients' participation in treatment planning is being increasingly advocated in mental health [23]. "Shared decision making" was an early contribution of the recovery movement to clinical care, and is becoming gradually a valued tool in person centered medicine. It is considered a promising method of engaging patients in medical decisions and improving health-related outcomes [29, 62]. The concept of "shared decision making" serves as a clinical tool towards enhancing communication and optimizing treatment planning as well as implementing respect for the autonomy, responsibility and dignity of every person involved. It is now a core concept applied in both recovery orientation as well as person-centered care, especially useful for chronic patients. The patient or client, an expert by experience, and the practitioner, an expert by training, are now expected to contribute from their own perspectives and determine collaboratively a course of treatment.

A comparison of the essentials of recovery orientation and person-centered care identified unique characteristics for each approach as well as substantial elements of convergence. Recovery orientation is primarily centered within the mental health and psychosocial fields while the person-centered approach covers general medicine and health care at large. Their points of convergence encompass a holistic theoretical perspective, an emphasis on contextualization and establishing a common ground for understanding and action, development of person-centered procedures for clinical care and health promotion, and, last but not least, an ethical commitment [60].

1.3 From Psychiatry for the Person to Person-Centered Medicine

The organized and institutional development of person-centered care in the psychiatry and mental health field has been unfolding in two phases. The first one from 2005 to 2008 took place in the form of an Institutional Program on Psychiatry for the Person within the World Psychiatric Association (WPA). The second one, since 2008 to date, evolved from the first one by extending its domain from psychiatry to medicine at large and progressing institutionally through collaboration with a large number of top global institutions in medicine and health.

1.4 WPA Institutional Program on Psychiatry for the Person

The Institutional Program on Psychiatry for the Person (IPPP), established by the 2005 General Assembly of the WPA, involved an organization-wide initiative affirming the *whole person of the patient within his context* as the center and goal of clinical care and health promotion, at both individual and community levels. This was set to involve the articulation of science and humanism to optimize attention to the ill and positive health aspects of the person. As care is basically a partnership experience, the program involved the integration of all relevant health and social services. Furthermore, the program also involved advancing appropriate public health policies.

Historians Garrabe and Hoff [27] have noted that the principles behind psychiatry for the person could be already detected at the very beginnings of the WPA in 1950. As a conceptual introduction to the whole Institutional Program, two editorials were published, one broadly focusing on articulating medicine's science and humanism [42] and another on the dialogic basis of the profession [43].

The work of the Institutional Program was organized in four components: Conceptual Bases, Clinical Diagnosis, Clinical Care, and Public Health. These are summarized next.

1.4.1 Conceptual Component

This component dealt with analyses and delineations of the conceptual bases of psychiatry for the person. It produced an editorial and a regular article in international journals presenting the objectives of this component [15, 44, 49].

Additionally, a monographic set on the conceptual bases of psychiatry for the person was prepared and eventually published with the following table of contents: Introduction [44, 49], Historical perspectives [27], Philosophy of science perspectives [65], Ethics perspectives [26], Biological perspectives [18], Psychological perspectives [9], Social perspectives [57], Cultural perspectives [25], Spiritual perspectives [20], Users perspectives [68], and Literature and art perspectives [64].

1.4.2 Clinical Diagnosis Component

There were two work objectives in this component. The first one involved collaborating with WHO toward the development of ICD-11. There was a preliminary background phase in this process during the first half of the preceding decade involving principally the WPA Classification Section and the WHO Classification Office and leading to two monographs [5, 52]. A full development of the ICD-11 Mental Disorders Chapter started in early 2007 under the direction of the WHO Mental Health Department.

The second and main work objective of the IPPP clinical diagnosis component was the development of a person-centered integrative diagnosis (PID) model. At its heart was a concept of diagnosis defined as the description of the positive and negative aspects of health, interactively, within the person's life context. The PID would include the best possible classification of mental and general health disorders (expectedly the ICD-11 classification of diseases and its national and regional adaptations) as well as the description of other health-related problems, and positive aspects of health (adaptive functioning, protective factors, quality of life, etc.), attending to the totality of the person (including his/her dignity, values, and aspirations). The approach would employ categorical, dimensional, and narrative approaches as needed, to be applied interactively by clinicians, patients, and families. A starting point for the development of the PID was the schema combining standardized multiaxial and personalized idiographic formulations at the core of the WPA International Guidelines for Diagnostic Assessment (IGDA) [73].

As an introduction to this IPPP component's work, a broad ranging volume on psychiatric diagnosis: challenges and prospects [58] was prepared. A paper on "Towards innovative international classification and diagnostic systems: ICD-11 and person-centered integrative diagnosis" was published by Mezzich and Salloum [45] as an invited editorial in *Acta Psychiatrica Scandinavica*. Other papers pertinent to this developmental work included an editorial on Clinical Complexity and Person-centered Integrative Diagnosis [47] and On Person-centered Integrative Diagnosis [46].

1.4.3 Clinical Care Component

The thrust of the work of this component encompassed educational efforts towards achieving person-centered care. The two main developments which were outlined were an approach to person-centered clinical care and a curriculum to carry out training on the above-mentioned approach.

It was noted that the teaching of medicine and that of psychiatry in particular was experiencing many changes. There was a time when the core curriculum in psychiatry, written by the WPA together with the World Federation for Medical Education, became a landmark because it not only defined the competencies in psychiatry that every physician should be taught, but mainly because it called attention to prevention of illness and promotion of health.

1.4.4 Public Health Component

Public health in modern times has a broad scope as the organized global and local effort to promote and protect the health of populations and reduce health inequities. This ranged from the control of communicable diseases to the leadership of intersectoral efforts in health [7]. It was noted that evidence had been growing on the value of integrating mental health in general health and public health practice

[31, 56]. Despite this, it was also noted that public health programs in many countries around the world have yet to recognize and include mental health and mental illness as areas of relevant action.

Psychiatry for the person became a basis for advocacy that emphasizes the value and dignity of the person as essential starting points for public health action. This includes development of policies and services, and research and evaluation supporting these. Failure to recognize the humanity and dignity of citizens living with mental illness as well as the value of mental health to the individual and community have resulted in abuse and neglect of the former and lost opportunities to improve mental health through population-based and person-based initiatives. The neglect of individual needs and the fragmentation and inadequacies of health and social services undermine policy development [63, 71]. Public health actions to promote mental health, prevent illness, and provide effective and humane services benefit from and contribute to the development of psychiatry for the person.

1.4.5 IPPP Events

1. *London Conference on Person-centered Integrative Diagnosis and Psychiatry for the Person:* It was organized on October 26–28, 2007 by both the WPA IPPP and the Health Department of the United Kingdom. It represented a path-opening opportunity for synergism between person-centered care and Britain's Shared Vision Project.

2. *Paris Conference on Psychiatry for the Person:* This was organized on February 6–8, 2008 by the WPA IPPP, the French Member Societies of WPA, and the five WPA European Zonal Representatives. The city and the professional community that served 58 years earlier as the cradle of WPA offered a special type of conference, focused and interactive, without commercial accompaniments.

3. *Philippe Pinel Prize on Psychiatry for the Person: Articulating Medicine's Science and Humanism:* In 2007, the WPA Executive Committee established this Prize to honor Philippe Pinel, a pioneer in the systematization of clinical psychiatry and an inspiring humanist who broke the chains of his hospital's mental patients. The awardee was Prof. Yrjo Alanen of Turku, Finland, world-acclaimed for his innovative work on *Need Adaptive Assessment and Treatment* integrating scientifically valid therapeutic techniques with attention to the experience and views of patients with psychotic disorders.

1.5 Development of Person Centered Psychiatry Within the Framework of Person Centered Medicine

Around 2008, contacts between the leaders of WPA and those of other important organizations such as the World Medical Association, the World Federation of Neurology, the World Organization of Family Doctors (Wonca), the International Council of Nurses, and the international Alliance of Patients' Organizations, among others, revealed wide interest for placing the person at the center of general medicine and health care. This led to the collaborative organization of the first Geneva Conference on Person Centered Medicine at Geneva University Hospital. This started a process of annual Geneva Conferences. Of note, the World Health Organization joined in formally co-sponsoring the Conferences since its third edition in 2010 to date. From this process emerged the International Network, now International College, of Person-Centered Medicine [50].

Within the framework of this broader conceptual scope and wide inter-institutional collaboration, work on person-centered psychiatry has continued with greater vigor and reach. Illustrative of these efforts are the following projects.

1.5.1 The Person-Centered Integrative Diagnosis (PID) Model

This work has involved the publication of a consolidated structural model for Person-centered Integrative Diagnosis (PID), following-up on the work on person-centered clinical diagnosis initiated during the period of the Institutional Program on Psychiatry for the Person mentioned above. Thus, most immediately, this is a model for person-centered psychiatric diagnosis, but potentially extensible to medicine at large.

The PID model [48, 51] articulates science and humanism to obtain a diagnosis *of* the person (of the totality of the person's health, both its ill and positive aspects), *by* the person (with clinicians extending themselves as full human beings, scientifically competent and with high ethical aspirations), *for* the person (assisting the fulfillment of the person's health aspirations and life project), and *with* the person (in respectful and empowering relationship with the person who presents for evaluation and care). This notion of diagnosis goes beyond the more restricted concepts of nosological and differential diagnoses.

The Person-centered Integrative Diagnosis model is defined by three key features: (a) broad informational domains, covering both ill health and positive health along three levels: health status, contributors to health, and health experience and values, (b) pluralistic descriptive procedures (categories, dimensions and narratives), and (c) evaluation partnerships among clinicians, patients, and families. Evolving research on the PID includes a conceptual validation of its basic elements [59].

1.5.2 The Latin American Guide of Psychiatric Diagnosis

The Latin American Psychiatric Association Section on Diagnosis and Classification has prepared and published the Latin American Guide of Psychiatric Diagnosis, Revised Version [4]. It was built as a revision of the original GLADP [3] and largely incorporating the basic elements of the Person-centered Integrative

Diagnosis (PID) model [48, 51]. For coding disorders, it uses categories and codes of the WHO International Classification of Diseases.

The GLADP-VR is being increasingly used throughout various Latin American countries. It is the official guide published by the Latin American Psychiatric Association for the use of health professionals in the region.

There are also plans to develop under the auspices of the International College of Person Centered Medicine a PID practical guide intended for use in general medicine.

1.6 The Person-Centered Psychiatry Book

The remainder of this introductory chapter attempts to delineate the purpose, authorship and organization of the Person-Centered Psychiatry book.

The experience of its five editors ranges from genetics to behavioral sciences to clinical care to public health. They are among the earlier and more consistent contributors to person centered psychiatry. Virtually all the book chapters are multi-authored to foster comprehensive, authoritative, and consensus presentations. The 83 chapter authors, all prominent scholars and clinicians come from 30 different countries from across the world. The countries involved from the Americas are Argentina, Brazil, Canada, Cuba, Peru, United States of America, and Venezuela. From Europe, they are Austria, Belgium, Bulgaria, Croatia, Denmark, France, Germany, Greece, Iceland, Italy, Norway, Portugal, Russia, Serbia, Spain, Sweden, Switzerland, and United Kingdom. From Africa they are Egypt and South Africa. And from Asia/South Pacific they are Australia, India, and New Zealand.

The chapter authorship includes representatives from 18 different Scientific Sections of the WPA, i.e., Anxiety and Obsessive Disorders, Biological Psychiatry, Child and Adolescent Psychiatry, Classification and Diagnostic Assessment, Education, Intellectual Disability, Military Psychiatry, Quality Assessment, Philosophy and Humanities, Preventive Psychiatry, Psychiatry and Human Sexuality, Psychoanalysis, Psycho-Oncology and Palliative Care, Psychotherapy, Public Policy and Psychiatry, Religion, Spirituality and Psychiatry, Schizophrenia, and Transcultural Psychiatry.

The book is institutionally sponsored by the International College of Person-Centered Medicine, and is formally co-sponsored by the WPA and the World Federation for Mental Health. The 40 chapters of the book encompass an introduction and 39 chapters clustered into the following five sections: (1) Principles (nine chapters), (2) Diagnosis and Assessment (five chapters), (3) Person-centered Care Approaches (seven chapters), (4) Person-centered Care for People with Specific Mental Conditions (11 chapters), and (5) Special Topics (seven chapters).

1.7 Colophon

This book emerges from a broad conceptual and collaborative process. Its authorship and structure reflects these features. Editors and chapter authors, alike, hope this volume will prove to be sound, innovative, and helpful to advance the science and practice of psychiatry in a manner faithful to its soul and highest aspirations.

References

1. Alanen YO. Schizophrenia: its origins and need-adaptive treatment. London: Karnak; 1997.
2. Anthony W. Recovery from mental illness. The guiding vision of the mental health service system in the 1990s. Psychosoc Rehabil J. 1993;16:11–23.
3. Asociación Psiquiátrica de América Latina, Sección de Diagnóstico y Clasificación. Guía Latinoamericana de Diagnóstico Psiquiátrico. Guadalajara: Asociación Psiquiátrica de América Latina; 2004.
4. Asociación Psiquiátrica de América Latina, Sección de Diagnóstico y Clasificación. Guía Latinoamericana de Diagnóstico Psiquiátrico, Version revisada (GLADP-VR). Lima: Asociación Psiquiátrica de América Latina; 2012.
5. Banzato CEM, Mezzich JE, Berganza CE, editors. Philosophical and methodological foundations of psychiatric diagnosis. Psychopathology. 2005;38(4):155–230.
6. Barber ME. Recovery as the new medical model for psychiatry. Psychiatr Serv. 2012;63 (3):277–9.
7. Beaglehole R, editor. Global public health: a new era. Oxford: Oxford University Press; 2003.
8. Botbol M. Du manifeste au subjectif: ce qu'est la médecine de la personne [from objectivity to subjectivity: what is person centered medicine]. In: Kipman SD, editor. Manifeste pour la médecine de la personne. Paris: Dion; 2012.
9. Botbol M, Alanen YO, Schmolke M. psychological perspectives on psychiatry for the person. Int J Pers Cent Med. 2011;1:134–6.
10. Botbol M, Lecic-Tosevski D. Person-centered medicine and subjectivity. In: Cornelius-White JHD, Motschnig-Pitrik R, Lux M, editors. Interdisciplinary applications of the person-centered approach. New York: Springer; 2013. p. 73–82.
11. Brundtland G. Preface to mental health: a call for action by world health ministers. Ministerial rounds at the 54th world health assembly. Geneva: World Health Organization; 2001.
12. Cassell E. The person in medicine. Int J Integr Care. 2010;10(Suppl):50–1.
13. Chamberlin J. On our own: patient-controlled alternatives to the mental health system. New York: McGraw-Hill; 1979.
14. Christodoulou GN, editor. Psychosomatic medicine. New York: Plenum; 1987.
15. Christodoulou GN, Fulford B, Mezzich JE. Psychiatry for the person and its conceptual bases. Int Psychiatry. 2008;5:1–3.
16. Cloninger CR. Feeling good: the science of well-being. New York: Oxford University Press; 2004. p. 374.
17. Cloninger CR. What makes people healthy, happy, and fulfilled in the face of current world challenges? Mens Sana Monogr. 2013;11:16–24.
18. Cloninger CR, Abou-Saleh MT, Mrazek DA, Möller H-J. Biological perspectives on psychiatry for the person. Int J Pers Cent Med. 2011;1:137–9.
19. Cloninger CR, Salloum IM, Mezzich JE. The dynamic origins of positive health and well-being. Int J Pers Cent Med. 2012;2(2):1–9.

20. Cox J, Verhagen PJ. Spirituality, religion and psychopathology: towards an integrative psychiatry. Int J Pers Cent Med. 2011;1:146–8.
21. Davidson L, Chinman M, Sells D, et al. Peer support among adults with serious mental illness: a report from the field. Schizophr Bull. 2006;32(3):443–50.
22. Deegan P. The independent living movement and people with psychiatric disabilities: taking back control over our own lives. Psychosoc Rehabil J. 1992;15:3–19.
23. Deegan PE, Drake RE. Shared decision making and medication management in the recovery process. Psychiatr Serv. 2006;57(11):1636–9.
24. Dyson M. Some problems concerning knowledge in Plato's *Charmides*. Phronesis. 1974;19:102–11.
25. Fabrega H Jr, Wintrob R. Ethnomedical and cultural foundations of psychiatry for the person. Int J Pers Cent Med. 2011;1:143–5.
26. Fulford KWM, Christodoulou G, Stein DJ. Values and ethics: perspectives on psychiatry for the person. Int J Pers Cent Med. 2011;1:131–3.
27. Garrabe J, Hoff P. Historical views on psychiatry for the person. Int J Pers Cent Med. 2011;1:125–7.
28. Greenhalg T. Patient and public involvement in chronic illness: beyond the expert patient. Br Med J. 2009;338:49.
29. Hamann J, et al. Shared decision making for in-patients with schizophrenia. Acta Psychiatrica Scandinavica. 2006;114:265–73.
30. Heath I. Promotion of disease and corrosion of medicine. Can Fam Physician. 2005;51:1320–2.
31. Herrman H, Saxena S, Moodie R. Promoting mental health: concepts, emerging evidence, practice. Geneva: WHO; 2005.
32. Herrman H, Stewart DE, Diaz-Granados N, Berger EL, Jackson B, Yuen T. What is resilience? Can J Psychiatry. 2011;56(5):258–65.
33. Hochmann J. Une histoire de l'empathie [A history of empathy]. Paris: Odile Jacob; 2012.
34. Ierodiakonou CS. The psychology of Aristotle, the philosopher. London: Karnak; 2011.
35. International College of Person-centered Medicine. Geneva declaration on person-centered care for chronic diseases. Int J Pers Cent Med. 2012;2:153–4.
36. Jouanna J. Hippocrates. Translated by M.B. Debevoise. Baltimore: Johns Hopkins University Press; 1999.
37. Keyes CL, Shmotkin D, Ryff CD. Optimizing well-being: the empirical encounter of two traditions. J Pers Soc Psychol. 2002;82(6):1007–22.
38. Kleinman A. The illness narratives. New York: Basic Books; 1988.
39. Lebovici S. L'arbre de vie—éléments de la psychopathologie du bébé [The tree of life—Principles of infant psychopathology]. Toulouse: Eres; 1999.
40. Mariátegui J. La concepción del hombre y de la enfermedad en el antiguo Perú. Revista de Neuropsiquiatría. 1992;55:156–66.
41. McWhinney IR. A textbook of family medicine. Oxford: Oxford University Press; 1989.
42. Mezzich JE. Psychiatry for the person: articulating medicine's science and humanism. World Psychiatry. 2007;6:1–3.
43. Mezzich JE. The dialogal basis of our profession: psychiatry with the person. World Psychiatry. 2007;6:129–30.
44. Mezzich JE, Christodoulou G, Fulford KWM. Introduction to the conceptual bases of psychiatry for the person. Int J Pers Cent Med. 2011;1:121–4.
45. Mezzich JE, Salloum IM. Towards innovative international classification and diagnostic systems: ICD-11 and person-centered integrative diagnosis. Acta Psychiatr Scand. 2007;116:1–5.
46. Mezzich JE, Salloum IM. On person-centered integrative diagnosis. Die Psychiatrie. 2007;4:262–5.

47. Mezzich JE, Salloum IM. Clinical complexity and person-centered integrative diagnosis. World Psychiatry. 2008;7:1–2.
48. Mezzich JE, Salloum IM, Cloninger CR, Salvador-Carulla L, Kirmayer L, Banzato CE, Wallcraft J, Botbol M. Person-centered integrative diagnosis: conceptual bases and structural model. Can J Psychiatry. 2010;55:701–8.
49. Mezzich JE, Snaedal J, van Weel C, Botbol M, Salloum IM. Introduction to person-centered medicine: from concepts to practice. J Eval Clin Pract. 2011;17:330–2.
50. Mezzich JE, Snaedal J, van Weel C, Heath I. The international network for person-centered medicine: background and first steps. World Med J. 2009;55:104–7.
51. Mezzich JE, Snaedal J, van Weel C, Heath I. Toward person-centered medicine: from disease to patient to person. Mt Sinai J Med. 2010;77:304–6.
52. Mezzich JE, Ustun TB, editors. International classification and diagnosis: critical experience and future directions. Psychopathology. 2002;35(2–3):59–201.
53. Patwardhan B, Warude D, Pushpangadan P, Bhatt N. Ayurveda and traditional Chinese medicine: a comparative overview. Evid Based Complement Altern Med. 2005;2:465–73.
54. Ricoeur P. Temps et récit [Time and narrative]. Paris: Le Seuil; 1983.
55. Rogers CR. On becoming a person: a therapist's view of psychotherapy. Boston, Houghton Mifflin; 1961.
56. Rutz W. Social psychiatry and public mental health: present situation and future objectives. Time for rethinking and renaissance? Acta Psychiatr Scand. 2006;429(Suppl):95–100.
57. Rutz W, Fernandez M, Trivedi J. Social perspectives on psychiatry for the person. Int J Pers Cent Med. 2011;1:140–2.
58. Salloum IM, Mezzich JE, editors. Psychiatric diagnosis: challenges and prospects. Chichester, UK: Wiley-Blackwell; 2009.
59. Salloum IM, Mezzich JE. Conceptual appraisal of the person-centered integrative diagnosis model. Int J Pers Cent Med. 2011;1:39–42.
60. Schmolke MM, Mezzich JE. Contrasting the essentials of recovery orientation and person-centered care. Int J Pers Cent Med. 2013;3:31–5.
61. Seyer J. Development of the health improvement card developed by the world health professions alliance. Paper presented at the 5th Geneva conference on person-centered medicine. International College of Person Centered Medicine, May 2012.
62. Stevenson FA, Barry CA, Britten N, Barber N, Bradley CP. Doctor–patient communication about drugs: the evidence for shared decision making. Soc Sci Med. 2000;50:829–40.
63. Strauss JS. The person—key to understanding mental illness: towards a new dynamic psychiatry, III. Br J Psychiatry. 1992;161(18):19–26.
64. Sukhanova E, Thomashoff H-O, Thoret Y. Literature and arts perspectives on psychiatry for the person. Int J Pers Cent Med. 2011;1:149–51.
65. Thornton T, Schaffner KF. philosophy of science perspectives on psychiatry for the person. Int J Pers Cent Med. 2011;1:128–30.
66. Tournier P. Médicine de la Personne. Neuchatel: Delachaux et Niestle; 1940.
67. Wagner P, Perales A, Armas R, Codas O, de los Santos R, Elio-Calvo D, Mendoza-Vega J, Arce M, Calderón JL, Llosa L, Saavedra J, Ugarte O, Vildózola H, Mezzich JE. Latin American bases and perspectives on person centered medicine and health. Int J Pers Cent Med. 2014;4:220–7.
68. Wallcraft J, Steffen S, Amering M. Service user and family perspectives on psychiatry for the person. Int J Pers Cent Med. 2011;1:152–4.
69. Warne C. Aristotle's Nicomachean ethics: reader's guide. London: Continuum; 2007.
70. World Health Organization. Constitution of the World Health Organization. Geneva: Author; 1946.

71. World Health Organization. The world health report 2001: mental health: new understanding, new hope. Geneva: World Health Organization; 2001.
72. World Health Organization. Global health status report on non-communicable diseases. Geneva: World Health Organization; 2012.
73. World Psychiatric Association (WPA). Essentials of the world psychiatric association's international guidelines for diagnostic assessment (IGDA). Br J Psychiatry. 2003;182(Suppl. 45):37–66.

Part I
Principles

The Person as Center of Health

2

Eric Cassell, MD and Drozdstoj S. Stoyanov, MD, PhD

2.1 Introduction

Increasing attention to the sick person and the movement for person-centered medicine require more consideration in medical education and practice. The definition of sickness that underlies this discussion is: "*Persons are sick who cannot pursue their purposes and goals because of impairments of function which they believe are in the domain of medicine. The goal of medicine is the well-being of the patient*" [1]. This definition is heavily dependent on an understanding of persons because only persons can know what purposes and goals are important to them, what functions are impaired and in what manner, and when they have achieved well-being. It does not matter that the sick person may not spontaneously know these things; it may take careful history taking and verbal interaction with the physician before they are clear enough to guide clinical action. Another critical facet to incorporate in clinical judgment thus is based on values, both intrinsic and external in respect to the person [5]. Values-based medical practice moves forward across the limitations of traditional twentieth century bioethics.

E. Cassell, MD
Emeritus Professor of Public Health, Weill Medical College of Cornell University, New York, USA; Adjunct Professor of Medicine, McGill University, Montréal, Canada; Attending Physician, New York Presbyterian Hospital, New York, USA

D.S. Stoyanov, MD, PhD (✉)
Professor, Department of Psychiatry and Medical Psychology, Faculty of Medicine, Medical University of Plovdiv, 15-A Vassil Aprilov Boulevard, 4002 Plovdiv, Bulgaria
e-mail: stojanovpisevski@gmail.com

J.E. Mezzich et al. (eds.), *Person Centered Psychiatry*,
DOI 10.1007/978-3-319-39724-5_2

The net effect of the impairments of function can be to make the person unrecognizable in his or her own eye. Each particular aspect—for example, sense of self, notions of future and past, life plans, pursuit of goals and purposes—can be specifically called up by the physician and restored even in the face of the most serious or fatal illness. This is a specific task of medicine.

In advance of the core sections of this chapter we should pose the fundamental question; what should be the relationship between the notions of person and ***personality***? Contemporary psychology has contributed extensively to understanding of personality as a complex multidimensional combination of temperament and character traits [2, 3, 4, 6]. Those traits interact permanently in a nonlinear manner with the dimensions of the context, e.g., psychological climate at workplace [13]. In our chapter, we have adopted the view that the person is a more general superstructure around personality in the meaningful connections of social life. In that sense person is not only a psychological and physical construct per se, but should be seen from ethical, aesthetical, communicative, and other perspectives as well.

2.2 The Person and Its Existential Being

A person is an embodied being, purposeful, thinking, feeling, emotional, capable of choosing, reflective, relational, responsible, very complex human individual of a certain personality and temperament, existing through time in a narrative sense, whose life in all spheres points, both outward and inward, and who does things. Each of these terms is a dynamic function, constantly changing, and requiring action on the part of the person to be maintained—although generally the maintenance is habitual and unmediated by thought.

Persons are always in action and never quiescent in the manner of inanimate objects. Persons are complex and can support contradictory thoughts and actions simultaneously, which, however, produce new thoughts and actions. Although fundamentally stable in personality and overall psychological and social being, persons are always changing perceptions, thoughts, and actions in a continuous manner. They are dynamically and interactively responsive to their inner and outer environment.

A person is a temporal as well as a spatial object. A person as a temporal object like a piece of music extends through time. As such **persons have an aesthetic dimension** where one can judge whether seeing or knowing about the person through time presents a harmonious aspect to consideration. This understanding of the esthetics of a life over time fits well with the use of the narrative to describe a person over time. As it has been emphasized by Musalek [9] social-aesthetical factors can influence in various ways the treatment, clinical course, and outcome of disease. One part of the story of a life or a part of a lived life generally fits with the preceding and the following parts of the narrative. Or its parts may be in discord or unbalanced. There can be no objective measurement of this idea of "fit," but it is not usually idiosyncratic; as with other things in the aesthetic domain there will mostly be agreement among observers. The general belief that the life as lived should be concordant allows us to say that what happened to someone does not seem to fit his or her life as lived.

The process of care can be carried out with active thought given to fitting into the aesthetic balance of the person's story and thereby reducing the ugliness of the illness and its care. This requires that clinicians acquire an aesthetic viewpoint of their patient's life and that requires conscious effort. All persons have an innate aesthetic sense, a sense of order, harmony, and beauty (as they know it). This does not mean, as Benedetto Croce explained almost a hundred years ago, that they can paint or make a poem that will bring tears to your eyes. Those are the artistic expression of an aesthetic impulse, not the aesthetic thought itself, which comes prior to its expression.

A person is a being who has a sense of self, a notion of a future and past, can hold values, make choices, and who can adopt life plans. To have these capacities a person must be a being with its own point of view on things. A person is a being who in most states (but not when unconscious, anesthetized, or similarly impaired) can be addressed and who can reply. It is these features of persons that underlie the fact that they have goals and purposes and that the fulfillment of the person's purposes leads to a feeling of well-being [14]. **Persons act on the basis of the meanings** of things, not on things themselves. Meaning as used here is about the implied or explicit significance of the thing, what a thing is considered to represent or to be. There is perhaps no object, event, or relationship which does not have or will not acquire meaning. Meaning as used here is more than the denotative meaning or even connotative meaning. Meaning also has emotional, physical (bodily response), and spiritual dimensions.

All persons are different in virtually every feature of their existence. Biological, physical, psychological, and spiritual and this as fundamentally true as the communal nature of human life.

2.3 The Person as Psychological Functioning

All persons have a subjective dimension. "Relating to the thinking subject, proceeding from or taking place within the individual consciousness or perception." [11]. All the information from the senses is subjective—it happens to the person, the subject. The information from the major senses is in part a result of not only a sensory function but also a cognitive function because it is given meaning as it is sensed. An indistinct speech utterance may take several moments before it is sorted out into words that the listener hears. The remainder of the senses such as interior sensations from the gut, joints, skin, and so on are also supplying information which is given meaning if it reaches consciousness. Further, the meaning applied to one group of sensations influences the meaning assigned to other sensory responses. It appears to be possible to retrieve the original unmediated sensory information under certain circumstances. The assignment of meaning is coherent with general attitudes and understandings of the person's world and these are sometimes referred to as ideologies or general attitudes toward the world, or general understandings so that information received is seen as a this or a that and confirms the persons previous beliefs. Mostly these subjective dispositions toward the world are uniform in the person, however, a person may have more than one general attitude that shows itself in different circumstances. These attitudes are learned and may be present from early childhood.

Persons generally have more than one self. A self is an enduring set of cohesive personality and behavioral characteristics (including, sometimes differences in appearance, stance, gait, and speech) that exist over time and that may be public, private, or even secret. Selves arise as a result of occasional differences or even conflict between the manner of life someone must live in a family, group or community and that person's individual inborn nature and behaviors. There are usually only a few such selves each emerging in situations similar to those that originally evoked them, usually in childhood. This implies, correctly, we believe, that whatever other selves a person has, if any, all persons have an authentic self—an inborn and lifetime enduring constellation of personality and physical characteristics—whether it ever reveals itself fully or not. No one would confuse different selves with being a different person; executive control remains with the dominant self. (This distinguishes the phenomenon of different selves from the pathologic entity multiple personality disorder.) Despite the occurrence of different selves there is good evidence that personality is enduring over a lifetime.

Emotion is a fundamental aspect of mental activity. Just as there is a flow of thought where ideas seem to be central, there is a stream of thought where emotion and mood is the content. The list of human emotions is well over a hundred in number. Emotion may be experienced as transitory where one brief experience of emotion may follow another as the emotional reactions to thoughts and experiences. One emotion may last for hours. For example, if someone steps on your foot you might have a flash of anger which in its onset occurred too rapidly for you to identify a thought which preceded it or of which it is a component. The anger is the primary result of the emotive response to being stepped on; no thought beyond that is a necessary response. After being stepped on the anger may lasts all day long and you are still talking about the incident hours later. Then we think that the original flash of anger, a response to being stepped on, has been co-opted by another, more lasting idea, the idea that you are (say) commonly abused by other people. As noted above, emotion can take over the stream of thought, and you might be thinking about abuses and the things that have happened that reinforce that idea for hours to come.

Finally, an emotion such as anger may become the dominant mood. Then we might not say that the person is angry but that the person is an angry person. The dominant mood could as well be joy, despair, sadness, or love. In sick persons' emotiveness is blunted, just as cognition is impaired and executive control diminished. While there is experimental evidence of the impairments of cognition and executive control, the evidence for the impact of sickness on emotiveness is anecdotal. Patients report, for example, that although they know they should feel love for a family member visiting and they say the words, they do not feel the emotion.

All persons may experience fear, an emotion as universal in animals as is desire. Generally fear is described as an aversive emotional response to a specific stimulus—persons know what, in the situation, they are afraid of. Sometimes the fear is momentary, perhaps in response to an impending needle-stick. Fear may, however, become a pervasive emotion that invades everything; the fear of the hospital, for example. Sometimes fears seem to be less specific such as about dying, unfamiliar situations, loss of control, or dependency. When that is the case it is often possible to track down what the patient is afraid of about hospitals or surgery; loss of control or dependency. If the exact details of the fear can be elicited it can often be laid to rest.

The most effective antidote to fear is information; however, in order to be useful, the information should be focused around the particular concerns of the patient, at a level the patient can understand. Too much information, or undesired information, can lead to more fear. Information is transmitted in the context of a therapeutic relationship and for the information to be accepted and to do its job the relationship must be trusting. Trust is not blind trust. Herein lies the importance of truthfulness and honesty.

People in strange and threatening settings such as, for some, hospitals or other medical situations, can be expected to be frightened. Sometimes people have fears that seem understandable, but on further questioning the fear is not what it first appeared to be. The fear of death is very common, but often—perhaps most often—the real fears are not death but the fear of separation from others or from the group, or fear about the dying process.

All persons may experience anxiety, which like fear, is a normal response to certain kinds of threatening situations. Anxiety is, however, more complex than fear. It is important to distinguish the kind of anxiety that can occur in anybody as distinct from the psychological anxiety disorders such as generalized anxiety disorder, posttraumatic stress disorder, panic disorder, and social anxiety disorder. Whereas, fear has an identifiable object, anxiety is vaguer and it is less easy to identify what is at the root of the anxiety. When anxiety is present it is experienced as variable feelings of dread, tenseness or jumpiness, restlessness and irritability. There may be an anticipation of bad things or general apprehension. Restlessness, trouble concentrating, anticipating the worst, and waiting for the ax to drop are characteristic, as are nightmares and bad dreams. The anxious person's world threatens but what is actually the source of the threat is not obvious. Physical manifestations are almost universal and can be quite extreme; heart palpitations, shortness of breath, and chest pains which may seem like a heart attack. Fatigue, nausea, stomach aches, headaches, diarrhea, or other physical symptoms may make the anxious person sure he or she is physically ill. Physiological manifestations are common such as elevated blood pressure, increased heart rate, sweating, pallor, and dilated pupils. However, anxiety can make itself known by mild feelings of unease, irritability, and apprehension without obvious physical symptoms or go all the way to a full blown panic attack where the person is sure that death is imminent.

The source of the conflict that is always present in anxiety may be simple or more complex. For example, a person may seem to be very anxious in response to the threat of death, but it is really not death itself, but conflict about it that is evocative. A very sick person has come to terms with his impending death, but his wife is extremely upset at the idea of his death and he feels that his acceptance of death is a betrayal of his intense love and loyalty. He is afraid of what will happen to his wife when he dies, but he is tired of fighting an illness when the inevitability of death seems to offer surcease. As a consequence of this conflict of which he is unaware he becomes anxious and his anxiety is wrongly interpreted by observers as evidence of his fear of death. There was a period where great credence was given to something called "death anxiety" which was believed to be nearly universal. More careful recent research has failed to support the concept and its universality [7, 8].

Anxiety is sometimes aroused in situations where different selves in the same person come into conflict. An older woman found herself anxious in situations where she kept asking herself, "which me am I supposed to be, the compliant, hard working, but resentful me, or the hardworking but interested and creative me?" Without being aware of such a conflict, anxiety is evoked which resolves when the conflict is made clear. Anxiety is extremely common, especially in the medical setting. There are effective anti-anxiety drugs, but they do not expose, clarify, or generate understanding of the conflict that always exists. It may not require sophisticated psychotherapy to uncover and resolve the conflict. That is preferable to medication and but anything that works is better than allowing someone to endure chronic anxiety in serious illness, for example, wanting to live but not wanting to suffer, wanting to be cared for but feeling guilty about it; the anxious person is often of two minds, ambivalent and conflicted, and these feelings are commonly sources of anxiety. There may be partial awareness of these feelings of conflict, or even perhaps clarity about them, but the tension that creates the anxiety is not being able to have both desired outcomes even when they are known.

In all persons emotive thought also operates on content from perception and memory producing specific instantaneous evaluations which are felt as emotions. Emotions are feelings, affections such as, pleasure, love, amusement, amazement, anger, sadness, dejection, or joy. Pain is spoken of as an emotion by some, but it regularly evokes emotion. Much less is known about emotion and emotiveness than about ideas and reasoning because from antiquity emotions were thought to contaminate thinking and interfere with reasoning. Sometimes, even in contemporary writing about cognition, emotions are dismissed as lesser than or contaminations of thought. They are not; they are a central and essential element of the mental life. The emotions that sick patients have about their sickness are as much a part of the sickness as are the symptoms.

Persons are thinking all the time. They are mostly constantly aware of thought while awake, but mental quietude can be trained The mind is always occupied by and aware of a stream of thought—of cognitive activity usually in the form of language—that varies from moment to moment as focus, interests, occupations, and preoccupations shift. Content of the stream of thought also arises from memory as the information from the world evokes ideas and associations that have been stored in both distant and recent memory. The stream of thought is personal and it provides for further thought. That thought influences the focus of the subsequent mental activity which may change what is of interest and further change the direction of thought, and so on. The train of thought is also a commentary on the person's activities so that it may offer a meaning to explain something that happens, such as some difficulty lifting a weight. The focus of thought can become captured by one subject—for example, a fear or love so that all these aspects of thought are in the service of what can become monomania. This can happen when sickness occupies the person. Then all the facts generated by the various modalities of thought are interpreted in the light of the sickness—e.g., shortness of breath previously interpreted a result of steep stairs now becomes evidence for heart failure. Thought is also occurring below awareness as problems, including technical, mathematical, or others are solved and come to awareness in various forms. The nature of this kind of thought including how, when, and why it takes place is a matter of present speculation and investigations.

All persons understand their world, it is generally believed, by two kinds of thought; reasoning and emotiveness. Reasoning is based on what are believed to be facts and is able to follow ideas to their ends, take them apart, combine them to form new ideas, and generally go beyond the information given. Reason is a method of thinking which can be used to understand and follow any set of ideas whatever their subject. If the ideas are faulty—internally incoherent, or such as cannot be logically connected with other ideas, then the reasoning will be faulty, but its subject will not have been irrational. The mind also employs intuition to know things from objects or events apparently without the intermediary of reasoning. Conventional ideas about intelligence are now being challenged. The combination of new technologies in neuroscience and increased attention by psychologists to the operations of thought are leading to a reappraisal of older concepts about thinking. Ideas are probably generally in the form of words, but artistic, sculptural, or musical ideas (which may be called motifs) are in the form of the art in which they occur—sketches or musical notes, for example.

Persons are adaptive. Starting in very young childhood, the necessity is that persons must conform to a greater or lesser degree to the demands of their physical, emotional, and social circumstances and to the significant persons who are part of their context. Different selves are a manifestation of that adaptability. Children must accommodate to or attune themselves to the family of their birth (or developing years) even if they are, by nature different. The original inborn self, which may not fit in the family, then fades into the background and may not show up except in congenial environments. Persons are more or less aware, involved in, and largely influenced by the surrounding environment physically as well as cognitively, socially, and morally. An example of this last is that where all around the person others are talking from a specific frame of reference—for example, the oncology care environment where patient survival and response to chemotherapy is the dominant frame of reference—that is the set that will also frame the person's response to the actions and words of others as well as his or her own. Persons in such a context may experience themselves in such terms even though doing so may be against their interests as they know them They will often be unaware of the presence and impact of the frame of reference.

Events in childhood back to infancy may form the basis for adult behaviors. These events, even though they have this impact, may not come to awareness. Events in this sense are not restricted to brute facts but are also the person's emotional response to recall of early relationship with parents, siblings, caretakers or others. These memories may not be actively repressed. Even actively repressed early memories or their emotional content—memories that are not in and cannot be brought to consciousness—may have an impact on behaviors, including speech and bodily responses to stimuli (including sexual stimuli) which seem to come out of the blue or seem completely unexplainable. (This is what is usually meant by reference to the unconscious or "the Freudian Unconscious.") All of this may be particularly important in illness in which things happen which are in themselves reminiscent of childhood. When that happens, the door may be opened for the effect of childhood events and their emotional content, remembered (dissociated, incomprehensible and therefore shoved aside before even being remembered), or repressed (remembered but hidden from consciousness), to have an impact on the course of the illness.

All persons have the ability to evaluate themselves. As persons judge others they also judge themselves and their behaviors. This is an aspect of the fact, described above that everything from how and what they do to how brave or cowardly they have been is both shown outwardly and known inwardly. Persons are not always aware of what feelings or behaviors they have displayed to others. They may also evaluate themselves in a manner that does not reflect how they are actually seen by others.

All persons have a past, a present and a future. The neurobiology of memory is complex—more than one kind of memory and more than one perspective on past events. Further it depends to a great extent on some phenomenological features of time experience which transcend biological explanations, such as autobiographical memory; the phenomenon of "frozen" time in schizophrenia [10], etc. The past is often in terms of the things that matter personally. Persons are capable of great detail if prompted or otherwise helped to remember. As they go further into the past, unsupported memory becomes less reliable—particularly for unpleasant or unhappy events or circumstances Traumatic events in the past may stand out in memory or may be selectively forgotten. The experiences gathered during living one's life are a part of today as well as yesterday. Events of the present can be checked against the past, and events of the past contribute to the meanings assigned to present happenings. Memory can be evoked by sensory experience.

Life experiences—previous illness, experiences with doctors, hospitals, medications, deformities and disabilities, pleasures and successes, or miseries and failures—form the background for illness. The personal meaning of the disease and its treatment arise from the past as well as the present. The future is always uncertain; it cannot be otherwise. People tend to have enduring ideas about what the future will bring and how they will make it happen. Everybody indulges in hoping—formed by both desire and expectation—and their hopes are part of their ideas of the future. Hope is of concern in medicine where the dangers of hopelessness and of losing hope are emphasized.

People generally consider themselves unitary beings. Despite this belief, below the surface of consciousness there are other entities that in certain circumstances (for example, in hypnotic states) can openly voice opinions that are not necessarily the same as those expressed in ordinary everyday consciousness. This has been known for at least 150 years, demonstrated in the famous French neurology clinics of Jean Martin Charcot and Pierre Janet. These other, inner, voices are not ruled by dailiness. On the other hand, as experienced using hypnosis, or even by persons as inner "voices" they are usually shy and hesitant. They are easily dismissed and they are overridden by doubt and/or anxiety. More than one inner voice, however, is not uncommon. These voices rarely speak in full sentences or paragraphs, instead they are cryptic. (EJC Personal experience.) This inner world and the inner voices come to consciousness and are not what is usually meant by reference to the unconscious, or the Freudian unconscious (see below).

All persons have an inner negative voice. It is the voice of caution, of damping down expectations, suggesting that given the positive or negative possibilities, the negative will win out: so the inner voice suggests being prepared. It seems to serve the purpose of keeping the person from taking chances. The inner negative voice is not the same as optimistic versus pessimistic personality profiles. The problem for the person is that the negative voice points out evidence in support of its position. These "voices", selves, inner expressions are directly experienced by everyday persons and not as pathological events. Their presence has been encountered regularly by one of the authors (EJC) using hypnosis for more than 35 years in working with persons with life threatening illness. This experience is thus far unpublished.

All persons have a secret life. Sometimes it takes the form of fantasies and dreams of glory, and sometimes it has a real existence known to only a few. Within that secret life are fears and desires, love affairs of the past and present, hopes or fantasies, and ways of solving the problems of everyday life known to only the person. Disease may not only destroy the public person but the secret person as well. A secret beloved friend may be lost to a sick person because he or she has no legitimate place by the sickbed. When that happens, the sick person may have lost that part of life that made tolerable an otherwise embittered existence. The loss may be of only the dream—the wish or fantasy (however improbable) that one day might have come true. Such loss can be a source of great distress and intensely private pain.

All persons can dissociate themselves partly or completely from events, experiences, memories, or bodily sensations. Dissociation is defense psychological mechanism described by Freud (*abwehrmechanismen*), which is different from simply not remembering or forgetting, where a memory can be jogged back into existence by a clue or someone actively helping. Dissociation is an active process that selectively bans the dissociated material from consciousness or conscious recall. The memory of traumatic events may be hidden by dissociation, as may dreams, unpleasant conversations, or things people have been told that they did not want to know. Clinicians learn this when they tell a patient bad news and shortly the person behaves as if, or even says that they have never been told. People are also able to dissociate themselves from the experience of physical pain as though they cannot feel the sensation. One self may dissociate itself from other selves as though they or their behaviors did not exist.

2.4 Persons and Their Relationships with Others

All persons require recognition of their existence from others. Imagine a person in an environment in which he or she is absolutely and completely unnoticed. No one turns around or turns aside, no one looks up, no one speaks, all acted as if the person is nonexistent. Rage and impotent despair would soon well up. Imagine such person on a gurney in an emergency ward, in the hallway outside an operating room, in a hospital bed. Then when things were done to the person's body even if unexplained, uncomfortable, or painful the person might be grateful for the attention. With these painful scenes in mind you will understand the almost animal gratitude such persons will have for personal voices, little pleasantries, answered questions from even total strangers.

Relationships may be very difficult to understand. Nowhere is that mystery more important than in clinical medicine, where relationships abound, waiting to provide information and aids or barriers to the attentive clinician. How odd is this? A person can go to see a physician who is a stranger and within minutes the physician has a finger in the patient's rectum. And the person (now a patient) says "thank you." What made that otherwise inexplicable event possible? The name, the doctor–patient relationship, labels but does not explain it. What happened was guided by a complex set of rules and entitlements that applied to both patient and physician. We might guess that the doctor learned those rules and entitlements (not called such) during the long years of training. The physician's behavior is expected to be as described. Why did the patient bend over to expose the reluctant anus to the finger's penetration, something almost universally abhorrent? Perhaps the patient contains the same rules and entitlements (or their mirror image). This suggests that role behavior (for they were playing the parts required by their respective roles) resides in both of them. In fact, each of us has a library of roles that we follow throughout the living of daily life and which are quite detailed. They make daily life possible. But they also imply that even when we are complete strangers our behaviors are not strange. The degree to which our daily behaviors are rule guided is startling since we generally believe our behaviors are spontaneous and responsive to our chosen purposes.

All persons have a capacity to love to a greater or lesser extent. All seem to be captivated by the idea of love. Except for the most unfortunate, love—flowing in both directions—is a fact of infancy and young childhood. From that young experience we get the basic characteristic of the feeling of love; a merging of two people. Under even the best of circumstances the merging of loving persons (or at least the feeling of merging) is of relatively short duration but their belief in their love may be enduring. The feeling of merging, attachment, or connection can occur in the absence of recognition of the feeling of love and it is usually pleasant, but sometimes threatening as it may be accompanied by frightening awareness of vulnerability.

All persons have a capacity for trust. "Trust is confidence or reliance on some quality or attribute of a person or thing, or the truth of a statement" [11]. Trust in their care or the caregivers is necessary for sick persons because they live in a world of unknowns and uncertainty. The enhancement of trust is a necessary activity of clinicians. Some persons are unable to trust and their world is necessarily experienced as dangerous.

All persons have a variable capacity to merge with others. The *capacity* to merge with others seems to be accompanied by a *desire* to merge that is greater in some people than others, occasionally being extreme. When people are sick, especially very sick, their ability to connect to others—particularly caregivers—is greater than at other times. This may be the source of the sometimes very strong attachment of the very sick to their clinicians. This is a situation when the fact and the manner of the attachment of sick persons to their caregivers are reminiscent of the attachment of these persons to their mothers in infancy. Psychoanalysts generally believe that these attachments by the sick are similar to the phenomenon of transference in general where the patients react to the psychiatrists as they reacted to their mother or father. Not surprisingly, persons who care for the sick also seem to have more than the usual ability to form connections. In general the loving attachment seems to be a conduit to the feelings, thoughts, and even the body of the merged persons. Little is known of this because it is so difficult to study and because it shares in the disbelief in the everyday world of such things.

There is little doubt, judging from ordinary experience, that some degree of knowing what others are thinking is a commonplace. It is possible to feel the feelings of another person and that capacity is not uncommon among experienced clinicians, especially psychiatrists and psychotherapists.

All persons have sexual feelings and desires to one degree or another. In the past, physicians in general were often not good at taking a sexual history from patients because of embarrassment. With the emergence of the HIV/AIDS epidemic a sexual history became important and clinicians learned that it was not difficult once the questions were learned. Very sick patients usually lose sexual desire and do not have sexual thoughts until they start to recover. On the other hand, patients who are chronically ill, even if dying, may experience sexual thoughts and sexual desire. For that reason, questions about sexuality should be part of taking a history, even in a dying patient. Sexuality is not simply about physical desire and orgasm even in healthy persons; intimacy is an integral part of the human experience and may be vitally important to a patient even in the absence of normal erectile or vaginal function. Clinicians show their recognition of these and other intimate problems by asking simple and unembarrassed questions.

All Persons want to be accepted, admired, and valued by others (and themselves) and they want to be like those that they admire.

2.5 The Person and Its Context

All persons behave in a manner that is responsive to context. Whatever the behavior and whatever the context the self experienced now, that was experienced a few minutes and more time ago, that might emerge in different circumstances and that might be expected (without awareness of the expectation) to be experienced as time unrolls is what the person calls me. The person will not be aware, usually, that he or she is behaving like a different self than (say) in the doctor's office just minutes before. This me has a frame of mind and a bodily state of feelings, both of which the person is more or less aware, and is involved in some purposeful activity with some subsidiary goal in mind. Dailiness, the occurrences and settings of everyday life, is the overriding context in which life is lived and is a major source of the behavioral rules by which people are guided. Further, especially in psychiatry, it is of utmost importance to acknowledge the contextual factors, which impact both person's narrative behavior and professional judgment. This is probably the one essentially context-dependent area of medical expertise. Imagine for instance a person who is walking through the lobby of a luxurious hotel in a bath towel. This outfit can well be understood as normal in the context of a SPA hotel in some health resort and judged as abnormal (psychopathological) if it takes place in a business hotel downtown in New York. Overall the process of inference is governed by the so called logics of practice [12].

2.6 Persons Live Continuously in a Context of Relationships with Other Persons

Some relationships are close while others are formal. Close or formal persons are all separate beings. A variable degree of trust in both the self and others is necessary for the initiation and maintenance of relationships. In every thought, feeling, and action and in virtually every idea about oneself and in every dream, fantasy, and fear the presence of others is reflected. In everyday life, physical appearance, dress, walking and other bodily movements and actions, language, speech, and gesture, everything is tuned to others (even facial expression is a social construction). The same is true of ideas and beliefs—even ideas about how the world works. Humanity is divided into cultures, subcultures, and ever smaller groups—but always groups. The same is true about language groups consisting of shared language and meanings from large ones like national groups to small individual groups such as airline pilots, golfers, or doctors. Where there is common language there are common beliefs and prevalent sentiments. Part of the molding of individuals to each other must necessarily be physiological although the extent of such conforming is unknown.

Persons live in a figurative public space. The idea of human relationships is not exhausted by speaking of direct relationships of persons to each other or with groups. Persons also live in something that has been called a figurative public space, not an actual physical public space. An example might be or sitting side by side on a bus and one says to the stranger along side, "really crowded, isn't it." Here the person acknowledges he or she and the respondent (and perhaps others) are in the relationship of *immediate understanding* without further explanation. Similarly a patient might say, "I'm really sick," and we would understand not what sickness the person has or even that he or she is sick in the doctor's sense of the word but in the public social sense.

All persons have a family. The intensity of family ties cannot be overemphasized; people frequently behave as though they were physical extensions of their parents. Things that might cause suffering in others may be borne without complaint by someone who believes that the disease is part of the family identity and thus inevitable. Many diseases where no heritable basis is known may be acceptable to an individual because others in the family have been similarly afflicted.

All persons have a cultural background. It is well known that socially determined factors, such as diet, environment, and social behaviors, contribute to disease patterns. Because culture also contributes to beliefs and values, cultural factors play a part in the effects of disease on a person. Culture defines what is meant by masculine or feminine, what clothes are worn, attitudes toward the dying and the sick, mating behavior, the height of chairs and steps, attitudes toward odors and excreta, where computers sit and who uses them, bus stops and bedclothes, how the aged and the disabled are treated. These things, mostly invisible to the well, have an impact on the sick and can be a source of untold suffering. They influence the behavior of others toward the sick person and that of the sick toward themselves. Cultural norms and social rules regulate whether someone can be among others or will be isolated, whether the sick will be considered foul or acceptable, and whether they are to be pitied or censured.

All persons have a spiritual dimension. Spiritual and spirituality are words most often applied in a religious context. The meaning that has been assigned to spirituality is primarily a result of the history of the idea. Spirit and spirituality refer to matters which transcend the individual. Patriotism and team spirit are topics in the spiritual realm since the feelings transcend the boundaries of individuals.

2.7 Persons and Their Social Responsibility

All persons have a sense of responsibility to and for self and to and for certain others. Persons seem to accept that they a have responsibility to be who and what they are. Who they are in the sense of their presentation to the world and to some degree for their spoken words, their actions, and their appearance. Most people acknowledge their responsibility for their behaviors, actions, and responses to events, circumstances, and other persons. This fact of responsibilities accepted arise from the same roots as the aspects of persons that make them always in relationship to others. They usually hold themselves responsible also for their expressions of emotion even though they may not know why they responded in a particular way [14].

All persons have some choice in the kind of person they want to be. Persons have with limits an ability to choose how others see and behave toward them. Persons can also choose their goals and purposes. They can choose and work to accomplish being other than they are now. Within limits that vary from population to population, and may be at least partially determined by socioeconomic status, education, and other social and personality characteristics, they can choose what future they want to inhabit. The freedom to make such choice is characteristic of the egalitarian societies of Western democracies. To make a choice implies the responsibility to stand and accept the consequences of your actions and not to attribute them to external factors and circumstances. Persons do not always assume or act on the consequences of their choices.

2.8 Person and Body

All persons have a body. This person's body is different than any other person's body because it is this person's body. The body is an aspect of person. Person and body are integrated and in constant interplay. They can never be separated except in death. The body can do some things and not others. People become habituated to their body's enormous range of abilities and incapacities. They generally know exactly what every part can do (of which they are or can be conscious). These capacities become accepted as a part of their person ("me"). This physical view of persons has been partly hidden by the cultural importance of and attention to individuality developed over the past number of centuries in Western European and American societies. Individuals sometimes presented themselves as though they were not also bodies. It sometimes seems as though the body has its own intentions that are not the known intentions of the person. People also generally know when parts are not working properly and these impairments of function—if they come on quickly enough to be noticed and are lasting and important enough—become symptoms as they are joined to other incapacities. On the other hand, if impairments of function emerge only slowly, are easily accommodated, or are deemed unimportant, even quite impressive impairments will soon be adapted to or dismissed. This is particularly so because of the importance of impairments of social, psychological and spiritual function that is part of the understanding of sickness where the person is the object of concern, not merely the body.

The truth about bodies is that things happen to them—they can be injured or get sick. Bodies sometimes bleed, smell bad, make embarrassing sounds, have embarrassing functions, make inopportune demands, create strong desires, sometimes look bad, and become old and slow, and sometimes ugly. (These facts are frequently denied or hidden in everyday life.) Persons grow up with profound ignorance about how the body works even though most people learn about it in school. Unfortunately, clinicians can have considerable knowledge about diverse diseases but be quite ignorant about the body's everyday functions. This limits their ability to ask questions in the hunt for impairments of patients' functions. It also reduces their ability to make things function better.

All persons who are experiencing themselves include an awareness of the body and many of its functions. The function of the special senses and the somatic senses are generally within the awareness of the individual so that if they develop abnormalities, the functional loss reaches awareness. Muscle strength, walking speed, pulmonary capacity, bowel and bladder function, and others are part of what persons know of themselves. This is true of healthy as well as sick persons although persons will adapt to slowly losing function and sometimes be unaware of significant impairment until it is pointed out to them. This same adaptiveness allows persons to change the way they carry out tasks or the manner in which certain actions are performed so that they can do things despite major losses in function in virtually every system from the cognitive to the hand and other extremities. On the other hand, as impairments in function develop, particularly in systems such as bowel and bladder that impact on social function persons may change their habitual behavior to avoid embarrassment.

Psychological conflicts might also be converted into physical symptoms.

All persons die. The inevitability of death, mourning, and grief entailed present one significant issue to manage in health care delivery both from ethical and psychological perspectives.

In Summary a person is an embodied being, purposeful, thinking, feeling, emotional, capable of choosing, reflective, relational, responsible, very complex human individual of a certain personality and temperament, existing through time in a narrative sense, whose life in all spheres points both outward and inward and who does things. Each of these terms is a dynamic function, constantly changing, and requiring action on the part of the person to be maintained—although generally the maintenance is habitual and unmediated by thought.

2.9 Conclusions

This chapter presented a multidimensional perspective on what a person is and how it should be understood in the many different facets of its existence. Virtually nothing about persons that we have discussed in this chapter is unaffected by sickness. What sickness does is impair function but the functions that it limits may be found in every sphere of a person's life as it is lived. The knowledge of this provides an opportunity to understand sickness, but it also creates therapeutic opportunities that are far greater than are usually considered. The fundamental understanding that must not be forgotten diagnostically or therapeutically is that whatever happens to one part of a person happens to the entire person. Also, however, whatever is done for one aspect of a person has an impact on the whole person.

References

1. Boudreau JD, Cassell EJ, Fuks A. Healing curriculum. Med Educ. 2007;41:1193–201.
2. Cloninger CR, Svrakic DM, Przybeck TR. A psychobiological model of temperament and character. Arch Gen Psychiatry. 1993;50(12):975–90.
3. Cloninger CR, Zohar AH. Personality and the perception of health and happiness. J Affect Disord. 2011;128(1):24–32.
4. Eysenck HJ. Eysenck personality inventory. San Diego: Educational and Industrial Testing Service; 1968.
5. Fulford KWM. Ten principles of values-based medicine (VBM). In: Radden J, editor. The philosophy of psychiatry. New York: Oxford University Press; 2004.
6. Hathaway SR, McKinley JC. A multiphasic personality schedule (Minnesota): I. Construction of the schedule. J Psychol. 1940;10(2):249–54.
7. Irish DP, Lundquist KF, Nelsen VJ, editors. Ethnic variations in dying, death and grief: diversity in universality. Abingdon: Taylor & Francis; 2014.
8. Lonetto R, Templer DI. Death anxiety. Washington, DC: Hemisphere Publishing Corp; 1986.
9. Musalek M. Social aesthetics and the management of addiction. Curr Opin Psychiatry. 2010;23(6):530–5.
10. Musalek M. Meanings and causes of delusions. In: Fulford KWM, Moris KJ, Sadler JZ, Stanghellini G, editors. Nature and narrative. An introduction to the new philosophy of psychiatry. Oxford: Oxford University Press; 2003. p. 156–69.
11. OE Dictionary. OED online. Oxford: Oxford University Press; 1989. http://www.oed.com. Accessed 30 Nov 2006.
12. Stoyanov D, editor. Psychopathology: theory, perspectives and future approaches. New York: Nova Science Publishers; 2013.
13. Stoyanov DS, Cloninger CR. Relation of people-centered public health and person-centered healthcare management: a case study to reduce burn-out. Int J Person Centered Med. 2012;2 (1):90.
14. Taylor C. The concept of a person. Human agency and language: philosophical papers. vol 1. Cambridge: Cambridge University Press; 1985.

Ethics in Person-Centered Psychiatry

3

George N. Christodoulou, MD, PhD,
C.W. Van Staden, MBChB, MMed (Psych), MD,
D. Jousset, MD, PhD, M. Schwartz, MD
and A. Mishara, PhD, PsyD

3.1 Introduction

This chapter outlines the ethics of person-centered psychiatry (PCP). Doing so may seem superfluous considering that attention to the person is a *sine qua non* condition for the ethical practice of psychiatry. Almost all ethical codes for the practice of medicine and psychiatry underscore the importance of attention to the person and profess priority to the well-being of the patient in the clinical encounter above the well-being of the therapist's own self.

We should, however, consider the ethics of PCP since the ethical commitments expressed in the concept and practice of PCP need to be made clear [21]. What does the ethical commitment to a PCP entail and how does that contrast with positions that are not committed ethically in this way? For example, PCP may mistakenly be assumed to

G.N. Christodoulou, MD, PhD (✉)
Emeritus Professor of Psychiatry, University of Athens, Athens, Greece; Hellenic Psychiatric Association, 11 Papadiamantopoulou str., 11528 Athens, Greece
e-mail: profgchristodoulou@gmail.com

C.W. Van Staden, MBChB, MMed (Psych), MD
Nelson Mandela Professor of Philosophy and Psychiatry,
University of Pretoria, Pretoria, South Africa

D. Jousset, MD, PhD
University Lecturer, Director of Research, Program on Ethics, Professionalism, and Health, Department of Philosophy, University of Brest, Brest, France

M. Schwartz, MD
Clinical Professor of Psychiatry, Texas A & M Health Science Center,
College of Medicine, Round Rock, TX, USA

A. Mishara, PhD, PsyD
Full Professor, Department of Clinical Psychology, Chicago School of Professional Psychology, Southern California Campus, Los Angeles, CA, USA

J.E. Mezzich et al. (eds.), *Person Centered Psychiatry*,
DOI 10.1007/978-3-319-39724-5_3

incur necessarily a commitment to individualism, or liberalism. It may be mistakenly thought of as being exclusive of societal and public health interests or as nothing more than a commitment to the principle of respect for personal autonomy.

The ethics of PCP puts the person and his or her interests central in psychiatric practice [32], guarding against too narrow a focus or exclusive attention to his or her disorder, treatment, brain, mind, or ill health. The concern of what is good for the patient's disorder is one thing and a legitimate concern of psychiatry, no doubt. The broader concern of PCP is with what is good for the person (and not merely his disorder, treatment, brain, or mind).

The person is neither confined to a mere patient role, but all social capacities of the person matter in PCP—hence "person-centered" and not merely "patient-centered". Appreciating the patient in all his other capacities too, makes him not merely a receiver, user, or consumer of healthcare but an active participant who may contribute to the diagnostic understanding of his difficulties, his treatment, and the decisions made in his healthcare [4]. As a participant, the people of the clinical encounter may draw on the resilience that each brings (as expert by training and/or expert by experience) in joint pursuit of well-being and not merely the absence of illness. PCP also recognizes not only the patient as a person, but also the people in the patient's life [18] including the psychiatrist.

PCP neither escapes tensions between individual interests and those of society, nor does it necessarily side with the individual's interest. PCP recognizes the person in the singular and the plural (i.e., people in society) amidst these tensions [4].

PCP thus provides for that person who ascribes to individualism, or liberalism, but not exclusively so. PCP also provides for a communitarian ethic in which the person is held in high regard whether as an individual or in the society. But PCP is not necessarily committed to either individualism or communitarianism [33].

PCP so understood resonates nonexclusively with the utilitarian ethics theory of Jeremy Bentham in which an act is considered ethical if it gives pleasure to **most** people ("the greatest good for the greatest number") [7]) thus implicitly supporting societal interests. There are also utilitarian approaches that insist on the well-being of the individual vis a vis benefit to society as a whole. For example, in various parts of the Helsinki Declaration (the Ethical Principles for Medical Research of the World Medical Association) [36], the well-being of human subjects is of greater priority than the presumed benefit to society from the research results (articles 3, 4, and 8).

3.2 Ancient Greek Perspectives

Aristotle (384-322 BC) one of the best-studied and most prominent Greek ethicists of his time insisted on the attention to the needs of each particular person, a stance akin to the person-centered approach of our times [15]. He made various parallelisms between Medicine and Ethics and insisted on the individuality of each person by stating that what is good for one person may not be as good for another person ("a physician can take the best care for a patient when he knows the general rules of what is good for everyone but also what is good for the particular individual…." 1106b, Nicomachean

Ethics, Loeb's Edition, quoted by [15]). In another passage he makes human diversity even more explicit by explaining that "the natural inclination of one man is different from that of another" (1109b, Nicomachean Ethics).

As a consequence of the above advice of Aristotle pertaining to individuality, he professed contention with the **Approximate** rather than with the mathematically **Exact**. In his own words: "...for a well-schooled man is one who searches for that degree of precision in each kind of study which the nature of the subject at hand admits" (1094b, Nicomachean Ethics).

Aristotle underlined his individuality approach by providing the well-known paradigm of wrestler Milon, a heavy muscular athlete. He stated that while the standard portion of food provided by his trainer would be too little for Milon, the same portion would be too much for someone who has just started training.

However, even before Aristotle, a century earlier, in the era of Hippocrates, physicians "were concerned with the application of general knowledge to particular cases since most of them took the view that the individuality of each case and each patient had to be taken into consideration" [6]. These views are certainly in line with the modern idea of person-centered medicine [23].

3.3 Modern Perspectives on Personhood

In modern perspectives, the first principle of ethics is the respect of the autonomy, which stands for the very dignity of the human person. Thus, Kantian deontologism denounces the treatment of a person's humanity as only a means and no longer also an end in itself. The ethics of PCP represents a significant shift here, since Kant formulated the principle of respect for 'the rational being' as an end in itself ("[a]ct with reference to every rational being (whether yourself or another) so that it is an end in itself in your maxim") Kant [19]. However, psychiatry cannot focus on the rational being (in German, "jedes vernünftige Wesen"), but rather on the person and ultimately his deviation from the normal, or his temporary or irreversible inability to conform to a universal norm. It is no longer the legislative ability of reason that demands respect, but any person, regardless of the boundary between reason and deviation from it.

3.4 Phenomenological Contributions to a Person-Centered Ethics in Medicine

By virtue of its capacity to provide a provisional definition of the person as an embodied self in relation to others, and further its capacity to characterize how this relationship is structured, phenomenology can contribute to a person-centered ethics in medical practice. The clinical relationship—as any other relationship—is a relationship between embodied persons with their own perspectives—both in the current situation and in relation to the world generally. The perspective of each participant mutually shapes the perspectives of the other participants in an unfolding process. In clinical situations, this becomes particularly evident. Doctor and patient take reciprocal attitudes to one another in their common goal of treatment (as articulated by phenomenological clinicians or thinkers, including Binswanger,

Blankenburg, Buber, Gadamer, and von Weizsäcker). Through conveying an openness to affirmation of the patient as an autonomous person, the clinician empowers the patient to participate in the healing process.

A brief review of phenomenological contributions will follow, emphasizing the overlap between phenomenological approaches and person-centered medicine, and indicating how, given this overlap, the phenomenological approach may be applied to a person-centered medicine.

3.5 Max Scheler: Value Theory of the Person

The philosopher Max Scheler (1874–1928) employed the phenomenological method to define the concept of person and how we experience the personhood of others, which, as will be indicated, has relevance to clinical practice.

Scheler's concept of the person is complex. Here we only present its possible application to person-centered medicine. Scheler proposed an ethics based on value theory (Wertethik) and specifically the incontrovertible value of the person, to counter the formalism of Kant's ethics [27]. Our experience of the humanity of the other person whom we encounter is not given simply through adhering to any formal principle. Something more is required. Instead, there is a way in which the other person—and our feelings regarding their vulnerability or our empathy with their situation—touches us, and moves us to act compassionately.

For Scheler, it is not possible to grasp another person by taking an objective or neutral approach to another. The "perception" of another's value is only accomplished by an engaged commitment on our part to experience their value—which is given through emotional cognition. That is, each person has inherent value and this value can only be grasped through compassion, an act of openness to the other's transcendence as exceeding one's current perspective.

The value of each individual person is incontestable in Scheler's Wertethik. One only needs to open oneself to other(s) in an act of compassion. Furthermore, for Scheler, this absolute value of the individual persons we encounter is given us *a priori* as an emotion of love or compassion, which is a direct experience of their personhood. The other, in their mental activity, which can be understood but not objectified, remains transcendent.

Furthermore, for Scheler, "any objectifying attitude makes the person immediately transcendent" [27] and this is the case both for oneself as well as for others. This should be self evident, since no act can become the object of another act. And furthermore, such mental activity in itself can never become an object in a subsequent reflection, which tries to call it back to mind: "an act is never an object" [27]. Hence, the person as source of own mental activity cannot be objectified by oneself or another [27]. The person as the executor of acts is "...the most hidden of all phenomena" [27]. "The person lives…existence precisely in the experiencing…"

The person is embodied self as being a world inhabited by other persons. However, we do not directly experience the person through our perception of their body but only through our own emotive experiences of their value or dignity as persons. That is, we need to be open to experiencing other's value to be able to experience it emotively (for the role of empathy in our experience of other persons), see [29].

Furthermore, for Scheler, the cognitive act of perceiving the personhood of a fellow human being is an act of love, but love here is meant in a special sense. It is the affirmation of the other person as other, as transcendent, as a value in themselves which is given to me in emotional acts. Only recently has cognitive neuroscience started to accept the view that emotions and feelings convey information about the world and our relationship to others in this world (e.g., [12, 26]). It is only through love that we are able to "perceive" the other as person, to affirm their core of humanity as a continued process of becoming self.

In summary, once again in contrast to Kant's formalistic ethics, the phenomenological philosopher Scheler countered that ethics in its application to human relationships should be embodied based on feeling. The value of each individual is incontestable. One needs to only open oneself to other(s) in an act of compassion. Certainly, many are made uneasy by Scheler's basing ethical action on feelings, as this is precisely how bias enters. But it is not so much our feelings toward the individual, but our openness to the person's "thouness" in a mutual unfolding that is relevant.

Emphatically, it is not required that we agree with Scheler. Hartmann [14] or other value theorists state that these values are given as "existing in themselves, a priori givens." [10]. It is enough to acknowledge that the person, each person, has incontestable value in one's self. Still, it is in fact the emotion of compassion or love that is the sole assurance that we will not dehumanize others often in implicit bias [13] but see their incontestable value as persons. This requires an openness to the other that goes beyond our efforts to be neutral or objective. For the phenomenological philosopher, Levinas (e.g., [20]) it is the vulnerability of the other before us, as betrayed in the other's face, that calls for us to respond with caring for their suffering as an ethical imperative.

3.6 Hans-Georg Gadamer: The Transcendence of the Thou (a Hermeneutic Circle of Interpretation)

Following Scheler, the philosopher Gadamer (1900–2002) emphasized that the other's worth is not given through perception or what is called cold cognition but instead engages the embodied response of openness to the other in an unfolding dialog [11].

Gadamer proposes that open dialog anticipates a totality which both conversants share but to which neither has full access. In a similar vein, following Plato, thinking is a dialog with oneself in which totality or closure is anticipated, but never fully accomplished in what Gadamer calls a "hermeneutic circle" (see e.g., [8], p. 262). And, as emphasized by the phenomenologically oriented Heidelberg psychiatrist Beringer, "In healthy individuals there is the always unconscious heading towards a totality, an intuitive knowing where the thought is going which is missing…in thought disorders" of schizophrenia [1]. Similarly, Gadamer [9] describes how we apply in our understanding of others, a preliminary or anticipatory grasp of completeness (die Anwendung des Vorgriffs der Vollkommenheit). From a Bayesian perspective (and in conformity with the phenomenology), we tend to see or interpret our experiences of other persons, including clinical diagnosis or treatments, in terms of what we already expect or anticipate, updating these anticipations with new information only after they have been challenged (Mishara and Sterzer, in press). Citing Melancthon (1497–1560), Gadamer states that the proper *application* of the law to situations is that "therefore an interpretation should be applied to every law that would bend it to more humane and lenient decisions" [9, p. 324]. Similarly in diagnosis and treatment, we should consider and respect the totality of the person embedded in their situation, thus informing our clinical application with the most humane approach. In this sense, Gadamer continues the early Greek concern "with the application of general knowledge to particular cases" described above.

3.7 Karl Jaspers: Anticipation of a Person-Centered Medicine

The psychiatrist and philosopher Jaspers (1863–1969) was the first to apply phenomenology as a formal method to psychiatry and thus clinical situations. Mishara and Fusar-Poli [24] indicate that Jaspers' work anticipated a person-centered medicine: "When writing the Allgemeine Psychopathologie [17]; [General Psychopathology], Jaspers finds himself in the middle of a debate carried over from the 19th century. In this debate, which concerns the opposed methodology of the natural versus the human historical sciences, Jaspers emphasizes psychological or historical understanding". In psychiatry, the psychological understanding of the patient occurs in the interactive context of the diagnosis and treatment of mental disorders. This understanding is narrative-based; holistic; sensitive to ethnic, cultural, and individual differences; and ultimately oriented to patient strengths. In this sense, Jaspers' work anticipates a person-centered medicine. Jaspers [16] writes: "We experience in the other a unity which we cannot define but only experience" [16, p. 115]. Therefore, Jaspers underscores the importance of the contextuality in the developing expertise of diagnostic practice (for Jaspers' affirmation of diversity before his time, see [28].

3.8 Paradigm Shift for Medicine

Mezzich et al. [22] describe a progression from the current biomedical model to a more "person centered medicine." Citing the existential-phenomenological philosopher Ortega y Gasset, "I am I and my circumstance," they write, "Respect for the patient's autonomy, values, and dignity represents a fundamental recognition of his or her personhood, and an ethical imperative. Slowly these concepts are finding their way into evidence." In this sense, ethics underpins person-centered Medicine and Psychiatry and is at the foundation of its practice.

3.9 The Person-Centered Perspective in Psychiatry

Mental health is an area where ethics considerations are pressing, and often more pressing than in physical health. One reason for this is that patients with mental health problems are more vulnerable to abuses of various kinds and are less well-protected against these abuses. There are historical paradigms of unethical behavior towards patients with mental illness committed by relatives, professionals, governments, and society as a whole. Abuse is not only physical but also psychological and can occur not only by doing something harmful but also by not doing something that ought to be done (harm by neglect).

The person-centered approach is a prerequisite for the good practice of clinical psychiatry and in this sense it is in line with professional ethics. It is necessary for the development of a good interpersonal relationship and for the therapeutic impact this relationship is expected to have for the patient's health and well-being. This is especially relevant in the current time when over-dependence on modern laboratory technology has reduced clinical care to a seemingly secondary role.

Clinical psychiatry, by its very nature requires a close interpersonal relationship between two persons, the person of the therapist, and the person of the patient (provider and recipient of services). The interaction between these two persons determines to a great extent the outcome of the intervention. If the sensitive balances of this interaction are violated, then not only benefit may not be achieved but harm may be produced the non nocere principle of Hippocrates is violated.

Furthermore, in response to the alienation of health actors, PCP refers to the **empowerment** of "service users and carers" in the mental health system. This political concept should be evaluated at the ethical level by estimating the risk of making the actors overly responsible and by conceiving this power to act (*empowerment*) in the wider concept of **cooperation,** which implies a real sharing of the power of decision-making, a decentralization, and a valued application of individual and local experiences.

3.10 The Declaration of Madrid

The Ethics Code of the World Psychiatric Association (WPA) is the Declaration of Madrid. This Declaration was approved by the WPA General Assembly on August 25, 1996 and was amended in 1999 and 2002. Since then there have been no further revisions but certain guidelines for specific situations have been added in 1996, 1999, 2002, 2005, and 2011.

The importance of the **individual** sense of responsibility of each psychiatrist is underlined in the preamble of the Declaration. This is in line with two Ethics considerations. First, with the moral obligations of the provider of psychiatric services (Psychiatry **by** the Person) and, second, with the predominance of **principles** over legalistic codes and rules. Indeed, it is the principles (like the individual sense of responsibility) that provide the basis for the rules and also provide the ethical stance of each practitioner through whom the rules are filtered and implemented. Without the principles, the rules would be without reason, relevance and ideology. Even the most fundamental code of Ethics, the Hippocratic Oath would be nonsensical if it was not based on principles [3]. This point is made quite clear in the Madrid Declaration when it is explicitly stated that legalistic constructs do not guarantee the ethical practice of Psychiatry.

The Freedom of the patient is considered in paragraph 1 of the Declaration where it is stated that therapeutic interventions should be the least restrictive concerning the patient's freedom. **Autonomy** is the ethical principle that is observed in this paragraph.

The principle of autonomy of the patient is further stressed in paragraphs 3 and 4. In paragraph 3, it is underlined that the decisions of the patient should be free and informed and should be made on the basis of the personal values and preferences of the patient. In paragraph 4, safeguarding of the human dignity and rights of the patient and his or her right to accept or refuse treatment are underlined.

Paragraph 5 deals with a delicate albeit important person-centered mental health ethics issue, namely the obligation of the psychiatrist to inform a person being assessed about the purpose of the assessment. The fact that such an obvious obligation (arising from the well-known "double agent" issue) had to be included in an Ethics code suggests that psychiatric practice is not always consistent with this ethical obligation.

Paragraph 6 deals with a fundamental person-centered ethical issue, that of confidentiality and paragraph 7 emphasizes that psychiatric patients are vulnerable research subjects in need of special protection. From the person-centered ethics perspective, safeguarding the autonomy of the patient is once again emphasized.

In conclusion, the ethics principles that are more prominently highlighted in the Madrid Declaration are the principle of **autonomy** and the Hippocratic principle of "**μη βλάπτειν**" (non nocere). Both these principles are strongly person-centered.

3.11 Values and Ethics

One of the basic goals of PCP is to adjust the application of objective science to the values of the patient and each of the people involved in his or her care [2, 30, 31]. PCP puts thus the person in the center of clinical activities through an active engagement with the values of all the people that have bearing on the situation: the values of the patient, the family, the psychiatrist, and the community [4]. Some of the values may be shared among the role-players, yet other values may be diverse [34]. PCP seeks to engage with both the shared values, as expressed in, for example principlism, and the diverse values that the patient or his/her family bring to the clinical encounter.

To this end, Values-Based Practice (VBP) is a practical and theoretical resource that is derived from analytic ethics [34].

Fulford et al. [7] distinguish between **substantive** and **analytic ethics**.

Substantive ethics defines the guiding principles that provide substantive responses to ethical problems. Utilitarianism, deontology and principlism are examples of them. Analytic ethics on the other hand focuses on the meanings of the terms in which ethical issues are presented. This approach is concerned with unpacking the standards of reasoning as a basis for answering problems rather than providing the answers to problems as such.

The authors believe that ethical challenges should be approached with a combination of the substantive and the analytic approach. This complementary approach will allow the consideration of the different moral arguments that are relevant in every single case and in this way, optimal clinical decisions can be reached. To support this conclusion, the authors argue that the Guiding Principles, consistently with their status as *prima facie* principles may conflict. For example, in the case of Compulsory Admission, the "purpose principle" which covers safety may conflict with the principle of "autonomy" which is related to the patient's wishes. In this case, values-based practice can be used to support a process of balanced individualized (person-centered) decision-making [34].

Ultimately, one may ask if respect of the person is a higher or priority principle, justifying a transgression or suspension of the application of other principles. This is relevant to the debate on the ethical justification of coercive treatment, of psychiatric treatment without consent, in the name of "best interests of the patient" as pointed out in the Declaration of Hawaii, World Psychiatric Association [5] or by respect to the expressed volition of the patient. Ethical questioning resulting from practice relaunches the problematization of the foundations of the ethics of medical care.

3.12 Conclusions

Person-centered Psychiatry is closely associated with Ethics. This relationship provides fertile ground for an interaction of clinical and philosophical perspectives.

The Ethics of Person-centered Psychiatry regards the person as central in Psychiatric practice but considers it not only in the singular but also in the plural (i.e., people in society).

Many ethical questions in person-centered Psychiatry certainly remain unanswered and one of them is the issue of ethical priorities in clinical psychiatric practice. Further consideration of these issues would be very productive. The aim should be to harmonize the various points of view to reach conclusions that are theoretically valid but also clinically useful.

References

1. Beringer K. Beitrag zur analyse schizophrener Denkstörungen. Zeitschr. f.d. ges. Neurol. u. Psychiat. 1924;93:55–61.
2. Christodoulou GN, Fulford KWM, Mezzich J. Psychiatry for the person and conceptual bases. Int Psychiatry. 2008;5:1–3.
3. Christodoulou GN, Christodoulou A. Person-centered perspective in the madrid declaration. Int J Person-centered Med. 2013;3:266–9.
4. Crepaz-Keay D, Fulford KWM, Van Staden CW. Putting both a person and people first: interdependence, values-based practice and African Batho Pele as resources for co-production in mental health. In: Sadler JZ, Van Staden CW, Fulford KWM, editors. Oxford handbook of psychiatric ethics. Oxford: Oxford University Press; 2015.
5. Declaration of Hawaii (1983) World Psychiatric Association, 1977 (amended 1983). http://www.codex.vr.se/texts/hawaii.html.
6. Frede M. Philosophy and medicine in antiquity. In: Frede M, editor. Essays in ancient philosophy. Minneapolis: University of Minneapolis Press; 1987.
7. Fulford KWM, Christodoulou GN, Stein DJ. Values and ethics: perspectives on psychiatry for the person. Int J Person-centered Med. 2011;1:131–3.
8. Gadamer H-G (1975) Truth and method. 2nd ed. (Tran. Ed. G. Barden and J. Cumming). New York: Continuum Publishing Corporation.
9. Gadamer H-G (1990) Hermeneutik I. Wahrheit und Methode. Grundzüge einer philosphische Hermeneutik. Gesammelte Werke, Bd. 1. Tübingen: J.C.B. Mohr (Paul Siebeck).
10. Gadamer H-G (1999) Hermeneutics, religion and ethics. Trans. J Weinsheimer. New Haven: Yale University Press.
11. Hahn LE, editor. The philosophy of Hans-Georg Gadamer, library of living philosophers XXIV. Chicago: Open Court; 1997.
12. Harmon-Jones E, Winkelman P. Social neuroscience, integrating biological and psychological explanations of behavior. New York: The Guilford Press; 2007.
13. Harris LT, Fiske ST. Perceiving humanity or not: a social neuroscience approach to dehumanized perception. In: Todorov A, Fiske S, Prentice D, editors. Social neuroscience toward understanding the underpinnings of the social mind. Oxford: Oxford University Press; 2011. p. 123–34.
14. Hartmann N (1932) Ethics. London, George Allen & Unwin. Reprinted with a new introduction by A. A.M. Kinneging, New Brunswick, Transaction Publishers, 2002–2004.
15. Ierodiakonou CS. Medicine as a model for Aristotle's ethics and his person-centered approach. Int J Person-centered Med. 2014;4:31–4.
16. Jaspers K. Eifersuchtswahn, ein beitrag zur frage: entwicklung oder prozeß [Reprinted in Karl Jaspers, *Gesammelte Schriften zur Psychopathologie,* Berlin/Heidelberg/New York, Springer; 1963:85–141]. Z f ges Neur Psychtr. 1910;11:567–637.
17. Jaspers K. Allgemeine psychopathologie. Berlin, Germany: Springer; 1913.

18. Jousset D. An ethical analysis of person centered psychiatry. Int J Person-centered Med. 2014;4:228–33.
19. Kant I (1785) Foundations of the metaphysics of morals. Trans. Lewis WB (1990). New York: MacMillan.
20. Levinas E (1999) Alterity and transcendence. Trans. M.B. Smith. New York: Columbia University Press.
21. Mezzich JE, Christodoulou GN. Psychiatry for the person and its ethical perspectives. S Afr J Psychiatry. 2007;13:71–3.
22. Mezzich J, Snaedal J, van Weel C, Heath I. Toward person-centered medicine: from disease to patient to person. Mt Sinai J Med. 2010;77:304–6.
23. Mezzich JE, Christodoulou GN, Fulford KWM. Conceptual bases of psychiatry for the person. Int J Person-centered Med. 2011;1:121–4.
24. Mishara AL, Fusar-Poli P. The phenomenology and neurobiology of delusions: Jaspers, Truman signs, aberrant salience. Schizophr Bull. 2013;39:278–86. doi:10.1093/schbul/sbs155.
25. Mishara AL, Sterzer P. Phenomenology is Bayesian in its application to delusions (a commentary). World Psychiatry, in press.
26. Panksepp J. Affective neuroscience: the foundations of human and animal emotions. Oxford: Oxford University Press; 2004.
27. Scheler M (1973) Formalism in ethics and non-formal ethics of values: a new attempt toward the foundation of an ethical personalism. Trans. M Frings and R Funk. Evanston, Illinois: Northwestern University Press.
28. Schwartz M, Mishara AL, Wiggins O (2012) The biopsychosocial model is not a "straw man": how Jaspers' phenomenology opens the way to a paradigm shift in psychiatry. Existenz Int J Philos Religion Polit Arts, 6/1. http://www.bu.edu/paideia/existenz/index.html.
29. Stein E (1989) On the problem of empathy. Trans W Stein, from The Collected Works of Edith Stein, Volume 3. Washington, DC: ICS Publications.
30. Van Staden CW. The need for trained eyes to see facts and values in psychiatric diagnosis. World Psychiatry. 2005;4:94.
31. Van Staden CW. Facts and values in psychiatric practice: the theme of the 2006 14th National Psychiatry Congress. S Afr J Psychiatry. 2006;12:40.
32. Van Staden CW. Person-centred psychiatry: the recent 10th international conference on philosophy, psychiatry and psychology. S Afr J Psychiatry. 2007;13:124.
33. Van Staden CW. African approaches to an enriched ethics of person-centred health practice. Int J Person-centered Med. 2011;1:11–7.
34. Van Staden CW, Fulford KWM. The indaba in African values-based practice: respecting diversity of values without ethical relativism or individual liberalism. In: Sadler JZ, Van Staden CW, Fulford KWM, editors. Oxford handbook of psychiatric ethics. Oxford: Oxford University Press; 2015.
35. The Madrid Declaration. World Psychiatric Association website (www. wpanet.org).
36. WMA Declaration of Helsinki—Ethical Principles for Medical research involving Human Subjects, amended by the 64th General Assembly, Fortaleza, Brazil, October 2013.

Holistic Framework for Ill Health and Positive Health

4

C. Robert Cloninger, MD, PhD, Kevin M. Cloninger, PhD and Juan E. Mezzich, MD, MA, MS, PhD

4.1 A Holistic Approach to Health

Effective health care and promotion require growth in the complete health of the whole person [75]. A whole person is an inseparable component of a much larger psychosocial context, including the person's community, planet, and ultimately the universe as a whole [10]. In practice, the assessment of the healthy functioning of a person is most thoroughly based on a comprehensive description of their personality, as can be done with the temperament and character inventory [16, 19, 21]. It is also possible to describe the state of their functioning using measures of subjective well-being [25–28], but all such subjective measures are largely expressions of how happy or satisfied a person is and do not describe the components of the developmental processes leading to health and happiness [9, 46].

In order to be effective, health promotion of the person must increase knowledge and awareness of how to live and function well. Health promotion with the person helps a person to identify and accept valued goals. It teaches self-regulatory skills

C.R. Cloninger, MD, PhD (✉)
Department of Psychiatry, Washington University School of Medicine,
660 South Euclid Avenue, Campus Box 8134, St. Louis, MO 63110, USA
e-mail: clon@wustl.edu

K.M. Cloninger, PhD
President, Anthropedia Foundation, St. Louis, MO, USA

J.E. Mezzich, MD, MA, MS, PhD
Professor of Psychiatry, Icahn School of Medicine at Mount Sinai, New York, USA;
Secretary General, International College of Person Centered Medicine, New York, USA;
Editor in Chief, International Journal of Person Centered Medicine, New York, USA;
Former President, World Psychiatric Association, Geneva, Switzerland

J.E. Mezzich et al. (eds.), *Person Centered Psychiatry*,
DOI 10.1007/978-3-319-39724-5_4

that enhance self-efficacy in functioning. Health promotion by the person supports the integration of this factual knowledge and personal values to support a commitment to change that cultivates plasticity. Health promotion for the person assures that values are directed toward enhanced personal and collective well-being. Values that are optimally healthy and prosocial are self-transcendent and virtuous because social inequality and personal vices are unhealthy for individuals and the social groups in which they live [59]. Thus, person-centered health promotion works by activation of synergy among healthy functioning, plasticity, and virtue [16, 17] (see Chapter on Integrative Approach to Person-centered Therapeutics).

4.2 Why Are the Individual Components of Health Promotion Only Weakly Effective?

Self-transcendent values (i.e., virtue) guide a person to function in ways that promote both individual and collective well-being [16]. In turn, healthy functioning promotes a person's plasticity, which allows him or her to be resilient, flexible, and free in the choice of valued actions to which they commit. Plasticity allows the flourishing of the "good life" that is healthy, happy, and virtuous. Thus, person-centered medicine promotes healthy functioning, plasticity, and virtue, which are synergistic in their promotion of well-being with strong and consistent effects [18]. If any one of these crucial components of health care promotion is blocked, a person's health is vulnerable, does not flourish and begins to deteriorate in the face of daily life challenges [18]. When health promotion efforts address only individual components of well-being, then the other indispensable components may be unhealthy, resulting in interventions and treatments that are weak and inconsistent in their efficacy. Treatments and interventions may work weakly or sometimes in those people in whom the other neglected components already happen to be healthy.

Physical, mental, and social aspects of well-being are all strongly dependent on the TCI character traits of self-directedness, cooperativeness, and self-transcendence [20, 45]. The development of these personality traits over the life course is a complex adaptive process that allows a person to adapt one's outlook, goals, and values to social norms and individual life experiences in a meaningful and satisfying way [10, 46].

Personality provides a reliable way to assess the quality of a person's functioning in the general population as well as with psychiatric and other medical patients with physical disorders [19, 22]. In order to promote physical, mental, and social well-being, it is necessary to promote the healthy personality development that underlies healthy living. Perhaps the inadequacies of past efforts at health promotion can be explained by the need to more fully accept the fact that the well-being depends on the development and maintenance of a healthy personality, not just knowledge, external support, and encouragement although those things represent part of the necessary resources. So, we need to know what is a healthy personality?

4.3 What Is a Healthy Personality?

Three key practices have consistently been shown to lead to the development of well-being: (1) letting go, (2) working in the service of others, and (3) growing in awareness [10, 12]. Letting go involves acceptance of who you really are so that you can develop realistically and calmly without fighting or worry. Acceptance and letting go are expressions of hope, rather than giving in to excessive or insatiable desires. Working in the service of others is expressed as genuine acts of kindness, which are satisfying even when it involves personal sacrifice. Serving others is an expression of love, rather than giving into fear and selfishness. Growing in awareness is the result of using our intelligences to listen to all aspects of our being. Through reflection, meditation, and contemplation a person can discover more about one's self and the mysteries of one's inseparable relations to others and the world as a whole. Awareness is the actualization of the benefits of faith. Such faith is based on the insight and conviction that comes from intuitive understanding, rather than blind acceptance of dogmatic assertions by external authorities.

Each of the practices that lead to well-being is functional expressions of the character traits of self-directedness, cooperativeness, and self-transcendence. Self-directedness (i.e., being resourceful, purposeful, self-accepting, responsible, and foresighted) leads to confidence about one's ability to accomplish valued goals, and such self-confidence is a way of describing hopefulness. Consequently people who are highly self-directed accept who they are really and can admit to faults and weaknesses, whereas others are too proud or ashamed to admit their faults [10].

Cooperativeness (i.e., being tolerant, helpful, empathic, principled, and compassionate) is an indicator of a person's disposition toward kindness and compassion for one's fellow human beings. Such loving kindness and compassion motivates a person to work in the service of others, rather than for personal gain [10]. Acts of kindness are satisfying and enhance physical, mental, and social aspects of well-being [24, 55, 77]. Acts of kindness make people happy [55], and happy people experience less pain [77], have improved cardiovascular health and resilience [24], fewer accidents and suicides, and live longer [32].

Self-transcendence (i.e., being intuitive, imaginative, easily absorbed and engaged in what is valued, and spiritually accepting) indicates capacity for insight from meditation and contemplation. Such contemplation leads to enhanced awareness, self-knowledge, and peak experiences of the inseparability of all things [10]. Mindful meditation has been shown experimentally to reduce stress and enhance objective indicators of well-being [40, 41].

Meta-analysis of longitudinal studies and experimental interventions show that increases in subjective well-being are predictive of reduced morbidity and mortality and of improved objective health and longevity [40, 41]. The effect size of the correlation between changes in subjective well-being with changes in objective physical health is weak ($r = 0.14$ to 0.16) in both longitudinal studies and in experimental interventions [41]. An effect size of 0.15 corresponds to an odds ratio around 1.3 for improvement, which indicates that most people are not substantially improved in objective measures of physical health from changes in subjective well-being [8]. Medical morbidity and mortality in 7-year follow-up is more strongly predicted by the absence of positive well-being than by the presence of negative well-being, but the effects are still weak and inconsistent [42].

Personality traits are predictive of later health status and mortality in longitudinal studies using the personality questionnaires measuring three and five factor models [1, 44]. High neuroticism and low conscientiousness are often predictive of higher mortality, but the results have been weak and inconsistent [11, 44]. More consistent predictors of health outcomes can be identified using Ryff's measures of psychological well-being (such as autonomy and self-control) [2, 30] and the character measures from the TCI previously described here [20, 45, 63]. The TCI was the strongest predictor of clinical health outcomes among all 14 multidimensional personality inventories tested in a longitudinal study in the USA [37]. The average of the TCI's multiple correlation with six clinical indicators of psychopathology was $r = 0.53$ compared to the averages for other personality tests ($r = 0.27$ to 0.45). Hence the linear prediction of mental health outcomes by antecedent personality traits is moderate in strength.

Multidimensional personality profiles are the most consistent predictors of well-being because they specify synergistic nonlinear interactions. Specifically, the combination of all three TCI character dimensions (i.e., high self-directedness, cooperativeness, and self-transcendence) predicts greater physical, mental, and social well-being than any other profile or individual trait [20]. The profiles are more informative than the average (linear) effects of the same traits for both mental health and physical health outcomes [20, 63].

The synergistic quality of all three character dimensions is called creativity and the healthy personality configuration is called the creative character profile [16]. Creativity can be defined as the original, adaptive, and beneficial innovation that emerges from the combination of high self-directedness (i.e., resourceful, realistic, and self-accepting), cooperativeness (i.e., tolerant, helpful, and empathic), and self-transcendent (i.e., intuitive, imaginative, and spiritual). Creativity depends on all three of these components of character because it must be (1) original (i.e., using imagination or innovative ideas to solve problems or to invent new and better solutions to traditional approaches, as is characteristic of highly self-transcendent people), (2) adaptive (i.e., a realistic way to use available resources to make something suitable for a new use or purpose, as is characteristic of highly self-directed people), and (3) beneficial (i.e., being favorable, helpful, or advantageous for others so that it becomes adopted by the culture or social group, as is characteristic of highly cooperative people). There is no consensus about a single definition or test for measuring creativity despite much study of the topic, but there is agreement that creative processes are original, adaptive, and beneficial for one's self or others [58, 68, 72]. Sometimes the word "adaptive" is taken broadly to imply both realistic and beneficial. In any case, the importance of creative products being socially valued and benefiting others has been well-documented in studies of creative achievement [23, 33, 65]. Creativity has been shown to be strongly related to three facets of individual differences: differences in (1) intellectual abilities (e.g., divergent thinking, imagination, and aesthetic sensibility), (2) personality traits (e.g., tolerance of ambiguity, desire to grow, desire to work for recognition, and willingness to take risks and try to overcome obstacles), and (3) character style or style of mental self-government (e.g., a progressive legislative style, which finds enjoyment in creating one's own rules and ways of doing things, looking for new things to do and for new ways to do old things), and [69, 70, 72].

Overall, creativity is a process that occurs within creative people in particular states of mind in a particular psychosocial context [10, 23]. Specifically, the creative character profile (i.e., the combination of being highly self-directed, cooperative, and self-transcendent) facilitates a person getting in a creative state of mind (i.e., calm alertness with a flowing intuitive awareness that awakens automatic intelligences), thereby helping a person to discover original solutions that are adaptive for one's self and others.

Each of the three TCI character traits contributes to positive affect and life satisfaction regardless of the level of the other two traits, and the combination of all three has a stronger correlation with subjective well-being than expected from the sum of the three individual contributions [20]. In other words, the dynamic nonlinear interaction among these dimensions has a synergistic effect to enhance physical, mental, and social aspects of well-being.

The creative process emerging from the healthy character configuration has concrete and practical benefits. People with high Self-transcendence have a vivid imagination, and this leads to creativity when combined with realistic thinking typical of high self-directedness and with schizotypal or magical thinking when combined with low self-directedness [66]. In contrast, people who are high in self-directedness and self-transcendence, but low in cooperativeness, are generally regarded as "fanatics" and often act with hostility or in ways that are destructive for themselves and others, so they are not regarded as creative despite their ingenuity. People who are "organized" (i.e., high in self-directedness and cooperativeness, but low in self-transcendence) have often been considered to have healthy personalities, but they are still vulnerable to being self-centered, materialistic, and conventional unless they are also high in self-transcendence [14, 15]. Creative processes require a freedom of will and thought that is not constrained by past conditioning and traditional beliefs [49, 50].

Creativity must not be regarded as a rare capacity of exceptional individuals. Existential and phenomenological approaches to medicine recognize that each moment in life is a creative process in which all people are transforming their past experiences and future hopes into the more-or-less adaptive actualization of the present moment. Illness provides the opportunity for creative development by increased awareness of our all three aspects of our being (i.e., body, thoughts, and soul), but only if we allow ourselves to accept reality and to grow in its understanding [76]. Our pains and fears force us to enlarge our consciousness if we are to adapt adequately. From this adaptive perspective, health is adequate creativity and an illness is inadequate adaptation [61]. From this person-centered perspective, Victor von Weizsaecker, observed that illnesses revealed meaningful information about reciprocal psychosomatic interactions that create health. From his clinical observations in psychosomatic medicine and his experimental observations about the phenomenology of perception, thought, and movement, he suggested that we become sick when we are not in a creative dynamic state:

> The health of a human being is not just capital to be consumed; rather health is actually present only when it is created in each moment of life.
> If health is not being created, then a person is already sick [74].

Essentially, when we are not growing creatively, we are consuming what health we have until we become ill, unhappy, and empty. When we are healthy, we are energetic, happy, and fulfilled because we are living creatively in each moment.

4.4 The Importance of a Synthetic and Holistic Perspective

The idea that health is being created in each moment of life has been forgotten in Western allopathic medicine with its tendency toward specialization that regards different organs and systems as separate parts, rather than interactive components of the whole person. In contrast, osteopathic medicine follows the Eastern tradition of recognizing that there is an underlying unity of structure and function, which leads to four main principles:

1. "The body is a unit, and the person represents a combination of body, mind, and spirit."
2. "The body is capable of self-regulation, self-healing, and health maintenance."
3. "Structure and function are reciprocally interrelated."
4. "Rational treatment is based on understanding these principles: body unity, self-regulation, and the interrelationship of structure and function." [Tenets of Osteopathic Medicine, American Osteopathic Association, www.osteopathic.org].

Likewise the principles of holistic medicine are person-centered [www.webmd.com]. Holistic medicine emphasizes that the patient is a person, not a disease or separate organ. All people have innate healing powers. Healing takes a team approach involving the patient and doctor, and addresses all aspects of a person's life using a variety of health care practices, including diet, exercise, psychotherapy, relationship and spiritual counseling, and a variety of complementary and alternative treatments, such as acupuncture, homeopathy, massage, and naturopathy. Treatment is directed to the underlying causes of diseases, not just alleviating symptoms. Holistic medicine takes a person-centered approach to provide unconditional positive regard plus respect for each person being responsible for their own health and well-being.

The combination of mainstream Western medical therapy with complementary and alternative medical procedures is defined as Integrative Medicine by the National Center for Complementary and Alternative Medicine at the US National Institutes of Health. Integrative Medicine is a person-centered medical approach that recognizes that the whole person has three aspects (body, thought, and spirit). It emphasizes the person-centered therapeutic relationship and makes use of all appropriate therapies that promote health, both conventional and alternative [73].

All these holistic approaches are person-centered, whereas some patient-centered approaches are not really holistic and do not recognize the person as a creative force in his own healing. The very notion of "patient" suggests a person who must wait patiently for the expert to instruct them in what to do, which is a framework inconsistent with truly person-centered care.

The importance of a holistic perspective for the full expression of person-centered medicine becomes clear when it is remembered that in Traditional Chinese Medicine (TCM), the physician was paid to keep a person well by curing emerging diseases before symptoms occurred. If symptoms occurred, the physician had already failed at his job. In TCM, the diagnostician learned to detect energetic changes that would predispose a person to disease and the effort of the physician was to prevent illness by correcting the prescribing changes in lifestyle and correcting energetic imbalances using methods such as herbal therapy and acupuncture. In contrast, Western medicine is skilled at acute treatment of disease, but is strikingly ineffective in the prevention and management of chronic disease [14, 15].

4.5 The Range of the Benefits from Creative Living with a Holistic Perspective

Mental Well-being: It is well established that a creative way of living (measured by a creative TCI character profile) is linked with greater subjective well-being, including greater life satisfaction (cognitive aspect of subjective well-being) and a more positive balance between positive and negative affect (the emotional aspect of subjective well-being) [20]; Josefsson et al. [45]. However, higher self-transcendence can also lead to increases in negative emotions, particularly in secular societies where self-transcendent attitudes are in disfavor, but even then positive affect is greater than negative affect in adults [45]. During adolescence, the roles of self-directedness, cooperativeness, and persistence appear to be more important than self-transcendence [34, 35]. The role of self-transcendence becomes clear only when individuals must cope with ultimate situations, like suffering, personal death, or mass extinction, which may occur at any age but only are recognized fully in older adults [9, 14, 15, 43, 46].

Physical Well-being: Both personality profiles and heart rate variability are predictive of physical morbidity and mortality [6, 7]. The impact of personality is not fully explained by people's choice of healthy lifestyles, such as habits about diet, physical exercise, and health care utilization [78]. In order to explore the physiological pathways by which personality influences physical health, we have studied relations between personality profiles and heart rate variability, which is sensitive to a variety of emotional and physiological stressors. We found that creativity, measured as the product of the three character scores in the TCI, was significantly correlated ($r = -0.3$) with healthy autonomic balance with predominance of parasympathetic activity, as measured by the ratio of high frequency (sympathetic) activity to low frequency (parasympathetic activity) [78]. In contrast, other character profiles (in which any one of the character dimensions was low) were not significantly correlated with healthy autonomic balance [78]. Agreeability is associated with greater parasympathetic activity but does not reduce sympathetic activity, whereas forgiveness reduces sympathetic activity but does not increase parasympathetic activity [78].

Greater parasympathetic balance is characterized by a state of calm alertness; it is facilitated by slow, deep breathing and is disrupted by stress or defensiveness. Defensiveness (i.e., fight or flight responses, including both aggression or avoidance) is characterized by sympathetic hyperactivity. All three TCI character traits are correlated with greater parasympathetic activity individually, and the product of the three together was greater than their individual association, indicating that there is synergy among these traits that leads to autonomic balance. Experimental interventions show that psychophysiological training with slow, deep breathing, and cultivation of positive affect can enhance heart rate variability and thereby promote healthier outcomes [51, 52].

Dean Ornish has developed multimodal training programs including diet, emotional self-regulation, and meditation to prevent or reverse coronary heart disease. Ornish has found in longitudinal studies that they lead to improved well-being, including longer telomeres (a predictor of longevity) compared to others who do not change their lifestyle [53, 54, 60]. Nevertheless, personality has not been measured with the TCI in Dean Ornish's program of lifestyle change, and the directions of influence among the several changing processes involved in comprehensive lifestyle change remain uncertain. The interactions among the multifactorial processes will need to be considered as components of a complex adaptive system [18].

Social Well-Being: Creativity is associated with perception of warm and satisfying social relationships [20]. The processes underlying the prosocial benefits of creativity have been studied in detail in negotiation and conflict resolution [36, 62]. Stable and satisfying social relationships depend on emotional communication that combines assertiveness with mutual respect, thereby leading to innovative and nonviolent resolution of disagreements. Nonviolent communication must begin with establishing a context of mutual respect and shared goals. In order to be authentic, there must be the opportunity to express and assert what each person feels and thinks candidly. Yet to avoid violence and resistance, there must be a freedom and openness to change that involves innovative solutions emerging from respectful dialogue. The same principles of nonviolent communication can be applied to negotiation generally. Again in social aspects of health, we can recognize a complex adaptive system involving multiple reciprocal feedback systems, in which trust stimulates openness, which in turn reinforces change with increases in trust. Similar mechanisms are involved in the formation and maintenance of a helping therapeutic alliance [38, 39].

Spiritual Well-being: Studies of the benefits of spirituality show that there are positive benefits from spiritual acceptance that there is a divine order like justice in the cosmos [5, 29] because this conviction is a basis for hope and other self-transcendent virtues that are characteristic of people who recover from physical and mental disorders [3]. Meta-analyses show that intrinsic motivations like love, hope, and faith led to positive psychological adjustments, whereas extrinsic motivation (doing outwardly pious acts to be seen by others) and avoidance of dealing with one's problems by withdrawing into religious activities led to negative mental and physical outcomes [4, 48, 56, 57, 67]. Religious struggles (like feeling God had abandoned you) has been associated with slightly increased mortality [56]. The effect of spiritual acceptance as a single variable to reduce mental distress or to improve health is weak in large-scale meta-analyses ($r = 0.09$) [4, 67].

Intrinsic motivation is based in inner awareness of a connection with something beyond one's self, which inspires a sense of meaning and commitment to valued action [13]. Creativity is consistently characterized by intrinsic motivation and a sense of meaning in life. Self-transcendence involves awareness of what gives meaning and purpose to a person beyond the selfish acquisition of pleasure, power, and possessions [31, 43]. The spiritual aspects of health are often discussed in secular cultures by reference to the strong human needs for engagement and meaning, as emphasized in Seligman's model of psychological health based on positive emotions (i.e., feeling good), engagement (i.e., being completely absorbed in valued actions), positive relationships (i.e., being authentically connected to others), meaning (i.e., feeling your existence has a significant purpose), and accomplishments (i.e., feeling successful in what you have done) (PERMA) [64]. Engagement is one of the facets of TCI Self-transcendence; people frequently become so absorbed in doing something they value, that they lose track of time and place for a while, so it is labeled as "self-forgetfulness" in the TCI [10, 13]. When people are asked what has given them the most lasting satisfaction in their life, the feeling of accomplishment is one of the three most common experiences they report, along with satisfaction with warm social relations and discovery of what gives them meaning [10, 47]. All of these aspects of the good life arise from using intuition to grow in awareness of who you really are and what you truly value so that you can flourish (i.e., function with happiness, plasticity and virtue).

In psychoanalytic terms, healthy and wise people function using the mature defenses of sublimation (i.e., letting go of desire for personal pleasure to accomplish something meaningful or beautiful, like an artistic creation), altruism (i.e., serving others unselfishly), hopeful anticipation (i.e., anticipating and preparing for possible future adversity by living moderately) with a sense of humor and humility [71]. People with creative characters are the individuals who are most aware of their need for coherence and self-actualization, which leads them to work on the development of wisdom and integrity [10]. Hence the healthy life is good life, and the good life is also the happy life. Lives that are healthy, happy, and good all involve doing what you value with flexibility, integrity, and wisdom.

4.6 Conclusion—Person-Centered Medicine Has a Holistic Perspective

Holistic and integrative medical approaches are fundamentally person-centered. Some approaches to medicine that practitioners consider as person-centered are not holistic (e.g., many patient-centered approaches are highly specialized and not integrative). However, health is a state of physical, mental, social, and spiritual well-being, so full health requires a holistic approach. As the holistic framework is adopted, the benefits of person-centered care becomes increasingly strong and consistent, as expected with the traditional view that people create health in each moment of their life. Therefore, as person-centered medicine develops in its effectiveness, it becomes increasingly synthetic rather than analytical, holistic rather than reductive, and functionally integrative rather than specialized.

References

1. Abbott RA, Croudace TJ, Ploubidis GB, Kuh D, Richards M, Huppert FA. The relationship between early personality and midlife psychological well-being: evidence from a UK birth cohort study. Soc Psychiatry Psychiatr Epidemiol. 2008;43(9):679–87.
2. Abbott RA, Ploubidis GB, Huppert FA, Kuh D, Wadsworth ME, Croudace TJ. Psychometric evaluation and predictive validity of Ryff's psychological well-being items in a UK birth cohort sample of women. Health Qual Life Outcomes. 2006;4:76.
3. Amering M, Schmolke M (2009) Recovery in mental health. New York: Wiley.
4. Ano GG, Vasconcelles EB. Religious coping and psychological adjustment to stress: a meta-analysis. J Clin Psychol. 2005;61(4):461–80.
5. Bach P, Hayes SC, Gallop R. Long-term effects of brief acceptance and commitment therapy for psychosis. Behav Modif. 2011;36(2):165–81.
6. Bradley RT, McCraty R, Atkinson M, Tomasino D, Daugherty A, Arguelles L. Emotion self-regulation, psychophysiological coherence, and test anxiety: results from an experiment using electrophysiological measures. Appl Psychophysiol Biofeedback. 2010;35(4):261–83.
7. Carney RM, Blumenthal JA, Stein PK, Watkins L, Catellier D, Berkman LF, Czajkowski SM, O'Connor C, Stone PH, Freedland KE. Depression, heart rate variability, and acute myocardial infarction. Circulation. 2001;104(17):2024–8.
8. Chinn S. A simple method for converting an odds ratio to effect size for use in meta-analysis. Stat Med. 2000;19(22):3127–31.
9. Cloninger CR. Completing the psychobiological architecture of human personality development: temperament, Character, and Coherence. Understanding Human Development: Dialogues with Lifespan Psychology. U.M. Staudinger and U.E.R. Lindenberger. London, Kluwer Academic Publishers; 2003. p. 159–82.
10. Cloninger CR. Feeling good: the science of well-being. New York: Oxford University Press; 2004.
11. Cloninger CR. How does personality influence mortality in the elderly? Psychosom Med. 2005;67(6):839–40.
12. Cloninger CR. The science of well-being: an integrated approach to mental health and its disorders. World Psychiatry. 2006;5(2):71–6.
13. Cloninger CR. Spirituality and the science of feeling good. South Med J. 2007;100(7):740–3.
14. Cloninger CR. Person-centered health promotion in chronic disease. Int J Person-centered Med. 2013;3(1):5–12.

15. Cloninger CR. What makes people healthy, happy, and fulfilled in the face of current world challenges? Mens Sana Monogr. 2013;11:16–24.
16. Cloninger CR, Cloninger KM. Person-centered therapeutics. Int J Person-centered Med. 2011;1(1):43–52.
17. Cloninger CR, Cloninger KM. Development of instruments and evaluative procedures on contributors to health and illness. Int J Person-centered Med. 2012;3:446–55.
18. Cloninger CR, Salloum IM, Mezzich JE. The dynamic origins of positive health and wellbeing. Int J Person-centered Med. 2012;2(2):1–9.
19. Cloninger CR, Svrakic DM, Przybeck TR. A psychobiological model of temperament and character. Arch Gen Psychiatry. 1993;50(12):975–90.
20. Cloninger CR, Zohar AH. Personality and the perception of health and happiness. J Affect Disord. 2011;128(1–2):24–32.
21. Cloninger CR, Zohar AH, Cloninger KM. Promotion of well-being in person-centered mental health care. Focus. 2010;8(2):165–79.
22. Conrad R, Schilling G, Bausch C, Nadstawek J, Wartenberg HC, Wegener I, Geiser F, Imbierowicz K, Liedtke R. Temperament and character personality profiles and personality disorders in chronic pain patients. Pain. 2007;133(1–3):197–209.
23. Csikszentmihalyi M. Flow and the psychology of discovery and invention. Cambridge: Cambridge University Press; 1997.
24. Davis MC. Building emotional resilience to promote health. Am J Lifestyle Med. 2009;3(1 Suppl.):60S–3S.
25. Diener E, Emmons RA, Larsen RJ, Griffin S. The satisfaction with life scale. J Pers Assess. 1985;49(1):71–5.
26. Diener E, Larsen RJ, Levine S, Emmons RA. Intensity and frequency: dimensions underlying positive and negative affect. J Pers Soc Psychol. 1985;48(5):1253–65.
27. Diener E, Lucas RE, Scollon CN. Beyond the hedonic treadmill: revising the adaptation theory of well-being. Am Psychol. 2006;61(4):305–14.
28. Diener E, Wirtz D, Tov W, Kim-Prieto C, Choi H, Oishi S, Biswas-Diener R. New measures of well-being: flourishing and positive and negative feelings. Soc Indic Res. 2009; 39:247–66.
29. Ellermann CR, Reed PG. Self-transcendence and depression in middle-age adults. West J Nurs Res. 2001;23(7):698–713.
30. Fava GA, Tomba E. Increasing psychological well-being and resilience by psychotherapeutic methods. J Pers. 2009;77(6):1903–34.
31. Frankl VE. Man's search for meaning. Boston: Beacon Press; 2006.
32. Frey BS. Happy people live longer. Science. 2011;331(6017):542–3.
33. Gabora, L. Why blind-variation and selective-retention is an inappropriate explanatory framework for creativity: comment on "Creative thought as blind-variation and selective-retention: combinatorial models of exceptional creativity" by Prof. Simonton." Phys Life Rev 7(2):182–83.
34. Garcia D. Two models of personality and well-being among adolescents. Pers Individ Differ. 2011;50:1208–12.
35. Garcia D, Siddiqui A. Adolescents' psychological well-being and memory for life events: influences on life satisfaction with respect to temperamental dispositions. J Happiness Stud. 2009;10:407–19.
36. Gottman JM, Gottman JS, DeClaire J. Ten lessons to transform your marriage. New York: Crown Publishers; 2006.
37. Grucza RA, Goldberg LR. The comparative validity of 11 modern personality inventories: predictions of behavioral acts, informant reports, and clinical indicators. J Pers Assess. 2007;89(2):167–87.
38. Hilsenroth MJ, Cromer TD. Clinician interventions related to alliance during the initial interview and psychological assessment. Psychother Theory Res Pract Training. 2007;44(2):205–18.

39. Hilsenroth MJ, Peters EJ, Ackerman SJ. The development of therapeutic alliance during psychological assessment: patient and therapist perspectives across treatment. J Pers Assess. 2004;83(3):332–44.
40. Howell RT. Review: positive psychological well-being reduces the risk of mortality in both ill and healthy populations. Evid Based Ment Health. 2009;12(2):41.
41. Howell RT, Kern ML, Lyubomirsky S. Health benefits: meta-analytically determining the impact of well-being on objective health outcomes. Health Psychol Rev. 2007;1(1):83–136.
42. Huppert FA, Whittington JE. Evidence for the independence of positive and negative well-being: implications for quality of life assessment. Br J Health Psychol. 2003;8(Pt 1):107–22.
43. Jaspers K. The way to wisdom: an introduction to philosophy. New Haven: Yale University Press; 1954.
44. Jokela M, Batty GD, Nyberg ST, Virtanen M, Nabi H, Singh-Manoux A, Kivimaki M. Personality and all-cause mortality: individual-participant meta-analysis of 3,947 deaths in 76,150 adults. Am J Epidemiol. 2013;178(5):667–75.
45. Josefsson K, Cloninger CR, Hintsanen M, Jokela M, Pulkki-Raback L, Keltikangas-Jarvinen L. Associations of personality profiles with various aspects of well-being: a population-based study. J Affect Disord. 2011;133(1–2):265–73.
46. Josefsson K, Jokela M, Cloninger CR, Hintsanen M, Salo J, Hintsa T, Pulkki-Raback L, Keltikangas-Jarvinen L. Maturity and change in personality: Developmental trends of temperament and character in adulthood. Dev Psychopathol. 2013;25(3):713–27.
47. Kobau R, Sniezek J, Zack MM, Lucas RE, Adam B. Well-being assessment: an evaluation of well-being scales for public health and population stimates of well-being among US adults. Appl Psychol Health Well-being. 2010;2(3):272–97.
48. Koenig HG, Pargament KI, Nielsen J. Religious coping and health status in medically ill hospitalized older adults. J Nerv Ment Dis. 1998;186(9):513–21.
49. Krishnamurti J. The first & last freedom. Brockwood Park UK: Krishnamurti Foundation Trust; 1954.
50. Krishnamurti J. The awakening of intelligence. New York: Harper and Row; 1987.
51. McCraty R, Atkinson M, Lipsenthal L, Arguelles L. New hope for correctional officers: an innovative program for reducing stress and health risks. Appl Psychophysiol Biofeedback. 2009;34(4):251–72.
52. McCraty R, Atkinson M, Tomasino D, Goelitz J, Mayrovitz HN. The impact of an emotional self-management skills course on psychosocial functioning and autonomic recovery to stress in middle school children. Integr Physiol Behav Sci. 1999;34(4):246–68.
53. Ornish D, Lin J, Daubenmier J, Weidner G, Epel E, Kemp C, Magbanua MJ, Marlin R, Yglecias L, Carroll PR, Blackburn EH. Increased telomerase activity and comprehensive lifestyle changes: a pilot study. Lancet Oncol. 2008;9(11):1048–57.
54. Ornish D, Scherwitz LW, Billings JH, Brown SE, Gould KL, Merritt TA, Sparler S, Armstrong WT, Ports TA, Kirkeeide RL, Hogeboom C, Brand RJ. Intensive lifestyle changes for reversal of coronary heart disease. JAMA. 1998;280(23):2001–7.
55. Otake K, Shimai S, Tanaka-Matsumi J, Otsui K, Fredrickson BL. Happy people become happier through kindness: a counting kindnesses intervention. J Happiness Stud. 2006;7 (3):361–75.
56. Pargament KI, Koenig HG, Tarakeshwar N, Hahn J. Religious struggle as a predictor of mortality among medically ill elderly patients: a 2-year longitudinal study. Arch Intern Med. 2001;161(15):1881–5.
57. Pargament KI, Koenig HG, Tarakeshwar N, Hahn J. Religious coping methods as predictors of psychological, physical and spiritual outcomes among medically ill elderly patients: a two-year longitudinal study. J Health Psychol. 2004;9(6):713–30.
58. Pederson C, Seligman MEP. Character strengths and virtues: a handbook and classification. New York: Oxford University Press; 2004.
59. Pickett K, Wilkinson R. The spirit level: why greater equality makes societies stronger. New York: Bloombury Press; 2009.

60. Pischke CR, Frenda S, Ornish D, Weidner G. Lifestyle changes are related to reductions in depression in persons with elevated coronary risk factors. Psychol Health. 2010;25(9):1077–100.
61. Rimpau W, editor. A reader on viktor von Weizsaecker's why you get sick?. Suhrkamp: Frankfurt on Main; 2008.
62. Rosenberg MB. Nonviolent communication: a language of compassion. DelMar, CA: PuddleDancer Press; 1999.
63. Rosenstrom T, Jokela M, Cloninger CR, Hintsanen M, Juonala M, Raitakari O, Viikari J, Keltikangas-Jarvinen L. Associations between dimensional personality measures and preclinical atherosclerosis: the cardiovascular risk in Young Finns study. J Psychosom Res. 2012;72(5):336–43.
64. Seligman ME. Flourish. New York: Free Press; 2011.
65. Simonton DK. Creativity in science: chance, logic, genius, and zeitgeist. Cambridge UK: Cambridge University Press; 2004.
66. Smith MJ, Cloninger CR, Harms MP, Csernansky JG. Temperament and character as schizophrenia-related endophenotypes in non-psychotic siblings. Schizophr Res. 2008;104(1–3):198–205.
67. Smith TB, McCullough ME, Poll J. Religiousness and depression: evidence for a main effect and the moderating influence of stressful life events. Psychol Bull. 2003;129(4):614–36.
68. Sternberg RJ, editor. The nature of creativity. Cambridge: Cambridge University Press; 1988.
69. Sternberg RJ. A three-facet model of creativity. The Nature of Creativity. R. J. Sternberg. Cambridge UK: Cambridge University Press; 2004. p. 125–47.
70. Taylor CW. Various approaches to and definitions of creativity. The nature of creativity. R. J. Sternberg. Cambridge UK: Cambridge University Press. 2004; 99–121.
71. Vaillant GE. The wisdom of the ego. Cambridge, MA: Harvard University Press; 1993.
72. Vernon PE, editor. Creativity. Modern psychology readings. Baltimore: Penguin; 1970.
73. Weil A. The state of the integrative medicine in the U.S. and Western World. Chin J Integr Med. 2011;17(1):6–10.
74. Weizsaecker VV. Social disease and social recovery (volume 8 of collected works, 1986). Suhrkamp: Frankfurt on Main; 1930.
75. WHO. Definition of health: preamble to the constitution of the world health organization. Geneva: World Health Organization; 1946.
76. Wilberg P. The illness is the cure: an introduction to life medicine and life doctoring, a new existential approah to illness. Whitstable, Great Britain: New Yoga Publications; 2012.
77. Zautra AJ, Johnson LM, Davis MC. Positive affect as a source of resilience for women in chronic pain. J Consult Clin Psychol. 2005;73(2):212–20.
78. Zohar AH, Cloninger CR, McCraty R. Personality and heart rate variability: exploring pathways from personality to cardiac coherence and health. Open J Soc Sci. 2013;1(6):32–9.

Subjectivity, Intersubjectivity, and Psychological Functioning

5

Michel Botbol, MD and Dusica Lecic-Tosevski, MD, PhD

5.1 Introduction

Individual psychological development emerges in constant interaction with others, beginning with the infant–mother relationship. A gradual developmental process culminates in two critical separation-individuation phases—the first one in early childhood and the other during adolescence—and leads to increasing independence of the subject and more mature relationships with other persons [4].

From a psychological perspective, person-centered psychiatry (PCP) has then to consider both the intrasubjective and the intersubjective aspects of clinical situations whenever a person suffers from a psychopathological disorder not only when it results from a failure in the developmental process but also when it is due to any other determinants, because they contribute to the person's quality of life and healing process [3].

In line with a contextualized definition of the person ("I am I and my circumstance") [12], person-centered psychological approach has to focus both on the individual experience of the patient, including his subjectivity, and experience involving the family and the social environment.

M. Botbol, MD (✉)
Chief, Department of Child Psychiatry, Brest University Hospital,
University of Western Brittany, Brest, France; Professor, Service Universitaire de Psychiatrie Infanto Juvénile, CHU de Brest,
Hôpital de Bohars, 29820 Bohars, France
e-mail: botbolmichel@orange.fr; michel.botbol@chu-brest.fr

D. Lecic-Tosevski, MD, PhD
School of Medicine, Belgrade Institute for Mental Health, Serbian Academy of Sciences and Arts, University of Belgrade, Belgrade, Serbia

J.E. Mezzich et al. (eds.), *Person Centered Psychiatry*,
DOI 10.1007/978-3-319-39724-5_5

The PCP should not therefore be reduced to the individualization of care or the respect for patients' rights, as it aspires to something more: the recognition of the individual subjectivity of the whole person of the patient beyond what characterizes his or her illness or his status as patient [3]. What is of interest here is dealing with the inner world of a patient in his particular situation of suffering and dependence caused by illness, like in Aristotle's Nicomachean Ethics: "Cure of a unique person and not a generalized nosological case, in a specific situation, within a specific, unrepeatable period of one's life" [15]. What becomes crucial here is the commitment of the mental health professional to approach the patient's subjectivity in his singular vital situation.

5.2 Psychological Functioning and Subjectivity

To understand and assess psychopathology in PCP perspective one should take into account three psychological dimensions [4]:

- The patient' experience of an illness and the effects of an illness on his/her personal and social life: this aspect could be called the phenomenological dimension (which includes psychological suffering, quality of life and similar processes). It is certainly subjective and can be considered as a core aspect of the mental disorder, defining both the patient's clinical situation and his/her more global being in the world.
- The psychological functioning underlying a disorder and the global organization of psychological functions: this has to take into account not only the explicit symptoms but also the underlying normal or pathological personality within which they develop. This is not related only to the psychopathological elements but also to the overall organization of the patient's inner life. This aspect could be called the structural dimension.
- The conscious and unconscious meanings of symptoms and other life events and the embedding of disorders in the patient's narrative; we call this the metaphoric or symbolic dimension. This dimension is essential for the individual's appraisal of the disorder and for its treatment. In some cases, the elements of this dimension may have an etiological role. This specific subjective aspect should be considered in the design of the therapeutic approaches, as they may be crucial to the therapeutic alliance.

To these three psychological dimensions, Alanen et al. [1] adds a fourth one he calls the familial or environmental dimension including two groups of conditions that may require family- and environment-centered treatment. The first group is composed of acute crisis situations, especially when related to losses and other stressful life events in the family, including suicides and suicidal attempts that need empathetic support. The second group of conditions requiring family- and environment-centered treatment involves persons with increased dependence on their closest human network. "Children obviously belong to this group because of their dependence on the family. The same is also true for adolescents for whom a general goal of family therapy is often needed to support the individual development of the identified patient by clarifying the psychological boundaries between family members and to strengthen the adolescent's contacts outside the family" [4].

In adult psychiatry, this group of conditions may also include schizophrenia and other psychoses, substance abuse, severe eating disorders as well as borderline personality disorder. Elderly patients and other dependent individuals may also be included within this group.

Alanen considers that in "psychotic outbreaks, the general goals of family-centered treatment are usually twofold: to stimulate the individualized development of the patient and to support family members as they deal with the patient's disorders. The experiences of joint meetings of the treatment team with patient and family members have shown that they have both an important informative function and therapeutic significance" [1]. "In many cases, these joint meetings enhance the success of simultaneous or consecutive individual therapy" [4].

The consideration of the above-mentioned dimensions appears to be important for person-centered conceptual and practical approaches in psychiatry. However, they are often ignored by conventional disorder-centered psychiatry. Berganza et al. [2] has pointed out that the latter is one of the main limitations of the current standard classificatory systems on which much of modern psychiatry is grounded. Strauss [14] has stressed the problems of reductionist psychiatry by saying that "this has neglected attention to the importance of subjective factors such as feeling, meaning and will". "It has left us ignoring a major part of human experience, left us with half a science".

Unlike standard diagnostic criteria, these dimensions are not only subjective but also holistic. The recognition and assessment of these dimensions require improvements in the parameters and guidelines for the appraisal of evidence, beyond the rigidity and narrow scope of what is usually termed evidence-based medicine (EBM), because their holistic perspective implies constant interactions between ill and positive health aspects of the patient's health status and because their subjective components apply not only to the views of the patient and his family but also to those of the professionals.

For the psychiatry for the person perspective, one of the challenges is therefore to find a non-metaphysical way to give enough room to the above-mentioned psychological bases even though they can be accounted mainly through the patient's narratives and the subjective joint understanding of these narratives both by the patient and the professional in close interaction.

5.3 Subjectivity and Intersubjectivity in PCP Practices

In addition to the attention paid to the medico-biological aspects of the person's health status, a person-centered assessment needs then to give enough consideration to the patient's subjective feelings [5]. Whether or not we suspect a psychological or psychosomatic causality to the disorder that a patient brings to us, it is essential to keep in perspective the factors involved in the patient's health situation. Beyond reasserting this principle, we need to explicit the methodology for accessing these subjective dimensions among different partners involved in the diagnostic process and the therapeutic relationship. For the professionals, the only way to access these dimensions is through what the patient (and/or his carers) says in words or shows in acting, as long as these words or acts can trigger in the professionals enough empathy to approach the patient's subjective feelings to which these expressions are related.

Working on the diagnostic approach has become an important element to meet this methodological ambition. That is why on the basis of previous experience promoted with the World Psychiatric Association Essentials of the International Guidelines for Diagnostic Assessment [11], the PCP developed a Person-Centered Integrated Diagnostic (PID) model [10]. As it is developed elsewhere in this book, one of its main objective is to take into account the subjective aspects (positive and negative) of the health situation of persons seeking care, and not just an objective description of their illness. This diagnostic model includes, besides the objective elements about the patient and his or her context, the subjective elements reported by the idiographic formulations of the person who is being cared for, their carers and assisting professionals. This approach naturally led us to a closer examination of the role of the professional's empathy in the methodology to access the subjectivity of the patient, trying to go beyond the general assertions on the importance of this concept in therapeutic relationships and care activities [5].

At first considered as the professional's ability to listen sympathetically to the comments of the patient and to integrate his wishes and needs, the notion of empathy has gradually widened to include representations that the physician (or the health professional) makes of the clinical situation in which the person in need of care is involved. In short, these are representations that the professional makes of the health situation of the person suffering through his/her (the professional) own empathy, triggered by the words and the acts of the patients and of their carers. This mechanism is well described by the concept of "metaphorizing-empathy" proposed by Lebovici [9] from his work with babies and their mothers. It is also close to the notion of "narrative empathy" proposed by Hochmann [7] based on his work with autistic children and on the philosophical ideas brought by Paul Ricoeur, a famous French phenomenologist, in his book "Time and Narrative" [13]. It is also consistent with Kleinman's assumptions [8] on illness narratives. This important development in PCM marked the full recognition of the role of the physician's subjectivity as a diagnostic and treatment tool in the physician–patient relationship.

5.4 Concluding Remarks

The PCP has evolved from a PCP aiming to mirror the patient's opinion on himself or his health status to a PCP struggling to approach the subjectivity of the person (in both its conscious and unconscious aspects) [5]. This should be done through the personal commitment of the professional and his or her use of his or her metaphorizing empathy. This perspective is much more consistent with the reality of medical practice which, in one form or another, must deal with this vital dimension in every patient. Moreover, by establishing the subjectivity of the physician as a tool for understanding the patient and his disorder (and thus a meaningful encounter of two persons: a Buber's dialogue of I and Thou) [6] , the subjective involvement of the professional regains positive status which was lost with the progress of objective technical medicine. In this perspective the subjectivity of the professional can be properly included in practice and training if enough space is given to work it through. Rather than training the professionals to fight against their subjective movements or to deny it and to prevent them from getting closer to the patient's personal needs, the PCP proposes to train them to use these subjective movements as their best tool to access the patient's subjectivity. Thus, the PCP acknowledges relevance for clinical practice of the clinician's congruence in the relationship, (i.e., his or her access to experiences arising in resonance with the patient). A required condition is, for professionals, to be trained to work it through properly, and develop enough reflexive capacities. This would enable them to take subjectivity and intersubjectivity as one of the bricks of the therapeutic relationship, i.e., the interactive construction they should build with the patient and for him or her, involving all those who are contributing to their health care and health status [5]. The teamwork and peer supervision are crucial to enhance and sustain this interactive process.

References

1. Alanen YO, Lehtinen V, Lehtinen K, et al. The Finnish integrated model for early treatment of schizophrenia and related psychoses. In: Martindale B, Bateman A, Crowe R, Margison F, editors. Psychosis: psychological approaches and their effectiveness. London: Gaskell; 2000. p. 235–65.
2. Berganza CE, Mezzich JE, Pouncey C. Concepts of disease: their relevance for psychiatric diagnosis and classification. Psychopathol Spec Issue Philos Methodol Found Psychiatr Diagn. 2005;38(4):166–70.
3. Botbol M. Du manifeste au subjectif: ce qu'est la médecine de la personne [From objectivity to subjectivity: what is person centered medicine]. In: Kipman SD, editor. Manifeste pour la médecine de la personne [Manifesto for person centered medicine]. Paris: Dunod; 2012.
4. Botbol M, Alanen YO, Lecic Tosevski D, et al. Psychological perspective in psychiatry for the person. Int J Pers Centered Med. 2011;1(1):163–5.
5. Botbol M, Lecic-Tosevski D. Person-centered medicine and subjectivity. In: Cornelius-White JHD, Motschnig-Pitrik R, Lux M (eds) Interdisciplinary applications of the person-centered approach. New York: Springer; 2013. pp 73–82.
6. Buber M. I and Thou. Charles Scribner's Sons; 1937. Reprint Continuum International Publishing Group; 2004.
7. Hochmann J. Une histoire de l'empathie [A history of empathy]. Paris: Odile Jacob; 2012.
8. Kleinman A. The illness narratives. New York: Basic Books; 1988.
9. Lebovici S. L'arbre de vie—éléments de la psychopathologie du bébé [The tree of life—principles of infant psychopathology]. Toulouse: Eres; 1999.

10. Mezzich JE, Salloum IM, Cloninger CR, Salvador-Carulla L, Kirmayer L, Banzato CE, Wallcraft J, Botbol M. Person-centered integrative diagnosis: conceptual bases and structural model. Can J Psychiatr. 2010;55:701–8.
11. Mezzich JE, Berganza CE, von Cranach M, Jorge MR, Kastrup MC, Murthy RC, Okasha A, Pull C, Sartorius N, Skodol AE, Zaudig M. Essentials of the WPA International guidelines for diagnostic assessment (IGDA). Br J Psychiatr. 2003;182(Suppl. 45).
12. Ortega y Gasset J. Meditaciones del Quijote. Obras Completas de José Ortega y Gasset. vol 1. Madrid: Editorial Santillana; 1914, 2004. pp 745–825.
13. Ricoeur P. Temps et récit [Time and narrative]. Paris: Le Seuil; 1983.
14. Strauss JS. Diagnosis and reality: a noun is a terrible thing to waste. Psychopathol Spec Issue Philos Methodol Found Psychiatr Diagn. 2005;38(4):189–91.
15. Warne C. Aristotle's nicomachean ethics: reader's Guide. London: Continuum; 2007.

6 The Role of Communication

Marijana Braš, MD, PhD, Veljko Đorđević, MD, PhD,
Roger Ruiz-Moral, MD, PhD, Myriam Deveugele, MA, PhD,
Rodrigo Ramalho, MD, PhD and Peter Pype, MD, PhD

Everything is in human relationship
Homo homini remedium

6.1 Introduction

The doctor–patient relationship is central to the practice of health care and is essential for delivery of high-quality healthcare. The current model of the doctor–patient relationship is one of collaborative partnership. In this model, communication between patients and doctors is based on common understanding, and it occurs in a caring and dynamic relationship that must involve the family. Characteristic of the relationship should be the educated patient, confidence and level of guidance and leadership, with an educational and advocacy role on behalf of the doctor [13, 15]. However, this was not always the case, as the relationship between a patient and a doctor has changed throughout history and according to the evolving

M. Braš, MD, PhD (✉) · V. Đorđević, MD, PhD
Associate Professor, Department of Psychological Medicine, Clinical Hospital Centre Zagreb, School of Medicine University of Zagreb, Zagreb, Croatia; School of Medicine University of Zagreb, Salata 4, 10000 m Zagreb, Croatia
e-mail: mbras@kbc-zagreb.hr

R. Ruiz-Moral, MD, PhD
Professor of Medicine, Clinical Communication Skills Unit, School of Medicine, University Francisco de Vitoria, Madrid, Spain

M. Deveugele, MA, PhD · P. Pype, MD, PhD
Professor of Communication in Health Science, Department of Family Medicine and Primary Health Care, Faculty of Medicine, Ghent University, Ghent, Belgium

R. Ramalho, MD, PhD
Department of Social and Community Health, School of Population Health, Centre for Addiction Research (CFAR), The University of Auckland, Auckland, New Zealand

J.E. Mezzich et al. (eds.), *Person Centered Psychiatry*,
DOI 10.1007/978-3-319-39724-5_6

role of the doctor. Doctor–patient relationship is dependent on both the era and social culture, and the potentials and technological limitations of medicine in a particular period. Nowadays, we are witnessing an unprecedented development of the medical science and the medical profession. The development of nanotechnology, epigenetics, pharmacogenomics, functional imaging, and attempts to visually present human emotions are all examples of this development. However, all this technological superiority should not allow us to lose sight of the patient as a person in their physical, psychological, social, and spiritual totality [13, 15].

Communication has been defined as the transmission of information, thoughts, and feelings so that these are satisfactorily received and/or understood [17]. Communication is basic tool in building relationships as it allows people to share their interest, concerns, and support of each other; to make critical decisions and to cooperate better with each other. Communication in medicine is considered as a fundamental clinical skill and a way to successful diagnosis and treatment and to establish a relationship with the patient. Numerous studies have shown that communication skills are associated with the outcome measures, including patient satisfaction, treatment adherence, a lower incidence of complaints about medical errors, and to some extent health related outcomes [8, 11, 23, 27, 37, 38, 39]. Therefore, in recent decades great attention has been paid to the quality of communication in medicine. Communication is the most widely used clinical skill in medical practice, used hundreds of thousands of times in working life. Communication includes a large number of interactions with all participants in the health system, of which we mention only some: patient and doctor communication, communication between the patient and other members of the healthcare team (nurses, psychologists, teachers, social workers, medical technicians, physical therapists, etc.), communication between doctors and patients' family members, communication between members of medical teams and interdisciplinary teams, communication among health professionals within professional associations, doctors' communication with the local and national governments and intergovernmental organizations, communication with civil society organizations (particularly with associations of patients), communication with insurance companies, communication with pharmaceutical companies, the media, etc. Only good communication can provide and establish good relationship between the health professional and patient, and the most important aspect of communication is the medical interview, as a bridge from bench to bedside to community [13, 15]. Due to recent advances in neuroscience, we are now able to describe and discuss the neurobiology of the doctor–patient relationship [1]. Different physiological and biochemical mechanisms take part in complex functions, such as trust, hope, empathy, and compassion, which are all very important elements in the doctor–patient relationship. From a neuroscientific perspective, the doctor–patient relationship can be divided into at least four steps: feeling sick, seeking relief, meeting the therapist, and receiving therapy [2]. Although besides enabling an in-depth biological assessment of the doctor–patient relationship, the main advantage of a neuroscientific perspective is that doctors, psychologists, and other health professionals can better understand the kind of changes they can induce in their patients' brains, further boosting the professional's empathic and compassionate behavior [3]. This further supports the point that effective doctor–patient communication is a central clinical function not only in developing a therapeutic relationship, but also in the delivery of high-quality healthcare.

Person-centered medicine represents the novel paradigm of general well-being, and not merely absence of disease. In order for this to be successful, we must overcome numerous obstacles in our path, obstacles which dehumanize, so that we can find ourselves on a path that leads to the humanization of man, who has no earthly predator but himself, and the civilization to which he belongs [16].

6.2 Medical Interview

Modern healthcare professionals need to be educated on how to use their highly specialized knowledge when approaching an individual patient as a unique and whole person living in a given psychological, social, and material context. Such an approach combines the best of ancient medicine—which was individualized and person-oriented, yet not sufficiently scientific—and modern, scientific-oriented, highly efficient medicine, which, unfortunately, tends to disregard the person as a whole Đorđević et al. [13, 15]. In a series of talks given to students of the Harvard University School of Medicine, Francis W. Peabody said: "The practice of medicine in its broadest sense includes the whole relationship of the physician with his patient. It is an art, based to an increasing extent on the medical sciences, but comprising much that still remains outside the realm of any science. The treatment of a disease may be entirely impersonal; the care of a patient must be completely personal. One of the essential qualities of the clinician is interest in humanity, for the secret of the care of the patient is in caring for the patient" [25]. As there are no two identical genotypes or two identical DNAs, there are no two identical persons. Everyone is unique. We should accept the person seeking help as a whole, but that person should also accept the caregiver as a person who provides help and can be trusted. The stronger and more open this trust relationship, the better, faster, and more efficient the outcome. The treatment process exists only while the trust relationship exists [13, 15]. The medical interview provides a framework for exploring and understanding patients' concerns, fears, misconceptions, and how they experience their illness while taking into consideration their culture, availability of treatment options, and financial considerations [9]. Medical interview is a complex process of obtaining information for the purpose of making a diagnosis and it is an extremely important factor in establishing the relationship between health professionals and patients [9, 20].

Literature describes the medical interview as being 'physician-centered' or 'patient-centered'. The latter is advocated to replace the former. Physician-centered interview mainly includes asking specific questions in order to establish the diagnosis. The physician takes the lead during the whole consultation, defining the topics of the consultation along the interest of the doctor. This approach in most cases ignores important personal information about the patient, his or her personality, and emotions. Patient centered interview, on the contrary, focuses on the understanding the patient's perceptions of illness. Patient-centered communication style aims to identify the patient's needs. Likewise, the patient's open and clear presentation of his or her reasons for visit adds to an effective and efficient encounter, which makes the patient feel helped, empowered, and cared for [34, 35]. Moreover, this interview model includes the aspect traditionally connected to the physician-centered style (history taking, making diagnoses, giving information, and providing treatment). But even in these more strick medical aspects, the patient is seen as a whole person with his/her own preferences and with the ability to discuss the treatment options and to make the decision about treatment together with the caregiver. Patient-centered interview results in the most complete, accurate, and diagnostically powerful data set—the patient's biopsychosocial story, and strengthens the patient-physician relationship [35]. The essential elements of the patient-centered interview are to build a relationship, open the discussion, gather information, understand the patient's perspective, share information, reach agreement, and provide closure. Attentiveness and worth, empathy, respect, support, and partnership are basic relationship skills that help build physician–patient rapport [36]. Focused interventions, either with patients or their clinicians, enhance patients' involvement in decision-making [10, 18, 30].

In their book: 'Skills for Communicating with Patients', Silverman, Kurtz and Draper [33], provide the rationale for the importance of using good medical skills. They state that doctor–patient communication is central to clinical practice and is not an optional add-on. Communication turns theory into practice; how something is said is as important as what is communicated.

They describe three types of communicative skills:

Content skills—WHAT health professionals communicate; the substance of their questions and responses, the information they gather and give, the treatments they discuss. This includes the biomedical and patient's perspective; *biomedical perspective* refers to sequence of events, symptom analysis, past medical history, drug and allergy history, family history, personal and social history, review of systems, etc.; *patient's perspective* includes patient's illness experience, ideas and beliefs, concerning and feeling, expectations and effect on life;

Process skills—HOW health professionals communicate; this includes the way to communicate with patients, the strategy to discover the information and the medical history, which verbal and nonverbal skills are used, how the relation is developed and which structure is provided.

Perceptual skills—What does health professional think and feel. These skills include internal decision-making, clinical reasoning, and problem-solving at the one hand but also attitudes and personal capacities for compassion, integrity, respect, and flexibility of the healthcare provider on the other hand.

Content skills, process skills, and perceptive skills are linked and cannot be considered in isolation. As a result they need to be studied and taught as an inseparable whole. As communication is generally purposive, medical interview can be better understanding as a model of communicative activities, most of these activities can be taught as tasks. A number of well-established consultation models and recommendations list these tasks [21, 22, 26, 31, 30, 33] (Pendleton and Schofield 2003). An alternative is the Zagreb model of person-centerd medical interview (currently under development by its authors Đorđević et al. [15, 13]). This model focuses not only on the disease or illness but on patient's quality of life in the context of health and disease. Person-centered medical interview is an important bridge between personalized and person-centered medicine. In order to evaluate and influence communication in medicine and healthcare, trainers, researchers and providers increasingly monitor communication processes during healthcare encounters.

6.3 Teaching and Learning Communication Skills

Communication skills training is now internationally accepted as an essential component of medical education [12, 28]. Much of communication theory can be learnt through textbooks and guidelines that can provide a solid foundation and framework sufficient for the knowledge about communication or for understanding how to perform the medical interview. However, theory and knowing how is absolutely not sufficient to become skilled in the art of the medical interview, experiential learning is of crucial importance.

Fortunately during the last decades, much more attention is given to communication training when developing new medical curricula. Nevertheless, the implementation of communication training still deals with several problems. To name some: First, although good communication require generic skills, most curricula deal with specific topics like breaking bad news, genetic counseling, handling psychosocial problems, or smoking cessation. Generic skills (listening, empathy, negotiation, etc.) can be used more or less intensive, depending of the situation. In a good communication curriculum rehearsal and continuation throughout the whole curriculum is aimed for. Specific situations (like breaking bad news or smoking cessation) can then use the benefits of the skills trained earlier and be seen as an application of the generic skills learned. A second problem deals with the fact that training is limited in time and mostly not contextualized. As a result transfer from training to practice in the real world, is hard to achieve. A major problem is the role-models students get when they start their clerkship. Hospital care is diagnosis oriented, doctor centered, and often related to acute interventions. Students are seldom stimulated to look for patient's ideas, concerns and emotions at the bedside. Third, medical curricula often deal with teaching problems. It will be obvious that the specific didactical techniques are needed. Ex-cathedra lectures on communication will never be successful to teach communication skills [12].

Specific teaching methods for communication are needed, with an emphasis on skills, in order to achieve behavior change in participants. Cognitive learning (theory) and taking into account attitudes are certainly complementary approaches. Thus, it can be said that teaching communication skills is not to be considered optional and "supplement to other education" because proper communication is crucial to ensure effectiveness in every day medical practice. Communication bridges the barriers between evidence-based medicine and the individual approach to the patient [28]. It is nccessary to offer education in communication skills to both undergraduate and postgraduate education, for all health professionals. In communication skills laboratories students and professionals have a chance to practice with real-life and simulated patients using video cameras and scales, such as Roter Interaction Analysis System and Cambridge Guide to Medical Interview [4, 29]. This will give proper up-to-date tools to evaluate, modify, and adopt various aspects of communication processes [32]. Just a personal experience or talent is not enough for optimal physician–patient communication. Although some are more and some are less talented, it is encouraging to know that skills can be improved by training.

All health workers are primarily human, and to make errors is human. Only education can help us to reduce mistakes [5, 14].

Medical education is a critical component of the promotion of the culture of health, which requires a revised approach to the teaching of clinical and communication skills. *Ars medica* is as much "art in medicine" as it is "the medicine of art." It is a journey from a culture of illness toward a culture of health, from symptoms and diagnoses toward human beings and persons [16]. When we talk about different forms of communication in medicine, we must never forget the importance of communication through art. Although one of the simplest, art is effective way to approach the patient and produce the effect that no other means of communication can achieve. Art can be used as a therapeutic technique as well as a means of raising public awareness of some medical problems. Art can also be one of the form of educating medical professionals and others involved in treatment and decision-making [7]. Art influences people's emotions and forms an invaluable part of today's medicine. Creation is an act of survival, growth, and development of an individual and the community. There is no development without creativity. A doctor's approach is always unique and reflects us, as a person, and the context in which the meeting takes place. Each meeting is a new creation, a creation of a relationship that can be recorded or imitated, but never repeated in exactly the same way.

6.4 Communication in Interdisciplinary Team

Inter-professional communication is an important aspect in the treatment of patients, and all parties involved would benefit from proper inter-professional collaboration. The interdisciplinary team is one of the most widely accepted innovations in the delivery of health care and social services. In today's medicine and healthcare, patient outcomes are more than ever dependent on effective interdisciplinary teamwork. No single professional can deliver a complete episode of healthcare and there is a need for the division of labor among medical, nursing and allied health practitioners. Physicians, nurses, psychologists, social workers, physiotherapists, pharmacists, occupational therapists, technicians, chaplains, and volunteers must coordinate their activities, if safe and efficient patient care are to be a priority. Moreover, aging populations with growing multi-morbidity present with complex healthcare problems requiring inter-professional and interdisciplinary collaboration [41]. Inter-professional healthcare teams allow for health care providers to combine their individual competences and deliver an integrated high-quality patient care, leading to better health outcomes. Communication is one of the four core competences for inter-professional collaborative practice, besides values/ethics; roles/responsibilities and teamwork [19]. Communication is a core item in survey instruments measuring teamwork in healthcare settings [40]. Two major themes are subject to inter-professional team communication. First patient-centered care. Team members discussing patient care and treatment options need awareness of the value of every member's professional input and should strive for interdisciplinary shared decision-making on treatment plans. Frequent communication leads to shared knowledge creation, development of shared goals, and shared clinical decision-making [24]. Consequently the results of the team discussions can be communicated to the patient without conflicting messages, leading to higher patient satisfaction and better therapy compliance. Second, communication about the functioning of the team is important. Team meetings should also focus on individual members' roles, responsibilities and task description to avoid conflicts. Hierarchical differences between team members should equally be acknowledged and discussed to promote clarity.

To promote effective and efficient team communication, the Inter-professional Education Collaborative describes eight key recommendations [19]: 1. Use appropriate communication tools and techniques to facilitate interactions enhancing team function; 2. Avoid discipline-specific terminology; 3. Share your knowledge and opinions with team members to create common understanding of information and team decisions; 4. Listen actively and encourage ideas and opinions of other team members; 5. Provide feedback to other team members about their performance and be prepared to receive feedback from others; 6. Adapt your language to the requirements of the situation, e.g., respectful discussion in case of inter-professional conflict; 7. Acknowledge every team member's personal and professional identity and its impact on team functioning and inter-professional working relationships; 8. Be an advocate for teamwork in patient-centered care. Ideally, inter-professional communication should be part of undergraduate education to prepare the future healthcare workforce for collaborative practice [41].

The various practitioners benefit from this collaborative effort: as their role becomes clarified, they are viewed as an important member of the team, and their work becomes more streamlined and efficient.

6.5 Conclusion

The core of the medical profession has always been and will be the relationship between the health professional and the person seeking assistance. It is imperative, as individuals and families, as citizens and communities, and as healthcare professionals, that we view each person as a unique individual, whatever their biopsychosocial needs may be, and not as a disorder or the sum of their symptoms. Fortunately, the traditional relationship between the physician and the patient has changed and is greatly impacted by huge social, philosophical, economic, and scientific developments. Communication is an integral part of any relationship with patients and their families, and represents the key to the success of a medical team. The focus must be on stimulating healthy and creative forces in patients that are so important for their coping with disease, maintaining hope, fighting for life, and not giving up. An effort must be made to provide patients with the best humane healthcare and empathy as possible. Today is more than ever important to make a balance between humanism and medical sciences. The ability to communicate effectively is not innate; it is a skill that can be taught and learned. More importantly, the way in which this skill is taught determines how well the students and professionals learns to communicate. Experiential learning is important, with an individualized and interactive format of teaching. Health professionals must adhere to many of the principles of evidence-based medicine, but not forget to use person-oriented and person-centered approach. Human relationship is what matters most!

References

1. Benedetti F. How the doctor's words affect the patient's brain. Eval Health Prof. 2002;25:369–86.
2. Benedetti F. The patient's brain: the neuroscience behind the doctor-patient relationship. Oxford: Oxford University Press; 2010.
3. Benedetti F, Carlino E, Pollo A. How placebos change the patient's brain. Neuropsychopharmacology. 2011;36:339–54.
4. Brajković L. The CEPAMET approach to teaching communication skills to medical students. Int J Pers Centered Med. 2015;4(3):167–72.
5. Brajković L, Braš M, Đorđević V, Cvek M. In: Đorđević V, Braš M, Miličić D, editors Person in medicine: from bench to bedside to community. Zagreb: Medicinska Naklada; 2012.
6. Braš M, Đorđević V. Person-centered health education and training. Croat Med J. 2014;55: 79–80. doi:10.3325/cmj.2014.55.79.
7. Braš M, Đorđević V, Janjanin M. Person-centered pain management—science and art. Croat Med J. 2013;54:296–300.
8. Brown JB, Stewart M, Ryan BJ. Outcomes of patient-provider interaction. In: Thompson TL, Dorsey AM, Miller KI, Parrott R, editors. Handbook of health communication. London: Lawrence Erlbaum Associates, Publishers; 2003. p. 141–61.
9. Coulehan JL, Block ML. The medical interview: mastering skills for clinical practice. 5th ed. Philadelphia (PA): F.A. Davis Co; 2005. p. 3–21.
10. Deber RB. Physicians in health care management: 7. The patient-physician partnership: changing roles and the desire for information. CMAJ. 1994;151:171.
11. Detmar SB, Muller MJ, Schornagel JH, Wever LD, Aaronson NK. Health-related quality-of-life assessments and patient-physician communication: a randomized controlled trial. JAMA. 2002;288(23):3027–34.
12. Deveugele M, Derese A, De Maesschalck S, Willems S, Van Driel M, De Maeseneer J. Teaching communication skills to medical students, a challenge in the curriculum? Patient Educ Couns. 2005;58:265–70.
13. Đorđević V, Braš M, Brajković L. Person-centered medical interview. Croat Med J. 2012;53:310–3.
14. Đorđević V, Braš M, Milunović V, Brajković L, Stevanović R. The founding of the centre for palliative medicine, medical ethics and communication skills: a new step toward the development of patient oriented medicine in Croatia. Croat Med J. 2011;52:87–8.

15. Đorđević V, Braš M, Miličić D. Introduction. In: Đorđević V, Braš M, Miličić D, editors. Person in medicine and healthcare: from bench to bedside to community. Zagreb: Medicinska naklada; 2012. p. 43.
16. Đorđević V, Braš M, Kulić S, Demarin V. The founding of Zagreb's Institute for the Culture of Health: an important step toward a new medical paradigm. Croat Med J. 2015;56(1):1–3.
17. Gerteis M, Edgman-Levitan S, Daley J, et al., editors. Through the Patient's eyes: understanding and promoting patient-centred care. San Francisco: Jossey-Bass; 1993.
18. Holman H, Lorig K. Patients as partners in managing chronic disease: partnership is a prerequisite for effective and efficient health care. BMJ. 2000.
19. Interprofessional Education Collaborative (IPEC). Core competencies for interprofessional collaborative practice: report of an expert panel; 2011. Retrieved from http://www.aacn.nche.edu/education-resources/ipecreport.pdf.
20. Lazare A, Putnam SM, Lipkin M Jr. Three functions of the medical interview. In: Lipkin Jr M, Putnam SM, Lazare A, editors. The medical interview. NY: Springer; 1995. p. 3–19.
21. Makoul G. The SEGUE framework for teaching and assessing communication skills. Patient Educ Couns. 2001;45:23–34.
22. Makoul G. Participants in the Bayer-Fetzer conference on physician-patient in medical education. Essential elements of communication in medical encounters: the Kalamazoo consensus statement. Acad Med. 2001;76:390–3.
23. Mead N, Bower P. Patient-centered consultations and outcomes in primary care: a review of the literature. Patient Educ Couns. 2002;48:51–61.
24. Morgan S, Pullon S, McKinlay E. Observation of interprofessional collaborative practice in primary care teams: an integrative literature review. Int J Nurs Stud. 2015;52(7):1217–30. doi:10.1016/j.ijnurstu.2015.03.008 (Epub 2015 Mar 19).
25. Peabody FW. The care of the patient. JAMA. 1927;88:p877–82.
26. Pendleton D, Schofield T, Tate P, Havelock P. The new consultation. Oxford: Oxford University Press; 2003.
27. Rao JK, Anderson LA, Inui TS, Frankel RM. Communication interventions make a difference in conversations between physicians and patients: a systematic review of the evidence. Med Care. 2007;45:340–9.
28. Riley SC, Morton J, Ray DC, Swann DG, Davidson DJ. An integrated model for developing research skills in an undergraduate medical curriculum: appraisal of an approach using student selected components. Perspect Med Educ. 2013;2(4):230–47.
29. Roter D, Larson S. The roter interaction analysis system (RIAS): utility and flexibility for analysis of medical interactions. Patient Educ Couns. 2002;4246:243–51.
30. Ruiz-Moral R. The role of physician-patient communication in promoting patient-participatory decision making. Health Expect. 2010;13:33–44.
31. Ruiz-Moral R, Gavilán Moral E, Parras Rejano JM, Perula de Torres LA, et al. In: CICAA scale. Scale for assessing doctor-patient relationship in clinical encounter. Handbook. Barcelona: ESTEVE; 2006. http://www.doctutor.es/wp-content/uploads/2010/03/Escala_cicaa_2.pdf. Accessed on 06 June 2015 (published in Spanish).
32. Silverman JD, Kurtz SM, Draper J. Skills for communicating with patients. Oxford: Radcliffe Medical Press; 1998.
33. Silverman J, Kurtz S, Draper J. Skills for communicating with patients. 3rd ed. Radcliffe Publishing: London; 2013.
34. Smith RC. The patient's story integrated patient-doctor interviewing. Boston: Little Brown; 1996.
35. Smith RC. Patient centered interviewing. 2nd ed. PA: Lippincott Williams & Wilkins; 2002.
36. Snaedal J. Components of person-centered medicine in medical treatment and care. Int J Pers Cent Med. 2012;21:29–32.
37. Stewart MA. Effective physician-patient communication and health outcomes: a review. Can Med Assoc J. 1995;152(9):1423–33.

38. Stewart M, Brown JB, Donner A, McWhinney IR, Oates J, Weston WW, et al. The impact of patient-centered care on outcomes. J Fam Pract. 2000;49:796–804.
39. Travaline JM, Ruchinskas R, D'Alonzo GE. Patient-physician communication: why and how. J Am Osteopath Assoc. 2005;105(1):13–8.
40. Valentine MA, Nembhard IM, Edmondson AC. (2015). Measuring teamwork in healthcare settings. A review of survey instruments. Med Care. 2015;53(4):e16–30. doi:10.1097/MLR.0b013e31827feef6.
41. WHO. Framework for action on interprofessional education and collaborative practice. Geneva: World Health Organization; 2010.

7 Cultural Awareness and Responsiveness in Person-Centered Psychiatry

Laurence J. Kirmayer, MD, Rachid Bennegadi, MD
and Marianne C. Kastrup, MD, PhD

7.1 Introduction

Person-centered psychiatry aims to reorient clinical practice around understanding and engagement with the patient as a person. A crucial aspect of this reorientation is systematic attention to the social world in which the person lives—both in terms of individuals' developmental history and biography and their current life circumstances. Human beings are social and cultural beings: we are born unable to fend for ourselves and spend the first decades of life acquiring language and learning to navigate cultural constructed social worlds. Cooperative social activity is essential for human adaptation and flourishing. For millennia our environments of adaptation have been primarily humanly constructed and our biology and ways of life have undergone coevolution [14]. Hence, medicine and psychiatry must take culture and social context into account in understanding and responding to illness and promoting health and well-being. However, as our social worlds have changed with

L.J. Kirmayer, MD (✉)
James McGill Professor and Director, Division of Social and Transcultural Psychiatry, McGill University, Montreal, Canada; Director, Culture and Mental Health Research Unit, Institute of Community and Family Psychiatry, Jewish General Hospital, 4333 Cote Ste Catherine Rd., Montreal, QC H3T 1E4, Canada
e-mail: laurence.kirmayer@mcgill.ca

R. Bennegadi, MD
Director, Research and Teaching Pole, Centre Minkowska, Paris, France; Co-Director, University Diploma on Health, Disease, Care and Cultural Competence, University of Paris, Descartes, Paris, France

M.C. Kastrup, MD, PhD
Specialist in Psychiatry, Frederiksberg, Denmark

J.E. Mezzich et al. (eds.), *Person Centered Psychiatry*,
DOI 10.1007/978-3-319-39724-5_7

new technologies, forms of community, and global networks, so too has the nature of culture. Culturally informed psychiatric theory and practice must therefore consider the shifting meanings of culture in relation to new configurations of the social world.

In this chapter, we outline current thinking about the importance of culture in mental health and review approaches to integrating attention to culture in person-centered care. Although some anthropologists argue that culture is a concept that has outlived its usefulness and, indeed, may be a cloak under which various forms of discrimination hide, we believe that the construct of culture has utility in psychiatry, standing for a great variety of social determinants of health and illness experience that are crucial to effective mental health care. Moreover, while some who grant the importance of culture assume that adopting a person-centered approach will be sufficient for clinicians to elicit all they need to know about cultural and social context from the individual patient, we will argue that systematic attention to culture, guided by relevant conceptual frameworks is essential to obtain a comprehensive picture of patients' lifeworlds and respond appropriately to their health problems and concerns. In this light, we will review current approaches to integrating culture in health care systems and practice with particular attention to person-centered aspects. Finally, we will discuss some specific tools and strategies for culturally informed assessment and treatment and outline some issues for health care policy and mental health promotion [40].

Crucial to our approach is the recognition that culture is not simply a matter of discrete social factors, values or beliefs, but constitutes the matrix of meaning, discourse and practice through which structures of power, inequality and social position are constructed, legitimated and maintained [20]. As such, understanding the ways in which cultural identities are played out in a given society, community, or clinical setting must be central to any vision of a person-centered psychiatry that aims to provide equitable and effective care. Moreover, given that culture provides the language and the settings which people use to negotiate shared values and perspectives, attention to culture is an important bridge between person- and people-centered medicine, which aims to acknowledge the social determinants of health and address the political issues raised by inequalities at local, national, transnational, and global levels [15].

7.2 Thinking About Culture in Context

"Culture" is a broad term that covers all of the humanly constructed and socially transmitted knowledge and practices that constitute a way of life. The meanings of "culture" differ with social, geographic and political context, and have changed over time with the emergence of new technologies, forms of community, and networking. In any country, geographical region or clinical setting, there are specific historical, socioeconomic, and political factors that define major cultural groupings and highlight some forms of difference and diversity as relevant to the health care system, while others are ignored or rendered invisible. It is important to consider the specific contexts in which concepts and clinical approaches to culture emerge.

For example, much literature on culture and mental health has been produced in the U.S., where diversity is often discussed in terms of the five major ethnoracial blocs defined by the census based on language (Hispanic or Latino), geographic (Asian American or Pacific Islander), indigeneity (American Indian and Alaska Native), and racialized categories derived from the history of the slave trade (African American, Caucasia, or White). Of course, such broad groupings cannot capture the diversity within groups. Indeed, later changes in the U.S. census that allowed people to endorse multiple categories have revealed high levels of mixed identities or hybridity. When people are able to provide their own categories, the predefined categories are "shattered" resulting in a wide array of new identities constructed on many different bases including religion, sexual orientation, occupation, or vocation and illness [22]. However, epidemiological data, clinical studies and training materials from the U.S. continue to reference these broad categories, which simply do not make sense in other societies, which have other ways of framing difference and diversity [32].

In societies with a history of colonialism, for example, the identities of newcomers from former colonies may be framed in terms of categories that bear traces of the racism of the colonial past [18]. In other cases, ethnic identity may be suppressed in situations where political ideology sees it as a threat to national unity. The key issue for mental health is that cultural identities depend on local politics and are framed in terms of tensions and distinctions within and between communities. Hence, they are emotionally and politically charged and may be important influences on individual and population health.

Culture is often confused with ethnicity and we need to distinguish constructs of culture, ethnicity and race, which vary across societies with different histories, politics of identity and demographics. Culture generates local forms of identity, including concepts of race and ethnicity. The health implications of these categories must be understood in context. In most societies, culturally constructed categories of identity are associated with major health disparities due to ongoing structural violence [17]. However, these forms of collective identity, even when they are largely imposed by dominant groups within the society, may also constitute communities in ways that allow social support, solidarity and political agency.

Race refers to socially constructed notions of biological difference—usually based on superficial characteristics of appearance (skin color, facial features, hair) that are viewed as markers of intrinsic biological difference. In fact, the characteristics attached to race depend on cultural conventions that hide histories of colonization, slavery, and other forms of structural violence and institutionalized inequalities. Notions of race are commonly incorporated into stereotypes of others and used to maintain systems of racial discrimination and oppression. Hence, while race is a biological fiction, it is a social fact with major impact on physical and mental health [23, 53, 54].

Culture, race, and ethnicity then are not traits of individuals with a particular upbringing or an intrinsic characteristic of some group or community but are constituted by knowledge, practice, values, institutions that form social systems; in effect, culture is a name for a large number of inter-related social processes more than it is a discrete entity or object. The social processes that constitute culture vary at the level of local communities or neighborhoods, nations and transnational networks. At the level of local communities, for example, having neighbors of the same ethic background can promote the mental health of minority groups by improving their social supports and buffering some of the effects of racism [29, 59]. At the national level, recognition of minority rights and political voice can empower a community with positive effects on well-being. Internationally, the ways in which specific groups are framed and portrayed in mass media may have powerful impacts on the mental health and well-being of people throughout a global diaspora [57]. In each case, the health implications of identity for individuals depend on the interplay between individual psychology, family and community dynamics, and relationships with the larger society.

7.3 The Place of Culture in Person-Centered Psychiatry

The view of culture sketched above has implications for the place of culture in person-centered medicine and psychiatry. In particular, it suggests that many aspects of culture are expressed in very diverse ways among individuals, so that assumptions about patients based on aspects of their cultural origin or identity are likely to be unfounded. Hence, it is important to explore with each patient not only their cultural origins and background but specific aspects of their knowledge, ways of life and social identities, or affiliations relevant to their health care. Although it might be assumed that a thoroughly person-centered approach that explores the individual's perspective will be sufficient to uncover any and all crucial dimensions of culture, systematic attention to culture, and context can reveal important aspects of health and illness that may be missed by an approach limited to the individual's perspective. These hidden cultural dimensions include aspects of personal and collective identity, health and illness experience, social determinants of health, and the larger sociopolitical context of the clinical encounter and of population health. Uncovering these tacit dimensions of culture requires systematic inquiry guided by social science perspectives. In this way, the culturally informed clinician can develop a more complete picture of the patient's lifeworld and predicament. The impact of culture and social context should be explored in the clinical setting to clarify its relevance to the patient's own perspectives and concerns but the process may also uncover issues that enlarge the patient's self-understanding in ways that can be liberating.

Person-centered care begins by engaging patients as people on their own terms and this includes the ways that they understand their own identities. However, identity is not a monolithic construction, but is multistranded or variegated, involving multiple schemas and reference groups that vary with goals and context, including the setting and the perceived identity of the interlocutor. The answers a clinician gets in response to questions about identity will depend on how the question is posed and the aspects deemed relevant to the immediate concerns, as well as patients' perceptions of the clinician and the safety of the clinical setting. Appreciating patients' cultural background and current contexts requires engaging them at the level of their clinical concerns, which are related to the ways they understand symptoms and illness, their current predicaments, life trajectories, and social positioning. However, self-understanding has its own limits. People may not be aware of many of the social, cultural, and contextual factors that shape their identity and health problems.

Indeed the notion of personhood itself is a cultural construction, and there are important variations in what is viewed as central to the person, constitutive of identity and indicative of health or adaptive functioning, as well as positive social, moral, religious, and aesthetic values. Table 7.1 describes some broad cultural variations in personhood relevant to person-centered mental health care. These variations have implications for the assessment of identity, the impact of specific types of stressors, sources of resilience and healing, and the ways in which health, wellness, and recovery are conceived [3, 58].

The most common frameworks in psychiatry, clinical psychology, and psychotherapy employ an individualistic concept of the person that emphasizes the importance of self-direction, autonomy, and self-esteem [30]. On this view, persons are constituted by their individual history, goals, and aspirations. In contrast, sociocentric, familistic, or communalistic notions of the person give a more central place to relationships with others. People who understand themselves primarily in these terms will describe the self in terms of their lineage, family, clan, or community. They will privilege maintaining the harmony of these social groups and

Table 7.1 Cultural variations in concepts of personhood

	Framework for personhood	Health indicators	Illness indicators	Sources of resilience and healing
Individualistic egocentric	Individual agency, autonomy	Self-efficacy Independence	Lack of self-efficacy	Personality traits, knowledge, skills
Communalistic sociocentric	Collective agency, interdependence	Harmony of the group	Interpersonal conflict	Relationships to family, community, larger society
Ecocentric	Environment (animals, land, natural elements)	Vitality of the environment (biodiversity)	Degradation of the environment	Connection to land
Cosmocentric	Ancestors, spirits	Regular observance of spiritual or religious practices	Failure of observances	Rituals to restore respect and moral order

Adapted in part from Kirmayer [30]

emphasize collective agency and decision-making. Many indigenous peoples around the globe articulate ecocentric views of the person that point to the deep interconnections between the individual and the environment. From the ecocentric perspective, there may be no sharp boundary between the individual and the natural world. For example, Maori traditionally describe their identities not only in terms of clan (a sociocentric notion) but also in terms of the mountains and rivers to which they are connected [50]. Similarly, Inuit understand the physical and mental constitution of the person as deeply related to the consumption of country food as the source of the person's strength, integrity, and well-being [36]. Finally, many peoples have notions of the person as embedded in and constituted by relationships with spirits or ancestors in what might be termed a "cosmocentric" view of the self. This mode of being might lead people to see their own health and well-being as deeply connected to that of their ancestors and to consult the spirits or ancestors to determine the nature of health problems and to seek guidance when making important health-related decisions.

This list is not exhaustive and these versions of personhood are not mutually exclusive. Cultures, communities, and individuals differ in how often, when and where they employ particular modes of thinking about the self. Most people will have elements of each model available to guide their thinking about health and illness. Which schema is foregrounded at any given moment depends on the nature of the problem, the aspects of symptoms, health and identity they are thinking about, and other social contextual factors.

These versions of personhood are not just abstract conceptual schemas. They are grounded in bodily experiences, and overarching cultural frameworks that include notions about ontology (what the world is made up of), epistemology (how knowledge can be acquired and verified), and morality (what is the right way to live one's life). Because of this variation in concepts of the person, clinicians who aim to respect the patient's personhood cannot assume a completely shared understanding of what is at stake in an illness episode or experience. Health communication therefore cannot simply be a matter of conveying the correct biomedical perspective but must consider the significance for the person, their family, and community of differing ontologies, sources of knowledge, and conceptions of the good.

7.4 Culture and the Social Determinants of Health

A second key set of clinical issues concerns the ways that culture influences the social determinants of health. Table 7.2 lists some key social determinants of health that are shaped by culture. Research on social determinants of health has drawn attention to a broad set of factors related to social inequality, structural violence, and the political economy of health care [4, 66]. However, the forms of social life vary substantially across cultures. Consideration of this cultural variation can guide the clinician in identifying the particular social stressors or predicaments, causal processes, mediators, and mechanisms relevant to care. Understanding the cultural

Table 7.2 Cultural influences on social determinants of health

Social determinants	Influence of culture	Mediating process or mechanism
Ethnicity, religion Race Caste	Definitions of social groups Ontologies that essentialize socially constructed categories making them seem natural, necessary or inevitable	Belonging, solidarity Racism and discrimination Marginalization Subordination, disempowerment
Age Gender Sexual orientation Education Occupation	Links specific roles and identities to age, gender, sexual orientation, education, occupation, and other social statuses	Coherent identity Positively valued roles Social support versus isolation Opportunities to pursue education or find work
Social class	Ideologies that rationalize and maintain structure of communities and social stratification	Economic privation Income inequality

construction of identity and social position in terms of gender, race, ethnicity, caste, religion, or other categories can inform interventions aims to mitigate specific social determinants of health based on poverty, racism, discrimination, and marginalization. Moreover, there is evidence that cultural identity and other culturally configured dimensions of social relationships and environments can constitute determinants of health in their own right. Hence, current models of the social determinants of health need to be enlarged through systematic consideration of cultural diversity both within and between societies. This rethinking is essential for the translation of research on social determinants of health into culturally informed policy and practice both at the levels of population health and clinical services.

7.5 Culture in Clinical Assessment and Diagnosis

There is evidence that systematic attention to culture and context can impact on clinical assessment and reduce diagnostic error. Understanding symptoms in context may change their significance as indicators of psychopathology. For example, the comprehensive cultural assessment of patients referred by primary care and mental health practitioners to a cultural consultation service resulted re-diagnosis rates of 50–60 % across a wide range of patients and diagnostic categories [38]. In particular, there was evidence for a high proportion of re-diagnoses of patients with psychotic disorders [2]. In most instances, this reassessment was based on information about personal history, social context and cultural meaning [1]. Viewing symptoms in context led to reassigning some patients with apparent paranoid thinking, auditory hallucinations, or psychotic symptoms to diagnostic categories of affective disorder, dissociative disorder, and trauma-related conditions. Overall, when social context was considered, there were more frequent diagnoses of adjustment disorder, due to recognition of the importance of social stressors in patients' condition [38].

Systematic attention to culture and social context within a multidisciplinary team may also foster exchange of knowledge and perspectives among health and social service professionals [16]. In addition to better understanding the significance of symptoms and psychopathology, this leads to a more comprehensive assessment that includes of the patient's social context or predicament, resources, values, and treatment expectations.

7.6 Approaches to Culture in Mental Health Care

Given the central place of culture in person-centered care, it is essential to incorporate culture and context into clinical assessment, treatment planning, and intervention [40]. A variety of approaches have been developed to address the cultural dimensions of care and to understand the person in context [12, 33]; each approach has strengths and limitations as summarized in Table 7.3. Person-centered psychiatry can employ elements of each of these approaches.

Table 7.3 Strategies for integrating culture in clinical care

Strategy	Strengths	Limitations
Mental health literacy	• Educates individuals and communities to identify and respond to mental health problems; • Aims to reduce stigma and improve access to and appropriate use of services	• Assumes that cultural knowledge can be changed by simply providing new information or education • Does not consider local implications of specific explanatory models or practices • May not address structural barriers to care
Language interpreters	• Communication is fundamental to safe and effective health care • Trained interpreters observe ethical standards and provide accurate translation	• Need to go beyond linguistic interpretation to explore meaning of cultural context
Culture brokers or mediators	• Focus on cultural translation can go beyond language to include nonverbal, contextual and community dimensions of meaning and identify important stressors and sources of support and resilience	• Roles, training, and ethical standards for culture brokers not well-established

(continued)

Table 7.3 (continued)

Strategy	Strengths	Limitations
Ethnic matching	• Practitioners and institutions can present a welcoming face and make use of knowledge of the needs of specific groups to respond appropriately • May be addressed at level of intervention, practitioner or institution with specific benefits	• Matching usually imprecise • May not be able to find match for patients from smaller local communities • May not result in tailored services or intervention • May be stigmatizing for patient and for minority practitioner
Cultural adaptation of intervention	• Interventions can be tailored to be more acceptable and effective for individuals and to mobilize or integrate culturally grounded coping strategies	• Cultural adaptation is time-consuming and costly • Effectiveness of adapted intervention may be uncertain and require additional evaluation
Cultural competence of clinician	• Focus on clinician fits with professionals' emphasis on knowledge and skill acquisition • Generic skills can be used with diverse and changing population across different settings	• Tends to locate culture with the patient and expertise with the clinician • May not sufficiently emphasize issues of power, structural violence and inequality
Cultural competence of institution and health care system	• Organizations that make efforts to address culture may be seen as more receptive and responsive by ethnocultural communities • Can change local institutional culture in ways that foster competence at all levels of service delivery	• May emphasize form rather than substance in terms of structural organizational change • Requires resources for institutional reorganization
Cultural safety	• Addresses issues of power and inequality rooted in historical and structural violence • Focuses on safety of systems, institutions, clinical settings and encounter • Emphasis on power sharing and dialogue	• Framed in terms of vulnerability rather than strengths
Cultural formulation	• Use of specific tools and procedures to elicit and organize clinically relevant cultural information (e.g., DSM-5 Cultural Formulation Interview) • Emphasis on understanding context in systematic way • Relevant to all patients	• Issues of how to integrate information into clinically useful formulation

See: Kirmayer [33]

Mental health literacy approaches assume that lay people may have limited information or be misinformed about mental health and that this can be addressed by education which may include explanations about the nature of mental health problems, everyday coping strategies, mental health "first aid" and appropriate help-seeking. The notion is that if people are well-informed they will be better able to cope and to make appropriate use of the health care system [28]. Increasing the knowledge and skills of community members in general will enable them to respond more effectively to others who face mental health problems. The strengths of this approach include knowledge sharing, patient activation or empowerment, and engagement of the wider community in helping and guiding individuals toward appropriate treatment. Among the potential limitations of the mental health literacy approach is the tendency to view patients' knowledge and illness models mainly in terms of how well they fit the biomedical view, rather than in relation to their personal and cultural meaning and social implications. When patients' understanding is rooted in particular cultural systems of knowledge and practice, merely providing new information may be insufficient to change their values, attitudes and behaviors, and may have unintended negative consequences [35]. For example, efforts to promote a view of major mental health problems as biological diseases, while intended to reduce stigma, may have instilled pessimism about treatability [42]. Moreover, given that many barriers to help seeking are structural and economic, focusing primarily on patients' knowledge of mental health may be insufficient [46, 62].

Language skill may constitute a structural barrier in health care and limit the ability to deliver person-centered care. When patient and clinician do not share facility with a common language, communication will be limited and the quality of assessment and care can be severely compromised. In such situations, the use of professional medical interpreters is an essential strategy to improve clinical communication [43]. While limited language proficiency may suffice to express very basic health needs and concerns, greater skill is needed to convey the complexity of symptom and illness experience associated with mental health problems. Moreover, attention to language history and preference may allow the clinician to appreciate key aspects of patients' identity and social position. Language is key to patients' feelings of recognition, comfort and safety in the clinical setting, as well as the clinician's empathy, access to affect and memory, and ability to mobilize the patient's capacity for creative problem-solving.

While language is central to culture, not all of culture is directly encoded or expressed in language; for example, important aspects of culture reside in nonverbal communication and body practices, family structure and interaction, as well as social networks and community institutions. Understanding these dimensions of culture requires systematic inquiry with patients and others in their entourage or community. To address the broader aspects of culture, clinicians may work with culture brokers or mediators, who have knowledge of the cultures of the patient and the practitioner or institution [49]. The culture broker can act as a go-between, interpreting the meaning of statements and experiences to both patient and clinician by supplying missing or taken-for-granted cultural context and background knowledge. The clinician's ability to understand the patient's social world is crucial for clinical empathy [31].

The strategy of "ethnic match" assumes that addressing cultural dimensions of care can be accomplished by matching patients and services. However, matching can occur at different levels, including the institution, the provider, and the intervention itself. Each level of matching has its own benefits and limitations, which may vary for specific ethnocultural groups and contexts. Matching interventions to the patients' cultural background and expectations can allow them to make use of their own personal and family resources. For example, patients for whom mediation, yoga, or other practices are culturally familiar may approach such interventions with positive expectations and find them easier to integrate into their treatment.

Ethnic matching also has important limitations. There is usually wide variation in experience among people from the same ethnocultural group or geographic region. Hence, matching is usually very rough or imprecise and often cannot address all of the salient dimensions of patients' self-identified ethnicity, language, religion, gender, politics, and values. Patients from minority communities may find that matching makes them feel singled out in ways that seem racist or discriminatory or else threatens clinical confidentiality because the clinician is from the same small, local community. In some cases, migrants who have fled persecution may not trust others from their country, community, or ethnic group [39].

There are also issues for practitioners associated with ethnic matching. While practitioners from similar backgrounds may share some aspects of identity with patients, their education, and professional training often distance them from patients. Practitioners who are expected to work with patients from specific communities may feel typecast or marginalized because they want to be recognized primarily for their technical skills or other competencies rather than their cultural identity [63]. Moreover, practitioners who lack frameworks for incorporating cultural knowledge into their professional practice may not make optimal use of their own background knowledge. Finally, in settings with high levels of diversity and many small communities, matching may not be feasible.

Cultural adaptation approaches aim to modify existing evidence-based treatments to better fit the language, culture, expectations, and resources of patients from particular backgrounds [9, 26]. The adaptation process involves translation of language, concepts, and procedures in ways that balance fidelity to the original intervention and fit with the new population or context. There is evidence that such adaptation can improve treatment acceptability, adherence and outcomes.

Perhaps the most common framework for addressing diversity in mental health services is cultural competence, which is defined in terms of a set of practitioner attitudes, knowledge, and skills along with organizational policies and practices that facilitate effective intercultural care [10]. There is some evidence that cultural competence can improve the quality of care and health outcomes in general medicine as well as mental health [6, 11, 12, 56, 61]. For clinicians, cultural competence includes: (1) awareness of one's own identity, its potential meaning to patients, and how it affects clinical practice; (2) language and communication skills (including skill in working with interpreters); (3) knowledge of issues of racism, discrimination, structural violence, power, and privilege; (4) specific cultural knowledge relevant to the patient population (e.g., developmental processes, family structure, migration trajectories, explanatory models of illness, healing practices, local community institutions, resources, and social issues) [7, 25, 33, 55].

Cultural competence outlines a general approach that can be applied to every situation and can promote thinking about mental health problems in context in ways that are relevant to person-centered care for patients from any background. Generic cultural competence begins with professionals' awareness of their own cultural background and identity, assumptions, biases, and prejudices. To explore these personal dimensions of their own experience, professionals need safe training and practice settings that encourage self-reflection as well as learning about others' experience, communities, history, traditions, and concerns. Applied to institutions and health care systems, cultural competence aims to organize services in ways that respect the language, values, and priorities of people from diverse communities. At the institutional level, cultural competence includes establishing collaborative relationships with local cultural communities to identify their needs and concerns and ensure they have a voice in shaping systems and services [19].

Despite its popularity as a rubric under which to develop strategies to address diversity, as currently constructed cultural competence has a number of limitations [33, 64, 65]. Discussions of culture tend to locate culture primarily with the designated 'Other', ignoring the sense in which mental health practice itself is an expression of specific cultural values and attitudes. Cultural competence tends to construe culture mainly in terms of individual characteristics or traits rather than the structure and dynamics of social systems. Cultural competence training sometimes focuses on information about specific ethnocultural groups and this may inadvertently foster stereotypes. A further concern is that the emphasis on the clinician's competence treats the negotiation of values and perspectives as a technical issue outside interpersonal relationships and larger structures of power and domination. In the clinical encounter, the superficial application of principles of cultural competence may create the illusion of mastery rather than opening up a respectful relationship of dialogue, shared inquiry, co-learning, and collaboration in decision-making. A person-centered approach to culture and context in the clinical encounter would address this by insisting that the voice and perspective of the individual remain central throughout.

A critical advance in medical anthropology applied the methods of social science to studying the culture of biomedicine and psychiatry. This shift in focus revealed many of the tacit assumptions of biomedicine based on its specific cultural history and values [21, 45, 51]. Becoming of aware of these assumptions and potential biases opens up a space for recognizing the diversity of illness experience and can encourage the clinician to consider alternative approaches. This self-reflectiveness is the most general aspect of cultural competence. There is a more intimate, personal dimension to this self-reflection and openness that depends on clinicians' understanding of their own identity, both in terms of their own strengths and vulnerabilities, and in relation to how they are perceived by the patient. This will help the clinician develop the sensitivity needed to remain open to patients' perspectives and to address issues related to institutional context and social difference.

Concern about the risk of appropriating the other's cultural knowledge, and reducing culture to a set of impersonal "factors" led medical educators to the construct of cultural humility as corrective stance [60]. Cultural humility recognizes clinicians' necessarily limited knowledge of any patient's culture and lifeworld and focuses on remaining open to dialogue and learning from the patient in ways that allow mutual understanding and collaboration. Similar concepts have been framed as "intercultural opening" and "cultural safety."

The concept of cultural safety, developed by Maori practitioners in New Zealand [41, 52] and elaborated for other health care contexts, emphasizes the ways in which power disparities and histories of domination make institutions of the dominant society unsafe for minority groups [13, 27]. Safety may be especially salient for patients who have experienced silencing, marginalization, and discrimination due to gender, sexual orientation, minority status, or other aspects of their identity. But issues of safety are important for all patients who hope to have their unique personhood recognized and respected in health care. Such recognition requires knowledge of the historical and contemporary social, economic and political contexts that create health disparities, social inequities, and structural violence. In clinical practice, cultural safety involves building relationships with others based on recognition, respect, and inclusiveness. The goal is to create safe spaces for meeting, dialogue, and collaboration. As with cultural competence, this begins with becoming aware of and working through one's own stereotypes, biases, and assumptions. Establishing a safe communicative situation requires concerted listening to the voice of other, sharing power and control, and learning each other's conceptual language.

The strength of the cultural safety approach is that it recognizes the power differentials inherent in health care with ethnocultural minorities or other vulnerable groups and aims to make structural changes to health services and the clinical encounter to share power and promote patients' voice and agency. The main limitation of the cultural safety construct is that it frames the encounter in terms of vulnerabilities rather than strengths, viewing collective history in terms of conflict and domination rather than resilience. Nevertheless, the effort to foreground histories and enduring structures of inequality is crucial to developing what has been called "structural competence" as a basic component of ethical and effective care [46].

7.7 Implementing Culturally Responsive Person-Centered Psychiatry: Implications for Education, Policy and Practice

Sensitivity to cultural dimensions of the lifeworlds of patients, as well as their families and communities is an essential component of person-centered psychiatry. But the clinician and health care system must go beyond sensitivity to respond effectively in ways that meet patients' needs. Elements of each of the approaches described in the previous section can be brought together in forms of culturally responsive person-centered care that address the quality of the clinician–patient relationship, the safety of the clinical setting and practices, and the organization of health care systems and institutions [33]. Specific information about culture and context can then be elicited by practitioners and integrated into the process of comprehensive clinical assessment, case formulation, and intervention based on conceptual models of the place of culture in psychopathology, healing and recovery [38, 48]. The process of cultural formulation can be aided by frameworks like the outline for cultural formulation and cultural formulation interview in DSM-5 [44, 47]. Significantly, DSM-5 recognizes the cultural formulation interview as a part of a person-centered approach relevant to all patients, whatever their background [5].

With increasing globalization and migration, communities everywhere are becoming more diverse and policy makers must respond to changing demography. Addressing cultural diversity in population health is important for the effectiveness of health services, social justice and equity, and human rights [32, 34]. In most regions, policy-makers and administrators will need to consider changes in organizational culture within health care institutions to make services culturally accessible and responsive to the all minority groups [24]. Patients from diverse cultural and ethnic backgrounds do not represent a homogeneous group characterized by their "difference" from some taken-for-granted norms of the mainstream or dominant local groups, but present multifaceted needs that need careful consideration if person-centered care is to succeed.

The work of the Centre François Minkowska, which provides care for migrants and refugees in the Paris region, illustrates how cultural and person-centered perspectives can be usefully integrated. While the reflex of many clinicians, when confronted with a patient who is culturally or linguistically "different", is to focus on language barriers and cultural references that are unfamiliar, the person-centered transcultural psychiatry developed by the Centre François Minkowska is not centered exclusively on language or any other sociological consideration, but approaches each patient as a person in all his or her complexity. Social and cultural context is relevant to all patients, who deploy their own cultural meaning systems to make sense of and cope with illness and the clinician must consider these to determine the nature of patients' problems and healing resources. Of course, applying this person-centered approach requires effective communication. This begins with identifying the necessary resources: (1) if clinician and patient share a common language, the principles of person-centered care and culturally informed assessment can be applied directly; (2) if clinician and patient do not share a common language, it is essential to work with a skilled interpreter; and (3) whatever the linguistic situation, when cultural differences are substantial and resources allow, it is preferable to work with a cultural mediator with expertise in mental health care, who can function as a co-therapist [8].

The knowledge and skills needed for cultural competence must be incorporated into professional training and the elements of institutional cultural competence integrated into health care policy and accreditation standards for health care institutions [37]. With regard to treatment, service providers must strive to provide care that responds to the diversity of the populations they serve. This requires integrating person-centered services with culturally appropriate resources according to patient need. When establishing services, attention should be given to relevant sociodemographic factors affecting the physical and mental health of ethnic minorities, including employment, housing, education, and migration status.

Each of the social factors that affect health in the clinical setting has broader implications for social policy and prevention. In the case of migrant populations, policy-makers must allocate sufficient resources to support public mental health and education about migration and its consequences when developing culture sensitive, person-centered policies [39]. The goal should be to ensure cultural diversity and competence in all aspects of mental health care but also to emphasize that mental health issues are as important as physical health in the policy for social development and long-term integration. In this way, mental health services can facilitate adaptation and social integration for migrants as well as promoting the cultural capital associated with diversity [32].

7.8 Conclusions

Concepts of culture and context are central to the conceptual framework of person-centered medicine. Understanding patients as persons who live in social worlds configured by both local and global cultures provides a basis for developing modes of practice that can respond appropriately to each person's values and promote their health and well-being as members of communities. The meanings of culture are changing with both global and local forces, and psychiatry must evolve in response. Globalization has not eliminated cultural diversity but given rise to new hybrid forms. The networking made possible by information technologies has created new kinds of identity and community, new sources of resilience and healing, as well as new pathologies. Addressing these emerging forms of personhood, ways of life, and conflicts requires a broad program of ongoing research and clinical innovation [35].

The effort to recognize, respect and respond to cultural diversity in mental health care is not only a central pillar of person-centered medicine, it is an important issue for strengthening local and global civil society and human rights. People need to participate in meaningful cultural worlds to realize their capabilities. Addressing diversity through culturally responsive mental health care is therefore a contribution to population health at the levels of the person, family, community, and global society.

References

1. Adeponle AB, Groleau D, Kirmayer LJ. Clinician reasoning in the use of cultural formulation to resolve uncertainty in the diagnosis of psychosis. Cult Med Psychiatry. 2015;39(1):16–42. doi:10.1007/s11013-014-9408-5.
2. Adeponle AB, Thombs BD, Groleau D, Jarvis E, Kirmayer LJ. Using the cultural formulation to resolve uncertainty in diagnoses of psychosis among ethnoculturally diverse patients. Psychiatr Serv. 2012;63(2):147–53. doi:10.1176/appi.ps.201100280.
3. Adeponle AB, Whitley R, Kirmayer LJ. Cultural contexts and constructions of recovery. In: Rudnick A, editor. Recovery of people with mental illness: philosophical and related perspectives. New York: Oxford University Press; 2012. p. 109–32.
4. Allen J, Balfour R, Bell R, Marmot M. Social determinants of mental health. Int Rev Psychiatry. 2014;26(4):392–407.
5. American Psychiatric Association. Diagnostic and statistical manual of mental disorders (DSM-5®). Washington, DC: American Psychiatric Pub; 2013.
6. Beach MC, Price EG, Gary TL, Robinson KA, Gozu A, Palacio A, Smarth C, Jenckes MW, Feuerstein C, Bass EB, Powe NR, Cooper LA. Cultural competence: a systematic review of health care provider educational interventions. Med Care. 2005;43(4):356–73.
7. Bennegadi R. Cultural competence and training in mental health practice in Europe: strategies to implement competence and empower practitioners. Background paper. Brussels, Belgium: International Organization of Migration; 2009.
8. Bennegadi R. Compétence culturelle et migrations. In: Coutanceau R, Bennegadi R, editors. Résilience et relations humaines: Couple, Famille, Institution, Entreprise, Cultures. Paris: Dunod; 2014. p. 141–52.
9. Bernal G, Domenech Rodriguez MM. Cultural adaptations: tools for evidence-based practice with diverse populations. Washington, D.C.: American Psychological Association; 2012.
10. Betancourt JR, Green AR, Carrillo JE, Ananeh-Firempong O. Defining cultural competence: a practical framework for addressing racial/ethnic disparities in health and health care. Public Health Rep. 2003;118(4):293–302.
11. Bhui K, Aslam RHW, Palinski A, McCabe R, Johnson MR, Weich S, Szczepura A. Interventions designed to improve therapeutic communications between black and minority ethnic people and professionals working in psychiatric services: a systematic review of the evidence for their effectiveness. Health Technol Assess. 2015;19(31):1–174.
12. Bhui K, Warfa N, Edonya P, McKenzie K, Bhugra D. Cultural competence in mental health care: a review of model evaluations. BMC Health Serv Res. 2007;7:15.
13. Brascoupé S, Waters C. Cultural safety: exploring the applicability of the concept of cultural safety to Aboriginal health and community wellness. J Aboriginal Health. 2009;7(1):6–40.
14. Choudhury S, Kirmayer LJ. Cultural neuroscience and psychopathology: prospects for cultural psychiatry. Prog Brain Res. 2009;178:261–81.
15. Cloninger CR, Salvador-Carulla L, Kirmayer LJ, Schwartz MA, Appleyard J, Goodwin N, Groves J, Hermans MHM, Mezzich JE, van Staden CW, Rawaf Salman. A time for action on health inequities: foundations of the 2014 Geneva declaration on person- and people-centered integrated health care for all. Int J Pers Cent Med. 2014;4(2):69–89.
16. Dinh MH, Groleau D, Kirmayer LJ, Rodriguez C, Bibeau G. Influence of the DSM-IV outline for cultural formulation on multidisciplinary case conferences in mental health. Anthropol Med. 2012;19(2):261–76.
17. Fernando S. Mental health, race and culture. London: Palgrave Macmillan; 2010.
18. Fernando S. Race and culture issues in mental health and some thoughts on ethnic identity. Counselling Psychol Q. 2012;25(2):113–23.
19. Fung K, Lo HT, Srivastava R, Andermann L. Organizational cultural competence consultation to a mental health institution. Transcult Psychiatry. 2012;49(2):165–84. doi:10.1177/1363461512439740.

20. Gone JP, Kirmayer LJ. On the wisdom of considering culture and context in psychopathology. In: Millon T, Krueger RF, Simonsen E, editors. Contemporary directions in psychopathology: scientific foundations of the DSM-V and ICD-11. New York: Guilford; 2010. p. 72–96.
21. Good BJ. Medicine, rationality, and experience: an anthropological perspective. Cambridge: Cambridge University Press; 1994.
22. Good MJD, Hannah SD. "Shattering culture": perspectives on cultural competence and evidence-based practice in mental health services. Transcult Psychiatry. 2015;52(2):198–221.
23. Gravlee CC. How race becomes biology: embodiment of social inequality. Am J Phys Anthropol. 2009;139(1):47–57.
24. Graves DL, Like RC, Kelly N, Hohensee A. Legislation as intervention: a survey of cultural competence policy in health care. J Health Care Law Policy. 2007;10:339–61.
25. Hernandez M, Nesman T, Mowery D, Acevedo-Polakovich ID, Callejas LM. Cultural competence: a literature review and conceptual model for mental health services. Psychiatr Serv. 2009;60(8):1046–50.
26. Huey SJ Jr, Tilley JL, Jones EO, Smith CA. The contribution of cultural competence to evidence-based care for ethnically diverse populations. Annu Rev Clin Psychol. 2014;10:305–38.
27. Indigenous Physicians Association of Canada. Promoting improved mental health for Canada's indigenous peoples: a curriculum for psychiatry residents and psychiatrists. Winnipeg, Ottawa: IPAC-RCPSC Psychiatry Curriculum Development Working Group; 2009.
28. Jorm AF. Mental health literacy: empowering the community to take action for better mental health. Am Psychol. 2012;67(3):231–43. doi:10.1037/a0025957.
29. Jurcik T, Ahmed R, Yakobov E, Solopieieva-Jurcikova I, Ryder AG. Understanding the role of the ethnic density effect: issues of acculturation, discrimination and social support. J Commun Psychol. 2013;41(6):662–78.
30. Kirmayer LJ. Psychotherapy and the cultural concept of the person. Transcult Psychiatry. 2007;44(2):232–57.
31. Kirmayer LJ. Empathy and alterity in cultural psychiatry. Ethos. 2008;36(4):457–74.
32. Kirmayer LJ. Multicultural medicine and the politics of recognition. J Med Philos. 2011;36 (4):410–23. doi:10.1093/jmp/jhr024.
33. Kirmayer LJ. Rethinking cultural competence. Transcult Psychiatry. 2012;49(2):149–64. doi:10.1177/1363461512444673.
34. Kirmayer LJ. Culture and context in human rights. In: Dudley M, Silove D, Gale F, editors. Mental health and human rights: vision, praxis and courage. Oxford: Oxford University Press; 2012. p. 95–112.
35. Kirmayer LJ, Ban L. Cultural psychiatry: research strategies and future directions. Adv Psychosom Med. 2013;33:97–114. doi:10.1159/000348742.
36. Kirmayer LJ, Fletcher C, Watt R. Locating the ecocentric self: Inuit concepts of mental health and illness. In: Kirmayer LJ, Valaskakis G, editors. Healing traditions: the mental health of Aboriginal peoples in Canada. Vancouver: University of British Columbia Press; 2008. p. 289–314.
37. Kirmayer LJ, Fung K, Rousseau C, Lo HT, Menzies P, Guzder J, Ganesan S, Andermann L, McKenzie K. Guidelines for training in cultural psychiatry. Can J Psychiatry. 2012;57(3), Insert 1–16.
38. Kirmayer LJ, Guzder J, Rousseau C, editors. Cultural consultation: encountering the other in mental health care. New York: Springer SBM; 2014.
39. Kirmayer LJ, Narasiah L, Muniz M, Rashid M, Ryder A, Guzder J, Hassan G, Rousseau C, Pottie K. Common mental health problems in immigrants and refugees: general approach to the patient in primary care. Can Med Assoc J. 2011;183(12). doi:10.1503/cmaj.090292.
40. Kirmayer LJ, Rousseau C, Jarvis GE, Guzder J. The cultural context of clinical assessment. In: Tasman A, Maj M, First MB, Kay J, Lieberman J, editors. Psychiatry. 4th ed. New York: Wiley; 2015. p. 54–66.

41. Koptie S. Irihapeti Ramsden: the public narrative on cultural safety. First Peoples Child Fam Rev. 2009;4(2):30–43.
42. Kvaale EP, Haslam N, Gottdiener WH. The 'side effects' of medicalization: a meta-analytic review of how biogenetic explanations affect stigma. Clin Psychol Rev. 2013;33(6):782–94.
43. Leanza Y, Miklavcic A, Boivin I, Rosenberg E. Working with interpreters. In: Kirmayer LJ, Guzder J, Rousseau C, editors. Cultural consultation: encountering the other in mental health care. New York: Springer; 2014. p. 89–114.
44. Lewis-Fernández R, Aggarwal NK, Hinton L, Hinton DE, Kirmayer LJ, American Psychiatric Association. DSM-5 handbook on the cultural formulation interview. Washington, DC: American Psychiatric Publishing Inc.; 2015.
45. Lock MM, Nguyen V-K. An anthropology of biomedicine. Chichester, West Sussex; Malden, MA: Wiley-Blackwell; 2010.
46. Metzl JM, Hansen H. Structural competency: theorizing a new medical engagement with stigma and inequality. Soc Sci Med. 2014;103:126–33. doi:10.1016/j.socscimed.2013.06.032.
47. Mezzich JE, Caracci G, Fabrega H Jr, Kirmayer LJ. Cultural formulation guidelines. Transcult Psychiatry. 2009;46(3):383–405.
48. Mezzich JE, Salloum IM, Cloninger CR, Salvador-Carulla L, Kirmayer LJ, Banzato CEM, Wallcraft J, Botbol M. Person-centered integrative diagnosis: conceptual basis and structural model. Can J Psychiatry. 2010;55(11):701–8.
49. Miklavcic A, LeBlanc MN. Culture brokers, clinically applied ethnography, and cultural mediation. In: Kirmayer LJ, Guzder J, Rousseau C, editors. Cultural consultation: encountering the other in mental health care. New York: Springer; 2014. p. 89–114.
50. Murton B. Being in the place world: toward a Maori "geographical self". J Cult Geogr. 2012;29(1):87–104.
51. Napier AD, Ancarno C, Butler B, Calabrese J, Chater A, Chatterjee H, Guesnet F, Horne R, Jacyna S, Jadhav S, Macdonald A, Neuendorf U, Parkhurst A, Reynolds R, Scambler G, Shamdasani S, Smith SZ, Stougaard-Nielsen J, Thomson L, Tyler N, Volkmann A-M, Walker T, Watson J, Williams ACDC, Willott C, Wilson J, Woolf K. Culture and health. Lancet. 2014;384(9954): 1607–39. doi:10.1016/S0140-6736(14)61603-2.
52. Papps E, Ramsden I. Cultural safety in nursing: the New Zealand experience. Int J Q Health Care. 1996;8(5):491–7.
53. Paradies Y. A systematic review of empirical research on self-reported racism and health. Int J Epidemiol. 2006;35(4):888–901. doi:10.1093/ije/dyl056.
54. Priest N, Paradies Y, Trenerry B, Truong M, Karlsen S, Kelly Y. A systematic review of studies examining the relationship between reported racism and health and wellbeing for children and young people. Soc Sci Med. 2013;95:115–27.
55. Pumariega AJ, Rothe E, Mian A, Carlisle L, Toppelberg C, Harris T, Gogineni RR, Webb S, Smith J, American Academy of Child and Adolescent Psychiatry (AACAP) Committee on Quality Issues (CQI). Practice parameter for cultural competence in child and adolescent psychiatric practice. J Am Acad Child Adolesc Psychiatry. 2013;52(10):1101–15. doi:10.1016/j.jaac.2013.06.019.
56. Renzaho AM, Romios P, Crock C, Sonderlund AL. The effectiveness of cultural competence programs in ethnic minority patient-centered health care—a systematic review of the literature. Int J Q Health Care. 2013. doi:10.1093/intqhc/mzt006.
57. Rousseau C, Hassan G, Moreau N, Thombs BD. Perceived discrimination and its association with psychological distress among newly arrived immigrants before and after September 11, 2001. Am J Public Health. 2011;101(5):909–15. doi:10.2105/AJPH.2009.173062.
58. Ruiz-Casares M, Guzder J, Rousseau C, Kirmayer LJ. Cultural roots of well-being and resilience in child mental health. In: Ben Arieh A, Frones I, Casas F, Korbin J, editors. Handbook of child well-being. New York: Springer, p. 2379–2407.
59. Shaw RJ, Atkin K, Becares L, Albor CB, Stafford M, Kiernan KE, Nazroo JY, Wilkinson RG, Pickett KE. Impact of ethnic density on adult mental disorders: narrative review. Br J Psychiatry. 2012;201(1):11–9. doi:10.1192/bjp.bp.110.083675.

60. Tervalon M, Murray-Garcia J. Cultural humility versus cultural competence: a critical distinction in defining physician training outcomes in multicultural education. J Health Care Poor Underserved. 1998;9(2):117–25.
61. Truong M, Paradies Y, Priest N. Interventions to improve cultural competency in healthcare: a systematic review of reviews. BMC Health Serv Res. 2014;14(1):99.
62. Viruell-Fuentes EA, Miranda PY, Abdulrahim S. More than culture: structural racism, intersectionality theory, and immigrant health. Soc Sci Med. 2012;75(12):2099–106.
63. Weinfeld M. The challenge of ethnic match: minority origin professionals in health and social services. In: Troper H, Weinfeld M, editors. Ethnicity, politics, and public policy: case studies in Canadian diversity. Toronto: University of Toronto Press; 1991. p. 117–41.
64. Whitley R, Rousseau C, Carpenter Song E, Kirmayer LJ. Evidence-based medicine: opportunities and challenges in a diverse society. Can J Psychiatry. 2011;56(9):514–22.
65. Willen SS, Bullon A, Good MJ. Opening up a huge can of worms: reflections on a "cultural sensitivity" course for psychiatry residents. Harvard Rev Psychiatry. 2010;18(4):247–53. doi:10.3109/10673229.2010.493748.
66. World Health Organization and Calouste Gulbenkian Foundation. Social determinants of mental health. Geneva: World Health Organization; 2014.

8 Recovery, Empowerment, and Person Centeredness

Margit Schmolke, PhD, Michaela Amering, MD
and Alessandro Svettini, MD

8.1 Introduction

The topic "recovery" has been increasingly discussed in the last 15 years among professionals in the mental health field [3]. In comparison to the concept of Person-Centered Psychiatry [36], the Recovery concept has emerged from ex-patients or consumers of psychiatric services themselves, taken up and supported by mental health policy makers and professionals. At the beginning of the recovery area, one could find information about this topic almost only in the so-called gray literature, i.e., in Internet forums, special websites and brochures. Meanwhile, the interested reader can find high quality publications in international professional journals, books and readers—written by persons with a lived recovery experience and by professionals dealing with psychiatric rehabilitation, psychiatric treatment and policy. An impressive amount of articles and books can be found in the literature written jointly by authors with and without a lived experience of mental health problems and service use (e.g., [19, 59]).

The recovery movement has grown to an impressive number of activists, mainly in English-speaking countries all over the world, who exchange their experiences in forum groups, many of them offer additional services in the mental health field

M. Schmolke, PhD (✉)
Psychologist, Psychoanalyst and Director of the Munich Training and Research Institute of the German Academy of Psychoanalysis, Munich, Germany
e-mail: margitschmolke@aol.com

M. Amering, MD
University Professor, Department of Psychiatry and Psychotherapy, Medical University of Vienna, Vienna, Austria

A. Svettini, MD
Psychiatrist, Psychotherapist—Department of Psychiatry, Health Trust of Bolzano, Bolzano, Italy

J.E. Mezzich et al. (eds.), *Person Centered Psychiatry*,
DOI 10.1007/978-3-319-39724-5_8

based on their lived recovery experiences and participate and create own ideas in mental health research. International interest and implementation efforts are growing and discussed widely and controversially [50].

Discussions concern the scientific basis and requirements [5, 51] as well as how clinically useful the Recovery concept is being regarded up to date. Concerns by mental health professionals are often expressed in terms of fear of misunderstandings and illusionary hopes and expectations, lack of clear definition, and lack of scientific evidence [45].

Recovery from severe mental illness is to be seen as a continuous and interactive process, a personal journey of regaining the sense of self, the self-management of the illness, a feeling of belonging and of rebuilding one's own life in the community [18]. Differently from the concept of Person-Centered Psychiatry [36], Recovery as a concept emerged in the 70s and 80s from the movement of ex-patients or users of psychiatric services mainly in North America and continues to be used and developed at the international level by people with lived experience of mental illness [49]. In the last 15 years, the topic "recovery" has been increasingly discussed among professionals in the mental health field [3] and it is now is taken up and supported by mental health policy makers and professionals.

At the beginning of the "Recovery Era", one could find information about this topic almost only in the so-called gray literature, i.e., in internet forums, special websites, and brochures. Nowadays, the interested reader can find high quality scientific publications in international professional journals, books, and readers—written by persons with a lived recovery experience and by professionals involved in psychiatric treatment and rehabilitation as well as in policy making. An imposive amount of articles and books can be found in the literature written jointly by authors with and without a lived experience of mental health problems and service use (e.g., [19, 59]).

The recovery movement has grown to an impressive number of activists, mainly in English-speaking countries all over the world, who exchange their experiences in forum groups. Many of them offer additional services in the mental health field based on their lived recovery experiences and participate and create own ideas in mental health research. International interest and implementation efforts are growing and discussed widely and controversially [50].

Discussions concern the scientific basis and requirements [5, 51] as well as how clinically useful the concept of Recovery is being regarded up to date. Concerns by mental health professionals are often expressed in terms of fear of misunderstandings and illusionary hopes and expectations, lack of scientific evidence, and lack of clear definition [45].

In this sense, evidence from scientific research sheds some light on the subject. Long-term follow-up studies of patients who had schizophrenia for 20–40 years have consistently found recovery rates from 45 to 68 % [29, 34]. From the researchers' perspective, recovery is understood as an outcome. In order to achieve a specific definition in this sense, Liberman et al. [35] defined some operational criteria for Recovery.

The definition of recovery encompasses functioning within normal limits in those very same dimensions of life that are abnormal for disabled persons. To be considered *recovered* from a serious mental disorder, a person should continuously fulfill for 2 years the following criteria:

1. a sustained remission of symptoms that constitute the diagnosis at a subclinical level of frequency and severity;
2. full- or part-time engagement in an instrumental role activity, such as work or school, that is constructive, productive, and age-appropriate;
3. a life independent of supervision by family or other caregivers such that the individual is responsible for day-to-day needs in managing money, medication, appointments, shopping, food preparation, and personal possessions;
4. cordial family relations;
5. recreational activities in normative places and settings;
6. satisfying peer relationships characterized by participation in an active friendship, with companions or a social network.

The contribution of Liberman et al. [35] identifies also some predictive factors of recovery from schizophrenia: a supportive family/housing stability; the absence of substance abuse; a shorter duration of untreated psychosis; a good initial response to antipsychotics; the adherence to treatment; a supportive therapy with a collaborative therapeutic alliance; a good neurocognitive functioning; the absence of the Deficit Syndrome; a good premorbid history; the access to comprehensive, coordinated, and continuous treatment. Most of the factors that influence disability are malleable and hence can be modified through psychiatric rehabilitation practices to promote recovery. As they move from their starting point of disability toward their destination of recovery, patients experience increasing amounts of hope, empowerment, self-responsibility, dignity, and self-esteem. These attributes promote further progress on the continuum from disability to recovery.

We have now entered the "Recovery Era." In our view, the most exciting aspect of this development is the active involvement of service users in discussions, in clinical care settings and in planning and evaluating clinical interventions together with mental health professionals [55]. Professionals are gradually changing their attitude toward persons in need for clinical care: instead of passive, dependent, symptom-loaded, marginalized, and chronically ill patient, the individual is seen more as an active, cooperative person looking for solutions toward independent life in the community, being in his/her own unique recovery process with or without clinical symptoms. A new culture of direct communication, involvement, exchange of ideas and critical feedback and of concrete proposals of changes toward a more humane future psychiatry has emerged. This development entails a challenge for mental health professionals by opening themselves toward the additional and complementing input of the "experts by experience" and by their willingness to share power and responsibilities with service users in mental health care and policy.

Service users, advocates and researchers with a lived experience have voiced concerns along the lines of the "risk of professional colonization of this very special and very different knowledge-base" [24] and co-option of the recovery movement and dilution of its challenges by the mental health system [3].

Recovery and Empowerment are powerful concepts promoting more partnership relationship between service users and mental health professionals, displacing the paternalistic pattern of the hierarchical professional–patient relationship. The authors of this chapter will outline convergences and divergences of these two concepts with the Person-Centered approach to Psychiatry, the overall topic of this book.

8.2 The Concept of Recovery

The essential element of what started the recovery movement in the 1980s is the voice of the user movement, one of its prominent pioneers is Chamberlin [8] who gave her pertinent book the title "On our own." She argued that stigma and discrimination can only be overcome when those struggling with mental illness and society's injustices against them, regain control over their lives. The most frequently quoted definition of recovery "as a guiding vision" stems from William Anthony [6, p 13]: "… a deeply personal, unique process of changing one's attitudes, values, feelings, goals, skills and roles. It is a way of living a satisfying, hopeful, and contributing life even with limitations caused by the illness. Recovery involves the development of new meaning and purpose in one's life as one grows beyond the catastrophic effects of mental illness." However, Jan Wallcraft importantly reminds us of the second part of this prominent recovery definition: "*Recovery from mental illness involves much more than recovery from the illness itself. People with mental illness may have to recover from the stigma they have incorporated into their very being; from the iatrogenic effects of treatment settings; from lack of recent opportunities for self-determination; from the negative side effects of unemployment; and from crushed dreams. Recovery is often a complex, time-consuming process. Recovery is what people with disabilities do. Treatment, case-management and rehabilitation are what helpers do to facilitate recovery,*" [61].

The central idea of recovery is that people can recover even from the most severe types of mental disorders and related disabilities. Recovery implies that a person has the chance of a satisfying and fulfilling life, despite psychiatric symptoms. The path and the experience of recovery cannot be the same for two different individuals. Attitudes and values have a profound impact on the further course of recovery for each person. Recovery is more than the absence of symptoms. Recovery is a profound personal process. The expectation of recovery and the understanding about the kinds of things that help people regain control over their life, is a key aspect (e.g. [12, 16]). Essential in the recovery process is to maintain a sense of self, to remain a person, in midst of a severe mental illness [14]. Recovery is both a result and a process, where recovery "from" mental illness and "in the" illness are concepts to be considered fluid, that are not mutually exclusive [13].

Examplary for a consensus on key elements of recovery is the Scottish Recovery Networks work ([7]; www.scottishrecovery.net):

Hope: Without hope, recovery is not possible. There can be no change without the belief that a better life is both possible and attainable.

Meaning and purpose: People find meaning in very different ways, for example, some people may find spirituality important while others may find meaning through the development of stronger interpersonal or community links.

Potential for change: A recovery approach requires a fundamental belief that everyone has the potential for change. It challenges the traditionally pessimistic outlook of mental health professionals, which is influenced by a historical belief in the chronic nature of some mental health problems. It also proposes that episodes of illness, while clearly distressing, can in fact be developmental and educative experiences.

Control: It is central for recovery to have the subjective experience of having regained control over one's life. People who use mental health services are sometimes denied an adequate level of involvement in their own care and treatment.

Active participation: In contrast with being a passive recipient of services, recovery aims at active individuals who take personal responsibility for their care, often in collaboration with friends, family, supporters, and professionals.

Holistic and inclusive approach: Recovery needs that all elements of a person's quality of life are considered. It recognizes that the extent to which someone enjoys good health and well-being is influenced by a wide range of social, environmental, and individual factors: namely "recovery" is much more than the management of symptoms.

Environment: External factors such as stigma and discrimination, employment and training opportunities, housing, and social exclusion have a strong influence on recovery.

Optimistic and realistic approach: Recovery is rarely a linear process, people will have periods where their recovery is slowed by a bout of illness.

Creative risk-taking: Services are rightly concerned about managing risk, but the danger is that it becomes the overriding concern. For someone to overcome a disabling illness and to become actively involved in their community requires an element of creative risk-taking.

8.2.1 Recovery Orientation in Mental Health Services

The concept of recovery is fundamental in order to have services promoting interventions oriented in the same direction of what service users consider to be essential to their road toward recovery, in order to achieve the right match between evidence-based techniques and participatory research [22].

Literature on recovery has highlighted the importance of organizational culture in facilitating a new, recovery-oriented approach at all levels in mental health services: in order to have recovery really embedded into clinical practice, a culture that supports the values of recovery becomes essential, with the commitment to integrate its principles into all organizational processes [21].

As such, a "recovery-oriented" practice describes an approach to mental health which includes the principles of self-determination and individualized care; such an approach emphasizes the importance of values such as hope, social inclusion, setting goals, and self-management by the patient. These values should permeate the practices of services [31]. The concept of recovery implies therefore moving away from a view of mental illness merely as a pathology, as well as care as just maintenance or stabilization, toward a holistic approach to wellness that is based on individual strengths, on partnership, on change [15]. However, if on one side it is increasingly important for professionals to have a clear vision of the principles of recovery, on the other side this outlook is complicated by the heterogeneity of opinions about what recovery really means in the daily context.

A central question is how these elements could be realized and implemented in psychiatric services in a concrete manner and what exactly needs to be changed in mental health institutions. Marianne Farkas and Bill Anthony, both prominent researchers in the field of psychiatric rehabilitation at the Boston University, belong to those established professionals who have endorsed the recovery approach from its beginnings. In the era of evidence-based psychiatry, they have been pioneers in defining a recovery orientation for mental health services. Several of their publications have been coauthored with activists with lived experience, like Judi Chamberlin from the National Empowerment Center [22]. These authors formulate four key values for recovery-oriented services (see also [3, p 223]):

1. *Person orientation*: Person orientation implies that the services are primarily defined according to the needs of an individual, with all his/her strengths, talents, interests, and limitations. This is in stark contrast to the focus on an individual as a "case", along with the signs and symptoms of an illness, and a diagnosis which determine the services to be delivered. Many recovery concepts and plans place a major emphasis on the way people are being approached. Many authors [18, 14] have pointed out that people are always more than just patients and that it serves them well to be seen as whole human beings. They should not merely be viewed and understood in their patient-role, but rather in their many life-roles along with their possibilities and limitations. Deegan [18] underlines explicitly that professional service providers who are denying such a holistic view to the people they encounter as patients, are causing them harm.
2. *Person involvement*: Services are concentrating on the right to a partnership in all relationships pertaining to recovery. This means that the people who are supposed to be assisted by those services have the right to have input in the planning, organization and evaluation of those services. Rehabilitation research teaches us that people are more likely to be successful when they have been meaningfully involved in the organization and evaluation of their services. User involvement is increasingly seen as a benchmark for quality in organization, planning, and evaluation.

3. *Self-determination/choice*: The service places an emphasis on the rights of all people to make individual decisions and choices in all aspects of their recovery. This includes, among others, treatment goals, choice of supports that should assist in reaching these goals, and determining when and whether to make use of services. The literature has repeatedly cautioned that compliance, i.e., simply going along with interventions suggested by professionals, should not be overestimated. It might very well be that such compliance could weaken a person who found himself dependent on the decisions of others.
4. *Growth potential*: Services are focused on the inherent potential for recovery of every person—irrespective of whether he/she is currently overwhelmed by the illness or disability, is struggling with adversity or living with disadvantages. It cannot be stated too often: hope is an essential ingredient of any recovery orientation. Concentrating on the potential of every person to grow, implies a dedication to sustain hope on the part of the professional service providers as well as on the part of the recipients. For the services this means that they need to assess themselves according to the amount of hope and belief in possibilities that is being offered. This might require a fundamental change in the way services are being offered.

8.3 The Concept of Empowerment

Historically, empowerment emerged from the civil rights movement of the Afro-American population in the United States in the 50s. Martin Luther King inspired the movement toward self-organized actions of nonviolent resistance in order to protest against prevailing discrimination and disadvantages and to fight for social and political participation. The basic idea of the civil rights movement was that disadvantaged groups are able to take control over their own life with the power of their own strengths. Feminism in the 60s was a second movement in which the empowerment idea became visible. Up-to-date, there are various social movements under the flag of empowerment such as peace, disabled, and health movement including self-help groups, civic action groups, and neighborhood projects. Although they have different backgrounds their common goal is to fight for more political rights of participation, impact and decision on their immediate life circumstances and to counteract against risky social developments [56].

Empowerment has become an essential role for professionals in the psychosocial field focusing on the self-help forces, self-realizing power and resources of persons as counterforces against challenges in critical life situations—in contrast to demoralization and resignation. Empowerment as an attitudinal concept is an effective tool for professionals to reinforce often forgotten strengths and capabilities of their clients in order to regain autonomy in their life and active participation in the community [30].

A working definition of empowerment proposed by Chamberlin [9] lists a number of characteristics, as follows:

- Having decision-making power.
- Having access to information and resources.
- Having a range of options from which to make choices (not just *yes/no*, *either/or*.)
- Assertiveness.
- A feeling that the individual can make a difference (being hopeful).
- Learning to think critically; learning the conditioning; seeing things differently; e.g.,
    - learning to redefine who we are (speaking in our own voice).
    - learning to redefine what we can do.
    - learning to redefine our relationships to institutionalized power.
- Learning about and expressing anger.
- Not feeling alone; feeling part of a group.
- Understanding that people have rights.
- Effecting change in one's life and one's community.
- Learning skills (e.g., communication) that the individual defines as important.
- Changing others' perceptions of one's competency and capacity to act.
- Coming out of the closet.
- Growth and change that is never ending and self-initiated.
- Increasing one's positive self-image and overcoming stigma.

Like recovery, empowerment is a complex construct in mental health. Empowerment, self-determination, and self-efficacy are essential elements of recovery processes and empowerment can be defined as the process of gaining a sense of mastery and control over one's own environment and self [10, 11].

Laugharne and Priebe [32] come to a critical conclusion that empowerment seems to have impacted more at an organizational level than on individual care and suggest that this might reflect the fact that the power differential between service users and providers is an extremely stubborn phenomenon, with a tendency to persist even in "person-centerd" and consumer-led services. They warn that the ethical and the economic arguments for patient choice should not be confused, the latter possibly granting a person choice among different institutions offering the same paternalistic approach to treatment decision-making.

Closely connected to empowerment is the concept of shared decision-making [19, 27] and the advanced directives [4] which enables both clients and providers to come to partnership-based decisions in difficult and complex decision processes, for example, on the necessity of taking medication or possible inpatient treatment during which the client may not be able to make autonomous decisions.

In a chapter on "Recovery and Psychopharmacology" of the book of Amering and Schmolke [3, p 219f.], the meaning of shared decision-making is emphasized and the ideas of Pat Deegan on this topic are described. Deegan's own lived experience of using psychiatric medication ranges from "compliance" and progress in the eyes of the psychiatrist, which led to the tragic realization that "I lost years of my life in this netherworld, and although I was treatment compliant and was maintained in the community, I was not recovering," to an extremely different experience, namely that of "using medication as part of my journey of recovery" [17, p 63]. Deegan conceptualizes shared decision-making as:

- "a person-centerd alternative to traditional notions of medical compliance" [17, p 62];
- an ethical imperative;
- consistent with the tradition of building therapeutic alliances;
- a superior approach to medical paternalism and insistence on compliance [20];
- founded on the premise of two experts who "must share information in order to arrive at the best treatment decisions possible and bridge the scientific and the personal knowledge domains through this process";
- an emancipatory praxis breaking silence and enhancing dialogue [17, p 64].

"Shared decision-making" is a good example of a clinical procedure of both person-centered care and of recovery orientation, enhancing communication between patients and clinicians and optimizing treatment planning. Furthermore, it may increase the respect for autonomy, responsibility and dignity of every person involved in a clinical decision process.

Seen as above described, empowerment represents then one of the key elements involved in fostering the recovery process from severe mental illness [54].

8.4 Person-Centeredness in Medicine, Psychiatry, and Psychotherapy

There is no unique or single concept of person-centeredness, but there are many diverse concepts and traditions of person-centered clinical care coming from different roots, philosophies, traditions and disciplines.

The term "personalized medicine" or "individualized medicine" is presently being discussed in a specific pharmacological context. Biological medicine aims at investigating the human being with genetic studies in order to arrive at specific diagnoses and make specific prognostic statements concerning health and illness, risk of developing a particular illness, or having resistance concerning a specific disease due to healthy life style activities. Biological researchers promise with these new personalized medical methods the improvement of the health system and the perfectionism in medicine (e.g., [28, 33, 43]). These current research interests need to be considered with justified skepticism and vigilance. Urban Wiesing (quoted by [44]), chair of the central ethical board of the German federal organization of physicians, criticizes the current development and says that "personal traits do not manifest themselves on a molecular but on a personal level."

One of the main person-centerd concepts to which many psychotherapists refer is the client-centered therapy of Rogers [46] who conceptualized the person's basic nature as profoundly confidential, constructive, social and proactive. However, one must admit that Rogers refers to the basic nature of a person, but not to all the person's behavioral manifestations which can be extremely cruel, hostile, negative, and antisocial [53]. In general, the main idea is that person-centered psychotherapy considers these negative behavioral manifestations as reactive answers of the clients to their psychic misery. In that sense, the person-centered philosophy can be understood as optimistic but not as naïve [53]. One main characteristic of a person-centered clinical attitude is to reach under the surface or behind the scenes of a person and to look after so far undeveloped potentials, strengths and resources within a person. A main concept of Rogers [47] is the "tendency of actualization," that means the tendency, inherent in any organism and in any person, of the development of all possibilities which serve his/her maintenance and development. This includes the differentiation of a person's capabilities, enlargement in the sense of growth and striving for autonomy.

The authors of this chapter aim at the person-centeredness in psychiatry and psychotherapy in the sense that each person has his/her unique needs, life history, cultural roots, symptom expression, illness history, family background and needs for a specific treatment program, as well as unique ways of recovery from a psychiatric disorder and related disabilities. The person's unique needs should be the basic orientation for treatment and therapy goals (e.g., [3]).

In this chapter we refer explicitly to the concept of a person-centered psychiatry recently developed by Mezzich [36, 37] and his colleagues. This concept was originally realized as a "WPA Institutional Program on Psychiatry for the Person: from Clinical Care to Public Health (IPPP)" and was approved by the 2005 General Assembly of the World Psychiatric Association. "It involves a WPA initiative affirming the *whole person of the patient in context as* the center and goal of clinical care and health promotion, at both individual and community levels. This involves the articulation of science and humanism to optimize attention to the ill and positive health aspects of the person." [36, p 65] Service user and family perspectives have been considered in this program (e.g., [60]).

Since 2008 the original concept of person-centeredness in psychiatry has been expanded toward the whole field of medicine in which psychiatry is one part of the full range of medical disciplines [39, 40]. The concept of person-centeredness is oriented to various medical fields and related topics, for example, in primary care [57], oncology [41], nursery [23], communication skills [58] or chronically ill patients [26].

8.5 Convergences and Divergences Among Recovery, Empowerment and Person-Centered Care

Mezzich and Schmolke [38] made a comparison of the essentials of Recovery Orientation and Person-Centered Care and identified unique characteristics for each approach as well as substantial elements of convergence. Recovery Orientation is primarily centered within the mental health and psychosocial fields while the Person-Centered Approach covers general medicine and health care at large. Their points of convergence encompass a holistic theoretical perspective, an emphasis on contextualization and establishing a common ground for understanding and action, development of person-centered procedures for clinical care and health promotion, and, last but not least, an ethical commitment.

In general, it is possible to say that there are more general convergences than divergences between the Recovery approach, with Empowerment as a key element of it, and the Person-centered Medicine concept.

Among the *convergences*, the following aspects can be summarized:

- Person-centeredness is a key common characteristic of all three concepts.
- A confidential and partnership relationship between the professional and the service user is central in treatment programs. For example, the Need-Adapted Treatment approach [1] is a common reference framework for both the Recovery concept and the Person-centerd Medicine concepts.
- A specific diagnostic assessment going beyond standardized diagnostic categories for each individual patient looking for the person's problems, symptoms as well as strengths, needs, assets, resilience.
- The professionals' ethical attitude to and respect of the unique person's interests, values, and aspirations.
- The individual as a person (not a case) is important with his/her unique history, illness development and unique resources.
- Unique recovery processes with or without professional support (there is no standard recovery valid for everybody); for example, specific aspects or particular events or particular persons can be helpful in the recovery process.
- Respect for autonomous decisions of service users about a specific treatment in a specific context.
- Individualization and personalization of interventions is fundamental in order to consider adequately the person's age, intelligence and health literacy level, sociocultural background, ethnicity, environment, language and cultural barriers, strengths and weaknesses, life goals, mental status, type, severity and duration of the disorder.

Among the *divergences*, the following elements can be mentioned:

- There are different conceptual and historical backgrounds of the three concepts.
- While the Person-centerd Medicine concept has been conceptualized by professionals from various medical disciplines, the Recovery and Empowerment concepts have been developed by activists and service users through their immediate personal experiences, e.g., of negative experiences in psychiatric treatment settings or experiences of exclusion and discrimination in the community.
- In the Recovery approach, the active user involvement and participation in treatment planning and evaluation as well as in psychiatric research play a central role.
- Trialogue [2] and Open Dialogue [48] are essential innovative developments within the Recovery approach which facilitate communication beyond the static roles of professional and patient, including also family members.
- Peer support is one specific characteristic of the Recovery concept with the orientation toward "consumer-driven systems transformation," that is self-help groups, internet support groups, peer delivered services, peer run or operated services, peer partnerships, peer employees [42, 52].

8.6 Closing Remarks

We would like to close with the words of Helen Glover, eminent recovery activist, social worker and peer counselor in Australia, from her foreword of the book of Amering and Schmolke [25, xii]:

> No one else, whether they are family, friends or workers, can 'recover' a person, no matter how much they long for that to occur. What then, is the role of the 'other', if not to create recovery for them? The role of the 'other' is to be in genuine relationships with people and create environments of support in which a person can negotiate their sense of 'self-righting'. If we dare to name ourselves as a supporter of another, then we must adhere to a number of foci in our support. Firstly, we must believe that a person has the capacity to 'self-right' or recover. Secondly, we must work 'as if' recovery is always real, present and possible, even though we might never have the privilege of being a full witness to it. We have to ensure that the environments of support provided are sufficiently accessible for a person to be able to exercise their recovery effort within them, and we have to be mindful not to stand in the way of, nor to inhibit their unique efforts to overcome.

References

1. Alanen YO. Schizophrenia: its origins and need-adapted treatment. London: Karnac Books; 1997.
2. Amering M, Hofer H, Rath I. The 'First Vienna Trialogue'—experiences with a new form of communication between users, relatives and mental health professionals. In: Lefley HP, Johnson DL, editors. Family interventions in mental illness: international perspectives. London, Westport, CT: Praeger; 2002. p. 105–24.

3. Amering M, Schmolke M. Recovery in mental health. Reshaping scientific and clinical responsibilities. Chichester: Wiley-Blackwell; 2009.
4. Amering M, Stastny P, Hopper K. Psychiatric advance directives: qualitative study of informed deliberations by mental health service users. Br J Psychiatry. 2005;186:247–52.
5. Amering M. Recovery, science and human rights. Epidemiol Psychiatr Sci. 2012;22:1–3 (Invited Commentary).
6. Anthony W. Recovery from mental illness. The guiding vision of the mental health service system in the 1990s. Psychosoc Rehabil J. 1993;16:11–23.
7. Bradstreet S. Harnessing the 'Lived Experience': formalising peer support approaches to promote recovery. Mental Health Rev J. 2006;11(2):33–7.
8. Chamberlin J. On our own: Patient-controlled alternatives to the mental health system. New York: McGraw Hill; 1978.
9. Chamberlin J. A working definition of empowerment. 2009. http://www.power2u.org/articles/empower/working_def.html.
10. Corrigan PW. Recovery from schizophrenia and the role of evidence-based psychosocial interventions. Expert Rev Neurother. 2006;6:993–1004.
11. Corrigan PW, Mueser KT, Bond GR. Principles and practice of psychiatric rehabilitation: an empirical approach. New York: Guilford; 2009.
12. Davidson L, Harding C, Spaniol L, editors. Recovery from mental illness: research evidence and implications for practice. Boston: Centre for Psychiatric Rehabilitation, Boston University; 2005.
13. Davidson L, Roe D. Recovery from versus recovery in serious mental illness: one strategy for lessening confusion plaguing recovery. J Mental Health. 2007;16:459–70.
14. Davidson L, Strauss JS. Sense of self in recovery from severe mental illness. Br J Med Psychol. 1992;65:131–45.
15. Davidson L, Tondora J, O'Connell MJ, Lawless MS, Rowe M. A practical guide to recovery-oriented practice: tools for transforming mental health care. New York: Oxford University Press; 2009.
16. Deegan PE. Recovery: the lived experience of rehabilitation. Psychosoc Rehabil J. 1998;11:11–9.
17. Deegan PE. The lived experience of using psychiatric medication in the recovery process and a shared decision-making program to support it. Psychiatr Rehabil J. 2007;31(1):62–9.
18. Deegan PE. Recovery as a journey of the heart. In: Davidson L, Harding C, Spaniol L, editors. Recovery from severe mental illnesses: research evidence and implications. Boston, MA: Center for Psychiatric Rehabilitation, Boston University; 2005. p. 57–68.
19. Deegan PE, Drake RE. Shared decision-making and medication management in the recovery-process. Psychiatric Services. 2006;57(11):1636–9.
20. Deegan PE, Rapp C, Holter M, Riefer M. Best practices: a program to support shared decision-making in an outpatient psychiatric medication clinic. Psychiatric Services. 2008;59:603–5.
21. Farkas M. The vision of recovery today: what it is and what it means for services. World Psychiatry. 2007;6:4–10.
22. Farkas M, Gagne C, Anthony W, Chamberlin J. Implementing recovery oriented evidence based programs: Identifying the critical dimensions. Community Mental Health J. 2005;41(2). doi:10.1007/s10597-005-2649-6.
23. Ghebrehiwet T. Nurses and person-centred care. Int J Person Cent Med. 2011;1(1):20–2.
24. Glover H. Recovery based service delivery: are we ready to transform the words into a paradigm shift? Aust e-J Adv Mental Health (AeJAMH), 2005;4(3):1–4. http://www.auseinet.com/journal/vol4iss3/glovereditorial.pdf (28.08.08).
25. Glover H. Foreword. In: Amering M, Schmolke M, editors. Recovery in mental health. Reshaping scientific and clinical responsibilities (p. xi–xiii). Chichester: Wiley-Blackwell; 2009.

26. Goetz K, Campbell S, Willms S, Rochon J, Klingenberg A, Szecsenyi J. How do chronically ill patients evaluate their medical care? An observational study with 46919 patients in 676 primary care practices of direct relevance to person-centered medicine. Int J Person Cent Med. 2011;1(2):338–46.
27. Hamann J, Cohen R, Leucht S, Busch R, Kissling W. Shared decision making for in-patients with schizophrenia. Acta Psychiatr Scand. 2006;114:265–73.
28. Hamburg MA, Collins FS. The path to personalized medicine. N Engl J Med. 2010;363: 301–4. doi:10.1056/NEJMp1006304.
29. Harding CM, Brooks GW, Ashikaga T, et al. The vermont longitudinal study of persons with severe mental illness, II: Long-term outcome of subjects who retrospectively met DSM-III criteria for schizophrenia. Am J Psychiatry. 1987;144:727–35.
30. Herriger N. Empowerment in der Sozialen Arbeit. Eine Einführung. Stuttgart: Kohlhammer; 2006.
31. Jacobson N, Greenley D. What is recovery? A conceptual model and explication. Psychiatr Serv. 2001;52:482–5.
32. Laugharne R, Priebe S. Trust, choice and power in mental health: a literature review. Soc Psychiatry Psychiatr Epidemiol. 2006;41(11):843–52.
33. Levenson V, Mori Y. The era of personalized medicine: mechanistic or correlative biomarkers? Personal Med. 2014;11(4):361–4.
34. Liberman RP, Kopelowicz A. Recovery from schizophrenia: a concept in search of research. Psychiatr Serv. 2005;56:735–42.
35. Liberman RP, Kopelowicz A, Ventura J, Gutkind D. Operational criteria and factors related to recovery from schizophrenia. Int Rev Psychiatry. 2002;14:256–72.
36. Mezzich JE. Psychiatry for the person: articulating medicine's science and humanism. World Psychiatry. 2007;6:1–3.
37. Mezzich JE, Christodoulou G, Fulford KWM. Introduction to the conceptual bases of psychiatry for the person. Int J Person Cent Med. 2011;1(1):121–4.
38. Mezzich JE, Schmolke M. Contrasting the essentials of recovery orientation and person-centered care. Int J Person Cent Med. 2013;3(1):31–5.
39. Mezzich JE, Snaedal J, van Weel C, Heath I. The international network for person-centered medicine: background and first steps. World Med J. 2009;55:104–7.
40. Mezzich JE, Snaedal J, van Weel C, Heath I. Toward person centered medicine: from disease to patient to person. Mt Sinai J Med. 2010;77:304–6.
41. Milne D, Sheeran L, Dryden T, Mileshkin L, Aranda S. Care requirements of patients with advanced cancer within a specialist centre—moving to person-centered approaches. Int J Person Cent Med. 2011;1(1):167–76.
42. Peebles SA, et al. Recovery and systems transformation for schizophrenia. Psychiatr Clin North Am. 2007;30:567–83.
43. Personalized Medicine Coalition. The case for personalized medicine. 4th ed. Washington, D.C.: PMC; 2014.
44. Pytlik W. Die personalisierte Medizin kommt aus den Startblöcken. Biotech/Life Sciences Portal Baden-Würtemberg. 7 Feb 2011.
45. Roberts G, Hollins S. Consumers' perceptions of negative experiences and 'sanctuary harm' in psychiatric settings. Psychiatr Serv. 2007;56:1134–8.
46. Rogers CR. Client-centered therapy: its current practice, implications and theory (Newer edition: Constable & Robinson Ltd. 2003). Boston: Houghton Mifflin; 1951 (ISBN: 1841198404).
47. Rogers CR. Eine Theorie der Psychotherapie, der Persönlichkeit und der zwischenmenschlichen Beziehungen (Original 1959). Köln: GwG; 1959/1987.
48. Seikkula J, et al. Five year experience of first episode non-affective psychosis in open dialogue approach: treatment principles, follow-up outcomes and two case studies. Psychother Res. 2006;16(2):214–28.

49. Slade M. Personal recovery and mental illness: a guide for mental health professionals. Cambridge: Cambridge University Press; 2009.
50. Slade M, Amering M, Farkas M, Hamilton B, O'Hagan M, Panther G, Perkins R, Shepherd G, Tse S, Whitley R. Uses and abuses of recovery: implementing recovery-oriented practices in mental health systems. World Psychiatry. 2014;13(1):12–20.
51. Slade M, Leamy M, Bacon F, Janosik M, Le Boutillier C, Williams J, Bird V. International differences in understanding recovery: systematic review. Epidemiol Psychiatr Sci. 2012;21 (4):353–64.
52. Solomon P. Peer support/peer provided services underlying processes, benefits, and critical ingredients. Psychiatr Rehabil J. 2004;27(4):392–401.
53. Stumm G. Menschenbilder in der Klientenzentrierten Psychotherapie (Gesprächspsychotherapie). In: Petzold H (Hrsg.), Die Menschenbilder in der Psychotherapie. Interdisziplinäre Perspektiven und die Modelle der Therapieschulen (pp. 585–618). Wien: Edition Donau-Universität-Krammer; 2012.
54. Svettini A, Boggian I, Lamonaca D, Basso L, Conca A. What do we learn from users and carers to provide a recovery-oriented mental health care? The Italian Study on Recovery (S.I.R.)—phase 2. Psychiatr Prax. 2011;38:S01. doi:10.1055/s-0031-1277850.
55. Svettini A, Boggian I, Lamonaca D, Conca A. A qualitative and quantitative research on recovery from severe mental illness: the Italian Study on Recovery (S.I.R.). Schizophr Res. 2010;117(2-3):522.
56. Theunissen G, Plaute W. Handbuch Empowerment und Heilpädagogik. Freiburg: Lambertus; 2002.
57. Uijen A, Schers H, van Weel C. Person centered medicine and the primary care team—securing continuity of care. Int J Person Cent Med. 2011;1(1):18–9.
58. Van Dulmen S, van Bijnen E. What makes them (not) talk about proper medication use with their patients? Int J Person Cent Med. 2011;1(1):27–34.
59. Wallcraft J, Schrank B, Amering M. Handbook of service user involvement in mental health research. Chichester: Wiley-Blackwell; 2009.
60. Wallcraft J, Steffen S, Amering M. Service user and family perspectives on psychiatry for the person. Int J Person Cent Med. 2011;1(1):152–4.
61. Wallcraft J. Consumer models of recovery: can they survive operationalism? World Psychiatry. 2012;11(3):166–7.

9 Person-Centered Patient Perspectives

Joanna Groves, BSc, MSc

9.1 The Global Healthcare Environment

The global healthcare environment has been constantly evolving and changing for thousands of years and the role of patients, or people living with long-term chronic conditions, has also been changing.

In terms of health demographics, populations around the world are ageing and chronic conditions such as cancer, diabetes, heart disease and mental health conditions (such as depression, schizophrenia, intellectual and behavioural disabilities and others) are affecting the health and quality of life of an increasing number of people around the world. The World Health Organization [16] estimated that mental, neurological and substance use disorders accounted for a significant 13 % of the total global disease burden in 2004. Depression accounts for 4.3 % of this, making it one of the largest single causes of disability worldwide. The number of people surviving and living long term with mental health conditions is influenced by advances in science and medicine, increased availability of a broad range of healthcare and social services and higher educational levels.

However, as the number of people living with chronic conditions rises it is placing an ever-increasing burden on health systems, originally designed to address acute medical conditions. Healthcare services are becoming increasingly fragmented, hospital-based and disease-oriented. This fragmentation can lead to barriers to person-centered psychiatry. It means that the people whose needs should be at the centre of healthcare services are often not fully taken into account or even totally overlooked or overuled entirely. Patients experience this as poor quality care and a lack of continuity of care with limited opportunities for them to engage in the

J. Groves, BSc, MSc (✉)
Board member, International College of Person Centered Medicine,
Former Chief Executive Officer, International Alliance of Patients' Organizations,
6 Brockwell Park Row, London SW2 2YH, UK
e-mail: joanna.m.groves@gmail.com

J.E. Mezzich et al. (eds.), *Person Centered Psychiatry*,
DOI 10.1007/978-3-319-39724-5_9

management and understanding of their own health and healthcare. This often makes them unsatisfied with their healthcare experiences.

The motivation of professionals is an important factor in the practice of person-centered psychiatry. On a personal level, most psychiatrists and other members of the health and social care team, such as psychologists, psychotherapists and social workers, will have gone into their chosen profession because they want to improve people's health and well-being and strive to be person-centered. Sometimes, professionals who have the best intentions believe that they know what the patient wants and what is best for them and these individual attitudes affect behaviour. A patient would ask, 'how can you know what I want if you don't ask me and listen to me?'

There are also many factors that can make it difficult for professionals to be person-centered. The dissociation between healthcare which focuses on the condition and services that focus on other aspects of an individual's life are not useful. A person's health affects all aspects of their life and conversely their life affects their health and healthcare. Sometimes there is an overemphasis on clinical and cost-effectiveness (or reducing costs) for individual medicines or procedures rather than consideration of the bigger picture including what patients see as important measures of success. These might include that they had a good discussion with their psychiatrist and agreed how healthcare could help them achieve their overall goals for a better quality of life. There are also barriers caused by the structure of the healthcare system, for example, short consultation times, underfunding (or inefficient processes), insufficient staffing levels and low morale. These restrict the practice of a person-centered approach and it can be seen as expensive in an already overstretched service.

In terms of the role of people with mental health conditions, historically the '*disease*' and how to '*treat*' it has been the focus of treatment. The traditional biomedical management model involved '*paternalistic*' treatment where the health professional decided the appropriate course of treatment often without any patient involvement in the decision. In the past few decades, people have become much more interested in their health and have been taking more responsibility for their personal healthcare. In psychiatry, the importance of listening to the patient and trying to understand their experiences and how their mental health, physical health and life are intertwined is part of a person-centered approach though the empowerment of the patient in goal setting and decision-making is critical to really achieve person-centered care.

Patient groups have been calling for a patient- or person-centered approach for decades, as have some academics, health professionals and policy-makers. Now, though, there seems to be greater consensus from all stakeholders than ever before that person-centered care is not only what patients' want and therefore the right thing to do but it is essential. Systems need to re-orient significantly if they are to successfully and appropriately meet the needs of people with mental health conditions in this century. Central to this is the need for more personalized and integrated care models which include the active involvement of patients and family members as whole people in their care.

9.2 Principles of Person-Centered Psychiatry

Person-centered psychiatry is one of the terms that is currently used to describe this shift in care to focus on the needs and wishes of the whole person.[1] This section outlines some of the definitions in use and considers the principles they encompass and how relevant they are to patients.

9.2.1 Terminology

The terminology used to refer to individuals with mental health conditions and more broadly to those with chronic conditions is a subject of intense debate. People feel strongly about the language they use to describe their relationship with their illness and a term can be very empowering or disempowering to a person.

Historically, since the first known use in the fourteenth century, someone that is ill or has a long-term condition has been referred to as a patient [13]. This comes from the Latin "pati" which means to suffer and, of course, many people with chronic conditions do suffer with physical or emotional pain. In more recent times many other terms have been proposed and used as people have strong opinions 'for' and 'against' the use of the term, 'patient'. Some patients think it a useful term to differentiate them from people who only occasionally have an illness and self define themselves. Others feel that the term is inappropriate because everyone will be a patient at some point. The term 'patient' can be restrictive because it focuses on the treatment of disease whereas now, more than ever, there is a need to focus on the long-term management of conditions and more broadly on health promotion and prevention.

Some individuals who have or have had mental health conditions are concerned that the terms used to define them can be disempowering and the term patient can imply that they are passive recipients of healthcare, a dependent with a lack of autonomy, rather than an active driver in managing their own health. Terms can reinforce negative public perceptions of mental illness which do nothing to overcome the significant challenges of stigma and discrimination towards those with mental health problems.

The Mental Health Foundation in the United Kingdom has defined 12 common terms used in mental health: clients; consumers; ex-patients; experts by/through experience; patients; people with mental health problems; people with experience of mental and emotional distress; people with mental illness; psychiatric survivors; service users; sufferers; survivors; and users. The terms can have positive and negative connotations [11]. Some emphasize the nature of the patient–health professional relationship as market-based (consumer) or imply choice in how people use services (e.g. consumer, client, service user, etc). Some people believe that the system will treat people better if they think of them as customers who have a choice

[1]There are numerous other terms in current use including, but not restricted to, person-centered medicine, patient-centered care, patient-focused care and people-centered care.

whether to use their service or not. This does not account for those that do not have a choice in whether or how they access services for whatever reason. Some terms may not allow the individual focus which recognises that people are individuals with different needs, values and preferences and not all 'generic' service users. Some are more empowering as they highlight the expertise of the person rather than their health status.

As people are individuals, it is unlikely that there will ever be one term that everyone can agree on but those with mental health conditions themselves must be involved in discussions as to what different terms resonate with them or whether they find them empowering or discriminatory and how they would like to define themselves on an individual level. The terminology should be regularly reviewed as language and the environment will not remain static.

9.2.2 Definitions of Patient-, Person-, and People-Centered Care

There is more than one term in current usage which aims to define and promote the approach to care which focuses on the whole person and is responsive to and addresses their needs, wishes and preferences for their health goals and living their lives. Definitions of some in common usage namely patient-centered, person-centered and people-centered care are considered in this section.

Patient-centered care

Patient-centered care became a common terminology in the 1990s with many academics proposing definitions of what patient-centered care could embody. One example, from a number brought together in Lutz and Bowers [10], states that patient-centered healthcare is, '*Health care that is closely congruent with and responsive to patients' wants, needs and preferences*'.

In 2001, the Institute of Medicine (IOM) in the United States of America proposed patient-centered care as one of its six aims for the twenty-first century healthcare system stating that healthcare should be, "*patient-centered—providing care that is respectful of and responsive to individual patient preferences, needs and values and ensuring that patient values guide all clinical decisions*" [9].

The first global definition of patient-centered healthcare developed and agreed by patients themselves is outlined in the International Alliance of Patients' Organization's (IAPO) Declaration on Patient-Centred Healthcare [5]. The Declaration identifies five principles of patient-centered healthcare which include the following elements:

- *respect* for patients, families and carers unique needs, preferences and values as well as their autonomy and independence;
- *choice and empowerment* whereby patients have a right and responsibility to participate to their level of ability and preference as a partner in making healthcare decisions that affect their lives;

- *patient involvement in health policy* at all levels and at all points of decision-making, to ensure that they are designed with the patient at the centre;
- *access and support* so that patients can access safe, quality and appropriate services, treatments, preventive care and health promotion activities with a commitment to equity and a holistic approach including health and non health factors for patients to achieve the best possible quality of life; and
- the need for accurate, relevant and comprehensive *information* to enable patients and carers to make informed decisions about healthcare treatment and living with their condition.

Person-centered care

The term person-centered care has become increasingly common, perhaps partly in response to the lack of consensus over other terms such as the word, 'patient'. This section outlines definitions proposed by health professionals, academics and patient/user groups.

For example, the International College of Person-Centered Medicine [7] state:

> Person-centered medicine is dedicated to the promotion of health as a state of physical, mental, socio-cultural and spiritual wellbeing as well as to the reduction of disease, and founded on mutual respect for the dignity and responsibility of each individual person.
>
> The conceptual bases of Person-centered Care include the following:
>
> a) Broad bio-psycho-socio-cultural-spiritual theoretical framework,
> b) Attention to positive-health and ill-health as components of a broad concept of health,
> c) Enhancement of person-centered communication, diagnosis, treatment, prevention and promotion of health,
> d) Respect for the autonomy, responsibility and dignity of every person involved,
> e) Promotion of person-centered relationships and partnerships at all levels, and
> f) Articulation of person-centered clinical medicine and people-centered public health.

The Health Foundation in the United Kingdom states that:

> Person-centred care sees patients as equal partners in planning, developing and assessing care to make sure it is most appropriate for their needs. It involves putting patients and their families at the heart of all decisions.
>
> Person-centred care aims to be user focused, promote independence and autonomy, provide choice and control and be based on a collaborative team philosophy. It takes into account service users' needs and views and builds relationships with family members.

They highlight essential components as: compassion, dignity and respect; shared decision making and collective patient and public involvement.

From a patient or user perspective, National Voices (the national coalition of health and social care charities in England) states that, "*person-centred care involves placing people at the forefront of their health and care. It ensures people retain control, helps them make informed decisions and supports a partnership between individuals, families and services*". They go on to outline some of the main components of person-centered care as being: supporting self-management;

supporting shared decision making; enhancing experience of healthcare; improving information and understanding; and promoting prevention.

People-centered care
At a global level, the WHO's World Health Report of 2008 on primary healthcare and subsequent resolution WHA62.12 called for service delivery reforms to make health systems more *people-centered* and *integrated*. In 2015, WHO will launch a Global Strategy on People-centered and Integrated Health Services to support the achievement of universal health coverage. WHO [15, 17] defines people-centered and integrated health services as, "*The management and delivery of health services such that people receive a continuum of health promotion, disease prevention, diagnosis, treatment, disease-management, rehabilitation and palliative care services, through the different levels and sites of care within the health system, and according to their needs throughout the life course". And "An approach to care that consciously adopts individuals', families', and communities' perspectives as participants in and beneficiaries of trusted health systems, that respond to their needs and preferences in humane and holistic ways. People-centred care also requires that people have the education and support they need to make decisions and participate in their own care. It is organized around the health needs and expectations of people rather than diseases*".

9.2.3 Principles of Person-Centered Psychiatry: Analysis and Discussion

There are many common principles in the definitions outlined in Sect. 2.2 of patient-, person- and people-centered care including:

1. Respectful of and responsive to individual's needs, wishes and preferences
2. Holistic/sensitive to non-medical or spiritual issues
3. Shared knowledge and decision-making
4. Continuity and integration of care
5. Involvement and empowerment of patients, their families and carers
6. Access to services, treatment and care

9.2.3.1 Respectful of and Responsive to Individual's Needs, Wishes and Preferences

In the majority of the definitions, respect for a person's dignity, needs, wishes and/or preferences in some form stands out as a core principle of person-centered care. This recognises that every person is an individual and has different needs and that the healthcare system should be able to be responsive to this. It should be able to balance encouraging people to be engaged and responsible to some extent for their mental health and care whilst recognizing and respecting the limits in people's ability of individual preferences.

This means that the required outcome of healthcare is a better quality of health *and/or life as defined by the patient themselves*. This is different from a professional working '*in the best interests*' of the patient as it is the patient that must determine whether the care is person-centered and respectful of their wishes and not the professional. This requires that the patient must be supported to be able, as far as possible, to determine what his or her wishes are which can be difficult with some mental health conditions and for other reasons. And, in mental health, it may sometimes be difficult to determine what the patient's wishes are. Professionals need to take time to understand the issues and problems that the patient is living with and their goals in addressing them. They need to '*put themselves in the patient's shoes*' and not project their own values and opinions onto the situation. This can be particularly difficult if the patient's wishes are different from those of the professional such as if a patient does not want to take a particular treatment. There is, of course, also a tension here as a balance must be sought between the conflicts of managing risk if a patient is considered to be likely to harm themselves (such as being at risk of attempting suicide) and enabling and empowering patients to their right to determine their own goals in terms of their health and health management and care so building up a dialogue and mutual respect and trust are critical.

9.2.3.2 Holistic/Sensitive to Non-medical or Spiritual Issues

It is well accepted that a person's quality of life does not solely depend on their disease but also encompasses how the disease impacts on their participation in society, and their physical and mental well-being such as that outlined in the WHO's constitution which states, "*Health is a state of complete physical, mental and social well-being and not merely the absence of disease or infirmity*". Mental and physical health and well-being may be influenced by diverse factors and a person's response will be shaped by their values, any spiritual or religious beliefs, their culture and environment. Therefore, all of these must be explored and only the individual can judge how a condition and treatment affects them and fits in with their values, beliefs and lifestyle. This information can make an important contribution to decisions relating to what the aims of the treatment should be and what a successful outcome would be for their personal situation.

It is, therefore, necessary to shift away from focusing just on the disease or condition, making a patient a member of a disease group and labelling them with general characteristics and to focus on the uniqueness of the personal experiences, considering what the disease means for the life and social participation of the individual. The key to understanding the whole person and addressing their needs is the health professional and patient relationship and how they communicate which is considered in the next section.

9.2.3.3 Shared Knowledge and Decision-Making

In the past century, the patient's role in healthcare was seen as receptive, a passive recipient provided with healthcare by their doctor or a health professional. The focus on scientific evidence and seeing the doctor as the expert led to the well known saying, "*The Doctor knows best*" and some people, including patients and doctors, still believe this to be the case. Many patients now consider that the doctor is still the medical expert whose advise is very important but that they are experts in how their condition affects their life. Shared decision making (SDM) has been defined as: "*an approach where clinicians and patients share the best available evidence when faced with the task of making decisions, and where patients are supported to consider options, to achieve informed preferences*" [3]. Therefore, a model of shared decision making which takes into account a person's abilities with respect to the level of involvement in decision-making and their health is necessary.

As a first step, professionals need to understand the experiences, needs and expectations of the patient; so communication becomes key. Too often communication is seen as a one way act, with professionals informing patients what their diagnosis is and what treatment they need to take. Real communication however is an interactive process, in which the act of listening is as important as the act of speaking. There is often a gap between what a patient wants and what the professional expects them to want.

The danger is that the professional may still be in charge directing the conversation. In addition, it will not always be easy for mental health professionals to know with certainty what a person's needs and expectations are. However, if the starting point is listening to a person's perspective and their experience with their health problems and in living their life before moving onto how they can meet their goals then they can be better guided in what care they want.

For real shared decision making and communication there need to be two well-informed partners (with their own particular expertise). Information in itself has no intrinsic power, but it is needed in order for patients and professionals to have the required information in order to have a constructive dialogue in an equal partnership where the balance of power is not with one party or the other.

Patients have to learn to articulate their needs in an understandable way and doctors have to take into account the differences in health literacy of the patients. There is not a '*one size fits all approach*' as people respond to different levels and types of communication. So, communication skills are necessary to ensure that patients' preferences, wants and need are considered and to facilitate an equal partnership where shared decisions can be made. This requires ongoing training of professionals, students and all others involved with patients. Patients need to be involved in the determination of communication skills but also may need training themselves so they can effectively communicate their needs and preferences in dialogue with health professionals.

There are many tools and programmes to promote and support shared decision making. The Health Decision Sciences Centre at Massachusetts General Hospital has created a streamlined process whereby doctors in primary and secondary care can 'prescribe' a patient decision aid through their electronic medical record. The patient can then access the tool outside of the consultation to facilitate better shared decision making [1].

Trust is essential in the professional–patient relationship because, despite regulations and practices to protect patient's personal information, patients may be concerned that sensitive information that they share with professionals may not be kept confidential and/or may be used against them.

9.2.3.4 Continuity and Integration of Care

Patients often feel that the system they find themselves in is not joined up. They are passed from one health professional to another (often in different centres at a distance from each other) and have to repeat their problem or situation multiple times. There are many areas which need integration in order for patients to feel that their needs are being recognised and that the system can competently and safely address them.

To a patient it does not matter whether the problems they are experiencing are considered to be in the field of psychiatry or whether they are healthcare issues or a social, educational or economic issues. Therefore, integration within the healthcare sector and between the healthcare sector and all other areas which will impact on their health such as education, employment and so on. It is important to them that there is integration on a personal level between themselves, their families, carers and professionals in the management of care. The involvement of family and friends can be very important for those with mental health conditions not just providing support but also, if desired by the patient, being involved in treatment planning and goal setting and health management. Team work is very important so that patients experience integrated care and patients should be considered part of the team, along with family, friends and carers where possible, desired and appropriate. Patients experience health and health problems in the living of their lives and so continuity of care for the patient throughout their journey as a person and patient throughout their lives is important.

The Geneva Declaration on Person- and People-centered Integrated Health Care for all [8] outlines six domains namely: (1) integrating the relations between the people seeking and delivering care; (2) that it is planned and delivered within the social network of each person; (3) ensuring coordination of health care over the trajectory of each person's life; (4) promoting vertical integration within the healthcare sector by planning and coordinating care among primary care-givers and specialists; (5) emphasizes horizontal integration of health care delivery across multiple sectors of society; and (6) for integration to succeed these values must become normative throughout society, that is, needs to foster common values and a shared vision of the future.

9.2.3.5 Involvement and Empowerment of Patients, Their Families and Carers

Healthcare policy decisions, at whatever level they are made, will ultimately affect patients' lives. There is, therefore, a moral imperative that they play a meaningful role in developing healthcare policies and, if done well, it helps to ensure that policies reflect patient and caregiver needs, preferences and capabilities.

The need to involve people in their own healthcare at an individual and community level in the design and delivery of healthcare systems is not a new concept. The WHO's Declaration of Alma-Ata [18] stated a commitment to it, "*The people have the right and duty to participate individually and collectively in the planning and implementation of their healthcare*". Patient groups have been advocating for involvement in *all* decision-making both at a personal and a policy level for many years now and the phrase (originally used by the disability movement), "*nothing about us, without us*" has increasingly become a mantra for patient groups from all over the world.

However, patient experiences and views are often not considered or valued in policy-making or practice. IAPO [6], states that, "*Patient involvement is often merely tokenism; its influence on policy-making can be restricted by practical and financial structures, differing knowledge bases, cultural barriers and personal attitudes. Patient involvement should not be dependent on the good will of individuals but institutionalised in policy frameworks in order to become the rule, rather than the exception*". For meaningful involvement, there need to be methods to ensure that the multiple opinions and patient voices are heard and acted upon. As patients are not a homogenous population with the same expectations and needs, this means ensuring that there are multiple patients involved in initiatives (just as we do other experts), recognizing what each person brings to the table and striving to be inclusive of underrepresented groups so that there are a balance of perspectives represented.

As we move away from a paternalistic provision of care to passive patients towards the empowerment of people so that they are active participants in their healthcare, we are talking about the patient's role in the co-production of their health. They should be the *driver* and an *equal* actor rather than as a participant who is still responding to the opportunities provided to him or her by the system.

Empowerment is not possible without having necessary information and opportunities for involvement but it is not merely that but the ability and confidence to take action based on the knowledge people have. The European Network for Patient Empowerment (ENOPE) says that an empowered activated patient is one which: understands their health condition and how to manage their lifestyle and condition; feels able to participate in decision-making and make informed choices about treatment and feels confident to challenge and ask questions of health professionals or where to find, evaluate and use the information they need. With the increased use of terminology regarding empowerment and person-centered care, it is important to ensure that this is not just rhetoric with the actual practice not changing in line with the language [4]. The All Party Parliamentary Group on Global Health in the UK [1] collected over 100 overseas examples of patient empowerment such as those relating to self-care, patients as experts, shared decisions and choice. They concluded that by giving patients the opportunity to expand their role and equipping them to do so new models of care are possible.

9.2.3.6 Access to Services, Treatment and Care

Fundamentally, people want to have access to safe, quality care which respects them and their needs, preferences and wishes. One of the important opportunities for the development of person-centered care currently is the global commitment to the achievement of universal health coverage (UHC) with its three pillars of: equity in access to health services; high quality health services and financial-risk protection.

Access to treatment and care is not just about physically accessing services but also includes being able to access care that is affordable and does not put the person at financial risk or into a life of poverty. People should not be prevented from accessing services by their educational or socio-economic status. Emotional as well as physical support may be needed in order for people to access services and care. In the case of mental health, anxiety and fear may be a barrier to accessing care which may be compounded by the stigma that people experience or that they perceive others have towards their mental illness. People need to feel safe and welcome and that they are not judged if they are to access services and continue to use and benefit from them overtime. UK providers have been expanding access to mental health services through computerized self-help and peer-support. Services like beatingtheblues.co.uk, bigwhitewall.com and fearfighter.com are helping to educate people about mental health and expand access to group, talking and cognitive behavioural therapies at extremely low costs [1].

9.3 Evidence for Person-Centered Psychiatry

The question always raised about a person-centered approach is does it work? What effect does the practice of person-centered healthcare have on health outcomes? This is a valid question but despite an increasingly solid evidence base supporting many of the principles of person-centered care its worth continues to be questioned. In addition, it must be recognised that it is not just important to measure the physiological health outcomes such as blood pressure but outcomes that people themselves find important such as their well-being and quality of life, their healthcare behaviour (such as lifestyle and attitude to agreed treatment) and their satisfaction with care including whether it meets their particular needs and respects their values and preferences.

National Voices has considered 779 systematic reviews which demonstrate the evidence for person-centered care [12]. The reviews showed that engaging people as active participants in their own healthcare leads to four key outcomes: the improvement of people's knowledge; better experience of services; better outcomes and better use of resources. Specifically, they found that there is evidence that engaging people as active participants in their own healthcare can

- improve people's experience and the quality of consultations and care
- inform people about health and healthcare and build health literacy
- ensure that treatment is appropriately selected and tailored to the individual
- help people manage their own care and records
- build partnerships with health professionals
- promote public health and reduce health inequalities

- ensure that health systems are responsive and accountable to the people they serve
- reduce wastage and make better use of scarce financial resources

Studies also show that people do want person-centered care, for example, in 2013, mental health services users in England were surveyed [2] and the results showed that users thought improvements were needed including in the areas of communication and information, reviewing care, involvement in decisions and support and understanding with other areas of life. In US, a study [14] sought to understand if shared decision making and/or receipt of mental health care was associated with patient satisfaction for patients with depression. From a sample of 1317 patients they found that shared decision making and receipt of mental health care were both positively associated with patient satisfaction.

9.4 Conclusions

The dissociation between healthcare which focuses on the condition and services that focus on other aspects of an individual's life are not useful. A person's health affects all aspects of their life and conversely their life affects their health and healthcare. It is therefore necessary to shift the focus of the entire healthcare system, to move away from focusing on the disease, making a patient a member of a disease group with general characteristics and to focus on the uniqueness of the personal experiences, considering what the disease means for the life and social participation of the individual.

Person-centered care can consider the best available evidence, the expertise of different professionals and patient's preferences and value them all. It recognises that patients are individuals and have different needs which the system can be responsive to, encouraging patients to take some responsibility for their healthcare whilst recognizing and respecting the limits in people's ability or their individual preferences.

There are different starting points for person-centered psychiatry around the world depending on national systems and economy, culture and attitudes and many different definitions and approaches being practised. What is important is that throughout the world, people understand about person-centered care and that people work in partnership to help shape health systems to focus holistically on respect for people's needs, preferences and wishes for their life and healthcare in the future.

There is a unique opportunity to move from the ad hoc practice of person-centered psychiatry to widespread practice. The starting point must be with the articulation of the patient's aspirations about what they want as an outcome in terms of their life which psychiatry and other health and social care services and options can support. The aim should be to improve the quality of life for people with mental health conditions, *as defined by them*. In order to shape health and social care services for the future so that they can meet people's needs, values and preferences, they must be meaningfully engaged in all aspects of healthcare policy and practice on an individual level and collectively.

References

1. All Party Parliamentary Groups on Global Health; HIV/AIDs; Population, Development and Reproductive Health; Global Tuberculosis; and Patient and Public Involvement in Health and Social Care. Patient empowerment: for better quality, more sustainable health services globally. 2014. www.appg-globalhealth.org.uk.
2. Care Quality Commission. Community mental health survey 2014. 2014. www.cqc.org.uk/content/community-mental-health-survey-2014.
3. Elwyn G, Coulter A, Laitner S, Walker E, Watson P, Thomson R. Implementing shared decision making in the NHS. BMJ. 2010;341:c5146. doi:10.1136/bmj.c5146.
4. European Network for Patient Empowerment. www.enope.eu/patient-empowerment.aspx.
5. International Alliance of Patients' Organizations. Declaration on patient-centred healthcare. 2006. http://iapo.org.uk/sites/default/filesfiles/IAPO_declaration_English.pdf.
6. International Alliance of Patients' Organizations. Policy statement on patient involvement. 2005. http://iapo.org.uk/sites/default/filesfiles/IAPO%20Policy%20Statement%20on%20Patient%20Involvement.pdf.
7. International College on Person-Centered Medicine. 2011. http://personcenteredmedicine.org/about-us.php.
8. International College on Person-Centered Medicine. 2014. http://personcenteredmedicine.org/doc/2014_Geneva_Declaration_Released_May_27.pdf.
9. Institute of Medicine. Crossing the quality chasm: a new health system for the 21st century. Washington, D.C.: National Academy Press; 2001.
10. Lutz B, Bowers B. Patient-centered care: understanding its interpretation and implementation in health care. J Sch Inquiry Nurs Pract. 2000;14(2):165–82.
11. Mental Health Foundation. Terminology. www.mentalhealth.org.uk/help-information/mental-health-a-z/T/terminology/.
12. National Voices. Prioritising person centred care: the evidence. 2014. www.nationalvoices.org.uk/evidence.
13. Oxford English Dictionary. 2005. http://www.oed.com.
14. Swanson KA, Bastani R, Rubenstein LV, Meredith LS, Ford DE. Effect of mental health care and shared decision making on patient satisfaction in a community sample of patients with depression. Med Care Res Rev. 2007;64(4):416–30. www.ncbi.nlm.nih.gov/pubmed/17684110.
15. World Heath Organization. Global status report on noncommunicable diseases 2014. 2014. www.who.int/nmh/publications/ncd-status-report-2014.
16. World Health Organization. Mental health action plan 2013–2020. 2013. http://apps.who.int/iris/bitstream/10665/89966/1/9789241506021_eng.pdf.
17. World Health Organization. People-centred and integrated care strategy. 2014. http://www.who.int/servicedeliverysafety/areas/people-centred-care/en/
18. World Health Organization. Declaration of Alma-Ata. 1978. http://www.who.int/publications/almaata_declaration_en.pdf.

References

Person-Centered Family Perspectives 10

Alessandro Svettini, MD, Sigrid Steffen and Spyros Zorbas

10.1 Introduction

Years and years—on a *round the clock* basis—of living with and caring for a person suffering from a mental illnesson one side is a big existential challenge, but on the other it provides family members a vast knowledge base and experience which can be available for sharing with the whole care team. This is a prime reason why families must be considered as an integral part of the primary care system.

A more holistic model is needed, addressing all aspects of a patient's health; a more modern approach-fostering empowerment and oriented to recovery-brings new responsibilities to all parties and the roles of clinicians, patients and carers require updating. In order to fully consider care as 'person-centered', it is essential a common understanding to be first established and that certain central characteristics are identified. Person-centered care [14] should encompass the following principles:

A. Svettini, MD (✉)
Psychiatrist, Psychotherapist—Department of Psychiatry, Health Trust of Bolzano, Servizio psichiatrico di Bolzano—Via Lorenz Boehler, 5, Bolzano 39100, Italy; Member of Board of Directors, EUropean Federation of Associations of FAmilies of People with Mental Illness (EUFAMI), Bolzano, Italy
e-mail: alessandro.svettini@asbz.it

S. Steffen
Past President, EUropean Federation of Associations of FAmilies of People with Mental Illness (EUFAMI), Salzburg, Austria

S. Zorbas
Economist and Mental Health Advocate, Member, European Federation of Associations of Families of People with Mental Illness (EUFAMI), Athens, Greece

J.E. Mezzich et al. (eds.), *Person Centered Psychiatry*,
DOI 10.1007/978-3-319-39724-5_10

- adopting an individual approach
- taking into account the patient's preferences, needs, interests, life goals, priorities; age, intelligence and health literacy level; family context, sociocultural background, ethnicity, environment, language and cultural barriers, strengths and weaknesses, mental status; type, severity, and duration of the disorder
- treating the patient as a person and not merely treating the symptoms of the disorder
- being flexibly connected with the phase of illness: prodromal, acute/relapsing, stabilizing, stable, recovery, and refractory
- being compassionate toward the suffering experienced by the patient and his/her family
- creating a culture of mutual respect among stakeholders, building true partnership of professionals with patients and family members
- collaboration, with active involvement and informed, shared decision-making by patient and family
- ensuring continuity of care, which must involve engaging the family
- comprehensiveness, integration, coordination, and accessibility of services and interventions offered
- cooperation with family, community and other external agencies and supports.

10.2 The Role of Families

The family is not only affected by their loved one's illness, but it usually plays a central role in the patient's care. Family members are very often the ones to meet the chronically ill person's primary needs and represent the main source of companionship, involvement in activities and assistance in coping with day-to-day problems, ensuring continuity of support and advocacy for the ill person. Besides, they provide help when necessary whilst respecting the wish and need of patients to help themselves; they can recognize the healthy aspects, the skills, and the resources of the patient beside the illness and can still maintain the trust and confidence of the patient, even if his/her attitude is unpleasant [18].

The family's functioning, emotional atmosphere, and their involvement in the treatment process have a significant influence on compliance as well as on the patient's coping and quality of life, particularly when coping with chronic diseases. The role of carers becomes fundamental in case of individuals with reduced levels of independence as well as cognitive and emotional capabilities (children, elderly, people with mental retardation or severe mental illness), in particular in the communication encounters with doctors and other health providers [19].

During the past three decades, numerous factors have contributed to focus more on families that are coping with serious mental disorders [12]:

1. Deinstitutionalization, with reduced accessibility to hospitals for even floridly ill psychotic patients, and increased responsibilities for care and support of the mentally ill by their relatives.
2. Realization that while pharmacotherapy can reduce or eliminate symptoms, stress-related relapse and functional decompensation require psychosocial services, including the mobilization of families as a factor in achieving recovery.
3. Realization that families are not responsible for causing serious mental disorders and deserve the respect, support, attention, and education that they need to participate constructively in the management and treatment of their mentally ill relatives.
4. Recognition that the stress-induced dysfunctions in communication and problem solving within families are a consequence, not a cause, of mental disorders.
5. Empirical studies that have shown how families can serve to protect their ill relatives from relapse and dysfunctional lives if they are prepared to cope with the enormous challenges posed by the illness. On the other side, patients experience high rates of relapse when living or interacting with relatives who lack the skills and resources to constructively collaborate in the treatment.
6. Development of behavioral, cognitive, and educational methods for clinical problems in psychiatry that offer practical help for patients and families of all social classes and that supersede less applicable psychodynamic and insight therapies.
7. Availability of well-designed and evidence-based practices that can reliably strengthen the coping, communication, and problem-solving skills of patients as well as of their relatives.
8. Stress and burden experienced by families who are ill equipped to manage their mentally ill relatives at home. Families have become assertive in requesting information and training to deal with stress that can result in anxiety, depression, and demoralization.
9. Reduction of stigma of mental illness and increased public awareness about and acceptance of mental disorders as bona fide illnesses that deserve treatment. Reduced stigma has led to families "coming out of the closet" to seek professional assistance to become educated about their relatives' mental disorders, and to advocate for their relatives' treatment and rehabilitative needs.
10. Growth of vital advocacy and self-help movements by relatives of mentally ill persons that have organized at national and international level, in order to promote better care, have their voices heard and their rights respected.

Families of persons with schizophrenia and other disabling disorders [12] usually pass through 10 phases as they try to adjust to living with the uncertain prospects and life-changing challenges of a mentally ill relative. These phases are not always linear but can recur in cycles, depending upon the stability of their ill relative and the assistance they receive from psychiatrists, other mental health professionals, and self-help organizations. Having the competence and emotional resilience to assist families as they move through these phases is a major responsibility for clinicians caring for the ill relative. Bearing with the family through the phases requires continuity of collaborative care. The 10 phases are as follows:

1. Initial awareness that a problem exists—early signs of symptoms and abnormal behavior: "*Must be just a phase he/she is going through*"
2. Denial of a mental illness—attributing the symptoms to a temporary aberration, stress, or illicit drugs
3. Searching for a cure: "*Give me my son/daughter back again*"
4. Accepting the existence of a mental illness but frustrated by its inadequate, limited treatments
5. Demoralization, depression, anxiety, worry, anger: "*It's like losing a loved one, but there's no death and the person is still there but not the same person*"
6. Becoming educated and knowledgeable about the illness
7. Advocating for better treatment and rehabilitative services for the ill relative
8. Cycles of optimism and pessimism as new treatments appear promising and then fail to deliver sustained improvement or to prevent relapses
9. Cumulative know-how in coping with the illness—navigating with increasing confidence through the stormy seas of the inevitable ups and downs of the illness and facilitating access to services
10. Participating in self-help groups, advocating for better services, becoming active in fighting stigma—helping others through the phases of adaptation to long-term illness and disability.

Family associationism is at the same time catalyst, result, and promoter of empowerment processes. Worldwide there are two main examples of organized movements of families of mentally ill persons: National Alliance on Mental Illness (NAMI) in the United States and European Federation of Associations of Families of People with Mental Illness (EUFAMI) in Europe.

NAMI,[1] founded in 1979, is the largest grassroots mental health organization in the USA. Its mission is to improve the lives of the millions of Americans affected by mental illness and their families. NAMI advocates for access to services, treatment, supports and research and is steadfast in its commitment to raise awareness and build a community for hope for all of those in need. It also offers a wide array of support and education programs for people living with a mental illness, their family members, partners and friends, as well as for providers of mental health services, school professionals, and for the general public.

EUFAMI[2] is an international nonprofit organization registered in Belgium that primarily advocates on behalf of carers. Founded in December 1992, it is active in lobbying European Union bodies on behalf of its member organizations. EUFAMI is a federation of 46 family associations and has members in 27 European countries, representing more than 5 millions of European citizens affected by mental illness and their family members. Its mission is to represent all family members of persons affected by severe mental illness at European level so that their rights and interests are protected and promoted. EUFAMI activities are articulated in several areas: recognition of the role of the family, empowerment, representation, capacity

[1]www.nami.org

[2]www.eufami.org

building, and support for member associations across Europe, promotion of best practice and public awareness, development of partnership, defense of the human rights of people with mental illness and their families.

10.3 Needs and Challenges of Carers

Family members have needs which often are overlooked and neglected: they need to be informed and educated on the nature of the illness and its therapeutic possibilities, trained in order to develop skills to cope with symptoms and disabilities, supported in their caring role and given respite opportunities, involved and empowered in shared information and decision-making together with patient and professionals [4, 20].

There is already a general recognition that carers' needs are closely linked with those of the person they care for; however, burdens of carers themselves and circumstances of care still need to be more specifically researched.

The *Caring for Carers* (C4C) *Survey* is an international survey being undertaken by EUFAMI, in collaboration with LUCAS (Center for care research and consultancy of the University of Leuven, Belgium) to understand the needs and challenges faced by carers supporting those living with a mental health illness. The purpose of this study, the first of its kind, is to capture and document the experiences and well-being of family caregivers of persons living with schizophrenia, offering more insight into the caregiver's role in mental disease management.

The survey follows an exploratory study design, with no predefined hypothesis; the topics addressed are: socio demographic and illness-related characteristics, well-being, need for support, satisfaction with professional support. In addition to these topics, the questionnaire also gleans information on the basic profile of carers, their experiences, and financial, emotional, and physical burdens. The questionnaires are disseminated through EUFAMI's member organizations in 25 countries and administered on paper, by email, or online. The survey by the time of writing this chapter is ongoing in 25[3] countries, mainly in the EU, and will close by the end of 2014. The first results are based on responses from more than 400 carers in Australia, Canada, France, Germany, Italy, Spain, and the UK.

The focus is on members of families of people with severe mental illness (included are carers who take on acute care as well as long-term care), with around 90 % of respondents caring for someone with schizophrenia. Family members are the likely primary carers, and can spend an average of 6–9 h a day caring; they consequently experience high personal impact, which can threaten their own long-term well-being.

[3]Countries surveyed: Australia, Austria, Belgium, Canada, Cyprus, Czech Republic, Denmark, Finland, France, Germany, Greece, Ireland, Israel, Italy, Lithuania, Malta, Netherlands, Norway, Portugal, Russia, Slovenia, Spain, Sweden, Switzerland, United Kingdom.

The preliminary results show that approximately three out of four (72 %) carers of those living with schizophrenia are mainly (34 %) or solely (38 %) responsible for caring, placing a huge emotional and physical burden on them. Family members perform their caregiver role for an average of 16 years, are likely to have to do so for the rest of their lives—due to the undetermined and long-term nature of schizophrenia—and report an average of 23 h a week caring for a loved one.

The average age of the carers surveyed is 61 years, with the majority (84 %) caring for a son or daughter. Many express deep concerns about what will happen to their child when they are unable to care for them or will no longer be 'around.'

Although about 1/3 of the carers report positive experiences of providing care, the survey also indicates that almost 40 % battle with feelings of being unable to cope with the 'constant anxiety' of caring, and 1/3 feel depressed. With this constant level of pressure, a third of carers are reported to be reaching 'breaking point' and feeling they cannot carry on with things the way they are. More than 1 in 10 carers worry about feeling isolated and experience strains in their social network because of the care they give.

Positive caregiving experiences are eclipsed by the fact that there is a degree of dissatisfaction with the level of, or lack of, support from care professionals. 92 % of carers surveyed want more support on several domains. The survey highlights carers' desire to be more involved in treatment conversations and to be better equipped to influence care decisions. A lack of support and dissatisfaction are expressed by family carers: 38 % feel they are not taken seriously by medical/care staff and 44 % are not feeling satisfied with their ability to influence important decisions in treatment and care planning.

The final results of the C4C survey are published in 2015. Already these preliminary findings highlight the contribution of people caring for those living with schizophrenia, offering evidence of the immense and unspoken burden they carry and the overwhelming impact this condition has on their own lives.

Families fulfill a distinct and important role by providing support and advocating for their ill relatives as well as contributing to their recovery. Caring for someone with schizophrenia takes time, energy, financial and emotional resources [13]. Although caregiving may give rise to positive feelings and experiences, carers feel highly exposed and caring for a relative with mental illness is related to high personal suffering, feelings of guilt, helplessness, fear, vulnerability, anxiety, and anger [21]. When a mental illness 'enters' the family circle, family members tend to remove themselves from their natural support networks for a number of different reasons [10]. Additionally, at the age of onset of a child's mental illness, the age of family carers (40–60 years) and the possibility of separation or divorce mean that they are at a time of great family stress and pressure. Given that the frequency and intensity of psychotic episodes is unpredictable in those with schizophrenia, coping with such a condition poses ongoing challenges to family carers [13].

Caregivers often experience a financial burden due to their caregiving, trapped in a so-called *sandwich situation*: the obligations toward their family member and toward their own job produce a conflict. When there is not enough understanding on the part of the employer, some people even lose their job—which in return is also a loss of talent for society.

Carers for people affected by psychosis often feel undervalued. Despite the essential role that family carers perform, they are not fully recognized as crucial partners in care so far. The contribution of families must be acknowledged appropriately and they should have the right and opportunity to state their needs and to define the role they are willing and able to play [6]. Family members need to be fully recognized for their contributions, that their voices are heard and that they are supported in order to allow them to continue caring effectively and safely for their loved ones, without putting their own physical and emotional well-being at risk. Healthcare professionals need to acknowledge that family carers can play a much stronger role, integrate them in treatment decisions and work together to achieve better outcomes for the patient.

10.4 Improving Communication

The manner in which families and medical professionals approach life and issues is very different: families tend to be impatient and thus approach issues in a very pragmatic way, whereas professionals view an issue from an evidence-based perspective [18]. Different approaches may need a particular attention on the communication used among stakeholders. Clinical communication is fundamental in building a therapeutic doctor–patient relationship, as well as the partnership with the patient's family.

In these past years the medical model has evolved from paternalism to individualism. Information exchange is nowadays the dominant communication model, and the health consumer movement has led to the current model of shared decision-making and patient-centered communication [1, 9, 17].

Because family members take on caring tasks and also suffer as a consequence of the illness of the patient, communication between health care professionals and family members of the patient is important. Involving family members and carers through an adequate communication allows a better understanding of the clinical condition, improves interaction between patient and carers, reduces the emotional burden and the expressed emotion levels in the family.

There is increasing awareness and evidence regarding the importance of clear and effective communication between patients, families, and medical staff as a cornerstone of providing quality health care. It is very important to understand the perspectives, knowledge and expectations of the patient and his/her family, sharing the available information [2, 15]. This can enhance adherence to treatments and allows a real inclusion of all stakeholders, in a condition where responsibilities of the care are shared with the practitioner and the patient is fully empowered in the decision-making process.

How to communicate is then crucial. There is a profound difference between communicating *to* patients and families and communicating *with* them. An optimal patient and family communication is about conveying a message as well as establishing a connection. The three main goals of effective communication are: creating a good interpersonal relationship, facilitating exchange of information, and including patients and their families in decision-making [1, 3, 11, 16].

Patient surveys have demonstrated that when communication is lacking it is palpably felt and it can lead to patients feeling increased anxiety, vulnerability, and powerlessness. Research in a variety of settings [8, 22] has found that suboptimal provider-patient/family communication is common, with negative effects on patient/family-centered outcomes.

Patients and their families do better when they are involved, informed and engaged in the process. Patients who understand their providers are more likely to accept their health problems, understand their treatment options, modify their behavior and adhere to follow-up instructions [5]. There are evidence-based clinical and ethical guidelines for health care staff, patients, and families to promote the efficacy of and the satisfaction with communication and collaborative care. Systematic interventions of communication quality improvement result in better patient care and shorter hospital stays, improve the level of care, the clinical decision-making process and family outcomes [7].

10.5 A New Approach to Professional Training

With regards to current training and training methods for psychiatry, a major seed change is required to ensure that the emphasis is placed more on the patient rather than on the illness and secondly that 'family training' is recognized as part of the official training curriculum of professionals.

Family members have gained a great deal of experience and have much to teach the medical community. Their expertise should be acknowledged and valued. Families should be involved in education and training of medical staff working in mental health services. Involvement of carers in mental health training is a beneficial development for service users and professionals, but it requires further work. From the limited amount of feedback that is available where families have become involved in the training of professionals, mental health professionals have more positive attitudes toward families, use less jargon and become more optimistic about patients' recovery. Families and carers, on the other hand, are empowered, have a better relationship with mental health professionals and enjoy far more personal satisfaction and improved quality of life. Attitudes dramatically change and everyone benefits—especially the person with the mental illness. Barriers begin to come down [18].

New modules need to be introduced to cover human aspects related to the patient and the family. In the long run, the participation of all interested parties in the care team will evolve and will result in a better and easier life for all concerned—the patient will feel more involved and take ownership; the medical profession will feel more relaxed and life will be easier as there will be more dialogue; the family member will feel valued and less isolated.

10.6 Conclusions

When dealing with severe mental illness, families have been seen for too long as a potential or real problem. Families can become empowered through person-centered care, so that a sense of commitment and a feeling of being valued can be achieved. Family involvement can help to reduce stress (by listening and giving space to 'chill out' or 'let steam off'), can help to establish a regular routine and encourage adherence to the care plan and to medication. A person- and family-centered approach allows to set the premises in order to have carers become a great resource. Ultimately we all want good services, support, information, advice, training and advocacy, and an end to stigma and discrimination. This can only be achieved by putting the patient at the center of the system, integrating the family in the patient's treatment plan as well as in person-centered education and training of medical staff.

References

1. Arora N. Interacting with cancer patients: the significance of physicians communication behavior. Soc Sci Med. 2003;57(5):791–806.
2. Baile WF, Buckman R, Lenzi R, Glober G, Beale EA, Kudelka AP. SPIKES—a six-step protocol for delivering bad news: application to the patient with cancer. Oncologist. 2000;5 (4):302–11.
3. Brédart A, Bouleuc C, Dolbeault S. Doctor-patient communication and satisfaction with care in oncology. Curr Opin Oncol. 2005;17(14):351–4.
4. Dixon L, McFarlane W, Lefley H, et al. Evidence-based practices for services to families of people with psychiatric disabilities. Psychiatr Serv. 2001;52:903–10.
5. Epstein RM. Making communication research matter: what do patients notice, what do patients want, and what do patients need? Patient Educ Couns. 2006;60(3):272–8.
6. EUFAMI. Position paper on family carers' needs. 2013. Available from: http://www.eufami.org/publications/position-papers/eufami-s-position-paper-on-family-carers-needs. Accessed 20th Oct 2014.
7. Fawole OA, Dy SM, Wilson RF, Lau BD, Martinez KA, Apostol CC, Vollenweider D, Bass EB, Aslakson RA. A systematic review of communication quality improvement interventions for patients with advanced and serious illness. J Gen Intern Med. 2013;28 (4):570–7.
8. Fong Ha J, Longnecker N. Doctor-patient communication: a review. Ochsner J. 2010;10 (1):38–43.
9. Henrdon J, Pollick K. Continuing concerns, new challenges, and next steps in physician-patient communication. J Bone Joint Surg Am. 2002;84 A(2):309–15.
10. Jones K. Family carer education in mental health. In: WHO Regional Office for Europe, empowerment in mental health meeting—working together towards leadership, Leuven, Belgium, 27–28 Oct 2010.
11. Lee SJ, Back AL, Block SD, Stewart SK. Enhancing physician-patient communication. Hematology Am Soc Hematol Educ Program. 2002;1:464–83.
12. Liberman RP. Recovery from disability. Manual of Psychiatric Rehabilitation. Washinghton D.C.: American Psychiatric Publishing; 2008.
13. MacCourt P. Family Caregivers Advisory Committee and Mental Health Commission of Canada. 2013.
14. Mezzich JE, Christodoulou G, Fulford KWM. Introduction to the conceptual bases of psychiatry for the person. Int J Person Cent Med. 2011;1(1):121–4.

15. Parker SM, Clayton JM, Hancock K, et al. A systematic review of prognostic/end-of-life communication with adults in the advanced stages of life-limiting illness: patient/caregiver preferences for the content, style, and timing of information. J Pain Symptom Manage. 2007;3 (1):81–93.
16. Platt FW, Keating KN. Differences in physician and patient perceptions of uncomplicated UTI symptom severity: understanding the communication gap. Int J Clin Prac. 2007;61(2):303–8.
17. Sawyer SM, Aroni RA. Sticky issue of adherence. J Paediatr Child Health. 2003;39(1):2–5.
18. Steffen S. EUFAMI'S initiatives on person-centred care. In: 3rd geneva conference on person-centered medicine. Geneva, Switzerland, 3–5 May 2010.
19. Svettini A. Research on communication among professionals, patients and families. In: Abstract book 6th Geneva conference on person-centered medicine. Geneva, April 29–May 1, 2013 p. 25.
20. Svettini A. The role of families in person-centered and integrative care. In: Abstract book 7th Geneva conference on person-centered medicine. Geneva, April 27–30, 2014. pp. 28–29.
21. WFMH. Caring for the caregiver: why your mental health matters when you are caring for others. 2009. (Online) Available from: http://wfmh.com/wpcontent/uploads/2013/11/WFMH_GIAS_CaringForTheCaregiver.pdf. Accessed Apr 2014.
22. Wilz G, Meichsner F. Involving family members of chronically ill patients in physician-patient communication. Bundesgesundheitsblatt Gesundheitsforschung Gesundheitsschutz. 2012;55 (9):1125–31.

Part II
Diagnosis and Assessment

Person-Centered Integrative Diagnosis and Its Context

11

Juan E. Mezzich, MD, MA, MS, PhD, Ihsan M. Salloum, MD, MPH,
C. Robert Cloninger, MD, PhD and Michel Botbol, MD

11.1 Introduction

The implementation of person-centered psychiatry and medicine requires a suitable person-centered diagnostic model. The bases of a Person-centered Integrative Diagnosis (PID) model include therefore the principles of person-centered medicine, an institutional framework that could nurture its development, and the engagement of the most suitable and helpful diagnostic methodology. To present this concisely is the purpose of the first section of this chapter.

J.E. Mezzich, MD, MA, MS, PhD (✉)
Former President, World Psychiatric Association, Geneva, Switzerland; Professor of Psychiatry, Icahn School of Medicine at Mount Sinai, New York, USA; Editor in Chief, International Journal of Person Centered Medicine, New York, USA; Professor of Psychiatry, Icahn School of Medicine at Mount Sinai, New York, USA
e-mail: juanmezzich@aol.com

I.M. Salloum, MD, MPH
Professor of Psychiatry, University of Miami School of Medicine, Miami, FL, USA; Chair, Section on Classification, Diagnostic Assessment and Nomenclature, World Psychiatric Association, Geneva, Switzerland

C. Robert Cloninger, MD, PhD
Wallace Renard Professor of Psychiatry Genetics, and Psychology, St Louis, MO, USA; Director, Center for Wellbeing, Washington University School of Medicine, St Louis, MO, USA

M. Botbol, MD
Professor of Child and Adolescent Psychiatry, Western Brittany University, Brest, France; Chief of Child Psychiatry Service, University Hospital, Brest, France; Chair, Section on Psychoanalysis in Psychiatry, World Psychiatric Association, Geneva, Switzerland

J.E. Mezzich et al. (eds.), *Person Centered Psychiatry*,
DOI 10.1007/978-3-319-39724-5_11

The second one will outline the person-centered diagnosis model. Such presentation will include its informational domain in terms of standardized health status, health contributors (including risk and protective factors), and health experience and values (including expectations and preferences). It will also cover the descriptive instruments for diagnostic formulation and the interactive process among clinicians, patient, and family.

The third section will refer to practical guides for the implementation of the PID model. Particular attention will be given to the Latin American Guide for Psychiatric Diagnosis, revised Version (GLADP-VR), which has been published by the Latin American Psychiatric Association (APAL) for the use of health professionals in the region and beyond.

The final section will deal with important aspects of the context of the diagnostic effort. One are the conditions and requirements for effective diagnostic interviewing, data gathering and formulation. The other is the articulation of diagnosis with clinical care planning.

11.2 Background of Person-Centered Diagnosis

11.2.1 Conceptual Bases

The overarching framework of person-centered diagnosis is person-centered medicine (PCM). From the beginning of the construction of person-centered medicine, it has been referred to as an approach that places the person in context (and not organs or disease) at the center and as the goal of medicine and health care. It has also been emphasized that PCM seeks fundamentally to articulate science and humanism in medicine and health care and refocusing these on the whole person [38].

Furthermore, it has been posited that PCM is dedicated to the promotion of health as a state of physical, mental, sociocultural and spiritual well-being as well as to the reduction of disease, and founded on mutual respect for the dignity and responsibility of each individual person [15].

The purposes of the PCM have been also summarized as promoting a medicine *of the person* (of the totality of the person's health, including its ill and positive aspects), *for the person* (promoting the fulfillment of the person's life project), *by the person* (with clinicians extending themselves as full human beings with high ethical aspirations) and *with the person* (working respectfully, in collaboration and in an empowering manner) [25, 37].

Concerning the identification of key concepts underlying PCM, the one that seems to have been most emphasized is its ethical base. This is indicating that ethics is fundamental for all medical activities, including clinical care, education, and research [8, 32]. It has also been argued by two recent presidents of the World Medical Association that PCM represents an ethical imperative for the medical profession [17].

Along the lines of such inquiries, a recent bibliographic and consultation study to explore the systematic conceptualization of person-centered medicine [34], has elucidated the following key concepts: ethical commitment, holistic scope, cultural awareness and responsiveness, communication and relationship focus, individualized treatment, common ground for diagnosis and care, people-centered systems of care, and person-centered health education and research.

11.2.2 Institutional Bases

From the viewpoint of the institutional construction of person-centered psychiatry and medicine, it should be noted that the World Psychiatric Association (WPA), which was born from the articulation of science and humanism [19], established at its 2005 General Assembly an Institutional Program on Psychiatry for the Person [14, 25]. This initiative expanded into general medicine through a series of Geneva Conferences since 2008 in collaboration with the World Medical Association, the World Health Organization, the International Council of Nurses, the International Federation of Social Workers, the International Pharmaceutical Federation, the European Federation of Families of Persons with Mental Illness, and the International Alliance of Patients' Organizations, among a growing number of other international health institutions [26].

The process and impact of the Geneva conferences led to the emergence of the International Network (now International College) of Person Centered Medicine (INPCM, ICPCM) [27, 37]. The ICPCM launched in 2011 the *International Journal of Person Centered Medicine* in collaboration with the University of Buckingham Press [39].

11.2.3 Diagnostic Methodological Bases

The eminent historian and philosopher of medicine Lain Entralgo [23] has cogently argued that diagnosis goes beyond identifying a disease (*nosological diagnosis*) to also involve *understanding* of what is going on in the body and mind of the person who presents for care. Understanding an individual's clinical condition also requires a broader assessment of experience and life context. As health may be conceived as a person's capacity to continue to pursue his or her goals in an ever-challenging world [12] this encompassing perspective should be incorporated in a thorough diagnosis of health. There are indeed compelling reasons for including health-promoting or *salutogenic* factors [7] and positive health [24] under comprehensive diagnosis, bringing it to consistency with WHO's definition of health [49]. Diagnostic understanding also requires a process of engagement and empowerment that recognizes the agency of patient, family, and health professionals participating in a *trialogical* partnership [6].

In connection with the above, one should examine the concept of the *validity* of diagnosis as it denotes its value and usefulness. Traditionally, this validity has been anchored on the faithfulness and accuracy with which a diagnosis reflects and identifies a disorder, its nature, pathophysiology, and other biomedical indicators [43]. Recently, *clinical utility* has been proposed as an additional indication of the value of diagnosis for clinical care [21]. Schaffner [46] has delineated further the epistemology of these two forms of diagnostic validity under the terms of *etio-pathogenic and clinical validities.* Pointing out the significance of the latter, experienced clinicians suggest that treatment planning is the most important purpose of diagnosis [3].

Concerning the architecture of diagnostic formulations, there has been a progressive development of diagnostic schemas with increasing levels of informational richness particularly to support treatment planning. These have ranged from a simple, typological *single-label diagnosis* denoting a symptom, problem, syndrome, or illness to a more complex *multiple illness formulation,* listing all identified clinical conditions or disorders, including coexisting psychiatric and general medical diseases. Such schemas intend to provide a fuller portrayal of the nosological condition, as well as other aspects of clinical interest such as disabilities, contextual factors, and quality of life, thus attempting to enhance diagnostic understanding, treatment planning, and prognostic determination [11]. Multiaxial diagnostic formulations are key components of most contemporary diagnostic systems including ICD-10 [50, 51], DSM-IV [4], GLADP [10], GC-3 [42], the French Classification for Child and Adolescent Mental Disorders [40], and the Chinese Classification of Mental Disorders [13]. Of note, a multiaxial schema was not included in DSM-5 [5], despite that a broad APA Committee established to evaluate DSM multiaxial systems documented their usefulness [29].

Another approach to comprehensive diagnosis involves both standardized and idiographic components. One such model is at the core of the International Guidelines for Diagnostic Assessment (IGDA), developed by the WPA [30]. Its standardized multiaxial component includes four axes dealing, respectively, with clinical disorders, disabilities, contextual factors, and quality of life. Its idiographic and narrative component covers the clinician perspective, perspectives of the patient and family, and integration of the perspectives of all the above. Many of the methodological developments highlighted above have been discussed in a WPA Psychiatry for the Person volume [44].

11.3 The Person-Centered Integrative Diagnosis Model

11.3.1 Development of the Model

The suitability of the prospective elements of PID was examined through surveys and consultations. Building on its long experience in developing diagnostic models, the WPA Section on Classification, Diagnostic Assessment and Nomenclature conducted a survey among the members of the 43-country Global Network of National Classification and Diagnosis Groups [45]. The survey was constructed in consultation with network members and aimed at surveying the most important domains to consider in the development of future diagnostic classification for psychiatric disorders. Of the group 74 % responded. Treatment planning was most frequently chosen as the key role of diagnosis. Communication among clinicians and diagnosis as a means to enhance illness understanding were also identified as key roles of diagnosis. The survey also highlighted the areas of information judged important to be covered by psychiatric diagnosis. These included disorders (100 %), disabilities (74 %), risk factors (61 %), experience of illness (58 %), protective factors (55 %), and experience of health (52 %). The responses suggested that in addition to the recognized importance of nosological diagnosis, subjective explanatory narratives of illness and health are also quite valuable. The survey responses also highlighted the importance of utilizing a variety of descriptive tools including categories (81 %), dimensions (74 %), and narratives (45 %). It also revealed that 80 % of responders choose clinicians, patients, and carers together as key players in the diagnostic evaluation process as compared to clinicians alone (20 %).

A number of focus and discussion groups were organized in 2009 with a variety of health stakeholders (health professionals, patients, family members, and advocates) at international events in Athens (Greece), Uppsala (Sweden), and Timisoara (Romania) [45]. In an overwhelming manner, the participants in the three settings considered that diagnosis should go beyond disease. Participants unanimously responded that diagnosis should cover dysfunctions and a great majority of them felt it is very important to include positive aspects of health. Over 83 % of the participants endorsed the inclusion of experience of health as part of diagnosis. Furthermore, there was unanimous agreement on incorporating contributing factors (including risk and protective factors), and on the use of descriptive methods, including dimensions and narratives in addition to conventional categories. Participants also emphasized that diagnosis is a process and not only a formulation and highlighted the partnership between caregivers and service users as fundamental.

11.3.2 Structure of the Person-Centered Integrative Diagnosis Model

The delineation of the structure of the PID must take into account that diagnosis is both a formulation and a process. The presentation of the fundamental elements of the model is made here in terms of the following three defining conceptual pillars: (a) Broad Informational Domains, (b) Pluralistic Descriptive Procedures, and (c) Partnership for Diagnostic Evaluation.

The PID framework's first pillar, *Broad Informational Domains*, is depicted in Fig. 11.1. These domains cover both ill health and positive health along three structural levels: Health Status, Experience of Health, and Contributors to Health.

The broadness of the PID informational domains, including ill and positive health, is intrinsic to holistic person-centered health care. The domain level on *Health Status*, includes first illnesses or disorders of both mental and physical forms, which correspond to Laín-Entralgo's [23] nosological diagnosis. They may be assessed according to the international standard, WHO's International Classification of Diseases (ICD) or a pertinent national or regional version or adaptation

ILL HEALTH	***POSITIVE HEALTH***
I. Health Status	
Illness & its Burden **a. Disorders** **b. Disabilities**	**Well Being** **Recovery/Wellness** **Functioning**
II. Contributors to Health	
Contributors to Illness **(Intrinsic/Extrinsic: Biological, Psychological, Social)**	**Contributors to Health** **(Intrinsic/Extrinsic: Biological, Psychological, Social)**
III. Experience of Health	
Experience of Illness **(e.g. suffering, values, perception, Understanding and meaning of illness)**	**Experience of Health** **(e.g. identity, contentment, & fulfillment)**

Fig. 11.1 Key structural levels covering ill health and positive health in the person-centered integrative diagnosis model

[35]. Disabilities would be assessed through procedures such as those based on the International Classification of Functioning and Health (ICF) [52]. The assessment of the well-being aspect of Health Status could be conducted through standard scales such as the WHOQOL Instrument [41] and the Multicultural Quality of Life Index [33]. An update on this domain can be found in Salloum et al. in Chap. 12 of this volume.

The domain level on *Experience of Health* would appraise the patient's illness- and health-related values and cultural experiences, possibly with a guided narrative procedure built on world-wide experience with the Cultural Formulation [31]. More recently, this domain has been reformulated in terms of Health Experience and Values (Kirmayer et al. in Chap. 14 of this volume).

The third domain level on *Contributors to Health* would cover a range of intrinsic and extrinsic biological, psychological, and social factors of both risk and protective types. Their assessment may involve a combination of procedures aimed at assessing healthy and unhealthy life-style factors and related health contributors [47]. Update information on this domain can be found in Chap. 13 of this volume by Saavedra, Villar, and Botbol.

The PID model's second defining pillar, *Pluralistic Descriptive Procedures*, opens up the opportunity to employ categories, dimensions, and narratives for greater flexibility and effectiveness for the evaluation task at hand [20, 22]. Further information on PID descriptive tools can be found in Chap. 15 of this volume by Botbol and Salvador-Carulla.

The third defining pillar of the PID model is *Partnership for Evaluation.* Such partnership is a fundamental element of person-centered care, and involves the pursuit of engagement, empathy and empowerment as well as respect for the autonomy and dignity of the consulting person. In fact, it is crucial for achieving shared understanding for diagnosis and shared decision-making (SDM) for treatment planning [3].

Additional information on the elements of the PID model can be found in Mezzich et al. [36].

11.4 PID-Related Practical Diagnostic Guides

Models need to have applications in the forms of guides or manuals for generalized use and real-world evaluation of their applicability, reliability, and validity.

11.4.1 The Latin American Guide for Psychiatric Diagnosis, Revised Version (GLADP-VR)

An application of the PID model is at the core of the Latin American Guide of Psychiatric Diagnosis, Revised Version (GLADP-VR) [9]. Its cover is presented in Fig. 11.2.

This Guide represents a revised version of the first GLADP edition [10]. Both editions of the GLADP were published officially by the Asociacion Psiquiatrica de America Latina (Latin American Psychiatric Association) through their Section on Diagnosis and Classification for the use of health professionals in this world region. As both editions use WHO ICD diagnostic codes, categories, and descriptions, the GLADP can be considered an adaptation of ICD for Latin America, complemented with Latin American Annotations to facilitate the use of ICD categories in this part of the world.

The GLADP-VR incorporates the basic elements of the PID model. The main difference between the PID model and the GLADP-VR schema is that the former has Health Experience as the second informational domain level while the latter has Health Experience as the third level. Furthermore, the GLADP-VR third level is enriched in its content with health values and expectations, in line with growing concern for incorporating these perspectives in a basic diagnostic formulation [18].

The **key information domains or levels** of the GLADP-VR diagnostic schema are summarized below.

11.4.1.1 Health Status

The first component of this model corresponds to Health Status. This includes standardized coverage of both pathological and positive aspects of health. As shown on the GLADP-VR Personalized Diagnostic Formulation, The Health Status component starts with a listing of mental and general medical disorders and other significant clinical conditions. These disorders and conditions are to be coded according to the various chapters of ICD-10, including, in addition to standard disease codes, the Z codes for non-disease conditions that require clinical attention.

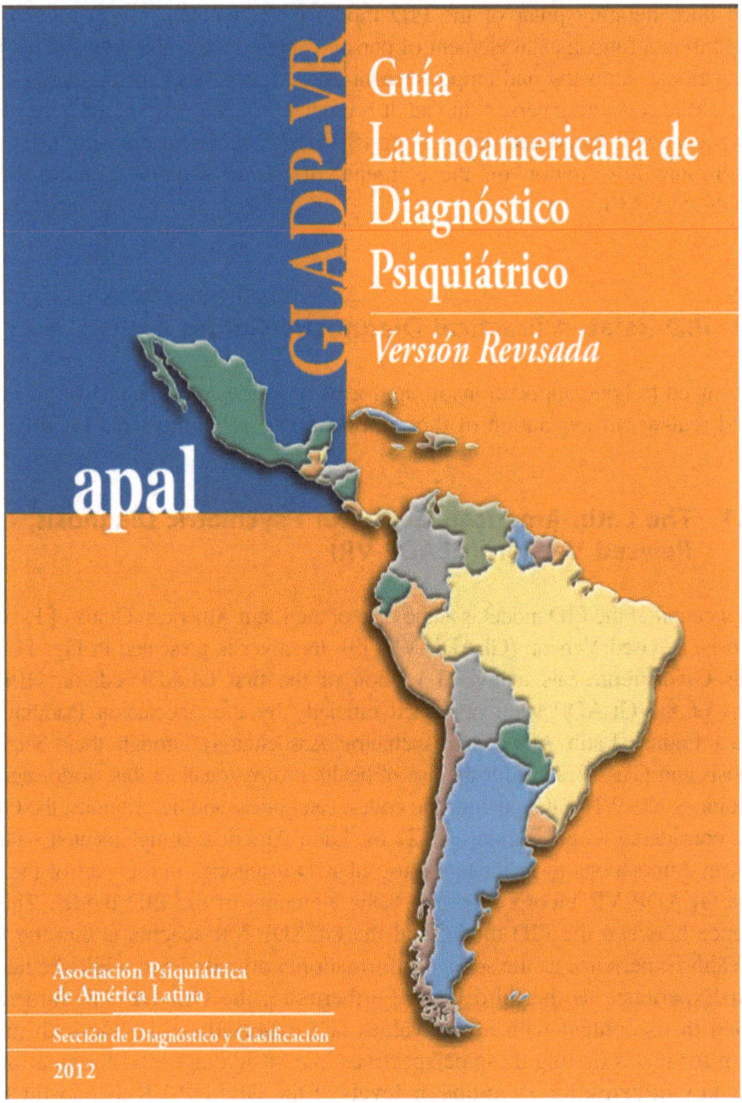

Fig. 11.2 Cover of the Latin American guide of psychiatric diagnosis, revised version (GLADP-VR)

Next in the Health Status component comes the evaluation of Personal Functioning in the areas of personal care, occupational, family, and social activities, each measured with a 10-point scale marked as follows: 0: worst functioning, 2: minimal functioning, 4: marginal functioning, 6: acceptable functioning, 8: substantial functioning, and 10: optimal functioning.

Finally, the Health Status component assesses degree of the person's well-being, from worst to excellent, by directly marking on the 10-point line displayed on the Formulation Form, with or without the help of an appropriate standardized instrument. This assessment is principally based on the judgment of the person involved, modulated collaboratively with perceptions by the clinicians and family.

11.4.1.2 Health Contributing Factors

The second component of the GLADP-VR Personalized Diagnostic Formulation corresponds to Health Contributing Factors. These include Risk Factors as well as Protective and Health Promotion Factors. Assessment in each case starts with the identification of relevant factors from the list presented on the form. These factors come from the Health Improvement Card prepared by the World Health Professions Alliance [47], supplemented by some factors particularly relevant to mental health. It continues with a narrative formulation of additional information about the identified factors and others that could also be elicited.

11.4.1.3 Health Experience and Expectations

The third component of the GLADP-VR Personalized Diagnostic Formulation assesses Experience and Expectations on Health. This is based on the combination of elements from the experientially described Cultural Formulation [31] and of patient's needs and preferences [18]. This assessment is obtained through narratives on the following three points: (a) personal and cultural identity (self-awareness and its potentials and limitations), (b) suffering (its recognition, idioms of distress, and beliefs on illness), and (c) experiences with and expectations and preferences for health care [28]. As mentioned before, further information on the conceptual bases for this level can be seen in Chap. 14 by Kirmayer, Mezzich and Van Staden in the present volume.

The actual layout of a personalized diagnostic formulation according to the GLADP-VR can be seen in Fig. 11.3.

11.4.2 Other PID Practical Applications

A full Second Edition of the Latin American Guide for Psychiatric Diagnosis (GLADP-2) is in the works as a priority project of the Diagnosis and Classification Section of the APAL. For covering mental and general medical disorders, it would be based on the categories and codes of the prospective Eleventh Revision of the International Classification of Diseases (ICD-11) which is expected to be completed around 2017. Its development would be based on the ongoing experience implementing, teaching, and studying the GLADP-VR.

There are also plans to develop under the auspices of the International College of Person Centered Medicine (ICPCM) other PID practical guides intended for use in general medicine.

I: HEALTH STATUS

Clinical Disorders and Related Conditions (as classified in CIE-10).

A. Mental Disorders (in general, including personality and developmental disorders, and related conditions):

	Codes:

B. General Medical Conditions:

	Codes:

Functioning of the Person (Use the following scale to evaluate each of the functioning areas)

Poorest		Minimal		Marginal		Acceptable		Substantial		Excellent
0	1	2	3	4	5	6	7	8	9	10

Functioning Areas		Score						
A	Personal care	0	2	4	6	8	10	?
B	Occupational (wage earner, student, etc.)	0	2	4	6	8	10	?
C	With family	0	2	4	6	8	10	?
D	Social in general	0	2	4	6	8	10	?

Degree of Well-being (Indicate level perceived by the person on the following scale, optionally using a suitable instrument).

Poorest										Excellent
0	1	2	3	4	5	6	7	8	9	10

II. HEALTH CONTRIBUTING FACTORS

Risk Factors: [ ] Abnormal weight [ ] Hyper-cholesterolemia [ ] Hyperglicemia [ ] Hypertensión [ ] Tabacco [ ] Alcohol [ ] Family psychiatric problems [ ] Severe child trauma [ ] Prolongued or severe stress

Additional information:..

Protective Factors: [ ] Healthy diet [ ] Physical activity [ ] Creative activities [ ] Social participation

Additional information: ....

III. HEALTH EXPERIENCES AND EXPECTATIONS

Personal and cultural identity: ....
....

Suffering (its recognition, idioms of distress, illness beliefs): ....
....

Experiences and expectations on health care: ....
....

Fig. 11.3 GLADP-VR personalized diagnostic formulation form

11.5 The Context of Person-Centered Diagnosis

While the context of person-centered diagnosis may be conceived to encompass also its conceptual, institutional, and methodological background (as presented in the first section of this chapter), this section of the manuscript will focus first on the diagnostic evaluation process and second on the articulation of diagnosis with clinical care planning.

11.5.1 Diagnostic Evaluation Process

The clinical assessment process is aimed at setting up the collaborative matrix for clinical care and obtaining effectively the information necessary to make a thorough diagnostic formulation. The diagnostic evaluation rather than a purely taxonomic exercise, represents the first step of the process of clinical care the main objective of which is the restoration and promotion of the health of the persons presenting for care and enriching their quality of life.

Thus, the first consideration in the planning of the diagnostic evaluation process should be awareness of its fundamental objectives and the engagement of the clinician as a person with the persons of the patient and the involved family. Conducting the diagnostic interview in a manner that is respectful and empowering of the person seeking help is a distinctive feature of person-centered care [37]. This requires the establishment of empathy and appreciation for the experience and feelings of the patient [2]. Highly relevant is attending to subjectivity and intersubjectivity, as discussed by Botbol and Lecic-Tosevski in Chap. 5 of the present volume. Adams [2] elaborates further on this as he argues for the importance of establishing a *common ground* among clinicians, patient, and family in order to achieve shared understanding of the clinical situation at hand.

Helpful from an organizational viewpoint are the steps for a thorough diagnostic evaluation proposed in the WPA International Guidelines of Diagnostic Assessment (IGDA) [30], as follows:

11.5.1.1 Patient Interview

The interview process should include a preparatory phase to ensure a quiet and reasonably comfortable environment where patients and their families are received cordially and respectfully.

The body of the interview should cover in an effective, smooth, and considered manner, the different areas of information relevant to the preparation of an adequate diagnostic formulation and an initial treatment plan. It should be emphasized in this process the importance of carefully listening to the patient and available family and the establishment of a close therapeutic relationship. This phase should conclude with the formulation of a jointly understood initial diagnostic assessment (which would continue later as the clinical care process unfolds), as well as shared decisions on what the next steps would be.

The closure phase of the interview should include a warm farewell connected to future visits or clinical activities. Regardless of the patient's socioeconomic status and attentive to cultural expectations, it is important to conduct the interview in a respectful, courteous, warm, and confidential manner.

11.5.1.2 Utilizing Additional Sources of Information

These sources can include family and other significant individuals, such as personal care workers, school teachers, and social workers, who have referred the patients or know them and their circumstances. The information from these sources can be obtained face to face, by telephone, or through documents. Whenever possible the patient's permission must be obtained before interviewing or contacting these additional sources of information. For children, it is important to also consider peers and friends as additional sources of information. It is also crucial to incorporate the family, including the nuclear and extended one as appropriate.

11.5.1.3 Symptomatic Assessment of Psychopathology

This assessment is aimed to systematically determining the presence and severity of psychopathology, both symptoms anamnestically explored as well as observable signs. These indicators of psychopathology are usually grouped into the following areas: sensorial, orientation, and cognitive functions, mood and affect, perception, thought process and content, and conative and behavioral aspects. Attention should also be paid to the somatic manifestations of mental syndromes.

11.5.1.4 Bio-psycho-social Complementary Assessments

These include detailed investigations, often using specific protocols or instruments that complement the basic psychopathological examination, according to perceived needs in each case and available resources. It is important to ensure that the procedures used are validated locally, particularly when they are from other world regions or cultures.

11.5.1.5 Comprehensive Diagnostic Formulation

It is recommended that this organizational phase synthesizing the information obtained through the above steps is completed according to a coherent and comprehensive diagnostic model centered on the person.

11.5.1.6 Articulating Diagnosis and Clinical Care Plan

The information contained in the different sections of the comprehensive diagnostic formulation should be organized into a list of problems as treatment goals and positive aspects of the patient are also considered to contextualize the care plan. For each problem or goal, an appropriate set of clinical interventions, including diagnostic, therapeutic, and health promotion activities should be arranged and the responsible professionals identified.

11.5.1.7 Clinical Chart Organization

The documentation of the different phases of the diagnostic evaluation, in particular, and the process of clinical care in general, should be presented in an organized and clear manner. It helps that the clinical history, as far as possible, includes structured and semi-structured components that facilitate that key elements are systematically covered and narrative spaces to accommodate descriptions in an individualized and flexible manner. Increasingly, such documentation may be organized electronically and trends are emerging to facilitate patients' access to their own clinical charts.

11.5.2 Articulation of Diagnosis with Clinical Care Planning

The ultimate purpose of a personalized diagnostic formulation, such as the one presented in Fig. 11.3, is to serve as an informational base for the preparation of a clinical care plan.

As in the previously mentioned case of the diagnostic evaluation process, it is crucial for person-centered care to establish first a *common ground* among clinicians, patient, and family as the basic collaborative matrix for treatment planning. The importance of this has been detailed by Adams and Grieder [3] and Adams [1]. They highlight in their recommendations the Wagner model of care [48], originally developed for the care of chronic illnesses and proposing as a keystone "productive interactions" between an "empowered, hopeful consumer" and a "receptive, capable treatment team."

A related conceptual and procedural development for the enhancement of person-centered treatment planning is *SDM*. Illustratively, Coulter et al. [16] reveal the increasing international experience with forms of SDM. These particular procedures may however limit their usefulness if employed mechanistically.

After proper attention has been given to the above conceptual considerations, it is helpful to consider organizational developments such as formats for treatment or care planning. Adams [1] highlights a generic format used in the health field and other sectors which focus on objectives, goals, and interventions (services, treatments, etc.). One can also consider, particularly for person-centered mental health treatment planning, the Clinical Care Plan included in the Latin American Guide for Psychiatric Diagnosis (GLADP-VR) [9]. It is organized around the identification of Problems (extracted from the GLADP-VR Personalized Diagnostic Formulation as targets for care), Interventions, and Observations. Its layout is presented in Fig. 11.4.

11.6 Conclusions

A review of conceptual, institutional, and methodological considerations provide a background for understanding person-centered diagnosis. Its refocusing diagnosis from disease to person has strong ethical and clinical effectiveness bases supported by major global institutions in clinical care and public health, and is consistent with contemporary developments in diagnostic methodology.

From such matrix emerges the PID model. Its informational domains (Health Status, Health Contributory Factors, and Health Experience and Values), pluralistic descriptive procedures (categories, dimensions and narratives), and diagnostic

Name: ______________________ Record No.: ____________ Date (d/m/y): ____________

Age: ________ Sex: ☐ M ☐ F Estado civil: ____________ Occupation: ______________________

Clinicians involved: ____

Service: ____

Instructions:

Under **Problems,** list important clinical disorders, idioms of distress, disabilities and contextual problems presented. Keep the list as short and simple as possible. Consolidate within an encompassing term all problems that share the same care plan.
Interventions would list diagnostic studies, treatments and health promotion activities pertinent to each problem. Specify as much as possible planned doses and schedules, amounts, and time references as well as clinicians responsible for each intervention.
The space for **Observations** may be used flexibly. It could include expected dates for the resolution of problems, dates for expected re-evaluations, or notes indicating that a specific problem has been resolved or has become inactive.

PROBLEMS	INTERVENTIONS	OBSERVATIONS

Fig. 11.4 GLADP-VR clinical care plan form

process engaging clinicians, patient, and family/carers in a *common ground*, attest to its relevance for person-centered care.

One of the first practical implementations of the PID model has been the Latin American Guide for Psychiatric Diagnosis (GLADP-VR), published recently by the APAL for the use of health professionals in Latin America and beyond. It uses WHO's ICD categories and codes and culturally informed Latin American Annotations for the identification and description of disorders, as well as a person-centered diagnostic process and formulation format.

Attention to the context of the PID model in terms of the diagnostic evaluation process and the articulation of diagnosis with the planning of care should enhance the PID effectiveness and usefulness.

References

1. Adams N. Treatment planning as a strategy for promoting person-centered care. Int J Person Centered Med. 2011;1:456–9.
2. Adams N. Finding common ground: the role of integrative diagnosis and treatment planning as a pathway to person-centered care. Int J Person Centered Med. 2012;2:173–8.
3. Adams N, Grieder DM. Treatment planning for person-centered care. Amsterdam: Elsevier; 2005.
4. American Psychiatric Association. Diagnostic and statistical manual of mental disorders, fourth edition (DSM-IV). Washington DC: Author; 1994.
5. American Psychiatric Association. Diagnostic and statistical manual of mental disorders, fifth edition (DSM-5). Arlington, VA: Author; 2013.
6. Amering M. Trialog—an exercise in communication between consumers, carers, and professional mental health workers beyond role stereotype. In: Conceptual explorations on person-centered medicine. Int J Integr Care. 2010;10(Supplement 10).
7. Antonovsky A. Unraveling the mystery of health. San Francisco: Jossey-Bass; 1987.
8. Appleyard J. Introduction to ethical standards for person-centered health research. Int J Person Centered Med. 2013;3:258–62.
9. Asociación Psiquiátrica de América Latina. Guía Latinoamericana de Diagnóstico Psiquiátrico, Versión Revisada (GLADP-VR). Lima: Asociación Psiquiátrica de América Latina, Sección de Diagnóstico y Clasificación; 2012.
10. Asociación Psiquiátrica de América Latina. Guía Latinoamericana de Diagnóstico Psiquiátrico. Guadalajara: Asociación Psiquiátrica de América Latina, Sección de Diagnóstico y Clasificación; 2004.
11. Banzato CEM, Jorge MR, Kastrup M. Multiaxial schemas for psychiatric diagnosis. In: Salloum IM, Mezzich JE, editors. Psychiatric diagnosis: challenges and prospects. Chichester, UK: Wiley-Blackwell; 2009.
12. Canguilhem G. The normal and the pathological (1966). New York: Zone Books; 1991.
13. Chinese Society of Psychiatry. Chinese classification of mental disorders, version 3 (CCMD-3). Jinan: Author; 2001.
14. Christodoulou GN, Fulford KMW, Mezzich JE. Conceptual bases of psychiatry for the person. Int Psychiatry. 2008;5(1):1–3.
15. Cloninger CR, Salloum IM, Mezzich JE. The dynamic origins of positive health and well being. Int J Person Centered Med. 2012;2:179–87.
16. Coulter A, Härter M, Moumjid-Ferdjaoui N, Perestelo-Perez L, Van der Weijden T. European experience with shared decision making. Int J Person Centered Med. 2015;5:9–14.
17. Deau X, Appleyard J. Person centered medicine as an ethical imperative. Int J Person Centered Medicine 2015;5:60–63.
18. Fulford KWM, Christodoulou GN, Stein DJ. Values and ethics: perspectives on psychiatry for the person. Int J Person Centered Med. 2011;1:131–3.
19. Garrabe J, Hoff P. Historical views on psychiatry for the person. Int J Person Centered Med. 2011;1:125–7.
20. Jablensky A. Categories, dimensions and prototypes: critical issues for psychiatric classification. Psychopathology. 2005;38:201–5.
21. Kendell R, Jablensky A. Distinguishing between the validity and the utility of psychiatric diagnoses. Am J Psychiatry. 2003;160:4–12.

22. Kirmayer LJ. Broken narratives: clinical encounters and the poetics of illness experience. In: Mattingly C, Garro L, editors. Narrative and the cultural construction of illness and healing. Berkeley: University of California Press; 2000. p. 153–80.
23. Laín-Entralgo P. El Diagnóstico Médico: Historia y Teoría. Barcelona: Salvat; 1982.
24. Mezzich JE. Positive health: conceptual place, dimensions and implications. Psychopathology. 2005;38:177–9.
25. Mezzich JE. Psychiatry for the person: articulating medicine's science and humanism. World Psychiatry. 2007;6:65–7.
26. Mezzich JE. The Geneva conferences and the emergence of the international network of person-centered medicine. J Eval Clin Pract. 2011;17(333–336):2011.
27. Mezzich JE. The construction of person-centered medicine and the launching of an International College. Int J Person Centered Med. 2011;2:6–10.
28. Mezzich JE. Towards a health experience formulation for person-centered integrative diagnosis. Int J Person Centered Med. 2012;2:188–92.
29. Mezzich JE, Banzato CEM, Cohen P, Cloninger CR, et al. Report of the American Psychiatric Association Committee to Evaluate the DSM Multiaxial System. Presented to the APA Assembly, Atlanta, 21 May 2005;2005.
30. Mezzich JE, Berganza CE, von Cranach M, Jorge MR, Kastrup MC, Murthy RC, Okasha A, Pull C, Sartorius N, Skodol AE, Zaudig M. Essentials of the WPA international guidelines for diagnostic assessment (IGDA). Br J Psychiatry. 2003;182(Suppl. 45).
31. Mezzich JE, Caracci G, Fabrega H, Kirmayer LJ. Cultural formulation guidelines. Transcult Psychiatry. 2009;46:383–405.
32. Mezzich JE, Christodoulou G. Psychiatry for the person and its ethical perspectives. S Afr Psychiatr J. 2007;13:71–73.
33. Mezzich JE, Cohen NL, Ruiperez MA, Banzato CEM, Zapata-Vega MI. The multicultural quality of life index: presentation and validation. J Eval Clin Pract. 2011;17:357–64.
34. Mezzich JE, Kirisci L, Salloum IM. Technical Report from the project on systematically conceptualizing and developing measures to assess progress towards person- and people-centered care. Technical Report, International College of Person Centered Medicine, New York;2015.
35. Mezzich JE, Salloum IM. Towards innovative international classification and diagnostic systems: ICD-11 and person-centered integrative diagnosis. Acta Psychiatr Scand. 2007;116:1–5.
36. Mezzich JE, Salloum IM, Cloninger CR, Salvador-Carulla L, Kirmayer L, Banzato CE, Wallcraft J, Botbol M. Person-centered integrative diagnosis: conceptual bases and structural model. Can J Psychiatry. 2010;55:701–8.
37. Mezzich JE, Snaedal J, van Weel C, Heath I. The international network for person-centered medicine: background and first steps. World Med J. 2009;55:104–7.
38. Mezzich JE, Snaedal J, van Weel C, Heath I. Toward person-centered medicine: from disease to patient to person. Mount Sinai J Med. 2010;77:304–6.
39. Miles A, Mezzich JE. Advancing the global communication of scholarship and research for personalized healthcare. Int J Person Centered Med. 2011;1:1–5.
40. Mises R, Quemada N, Botbol M, Burzsteijn C, Garrabe J, Golse B, Jeammet P, Plantade A, Portelli C, Thevenot JP. French classification for child and adolescent mental disorders (CFTMEA). Psychopathology. 2002;35:176–80.
41. WHO, QOL Group. The development of the world health organization quality of life assessment instrument (the WHOQOL). In: Orly J, Kuyken W, editors. Quality of life assessment: international perspectives. Heidelberg: Springer; 1994.
42. Otero AA. Tercer Glosario Cubano de Psiquiatría (GC-3). La Habana: Hospital Psiquiátrico de La Habana; 1998.
43. Robins E, Guze S. Establishment of diagnostic validity in psychiatric illness: its application to schizophrenia. Am J Psychiatry. 1970;126(7):983–7.

44. Salloum IM, Mezzich JE. Psychiatric diagnosis: challenges and prospects. Chichester, UK: Wiley-Blackwell; 2009.
45. Salloum IM, Mezzich JE. Conceptual appraisal of the person-centered integrative diagnosis model. Int J Person Centered Med. 2011;1:39–42.
46. Schaffner KF. The validity of psychiatric diagnosis: Etiopathogenic and clinical approaches. In: Salloum IM, Mezzich JE, editors. Psychiatric diagnosis: challenges and prospects. Chichester, UK: Wiley-Blackwell; 2009.
47. Seyer J. Development of the health improvement card developed by the world health professions alliance. Paper presented at the 5th Geneva conference on person-centered medicine. International College of Person Centered Medicine, May 2012.
48. Wagner E, Austin B, Davis C, Hindmarsh M, Schaefer J, Bonomi A. Improving illness care: translating evidence into action. Health Aff. 2001;20:62–78.
49. World Health Organization. Constitution of the world health organization. Geneva: Author; 1946.
50. World Health Organization. Multiaxial classification of child and adolescent psychiatric disorders. Cambridge, UK: Cambridge University Press; 1996.
51. World Health Organization. Multiaxial presentation of the ICD-10 for use in adult psychiatry. Cambridge, UK: Cambridge University Press; 1997.
52. World Health Organization. International classification of functioning and health (ICF). Geneva: Author; 2001.

Health Status: From Illness to Wellbeing

12

Ihsan M. Salloum, MD, MPH, C. Robert Cloninger, MD, PhD, Luis Salvador-Carulla, MD, PhD and Angel A. Otero, MD

12.1 Introduction

Health status, as concept that emphasizes the importance of the whole and the interdependence of its parts and not merely the presence of disease, has been a key concept in medicine since ancient times. Ancient traditions of medicines such as the Chinese, the Indian Ayurveda, as well as ancient Greek medicine, all embraced the holistic understanding of health and its ailments, emphasizing the concept of harmony and interdependence between the "part" and the "whole" [8, 18]. This understanding is also reiterated in modern times by the World Health Organization (WHO) constitution definition of health as "*a state of complete physical, emotional, and social well-being and not merely the absence of disease or infirmity.*" [25]

I.M. Salloum, MD, MPH (✉)
Professor of Psychiatry, University of Miami School of Medicine, Miami, FL, USA;
Chair, Section on Classification, Diagnostic Assessment and Nomenclature, World Psychiatric Association, Geneva, Switzerland
e-mail: isalloum@med.miami.edu

C.R. Cloninger, MD, PhD
Wallace Renard Professor of Psychiatry, Genetics, and Psychology, Washington University School of Medicine, St Louis, MO, USA; Director, Center for the Science of Wellbeing, Washington University School of Medicine, St Louis, MO, USA

L. Salvador-Carulla, MD, PhD
Professor, Centre for Disability Research and Policy, Faculty of Health Sciences, University of Sydney, Sydney, Australia

A.A. Otero, MD
Chair, Section on Classification, Diagnostic Assessment and Nomenclature, World Psychiatric Association, Geneva, Switzerland; Professor of Psychiatry, University of La Habana, Havana, Cuba

J.E. Mezzich et al. (eds.), *Person Centered Psychiatry*,
DOI 10.1007/978-3-319-39724-5_12

The focus of the assessment of health status in modern clinical medicine, however, has been the ascertainments of the presence or absence of ill health, while attention to positive aspects of health has received at best a cursory attention. It is not surprising that knowledge about etiology, risk factors, and vulnerabilities to ailments has exponentially expanded. On the other hand, development of knowledge regarding factors influencing positive aspects of health and recovery has been less extensive and has occurred, for the most part, outside the realm of clinical medicine.

Within psychiatry, the need to encompass a comprehensive view of the patient's problems and to enhance the clinical utility of psychiatric diagnoses, innovations such as the adoption of a biopsychosocial model for mental disorders have prompted the development of expanded diagnostic formulations for mental disorders. This is expressed in the various multiaxial schema included in national and international classification systems over the past few decades including the Mental Disorders Chapter of the International Classification of Diseases, 10th reversion (ICD-10), the various reiteration of DSM-III through DSM-IVTR, the Chinese Classification of Mental Disorders, the Latin-American Guide to Psychiatric Diagnosis and the International Guidelines of Psychiatric Diagnosis [1–5, 7, 13, 26]. Proponents of the multiaxial schema have highlighted their clinical utilities in treatment planning by providing an organized format to record and address key areas impinging on the care for the primary psychiatric disorder [12]. While some of these schemas included assessments of functioning or quality of life, these schemas were primarily focusing on the assessment of the presenting ill health problems and related factors. Thus, the inclusion of explicit assessment of health status as a concept emphasizing the importance of the whole and the dynamic interdependence of its parts have not been undertaken in clinical psychiatry or in general clinical medicine. This is not surprising; however, given that a disease-centered diagnostic and acute care intervention approach have been the dominated models of care in clinical medicine and psychiatry over the past half-century [22].

A disease-centered model, however, has multiple limitations for addressing recovery from multiple chronic, relapsing conditions, which constitute the vast majority of conditions worldwide. Chronic diseases involve an ongoing process of health support that requires the mobilization of multiple resources at the personal, family, care giver, stockholders, and community levels. For example, a disease-focused approach has been clearly inadequate at ameliorating one of the most common but complex problem frequently encountered during the management of chronic diseases which is adherence to care.

Management of chronic conditions highlight the importance of mobilizing the person's strengths and resiliency as preventative and health restorative effort relies primarily on the person's behavior and on their context as well such as on available support and partnership with other stakeholders. An acute care model, not based on a holistic concept of health and care, is not designed to address the treatment, health restoration and recovery needs of chronic and often multimorbid conditions. This narrow-focused care model has led to fragmentation, incoordination, and decreased access to care. The interconnectedness of health problems and the key role of behavioral determinants of health in both health and disease, strongly argue for an integrated approach to care encompassing the totality of health with strong emphasis on disease prevention and health restoration. This also calls for a reconsideration of the diagnostic process toward an integrated diagnostic assessment of the health status to include not only ill health, but also the other fundamental aspect of assessment of health that is of wellbeing and positive aspects of health.

12.2 Measures of Health Status and Well Being Predict Outcome

Different measures and conceptualizations have been advanced to define health status. The concept of health status has been seen as multidimensional domains that include symptoms and physiological states, physical, emotional, and cognitive functions, life expectancy and life expectancy along with perceptions about present and future [17]. Health-related Quality of Life (HRQOL) is another concept defined as "*an individual's or group's perceived physical and mental health overtime.*" HRQOL has been measured by the number of healthy days in work by the Center for Disease Control and Prevention [6]. HRQOL include aspects of life that are shown to affect physical and mental health. At the individual level, this includes physical and mental health perception, health risk, functional status, social support, and socioeconomic status. At the community level it compromises resources, conditions, policies, and practices that influence population health perception and functioning. Multiple disciplines are involved in the domains defining HRQOL, including sociology, psychology, social work, aging, disability, environment sustainability, economics, marketing, and urban planning among others. HRQOL has been found to be an acceptable measure of outcome. Self-assessed health status was found to be a more powerful predictor of mortality and morbidity than many objective measures of health [11].

Idler and colleagues examined 27 longitudinal studies of representative community samples examining global self-ratings of health as predictors of mortality. Global self-rated health was found as an independent predictor of mortality in most of these studies after controlling for other relevant predictors of mortality. The CDC highlighted a link between quality of life measures and prevention of chronic diseases (e.g., diabetes and hypertension, etc.) and also risk factors (e.g., overweight, smoking, and sedentary life style). Examples of commonly used HRQOL include the Medical Outcomes Study Short Forms (SF-12 and SF-36), the Sickness Impact Profile and the Quality of Well Being Scale [6]. Four questions proposed by the CDC as core healthy day measures. These include a question about the person's perception about their general health, rated from excellent to poor, and three questions about the number of days during the past 30 days were physical health (illness and injury), mental health (stress, depression, other emotional problems), and impairment in usual activities (self-care, work, or recreation) due to physical or mental health. More recent studies also highlighted the impact of health status as a risk factor in cardiovascular disorder. A review of 34 studies reported that poor physical health status was a significant predictor poor outcome in patients with congestive heart failure and coronary artery disease, although heterogeneity across studies was noted.

These consistent findings of the impact of health status on outcome have prompted calls for including health status assessment in regular clinical practice [19]. However, to date there have not been any concerted effort to critically examine the current model for diagnosis and to offer enhanced assessment and diagnostic process that is more person- and patient centered to include this key domain of assessment of health status. The need for improving the quality of care proposed by the Institute of Medicine Report on "*Crossing the Quality Chasm: A New Health System for the twenty first Century*" has identified "*patient centeredness*" among other specific aims of care which also included safe, effective, timely, efficient, and equitable [19].

12.3 Person-Centered Medicine and the Person-Centered Integrative Diagnostic Approach

The Person-centered Integrative Diagnosis model (PID) is an emerging model of diagnosis that highlight the importance of assessing health status in clinical care and public health. The PID model aims at putting into practice the vision of Person-centered Psychiatry and Medicine affirming the whole person of the patient in context as the center of clinical care and health promotion at the individual and community levels [15, 22]. The goals of Person-centered Psychiatry are to promote psychiatry of the person (of the totality of the person's health, both ill and positive health), by the person (with clinicians extending themselves as full human beings), for the person (assisting the fulfillment of the person's life project), and with the person (in respectful collaboration with the person who consults). The PID recognizes that the person of the patient and the person of the health providers are in a respectful and empowering partnership. The PID considers the totality of the person's health, including both ill health and positive aspects of health emphasizing prevention, recovery, health restoration, and wellbeing. Person-centered Psychiatry and the PID view the process of care as a partnership (equalitarian) approach, including the patient, family, caregivers, and other stakeholders and the health professionals forming a health support network.

The PID scheme is the only diagnostic model that explicitly incorporates the assessment of health status in clinical care. It provides a comprehensive and dynamic, multilevel assessment of the health status. The first level includes the assessment of health status, which includes the assessment of ill health (physical or mental disorders; functional abilities) and the assessment of positive aspects of health and wellbeing. Positive aspects of health and wellbeing are key to the recovery, health restoration, and health preservation efforts. The second level in the

PID is the assessment of contributors to the health status, including health promoters and health risks considered on a biopsychosocial continuum. Health contributors include diet, physical activity, creative activity, social involvement, and others which are those identified on the Health Improvement Card developed by the World Health Professions Alliance [24]. Health risks include overweight, elevated lipid, elevated glucose, high blood pressure, alcohol and tobacco use, family history, early trauma, and significant stress. The experience of health is the third level of the PID and includes the experience of wellbeing and the experience of ill health, which provides assessment of personal and cultural identity, suffering, and meaning of illness and expectations for the health care encounter. Inclusion of the experience of health provides idiographic narrative that is key for the processes of empowerment, engagement, partnership, and recovery [16, 21, 23].

As mentioned earlier, Health Status assessment in the PID model consider the assessment of the totality of health, including ill health and positive aspects of health to be at the core of the diagnostic process. The inclusion of positive aspects of health and the assessment of health status as perceived by the patient is supported by the empirical findings of being a robust predictor of outcome in addition to highlighting the patient-centeredness and of the partnership approach of the PID model.

12.4 Assessment of Health Status in the PID: Ill Health

The “Ill Health Status” domain of the PID encompasses both the presence of an illness or health problem either mental or general ill health condition as well as the presence of any related functional disabilities, such as in self-care, occupational functioning, functioning with family, and participation in community activities.

Thus, these levels may include any diagnostic entities or health conditions (based on ICD-10) such as mental disorder, substance use disorders, and general physical health such as diabetes, hypertension, thyroid problems, or obesity are recorded on this levels. Additionally, the ill health status will also asses for the presence of functioning/ disability. Several domains of functioning/disability are assessed using a dimensional scale of that ranges from very poor (disable) (0) to best functioning [10]. These domains include overall functioning, personal care, occupational care, functioning with family, and social functioning. The systematic recording of this domain will allow monitoring any potential disability issue which may become target for treatment intervention. For example, cognitive dysfunctions have been documented in many psychiatric and substance use disorders, such as alcohol use disorder and bipolar disorder; however, these dysfunctions are rarely recorded or taken into account in regular clinical care unless they are very prominent.

12.5 Positive Health: Health Status

The two domains that correspond to the positive health status include well-being and functioning/disability. Well-being is understood as a state of satisfaction, contentment, optimism, and happiness. Well-being may be characterized in four different ways [9, 10]. These include the presence of positive emotions and the absence of negative emotions or the presence of mature character traits, or the satisfaction with quality of life, or by virtuous conduct. Positive health encompass "*physical, material, emotional, social, ecological, and spiritual well-being*" and it "*promotes a satisfying quality of life, resilience despite stress, and recovery of positive emotionality*" [9, 10]. Positive emotions are more than the absence of negative emotions [9, 10], and the determinants of positive health are not the opposite of the determinants of ill health. Consequently, health is more than the absence of disease. The most recognized aspects of positive health include functioning (resilience), resources (supports), and quality of life [9, 10].

Well-being is assessed in the PID on a 10-point self-report scale, from 0 (very poor) to 10 (best). Furthermore, levels of functioning in the various domains discussed above also rated from 0 to 10 scale. Robustness and resilience are two notions conceptually related to functioning [14].

12.6 Conclusions and Future Directions

Assessment of health status as a holistic approach to the whole person is being reintegrated in clinical medicine because of the pressing needs created by chronic diseases and needs for more effective preventative approaches. The need for person-centered assessment has been recognized since ancient times and has been emphasized by definition of health in the WHO constitution. As a result of the prevalence and burden of chronic disease, there is a strong need for models that highlight health restoration and enhance prevention, recovery, and wellbeing. Measures of health status such as HRQOL have been found to be consistent predictors of outcome and have also been linked to the prevention of chronic diseases and to common risk factors; however, these assessments have not been incorporated into regular clinical practice and care.

The PID approach, embodying the vision of Person-centered Psychiatry and Medicine as expressed to a large extent in the various Geneva Declarations and proceedings of the International College of Person-centered Medicine (ICPCM) (http://www.personcenteredmedicine.org/), provides an overarching conceptual framework for an assessment of the health status in an integrated and dynamic framework converging on the person in context as the center and goal of care and public health. The PID model has been officially incorporated into the Latin-American Guide to Psychiatric Diagnosis-revised (GLADP), [20] an adaptation of the ICD-10 to Latin American Countries to enhance the patient- and person centeredness of psychiatric diagnoses. This new approach is being evaluated in terms of its usefulness and impact on the process and outcome of care.

References

1. American Psychiatric Association. DSM-IV-TR: diagnostic and statistical manual of mental disorders. Fourth edition, text revision. Washington, DC: American Psychiatric Association;2000.
2. American Psychiatric Association, A. P. Diagnostic and statistical manual of mental disorders, 3rd edition (DSM III). Washington, DC.: APA;1980.
3. American Psychiatric Association, A. P. Diagnostic and statistical manual of mental disorders (3rd edition, revised) (DSM III(R)). Washington, DC.: APA;1987.
4. American Psychiatric Association, A. P. DSM-IV: diagnostic and statistical manual of mental disorders. Fourth Edition, Washington, DC: American Psychiatric Association;1994.
5. Berganza CE, Mezzich JE, Jorge MR. Latin American guide for psychiatric diagnosis (GLDP). Psychopathology. 2002;35:185–90.
6. CDC. Measuring healthy days. Center for Disease Control and Prevention: Atlanta, Georgia; 2000.
7. Chen YF. Chinese classification of mental disorders (CCMD-3): towards integration in international classification. Psychopathology. 2002;35:171–5.
8. Christodoulou GN. Psychosomatic medicine. New York, NY: Plenum Press; 1987.
9. Cloninger CR. The positive health domain in person-centered integrative diagnosis. Int J Integr Care. 2010;10(Suppl):e026.
10. Cloninger CR, Salloum IM, Mezzich JE. The dynamic origins of positive health and wellbeing. Int J Person Centered Med. 2012;2:179–87.
11. Idler EL, Benyamini Y. Self-rated health and mortality: a review of twenty-seven community studies. J Health Soc Behav. 1997;38:21–37.
12. Mezzich JE. On developing a psychiatric multiaxial schema for ICD-10. Br J Psychiatry Suppl. 1988:38–43.
13. Mezzich JE. The WPA international guidelines for diagnostic assessment. World Psychiatry. 2002;1:36–9.
14. Mezzich JE. Positive health: conceptual place, dimensions and implications. Psychopathology. 2005;38:177–9.
15. Mezzich JE, Salloum IM, Cloninger CR, Salvador-Carulla L, Kirmayer LJ, Banzato CEM, Wallcraft J, Botbol M. Person-centred integrative diagnosis: conceptual bases and structural model. Can J Psychiatry (Revue Canadienne de Psychiatrie). 2010;55:701–8.
16. Mezzich JE, Snaedal J, van Weel C, Botbol M, Salloum I. Introduction to person-centred medicine: from concepts to practice. J Eval Clin Pract. 2011;17:330–2.
17. Patrick DL, Erickson P. Health status and health policy: quality of life in health care evaluation and resource allocation. New York: Oxford University Press; 1993.
18. Plato. Harmidis dialogue, 156 E. Athens: Papyros editions;1975.
19. Rumsfeld JS. Health status and clinical practice: when will they meet? Circulation. 2002;106:5–7.
20. Saavedra JE, Otero A, Salloum IM, Mezzich JE. The revision of the Latin American guide for psychiatric diagnosis (GLADP): a person centered approach to international classification. Int J Person Centered Med. 2011;1:446–55.
21. Salloum IM, Mezzich JE. Person-centered diagnosis. Int J Integr Care. 2010;10(Suppl):e027.
22. Salloum IM, Mezzich JE. Conceptual appraisal of the person-centered integrative diagnosis model. Int J Person Centered Med. 2011;1:39–42.
23. Salloum IM, Mezzich JE. Outlining the bases of person-centred integrative diagnosis. J Eval Clin Pract. 2011;17:354–6.
24. Seyer, J. Development of the health improvement card developed by the World Health Professions Alliance. In: ICOPC Medicine, editors. The 5th Geneva Conference of Person-centered Medicine. Geneva, Switzerland; 2012.

25. World Health Organization. WHO constitution. World Health Organization: Geneva, Switzerland; 1946.
26. World Health Organization. The ICD-10 classification of mental and behavioural disorders: clinical descriptions and diagnostic guidelines. Geneva: World Health Organization; 1992.

13 Health Contributory Factors

Javier E. Saavedra, MD, DrMedSc,
Eugenio Villar-Montesinos, MD, MSc
and Michel Botbol, MD

13.1 Health Contributory Factors and Diagnosis

Health is the most important factor for life satisfaction, particularly subjective well-being [26]. The study of the factors that determine the individual's health has been a main focus of research because of the implications on the countries' social policies in search of health equity. The World Health Organization (WHO) conceptualizes the factors that contribute to health and the determinants of health, as those factors that combined, affect or influence the public and communities' health. According to WHO, the determinants of health in general pertain to the social and economic environment, to the physical environment, and to the characteristics and the behaviors of the individual [57]. Similarly, from the mental health point of view WHO has summarized the factors that contribute to mental health in three main areas: (1) attributes and individual behaviors related to the ability of the individual to deal with emotional and social aspects of everyday life and genetic and biological factors; (2) social or economic determinants, linked to situations of personal support, academic achievement, level of income and socioeconomic status; and (3) environmental factors, related to health services, social policies, cultural beliefs,

J.E. Saavedra, MD, DrMedSc (✉)
Executive Director of the Specialized Research and Teaching Office, Instituto Nacional de Salud Mental "Honorio Delgado—Hideyo Noguchi" and Professor of Psychiatry, Universidad Peruana Cayetano Heredia, Lima, Peru; Chair, Section on Diagnosis and Classification, Latin American Psychiatric Association, Lima, Peru; Av. José Gálvez Barrenechea 274, Dpt. 402, San Isidro, Lima, Peru
e-mail: saavedra@terra.com.pe

E. Villar-Montesinos, MD, MSc
Medical Scholar, Geneva, Switzerland

M. Botbol, MD
Professor of Child and Adolescent Psychiatry, Western Brittany University, Brest University Hospital, Brest, France

J.E. Mezzich et al. (eds.), *Person Centered Psychiatry*,
DOI 10.1007/978-3-319-39724-5_13

prevalent discriminatory practices or conflicts of gender or structural violence [56]. As will be seen, later there is evidence that most of the determinants apply both to health in general and to mental health in particular.

Consequently, attention to health contributing factors forms an essential part in the interpretation of the underlying dynamics of health problems, factors that are involved in varying degrees in the etiological, physiopathological, and psychopathological processes. From this perspective the factors contributing to health should be fundamental part of the diagnostic process both for the importance that diagnosis gives to the understanding of the mechanism by which problems develop [19], as well for the understanding of the whole person who seeks attention which contributes to a proper treatment plan and a person-centered approach. At the same time the diagnostic process should be flexible and practical, and must be designed in such way that it can be used by the various clinical actors involved in the diagnostic evaluation process. Along this line, in a practical way, the Person-centered Integrative Diagnosis (PID) has considered that these contributing factors can be classified in two areas, the first from the ill-health as contributors to the disease or risk factors, and the second from the positive health as protective factors as contributors to health. In both cases, of an intrinsic or extrinsic nature, in regard to personal or environmental aspects, respectively, and they can be biological, psychological, or social [29].

As biological factors they are considered genetic factors and factors around birth, conditions affecting health or the course of health such as eating habits, physical activity, harmful habits (tobacco, alcohol or other drugs), and diseases background. In relation to psychological factors one can consider personality characteristics that have an impact on health, as well as children's experiences and family dynamics that have influence on personality. Finally, considered in relation to social factors are social support, socioeconomic status, education, occupation and cultural values that influence people's behavior (Table 13.1). The Latin American Guide for Psychiatric Diagnosis has included in its diagnostic formulation the PID model that comprises a specific level on health contributory factors. These include risk and protective factors for both physical and mental health (Table 13.2).

Some of the most important contributory factors will be reviewed next, noting that most of the supportive studies mainly involve significant statistical correlations which do not mean necessarily causality or determination. More studies, particularly of a more complex nature, will need to be conducted to reach more clearly determinant conclusions.

13.2 Health and Its Determinants

It is instructive to note that the Agency of Public Health of Canada specifies 11 key determinants of health: income and social status, social support, education, employment and working conditions, social environment, physical environment, personal practices of health, healthy child development, genetic and biological load, health services, gender, and culture [35]. From the point of view of public opinion, a

Table 13.1 Contributing factors to health

TYPE	BIOLOGICAL	PSYCHOLOGICAL	SOCIAL
INTRINSIC	**Genetic**	**Personality**	
	Prenatal	**Adaptability**	
	Perinatal	**Plasticity**	
	Postnatal	**Resilience**	
EXTRINSIC	**Dietary habits**	**Childhood experiences**	**Social Support**
	Harmful Habits	**Rearing styles**	**Economic conditions**
	Physical activity	**Family dynamics**	**Education**
	Pathological history		**Occupation**
			Cultural values
			Health system
			Psychosocial stressors

Table 13.2 GLADP's diagnostic formulation on health contributory factors [42]

II. HEALTH CONTRIBUTORY FACTORS
Risk Factors:
☐ Abnormal weight ☐Hyper-colesterolemia ☐Hyperglicemia ☐Hypertension ☐Tabacco
☐Alcohol Family psychiatric history ☐ Severe childhood trauma ☐ Severe enduring stress
Additional information:
....
Protective /promotional factors:
☐Healthy diet ☐Physical activity ☐Creative activity ☐Social participation
Additional information:
....

community study found that among the factors considered most important in hierarchical order were: physical environment, personal health practices, the health system, and the development of the healthy child [15]. These factors often contribute to the development of chronic diseases, like cancer, obesity, and depression which together cause the greatest burden of disease [14, 22]. However, these factors interact between themselves and many are mediators for the development of health problems as is the case with certain biological factors [60], like the genetic stock of the individual (through epigenetics). A constant question has been how much influence each of these factors has on health and the priority that must be set accordingly in public health [28]. Some authors have estimated that there is an inconsistency between the allocation of resources and the determinants of health since most resources are assigned to health care (especially to curative services) as the most significant contributors are patterns of behavior with a 40 % contribution to premature death, while the rest of the determinant contributions of the determinants have been calculated at 30 % to genetic predisposition, 15 % to social circumstances, 10 % to the health care system, and 5 % to environmental exposure [41]. In this sense, research has concluded that by far the factors of risk of individual practices or behaviors, as well as, the social factors make the biggest contribution to morbidity and mortality. Still more research is needed to clarify these associations [20].

Mokdad et al. [30] have reported that the main causes of mortality in the United States are tobacco (18.1 % of total deaths), poor diet and physical inactivity (16.5 %), and consumption of alcohol (3.5 %). In the same direction the 2010 Global Burden of Diseases study found that the major risk factors related to the Disability-adjusted lost life-years (DALYs) in the United States were: risky diet, tobacco, high body mass index, high blood pressure, high fasting blood sugar, physical inactivity, and alcohol use [45]. Taking together all countries involved in this study the top factors were arterial hypertension, tobacco, air pollution in the home due to solid fuels, diet low in fruit and high body mass index, alcohol use, high blood sugar in fasting, low weight at birth, exposure to environmental particulate matter, and physical inactivity [5]. Many of these factors interact amongst themselves to enhance their effects on health. For instance, lifestyles have a major impact on the use of leisure time and on the degree of mobility and physical activity, therefore influencing weight and the possibility of developing obesity which in turn predisposes to several of the factors mentioned [2].

It needs to be noted that according to the WHO Commission of Social Determinants of Health, all behavioral risk factors are at the same time closely linked to broader social factors in what are referred to as "structural determinants of health" [55]. It should also be kept in mind that some authors argue that it is not enough to identify and promote healthy behaviors because the majority of people who have unhealthy behaviors simply are not motivated to change and therefore suggest that in the assessment of health contributing factors it is important to pay attention also to the causes of these factors [6].

13.3 Personal Health Practices

These findings have led the World Health Professions Alliance (WHPA) to propose an initiative aimed at improving health through positive behavior and lifestyle changes focusing on chronic or non-communicable diseases considered to be reducible or preventable including cardiovascular disease, diabetes, certain types of cancer, and respiratory diseases [59]. For this purpose four factors are being considered related to lifestyle and behavior that are modifiable: an unhealthy diet, lack of physical activity, tobacco use, and harmful alcohol consumption, which in turn are related to metabolic or biometric risk factors such as hypertension, hyperglycemia, the increase of cholesterol and obesity. The following recommendations have been provided:

1. In relation to a healthy diet, the objective is the intake of five portions of fruit and vegetables a day. Less than five servings of fruits and vegetables is regarded as a sign for caution, and not eating fruits or vegetables is considered a high risk behavior.
2. In the case of physical activity, the aim is directed to the development of physical activity for at least 30 min a day. Less than 30 min of physical activity per day is pondered as a sign of caution and lack of physical activity as a high risk behavior.
3. With respect to tobacco, the objective is directed to quit its use completely as smoking tobacco in any proportion is considered a high risk behavior.
4. With regard to alcohol consumption, the WHPA suggests a consumption target of two or fewer glasses of wine (each 90 ml and 12 % alcohol by volume) a day. The consumption of 3–4 glasses of wine is a sign of caution, and the consumption of five or more glasses of wine a day or any consumption of five or more times a week is a high risk behavior. The equivalency of one 90 ml glass of wine to other drinks is: Beer 250 ml with 4 % alcohol by volume, whisky or vodka 20 ml.
5. With respect to metabolic risk factors the objective is to achieve a level of less than 100 mg/dl blood glucose; 126 mg/dl or above is considered high risk. As far as serum cholesterol the aim is to achieve a level below 200 mg/dl; 240 mg/dl or above is considered high risk.
6. With regards to the biometric factors, and specifically for weight, the aim is to achieve a rate of BMI (BMI) between 18.5 and 24.9 (kg/m^2); 30 or higher (kg/m^2) is considered to be considered high risk.

13.4 Relationship Between Contributors to Health and Mental Health Factors

From the point of view of mental health, WHO has established the importance of integrating the healthcare for mental disorders and other chronic medical conditions precisely because of their chronic nature and to address jointly determinants which coexist in an interdependent way or just coexist [58]. Most of the determinants referred to general health also apply to mental health and many of these determinants interact amongst themselves. These determinants of overall health are important because it has been shown that people suffering from mental disorders are more likely to suffer problems of obesity, hypertension, increase in cholesterol, and diabetes than the general population, which has an impact on the risk of premature death and can cause worse prognosis for individuals [51]. A meta-analysis performed through 17 community-based investigations and 204,507 participants found a significant positive association between depression and obesity, especially in women [12]. Another study carried out in communities of women between 40 and 65 found that the prevalence of moderate to severe depression increased from 6.5 to 25.9 % in women with mass index above 35, while the prevalence of obesity increased from 25.4 to 57.8 % in women who suffer from moderate to severe depression [43]. On the other hand, Wells et al. [49] studied the prevalence of eight chronic medical conditions in a sample of 2554 adult patients without or with psychiatric disorders and found out that the life prevalence for any of the chronic medical conditions concerning people with anxious, affective disorders or substance use was 61.4, 57.1, and 57.7 %, respectively, which were superior to the those without psychiatric disorders. In addition, studies have shown that people with mental disorders die at younger ages, for the same causes than the general population, in other words because of preventable diseases like diseases of the heart, cancer, accidents cerebrovascular, or respiratory diseases [9].

13.5 Specific Factors Influencing Mental Health

13.5.1 Biological Factors and Family History

From the genetic point of view, it has been shown that people with a family psychiatric history are more likely to suffer mental disorders. In this sense, there is a definite consensus that there is a genetic susceptibility to disorders such as bipolar disorder or schizophrenia, although it is also known that the environment might contribute to the onset of these disorders [31]. Evidence of genetic components has also been found in disorders such as borderline personality disorder [1] and other personality disorders. From a clinical point of view, the psychiatric family history can guide the clinician in the differential diagnosis, treatment plan and the assessment of the family dynamics in the context of potential risks and support systems [17]. Some authors have emphasized the importance of human neuroplasticity in the preservation of health or developing of illness and its associations with some personality aspects such as resilience [6]. In this sense resilience can be interpreted as a psychological and a biological characteristic that can influence health.

13.5.2 Individual Psychological Contributors

The holistic perspective in regard to person-centered care compelled the integration of clinical aspects with the identification of the environment and of the potential of the individual. Within this approach, it is highlighted the importance of considering the strengths of the person in the form of their knowledge, talents, abilities or skills, beside considerations like resilience [48], which is considered in the PID model as an important protective intrinsic factor [7]. Resilience is an important factor for the reestablishment of disease but at the same time plays an important role as a mediator between positive emotions and life satisfaction [8]. Cloninger has sustained that the psychological contributors factors for disease or health considerations must consider aspects that are synergistically involved along with neuroplasticity: auto-regulatory performance and virtue [6]. In relation to the first, he argues that it is not sufficient conscious reasoning for change in behavior and that it is necessary to pay attention to automatic and unconscious processes of a sociocultural nature that affect motivation to change. In relation to the second, the author argues that it is essential in consideration of the contributors to health and disease to have a values-based perspective, i.e., which are the principles or behavioral standards that establish what is important or desirable for the person in life and that guide final decisions.

13.5.3 Social Circumstances as Contributors

Poor people face many negative contextual factors and adverse environments such as inadequate housing conditions, overcrowding, unemployment, and underemployment, which create an atmosphere that could be detrimental to mental health [37]. This can easily lead to stress, despair, anxiety, or depression, although some authors consider that this is an indirect effect dependent on the circumstances surrounding poverty [13]. However, this situation not only increases mental health problems, but also puts at risk chances of accessing services and health care [40]. This relationship has been studied in various developed countries but has been less studied in developing countries [25]. This situation exposes people to social exclusion and deterioration of their social support networks that further affects their well-being and aggravates their mental disorders possibly leading to a vicious circle.

13.5.4 Children's Background as Risk Factors

From a lifetime perspective, it has been emphasized that certain experiences in the first years of life of the individual, such as use of substances during pregnancy, problems of violence or attachment in childhood, constitute risks for the development of mental health problems [56]. It has been shown that early trauma or severe stress in children are associated with adult mental disorders as has been shown by prospective epidemiological studies of adults who were separated from their parents in the second World War when they were kids [36]. From a biological perspective, early traumatic experiences have been associated with alterations in pituitary adrenal axis in response to adult psychosocial stress [34].

In regard to child abuse, it is presumed that there are a number of effects, such as emotional problems, post-traumatic stress disorder, participation in risk activities, problematic social relationships, and negative attitudes toward others that close a vicious circle, and that predispose a person to health problems in adulthood such as use of substances, obesity, suicide risk, or smoking [21]. In addition, population studies on physical child abuse found an association not only with an increase in depression and anxiety, but also with physical and more diagnostic medical symptoms in adulthood such as gastric ulcer, liver problems, asthma, allergy, arthritis, among others [44], as well as a greater experience of pain in health problems as adults [39]. Particularly important is the presence of child sexual abuse as a risk factor for the development of mental disorders in childhood and in adulthood, as has been shown by a 43 year follow-up study which concludes that the presence of child sexual abuse increases at 3.65 times the rate of contact with mental health in the future [11]. Other follow-up studies have shown the significant impact that domestic violence has in children's mental health, as well as displacements forced by social conflicts [33]. Also academic performance achievement during childhood and adolescence in women has been linked to health in adulthood, without knowing neither why this association exits nor the reason for the disparities between genders [24].

13.5.5 Stress and Health

Stress has been regarded as a central determinant factor and contributor to health, especially if persistent, through the action of cortisol and interactions in the serotonin circuits in the central nervous system, and plays an important role in alterations in the hippocampus that have an impact on the onset of psychiatric disorders [4]. In this regard, studies have found an association between job stress and the subsequent presence of depression or anxiety disorders, even with the further use of antidepressants [47]. However, stress is not only associated with the development of mental health problems but also with the predisposition to the development of physical problems such as gastrointestinal [27], cardiovascular, and endocrine problems [16, 23].

13.5.6 Social Support as a Promotional Factor Influential on Health

Within the promotional or protective factors of health, WHO has highlighted social support as one of the strongest determinants that contribute to health by virtue of providing people with emotional and material resources for their needs [50]. For example, studies have shown an inverse relationship between the degree of social integration and the mortality rate from any cause, in both men and women, still controlled by biomedical risk factors [18]. Bergman et al. [3] have proposed a model that links social integration and health in a cascade of events that determine final health outcomes. These events are initiated at the level of cultural and social structures such as culture conditions, socioeconomic factors, social policies, and social changes which affect the characteristics of the social networks. These in turn provide opportunities for the development of psychosocial mechanisms such as support, influence and social commitment, contact from person to person, and access to resources and material goods. Finally the latter give rise to healthy or non-healthy behaviors, the development of personal psychological resources such as self-esteem, self-efficiency, and the ability to deal with the problems which in turn influences the pathophysiological structure of the individual. In this line the Victorian Health Promotion Foundation has proposed social inclusion as key determinants of mental health, defining it as having relationships of support, and participation in group and civic activities [46]. Studies have found that relationships of trust are associated with a decline between 14 and 18 % in the occurrence of different diseases, including musculoskeletal problems, breathing problems, heart problems, diabetes, and anxious, or depressive problems [38].

13.6 Why and How Are Contributory Factors Linked to Person-Centered Psychiatry?

Three converging streams link contributory factors, especially the social determinants of health with person-centered medicine/psychiatry. On a normative perspective, the right to health was enshrined in WHO's Constitution of 1946–8 stating that health was a "fundamental right of all human beings" [52]. This mandate has been further developed by the "Right to Health" in 2000. It includes both the right to health care as well as to the "underlying determinants of health" [32]. It coherently links both aspects when states that the entitlements include provision of services of good quality, provided without discrimination, confidential, medically ethical, and culturally, scientifically, and medically appropriate. Furthermore, the report of the WHO Commission on the social determinants of health stated in 2008 that being included in the society in which one lives is vital to the material, psychosocial, and political empowerment that underpins social well-being and equitable health [10]. These aspects were further developed by a World Health Assembly Resolution in 2009 on the Social determinants of health which urged member states to increase awareness among public and private health providers on how to take account of the social determinants of health when delivering care to patients in order to reduce health inequities in and between all countries [53].

Finally in the same assembly in 2009, WHO's member states approved the renewal of the primary health care strategy approved 30 years before in Alma Ata which urged also members states to put people at the center of health care by adding as appropriate delivery models which provide comprehensive primary health care services including health promotion, prevention, and curative palliative care [54]. All those aspects, especially health prevention and promotion are closely related to addressing the social determinants of health, and by doing so contributing to reducing health inequities in the population at large.

13.7 Conclusions

The achievement of health as a state of physical, emotional, social, and spiritual well-being emerges from a complex network of genetic, social, economic, and environmental determinants that begin in childhood and interact with each other. Its identification as part of the diagnostic process will serve not only as an aid in the development of the therapeutic plan, but it may also enhance the well-being of the individual through comprehensive care directed not only toward reparative action but also toward preventive and promotional purposes. It also links the role psychiatrists play within and with overall society. The real challenge is how to move coherently from diagnosis and assessment of contributory factors in psychiatry to actual treatment and care by health professionals and society at large.

References

1. Amada A, Ramoz N, Thomas P, Jardri R, Gorwood P. Genetics of borderline personality disorder: systematic review and proposal of an integrative model. Neurosci Biobehav Rev. 2014;40:6–19.
2. Apostolopoulou M, Savopoulos C, Michalakis K, Coppack S, Dardavessis T, Hatzitolios A, Coppack S, Dardavessis T, Hatzitolios A. Age, weight and obesity. Maturitas. 2012;71:115–9.
3. Berkman LF, Glass T, Brissettec I, Seeman TE. From social integration to health: Durkheim in the new Millennium. Soc Sci Med. 2000;51:843–57.
4. Bremner JD. Does stress damage the brain? Biol Psychiatry. 1999;45:797–805.
5. Christopher JL, Murray MD, Lopez AD. Measuring the global burden of disease. N Engl J Med. 2013;369:448–57.
6. Cloninger CR, Cloninger K. Development of instruments and evaluative procedures on contributors to illness and health. Int J Pers Cent Med. 2011;1(3):456–9.
7. Cloninger CR, Salloum IM, Mezzich JE. The dynamic origins of positive health and wellbeing. Int J Pers Cent Med. 2012;2(2):179–87.
8. Cohn MA, Fredrickson BL, Brown SL, Mikels JA, Conway AM. Happiness unpacked: positive emotions increase life satisfaction by building resilience. Emotion. 2009;9(3):361–8.
9. Colton CW, Manderscheid RW. Congruencies in increased mortality rates, years of potential life lost, and causes of death among public mental health clients in eight states. Prev Chronic Dis. 2006;3(2):1–14.

10. Commission on Social Determinants of Health. Closing the gap in a generation: health equity through action on the social determinants of health. Final Report of the Commission on Social Determinants of Health., World Health Organization, Geneva; 2008.
11. Cutajar MC, Mullena PE, Ogloff JRP, Thomas SD, Wells DL, Spataro J. Psychopathology in a large cohort of sexually abused children followed up to 43 years. Child Abuse Negl. 2010;34:813–22.
12. de Wit L, Luppino F, van Straten A, Penninx B, Zitman F, Cuijpers P. Depression and obesity: a meta-analysis of community-based studies. Psychiatry Res. 2010;178(2):230–5.
13. Desjarlais R, Eisenberg L, Good B, Kleinman A. Salud Mental en el Mundo: Problemas y Prioridades en Poblaciones de Bajos Ingresos. Washington: OPS-OMS; 1997. p. 1–31.
14. DeVol R, Bedroussian A, Charuworn A, Chatterjee A, Kim I, Kim S, Klowden K. An unhealthy America: the economic burden of chronic disease. Santa Monica, California: Milken Institute; 2007.
15. Eylesa J, Brimacombeb M, Chaulkc P, Stoddartd G, Prangere T, Moasee O. What determines health? To where should we shift resources? Attitudes towards the determinants of health among multiple stakeholder groups in Prince Edward Island, Canada. Soc Sci Med. 2001;53:1611–9.
16. Hamedi V, Ameri A, Azamameri. Comparison of anxiety, depression, stress and anger in migraine, diabetic and cardiac patients and healthy people. Procedia Soc Behav Sci. 2013;84:1885–8.
17. Hirschfeld RMA, Bowden CL, Gitlin MJ, Keck PE, Perlis RH, Suppes T, Thase ME, Wagner KD. Practice guideline for the treatment of patients with bipolar disorder (revision). Am J Psychiatry. 2002;159(44 Suppl):1–50.
18. House JS, Landis KR, Umberson D. Social relationships and health. Science. 1988;241:540–5.
19. IGDA Workgroup, WPA. IGDA. 1: Conceptual bases—historical, cultural and clinical perspectives Br J Psychiatry 2003;182(suppl. 45):s40–s41.
20. Kaplan RM (2014) Behavior change and reducing health disparities. Prev Med. http://dx.doi.org/10.1016/j.ypmed.2014.04.014. Accessed 30 Oct 2014.
21. Kendall-Tacket K. The health effects of childhood abuse: four pathways by which abuse can influence health. Child Abuse Negl. 2002;26(6–7):715–29.
22. Kessler RC, Greenberg PE, Mickelson KD, Meneades LM, Wang PS. The effects of chronic medical conditions on work loss and work cutback. J Occup Environ Med. 2001;43:218–25.
23. Lazzarino AI, Hamer M, Gaze D, Collinson P, Steptoe A. The association between cortisol response to mental stress and high-sensitivity cardiac troponin T plasma concentration in healthy adults. J Am Coll Cardiol. 2013;62:1694–701.
24. Lê-Scherban F, Diez Roux AV, Li Y. Does academic achievement during childhood and adolescence benefit later health? Ann Epidemiol. 2014;24:344–55.
25. Lund C. Poverty and mental health: towards a research agenda for low and middle-income countries. Commentary on Tampubolon and Hanandita. Soc Sci Med. 2014;111:134–6.
26. Margolis R, Myrskyla M. Family, money, and health: regional differences in the determinants of life satisfaction over the life course. Adv Life Course Res. 2013;18:115–26.
27. Mayer EA. The neurobiology of stress and gastrointestinal disease. Gut. 2000;47:861–9.
28. McGinnis JM, Williams-Russo P, Knickman JR. The case for more active policy attention to health promotion. Health Aff. 2002;21(2):78–93.
29. Mezzich JE, Salloum IM, Cloninger CR, Salvador-Carulla L, Kirmayer L, Banzato CE, Wallcraft J, Botbol M. Person-centered integrative diagnosis: conceptual bases and structural model. Can J Psychiatry. 2010;55:701–8.
30. Mokdad AH, Marks JS, Stroup DF, Gerberding JL. Actual causes of death in the United States, 2000. JAMA. 2004;291(10):1238–45.
31. NIMH Genetics Workgroup. Genetics and mental disorders. Biol Psychiatry. 1999;45(5): 559–73.

32. Office of the United Nations High Commissioner for Human Rights. The right to health; 2008. Fact Sheet No. 31. UN, Geneve. http://www.ohchr.org/documents/publications/factsheet31.pdf. Accessed 10 Oct 2014.
33. Panter-Brick C, Goodman A, Tol W, Eggerman M. Mental health and childhood adversities: a longitudinal study in Kabul, Afghanistan. J Am Acad Child Adolesc Psychiatry. 2011;50(4):349–63.
34. Pesonen A-K, Räikkönen K, Feldt K, Heinonen K, Osmond C, Phillips DIW, Barker DJP, Eriksson JG, Kajantie E. Childhood separation experience predicts HPA axis hormonal responses in late adulthood: a natural experiment of World War II. Psychoneuroendocrinology. 2010;35:758–67.
35. Public Health Agency of Canada. What determines health? 2014. http://www.phac-aspc.gc.ca/ph-sp/determinants/index-eng.php#determinants. Accessed 10 Nov 2014.
36. Räikkönen K, Lahti M, Heinonen K, Pesonen A-K, Wahlbeck K, Kajantie E, Osmond C, Barker DJP, Eriksson JG. Risk of severe mental disorders in adults separated temporarily from their parents in childhood: the Helsinki birth cohort study. J Psychiatr Res. 2011;45:332–8.
37. Robichaud JB, Guay L, Colin C, Pothier M. Les lienss entre la pauvrété et la santé mentale: de léxclusion á léquite. Montreal: Gaëtan Morin Editeur; 1994. p. 93–8.
38. Rocco L. Trust me, you will be in better health. Health Policy. 2014;116:123–32.
39. Sachs-Ericsson N, Kendall-Tackett K, Hernandez A. Childhood abuse, chronic pain, and depression in the National Comorbidity Survey. Child Abuse Negl. 2007;31:531–47.
40. Salganicoff A, Wyn R. Access to care for low-income women: the impact of medicaid. J Health Care Poor Underserved. 1999;10(4):453–67.
41. Schroeder SA. We can do better—improving the health of the American People. N Engl J Med. 2007;357:1221–8.
42. Sección APAL de Diagnóstico y Clasificación. Guía Latinoamericana de Diagnóstico Psiquiátrico Versión Revisada, APAL, Lima; 2012.
43. Simon GE, Ludman EJ, Linde JA, Operskalski BH, Ichikawa L, Rohde P, Finch EA, Jeffery RW. Association between obesity and depression in middle-aged women. Gen Hosp Psychiatry. 2008;30(1):32–9.
44. Springer KW, Sheridan J, Kuo D, Carnes M. Long-term physical and mental health consequences of childhood physical abuse: results from a large population-based sample of men and women. Child Abuse Negl. 2007;31:517–30.
45. US Burden of Disease Collaborators. The state of US health, 1990–2010 burden of diseases, injuries, and risk factors. JAMA. 2013;310(6):591–608. doi:10.1001/jama.2013.13805.
46. Victorian Health Promotion Foundation. A Plan for Action 2005–2007. Promoting mental health and Wellbeing; 2005. http://www.vichealth.vic.gov.au/~/media/ResourceCentre/PublicationsandResources/General/VH%20action%20plan-web.ashx. Victorian Health Promotion Foundation, Carlton, Australia. Accessed 01 Oct 2014.
47. Virtanen M, Honkonen T, Kivimäki M, Ahola K, Vahtera J, Aromaa A, Lönnqvist J. Work stress, mental health and antidepressant medication findings from the health 2000 study. J Affect Disord. 2007;98:189–97.
48. Wallcraft J, Gayvoronskaya E, Salloum IM. Strengths and protective factors in person-centered integrative diagnosis. Int J Pers Cent Med. 2012;2(2):193–5.
49. Wells KB, Golding JM, Burnam MA. Chronic medical conditions in a sample of the general population with anxiety, affective, and substance use disorder. Am J Psychiatry. 1989;146:1440–6.
50. Wilkinson R, Marmot M, editors. Social determinants of health. The solid facts. Denmak: WHO; 2003.
51. World Health Organization (2004) Promoting mental health. Concepts, emerging evidence, practice. Summary Report. WHO, Geneva.
52. World Health Organization. Basic documents. 45th ed. Supplement, Geneva: WHO; 2006.

53. World Health Organization. Resolution WHA 62.12 reducing health inequities through action on the social determinants of health. WHO, Geneva; 2009. http://apps.who.int/gb/ebwha/pdf_files/A62/A62_R14-en.pdf. Accessed 10 Oct 2014.
54. World Health Organization. Resolution WHA 62.12 WHO's role and responsibilities in health research. WHO, Geneva; 2009. http://apps.who.int/gb/ebwha/pdf_files/A62/A62_12-en.pdf. Accessed 10 Oct 2014.
55. World Health Organization. A conceptual framework for action on the social determinants of health. WHO, Geneva; 2010. http://www.who.int/sdhconference/resources/Conceptualframe-workforactiononSDH_eng.pdf. Accessed 01 Oct 2014.
56. World Health Organization. Risks To mental health: an overview of vulnerabilities and risk factors. WHO discussion paper; 2012. http://www.who.int/mental_health/mhgap/risks_to_mental_health_EN_27_08_12.pdf. Accessed 10 Oct 2014.
57. World Health Organization. The determinants of Health; 2014. http://www.who.int/hia/evidence/doh/en/#. Accessed 10 Nov 2014.
58. World Health Organization, Calouste Gulbenkian Foundation. Integrating the response to mental disorders and other chronic diseases in health care systems. Geneva: World Health Organization; 2014.
59. World Health Professions Alliance (WHPA). Health improvement card. User guide for health professionals. France: World Medical Association; 2011. http://www.whpa.org/ncd_health_improvement_card_professionals.pdf. Accessed 01 Oct 2014.
60. Yuyan S, Sheng Z. From genomes to societies: a holistic view of determinants of human health. Curr Opin Biotechnol. 2014;28:134–42.

Health Experience and Values in Person-Centered Assessment and Diagnosis

14

Laurence J. Kirmayer, MD, FRCP(C), FCAHS,
Juan E. Mezzich, MD, MA, MS, PhD
and C.W. Van Staden, MBChB, MMed (Psych), MD

14.1 Introduction

Person-centered psychiatry aims to approach care through an integrative assessment of patients' mental health status, needs, and concerns as well as many factors contributing to resilience and vulnerability to illness [54]. Subjective experience is central to this assessment for fundamental ethical, conceptual, and pragmatic reasons. Mental health problems are felt through an array of symptoms, which include bodily sensations, emotions, and thoughts. These are organized in terms of social and cultural templates and communicated to others. Experience involves processes of embodiment and enactment [39]. Thus, while medical semiotics tends to treat the symptoms of illness as a more or less direct reflection of physiological processes, in

Juan E. Mezzich—Editor in Chief, International Journal of Person Centered Medicine.

L.J. Kirmayer, MD, FRCP(C), FCAHS
James McGill Professor and Director, Division of Social and Transcultural Psychiatry, McGill University, Montreal, Canada; Director, Culture and Mental Health Research Unit, Institute of Community and Family Psychiatry, Jewish General Hospital, Montreal, QC, Canada
e-mail: laurence.kirmayer@mcgill.ca

J.E. Mezzich, MD, MA, MS, PhD
Professor of Psychiatry, Icahn School of Medicine at Mount Sinai, New York, USA; Secretary General, International College of Person Centered Medicine, New York, USA; Editor in Chief, International Journal of Person Centered Medicine, New York, USA; Former President, World Psychiatric Association, Geneva, Switzerland

C.W. Van Staden, MBChB, MMed (Psych), MD (✉)
Nelson Mandela Professor of Philosophy and Psychiatry, University of Pretoria, Pretoria, South Africa
e-mail: werdie.vanstaden@up.ac.za

J.E. Mezzich et al. (eds.), *Person Centered Psychiatry*,
DOI 10.1007/978-3-319-39724-5_14

fact, all experience is mediated by cognitive and social interpretive processes involving metaphoric and narrative constructions and communication [36]. These interpretive processes are not neutral or “value-free” but guided by specific processes of valuation that lead us to experience some events as positive, good, desirable, and beneficial and others as negative, bad, undesirable, and harmful. In this chapter, we consider some of what is known about the nature of these processes of embodiment, interpretation, and enactment that contribute to subjectivity and outline an approach to clinical assessment that gives explicit attention to patients' experience and values through understanding the meanings of symptoms and suffering in social context.

14.2 The Importance of Health Experience

Understanding health and illness experience is crucial to person-centered psychiatry for several basic reasons:

1. Experience is central to what is of greatest concern to patients—whether that be symptoms of illness like pain, fatigue, and malaise, impaired functioning, or the pursuit of wellness; even health concerns involving other family members are felt as emotional distress and mental preoccupation in ways that may become problems in their own right. Hence, clinical empathy and understanding must begin with an engagement with patients' experience [39];
2. The experience of symptoms, distress, or impairment is a key motivator and determinant of help-seeking behaviors. People may cope with various forms of discomfort or accept them as part of the human condition, but when a symptom provokes concern or distress that exceeds the person's threshold of tolerance, that experience becomes the impulse for seeking help and, through its experiential quality, suggests particular targets for treatment;
3. Subjective reports of health status and distress are strong predictors not only of quality of life, but also of morbidity and mortality [31, 66]. Hence, most areas of medicine have recognized the importance of assessing self-rated health;
4. In the case of psychiatric disorders, alterations of experience in themselves may be crucial signs and symptoms of illness, indicating the nature of the problem and providing a target for intervention. Consider, for example, the *experience* of panic, fear, worry, and anxiety in anxiety disorders, the elation or hopelessness at the core of mood disorders, and hallucinations in psychosis. Thoughts and beliefs are at least in part also expressions of experiences, even when these are delusional or reflect the racing thoughts of mania or the cognitive deficits of dementia;
5. Ultimately, experience it is the medium through which the impact of illness and interventions is felt and outcomes of interventions are largely evaluated. Moreover, health itself is experienced as feelings of vitality, joy, satisfaction, or the ability to pursue one's goals and realize one's capabilities.

The centrality of experience in medical care is recognized in the social science distinction between *illness* and *disease*, with *illness* standing for the person's experience of affliction and *disease* for the constructs of biomedical explanations. Illness and disease have a complex and changeable relationship. Illness can occur without disease, when individuals present symptoms for which biomedicine has no disease explanation; and disease often occurs without illness, for example, when screening discovers physiological problems like hypertension or diabetes that the person was unaware of. But once a diagnosis is made, patients may experience the illness in new ways as a result of their knowledge and interpretation of the diagnosis, the effects of the treatment regimen, or the wider social meaning of the diagnostic label.

Experience has an added crucial role in psychiatry, because many psychiatric disorders involve alterations or disturbances in the basic processes that underlie experience itself. Accordingly, in psychiatric assessment and diagnosis, we must consider both the experience of health and illness and the dynamics of health and illness within experience. Teasing apart the contributions of underlying psychopathology, adaptive responses, and cognitive-social interpretive practices may be difficult in any given case. Indeed, psychiatry needs its own epistemology that recognizes the ongoing cycles or looping between neurobiological function, bodily and self experience, and interpretive processes [5, 74].

In practice, clinicians use multiple frameworks to think about the relationships between health, illness, and experience. In the following sections, we will briefly consider three broad perspectives on experience, each of which has implications for how we might understand and assess health experience and values, specifically: (1) phenomenology; (2) cognitive social psychology; and (3) cultural anthropology.

14.3 Phenomenological Approaches to Experience and Subjectivity

There is a long tradition in psychiatry, examining the texture of psychopathological experience through close phenomenological analysis of first-person experience [8]. This understanding of the subjective experience of illness lies at the root of the diagnostic nosologies of psychiatry, but it is also a crucial path to empathic understanding in the clinical encounter.

Phenomenological philosophy, in its various schools or versions, aims to understand the structure of experience from a first-person perspective, without referring to external reality, underlying mechanisms, or to a subject/object distinction [1]. However, as a clinical discipline, psychiatry must integrate phenomenological aspects of experience with naturalistic explanations of mental mechanisms [60, 63, 72]. In psychiatry, a phenomenological approach was advanced in the early work of Karl Jaspers who collected richly detailed analyses of various forms of psychopathological experience [29, 71]. The changes in diagnostic practice heralded by DSM-III reflected a dramatic simplification in phenomenological accounts of mental disorders, with the complexity of patients' illness experience mapped onto limited lists of symptoms and signs that constitute the diagnostic criteria for specific disorders. Clarity in diagnostic labeling was achieved at the cost of a great reduction in the richness of information present in patients' illness experience [3].

In recent years, there has been a resurgence of interest in phenomenological approaches as a way to explore the complexity of psychopathological experience. Tools have been developed to explore specific domains of experience. Psychiatrists have developed semi-structured interview protocols and methods of analysis that unpack psychotic experience [59, 61]. Ethnographic researchers have adapted phenomenological theories and methods to studying the nature of psychotic experience and other forms of psychopathology in social context [10, 11, 13, 14]. Philosophers have adopted more experimental methods working with larger samples and systematic content analysis to explore the fine-grained texture of experience [65]. However, the essential methods of phenomenology remain the openness and attentiveness of the observer to the structure of experience, combined with an effort to bracket off received or taken-for-granted categories and assumptions.

Phenomenology can be a path to advancing psychiatric science [16]. Careful studies of psychopathological phenomena including hallucinations, delusions, anxiety, and depressed mood have revealed the diversity of experiences labeled with a single term and can guide research on potential mechanisms of illness and recovery. Given the hypothesis that certain forms of psychopathology reflect distinctive alterations in brain functioning, we would expect to find correlations between changes in neural processing and illness experience. Psychiatric illness can affect the underlying machinery and dynamics of experience, and hence alter the relationship between physiology, symptom, sign, and behavior. Although research is still at an early stage owing to its complexity, neurophenomenological studies of functional brain imaging in psychopathology point toward specific neural substrates of self experience in psychiatric disorders [58]. However, all experience is filtered through attentional mechanisms and formulated in terms of conceptual frameworks that rely on cognitive-social interactions and cultural models [64]. Hence, we need a *cultural neurophenomenology* that encompasses both brain and social-historical context [40, 74].

Identifying the distinctive experiences associated with particular kinds of psychopathology is basic to clinical assessment. Phenomenology can also provide clinicians with a rich language to understand and engage with patients' experience. This can foster empathy and so strengthen the clinical alliance. However, patients' may also have experiences that are difficult to describe because they are subtle, unusual, and not recognized in folk psychology or in familiar cultural models. Phenomenological analysis can provide ways to describe these unusual experiences, refining assessment, but also allowing patient and clinician to co-construct a model or interpretation and reach a new level of mutual understanding [77].

Finally, close tracking of phenomenology is essential to insure that we assess outcomes in meaningful ways. Lack of attention to phenomenology may account for conflicts or disappointments in treatment settings when patients feel their experience is neglected, not adequately recognized, or discounted. For example, for many patients, currently available treatment with neuroleptics or other psychiatric medications, while alleviating some symptoms, leaves them with "side-effects" including alterations of ordinary experience and the sense of self that can be difficult and distressing. Recognizing the nature of these experiences (e.g. loss of libido with SSRI antidepressants; dyskinesias with neuroleptics; motor incoordination and proprioceptive disturbances with benzodiazepines) is essential for humane care, as well as for improving treatment adherence and outcomes.

14.4 Cognitive and Social Mediation of Experience

Medical semiotics tends to approach experience as a more or less direct outcome of physiological processes. Ideally, symptom reports should match experience and experience should parallel physiological events in the body. Patients who give accounts that do not accord with medical models of bodily processes are sometimes viewed as "poor historians" and this in itself becomes a symptom of problematic illness behavior or psychiatric disorder.

In reality, symptom experience and reporting are the outcome of a nested series of processes that include perception, attention, interpretation, and communication (see Fig. 14.1). Health and illness experience are embedded in processes of perception, attention, cognitive-interpretation, interpersonal interaction, and institutional practices, including those of the health care setting ([35, 38, 44, 56, 62]). All of these contribute to embodied experience. At the same time, illness experience is enacted and expressed through communicative action in ways that influence subsequent interpretation [35]. The feedback loops between embodiment and enactment at the levels of bodily processes, perception, attention, interpretation, and social interaction constitute "hermeneutic circles" in which the construction and negotiation of meaning reshapes experience [39].

Perception of bodily sensations, thoughts, and feelings varies across individuals and depends on past developmental experiences, cultural scripts or models, and social contexts [68]. From moment to moment, attention can be differentially directed to bodily experience, thoughts and feelings, one's own behavior, or the social environment. The focus of attention will influence what the person notices and foregrounds, which then demands interpretation or explanation. When worrisome or distressing, the experience can become a focus of coping efforts and requests for help. Novel or distressful experience like pain, nausea, or anxiety can grab attention, but attention can also select sensations from the constant background "white noise" of transient experiences. Focusing on a transient sensation makes it more salient, and when this leads to distress, one can contribute to vicious circles that maintain symptom persistence.

There is a large body of research on how cognitive-interpretive processes regulate symptom experience, coping, and the response to clinical interventions [38, 44, 45]. This work demonstrates that people have models of symptoms and illness that include: notions about the identity of their illness; causal attributions or explanations; temporal course; appropriate modes of coping, help-seeking, and treatment; and potential consequences. These models may initially be fragmentary or incomplete, leaving areas of illness experience uncertain, confusing, and inchoate. However, this uncertainty prompts a search for meaning and clarification

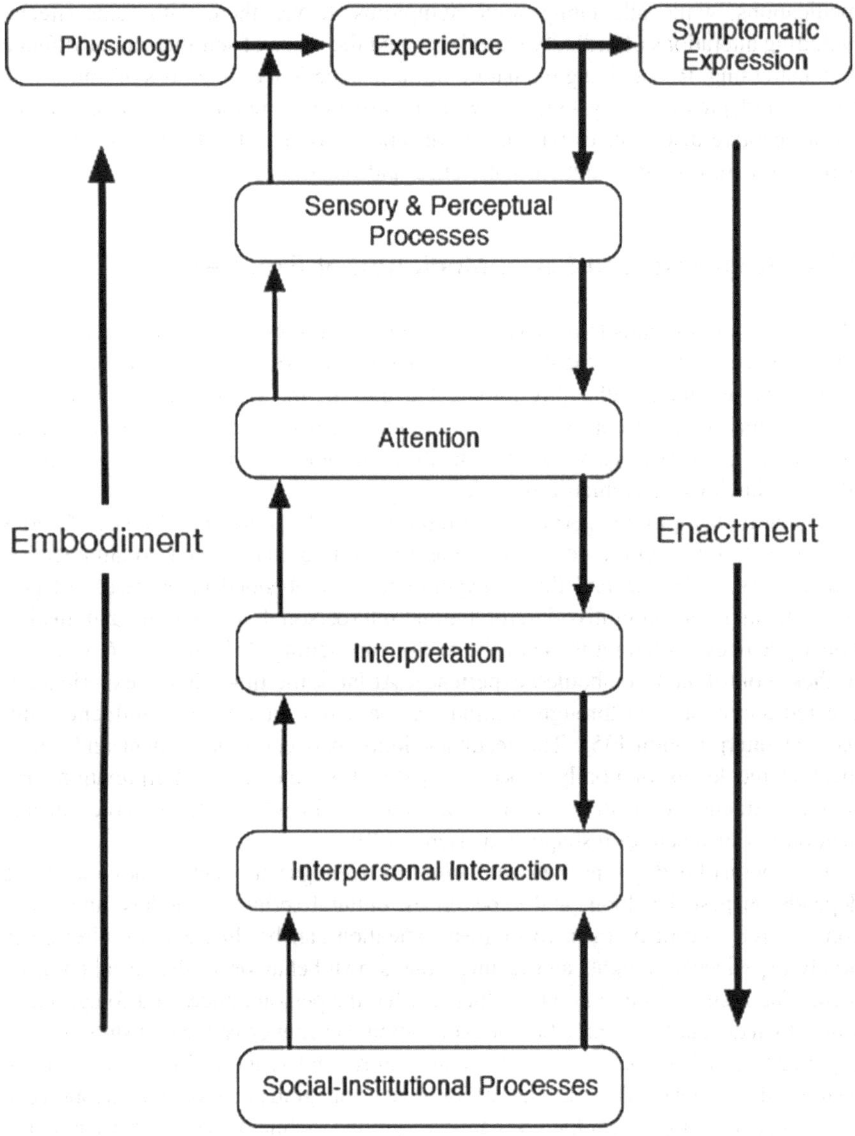

Fig. 14.1 Embodiment and enactment in health and illness experience. Illness experience is embedded in processes of perception, attention, cognitive-interpretation, interpersonal interaction, and health care settings. See text

and, over time, illness labels, explanations, and expectations become organized into stable and coherent schemas. Crucial for our discussion, these cognitive-interpretive processes and schemas are not simply a response to illness experience but actually may be constitutive of experience. For example, thinking that one has a common cold will lead to increased attention on potential nose and throat symptoms. Similarly, labeling one's state as anxiety or depression will lead to shifts in attention and modes of interpretation that may result in experiencing additional symptoms consistent with the person's model for anxiety or depression. Hence, the models that people engage reshape their experience from the first intimations that something is wrong to the long-term course of coping with chronic illness.

Contemporary cognitive science takes this emphasis on individual interpretive processes, further by emphasizing the ways in which experience is embodied and enacted in specific social contexts [21]. Individuals' interpretations of illness experience are influenced by their own previous experiences as well as by common models or prototypes available in their families and communities or from mass media. Health care providers and institutions contribute to building these models through their efforts at education and knowledge translation. In so doing, medical and psychiatric care influence subsequent illness experience.

14.5 Anthropological or Ethnographic Approaches to Subjectivity

Medical and psychiatric anthropology have used the methods of ethnography to explore the social embedding, meaning, and significance of illness experience and values [6, 13, 28, 30, 43]. These approaches understand experience not just as a bodily given, but as created within and through particular forms of subjectivity [48]. These forms of subjectivity and intersubjectivity are related to wider social and cultural systems of knowledge and practice involving notions of personhood, ontologies, epistemologies, moral orders, and politics of self-governance. From this perspective, modes of experiencing may be social, moral, or political acts. This has profound consequences for how we understand suffering itself, not just as something that medicine and psychiatry strive to eliminate but also as part of morally shaped forms of personhood and ways of being-in-the-world that have their own value and consequences [37].

Although basic elements of illness experience are embodied and may be difficult to put into words, most complex experience is elaborated and expressed through narratives. These narrative accounts are not only used to communicate but also provide internal frameworks for interpreting experience and clarifying our thoughts and understanding. Systematic exploration of illness narratives reveals the extent to which they are complex, multistranded, and reorganized in response to specific needs or contexts [34, 76]. The narratives that are presented in clinical settings reflect ongoing efforts at organizing illness experience that may be influenced by others in the patients' family or community. As they are reworked in the clinical encounter, they often change, leading to new ways of experiencing symptoms and afflictions.

This is illustrated by ethnographic research on illness experience and help-seeking with the McGill Illness Narrative Interview [26]. Interviews with people in the community about their medically unexplained symptoms revealed an evolving narrative that referenced past traumas as well as current social difficulties [24]. The meanings of the symptoms changed as people were encouraged to reflect on their significance. Although not intended to be an intervention, this process of exploration and re-narration of experience was viewed by many research participants as helpful or therapeutic, much as seen in narrative psychiatry and psychotherapy [27].

Consistent with contemporary phenomenology, ethnographic approaches to illness experience recognize that experience is inherently *intersubjective*—arising from and residing in the co-presence and interaction of self and others. This intersubjectivity involves both the bodily-felt aspects of empathy and the co-construction of shared narratives. When this process of co-construction of narratives fails or breaks down, patients may experience themselves as misrecognized and misunderstood by the clinician in ways that undermine clinical care and collaboration [35]. Mutual understanding depends on attentiveness, openness, and knowledge of patients' lifeworlds, which include their social position, relations with others, and participation in multiple systems of meaning and value.

14.6 The Location of Values

Some aspects of illness experience are intrinsically negatively valued—indeed, this is part of what makes them signs of illness. Pain, nausea, fatigue, and malaise are general experiences that people dislike, wish to avoid, and expend effort and resources to resolve. Although we do not need to learn to dislike pain and nausea, past experiences, and social and cultural meaning play a major role in most aspects of illness experience [23]. Moreover, most experiences of health and illness are multifaceted and the weight given to different facets and the ways they are assessed may differ substantially across individuals, communities, and cultures.

Experiences are constantly evaluated against particular frameworks of meaning. This occurs in highly valenced ways that attach a sense of good and bad, desirable or undesirable to experiences, which determines what is important and worth acting on, and what can be ignored. What makes an experience evidence of illness or health is essentially its value to the person and others in their family or community. Each person has his or her own implicit set of values, which are rooted in the ways that human biology valences certain experiences as distressing (e.g. pain, nausea, negative emotions, or cognitive confusion) but which also reflect the individual's past experiences, development, personal identity, goals, and plans. The individual's history gives rise to more elaborate systems of values that include how particular experiences or events fit with larger personal goals (e.g. one might positively value pain as evidence that one is getting better or view it as a personal challenge, trial or punishment). Finally, cultural background and social contexts frame these individual interpretive processes and give added meaning and value to specific experiences. Medicine and psychiatry as social and cultural institutions have their own systems of values, which may be consistent or conflict with those of patients and their families [22, 33, 35, 42].

For example, much of the theory and practice of psychiatry and clinical psychology is rooted in an individualistic concept of the person that emphasizes values of autonomy, self-directedness, and freedom of choice [37]. Well-being is then equated to the exercise of this freedom. In contrast, for people living in more communal or collectivistic contexts, maintaining the harmony and integrity of the family, clan, or community (from neighborhood to mankind) may be paramount and provide a crucial dimension of health and well-being [67]. This has implications for clinical ethics [75] and notions of recovery [2], as well as the practice of psychotherapy [37]. Even the experience of psychiatric medications is shaped by cultural values. Ethnographic research on the experience of adolescents taking psychiatric medications illustrates the ways in which moral discourse about personhood can interact with the embodied experience of biomedical treatment [9].

Although clinical care, borrowing from the individualistic ethos that dominates much professional mental health care, tends to frame values in terms of individual goals, in most instances the meaning of individual values must be understood in relation to social values shared by others in the person's family, community, or wider social circles [12]. Values are present both as explicit norms and standards embedded in moral codes, but also as implicit ideas, ontologies, notions of authority, commitments, and practices [20]. Even when people explicitly reject these values, they may be strongly influenced by them. In any event, the very rejection is driven by values. Exploring values therefore needs to take place on multiple levels: both explicitly in terms of the goals and tradeoffs the individual is willing to make and implicitly, in terms of what they find difficult, repugnant, or simply unimaginable.

Our domain of value therefore is not restricted to rational choice, but is equally connected to lived realities that the person may experience as external to them, or as deeply intrinsic to their identity and difficult to manage. Person-centered psychiatry needs a conceptualization of the person that allows us to understand value decisions and commitments that are essentially "irrational" or extra-rational. This may be informed by a variety of models, ranging from cognitive theories of judgment heuristics and biases [32], through psychodynamic theories of hidden or repressed conflicts and motivations, to social theories of the functions of the sacred or sacrosanct.

14.7 Assessing Health Experience and Values

Our discussion of different approaches to subjectivity has implications for how we might approach the assessment of health experience and values in clinical practice. Assessment of illness experience and values requires adequate time and a safe space, within which the clinician can make use of empathy, specific interviewing skills, and conceptual frameworks to elicit and interpret patients' verbal and nonverbal communication [15]. This process is fundamentally intersubjective, requiring that clinicians attend to and reflect on their own experience and intuitions in the process of exploring the patient's predicament and the co-construction of a shared understanding [79].

Illness experience is not fixed, static, or monolithic and is not located entirely within the patient but emerges in the context of the patient's lifeworld. Different facets of experience may be foregrounded in relation to the demands of specific social contexts and relationships including the clinical encounter. The ways in which experience is recognized, narrated, and handled in the clinical setting by both patient and practitioner will change the illness experience. In particular, medical or psychiatric interventions (including exploring specific symptoms, performing laboratory tests, assigning diagnostic labels and prognoses, and assessing outcomes) change illness experience. Staying alert to the ways in which clinical interaction shapes illness experience requires self-reflection on the part of the clinician.

Similarly, values are not primarily encoded as abstract, the person tries to live by general principles but practices and commitments are embedded in particular relationships, social contexts, and communities. The relationship between experience and values is complex with bidirectional influence and conceptual overlap. Many values are grounded in certain kinds of experience (developmental, social, illness history and help-seeking behaviors) and, in turn, influence the ways that symptoms and functional limitations are experienced. The implication for psychiatry is that we need to reflect on the significance and impact of the context of evaluation, and may need multiple assessments in different contexts to stay alert to how valuation changes across contexts.

Clinical empathy depends on the capacity to understand patients' feelings in context. This requires not only affective and relational skills, but also an appreciation of the complexity of the human condition in social context. Empathy for illness experience is informed by clinical knowledge of the nature of psychopathology, which must be complemented by awareness of the nature of the patient's personal history and social world. A pedagogy of empathy will cultivate the tolerance of strong emotion and ability to regulate one's own response to the other as well as providing the background knowledge necessary to appreciate diverse values and experiences of psychopathology, human development, social contexts, and lifeworlds ([18, 79]).

Training in phenomenological interviewing can enhance the clinician's capacity to elicit a detailed picture of the patient's experience and values. Table 14.1 lists some semi-structured interviews and questionnaires that have been developed for research on illness experience. Familiarity with these tools can help clinicians enlarge their repertoire of strategies to elicit illness experience. Specific questions can be employed and followed up by further probes to explore the quality of patients' experience. Innovative assessment methods including the use of expressive media like drawing or photography can help patients express aspects of illness that may be difficult to convey through language. Information elicited through interviews or other methods must be brought back to the clinical dialog to clarify how the clinician's model fits with patients' own self-understanding and illness experience. Too often, when patients' experience is inconsistent with clinical expectations it is simply discounted or taken as byproduct of their psychopathology.

Table 14.1 Tools for eliciting health and illness experience

Instrument	Format and structure	Domains of experience
Cultural formulation interview ((DSM-5 CFI) [46])	Semi-structured interview, open-ended questions	Definition of the problem; causal explanations; social stressors and supports; cultural identity; coping and help-seeking; expectations for care; supplementary modules on explanatory models, level of functioning, social network, psychosocial stressors, spirituality and religion, migration, developmental experiences
Examination of anomalous self-experience (EASE) [61]	Symptom checklist used by clinician trained in conducting a phenomenologically oriented interview	Disorders of self-awareness
Explanatory model interview catalogue (EMIC) [80]	Semi-structured interview, open-ended questions	General illness explanatory models
McGill illness narrative interview (MINI) [25, 26]	Semi-structured interview, symptom focused, open-ended questions	Initial symptom experience (temporal narrative); symptom or illness prototypes from self, others or media; explanatory models (label, causal explanations, expectations for outcome)
Clinical ethnographic interview (CEI) [70]	Semi-structured interview supplemented with social network map, body image map, and timeline of illness experience	DSM-IV outline for cultural formulation domains
Illness perception questionnaire (IPQ: Revised, IPQ-R) [57, 83]	Self-report questionnaire (likert scales)	Symptom experience, affective responses to symptoms, causal explanations, coping and treatment expectations
Multicultural quality of life index [47, 50, 53, 84]	Self-report scale	Physical well-being, psychological well-being, self-care functioning, occupational functioning, interpersonal functioning, social-emotional support, community and services support, personal fulfillment, spiritual fulfillment, global QoL
WHOQoL [81, 82]	Self-report questionnaire (Likert scales)	Physical, psychological, social, environmental, spiritual dimensions of health and well-being

A person-centered approach emphasizes recognition of patients' and clinicians' experiences and values as essential bases of collaboration, assessment, treatment negotiation, and the process of care [73, 78].

14.8 Incorporating Experience and Values into Person-Centered Assessment and Integrative Diagnosis

Informed by the phenomenological, cognitive-social, and anthropological-ethnographic considerations discussed above, in this section we outline some strategies for the incorporation and assessment of experience, values, and expectations as core elements of person-centered integrative diagnosis of illness and health.

Attempts to integrate experience and values in diagnostic systems were pioneered through the development of the Outline for Cultural Formulation for DSM-IV [51, 52]. More recent work on the Cultural Formulation is illustrated by the Cultural Formulation Guidelines [49], and the Cultural Formulation Interview for DSM-5 [46]. These methods and tools can help clinicians systematically explore patients' experience and understanding of their symptoms and health concerns as well as their values and priorities for care. Culturally oriented assessment is grounded in an understanding of experience as embodied and embedded in social contexts. Hence, it includes systematic inquiry into the illness explanations and responses of others in the patient's entourage, family, and community (see: Kirmayer et al., this volume). Moreover, it includes both diachronic (developmental) and synchronic (ecosystemic) dimensions that locate health and illness in their causal trajectories and current contexts. This work inspired the conceptual development of the Health Experience level of the Person-centered Integrative Diagnostic Model, which also includes as its other two core levels, Health Status and Health Contributors [54].

In addition to health experience, attention to values and needs is crucial to all decision making in health care [17]. To this end, values based medicine has been promoted both as a research domain and as a component of clinical practice. For example, current United Kingdom Health Department policies note the importance of health care decision making addressing the values of the patient but also of the practitioner (both professional and personal), the community, the society, and the health care institution [18, 79]. Accounting for the specific values that people experience in their individual capacities and communal roles is conceptually consistent with person-centered care [19]. Values based medicine has received broad international support [78], including from proponents of evidence-based medicine. Indeed, the originators of evidence-based medicine have stated expressly that patient values must be integrated into clinical decisions if these are to serve the patient [69].

Both Health Experience and Health Values/Expectations are concepts constituting the third informational level of the Person-centered Integrative Diagnosis model applied as a practical guide in the Latin American Guide of Psychiatric Diagnosis, Revised Version (GLADP-VR), published by the Latin American Psychiatric Association for regular use in clinical care, training, and research in the Latin American region [4]. The GLADP-VR Health Experiences and Expectations level covers three areas: [1] Personal and cultural identity; [2] Suffering (its recognition, idioms of distress, illness beliefs); and [3] Experiences and expectations of health care. Each of these areas is explored and summarized narratively. This use of narrative to capture key clinical information is in line with the importance of narrative in subjectivity and reflects the need to allow maximum flexibility for the description of the intricacy and complexity of illness experience [55].

14.9 Conclusion

Attention to personal experience and values is essential for clinical empathy, for accurate assessment of symptoms or states of health and illness, for understanding patients' values and concerns, and for communicating and intervening effectively in clinical settings. While the semiotics of medicine tends to assume that experience follows directly from underlying physiology or bodily events, in fact, cognitive-emotional and interpretive processes as well as social interaction and wider discursive practices all contribute to the person's experience of health and illness. Hence, person-centered care needs to integrate—both theoretically and practically—the multiple processes that contribute to subjectivity and values. This core concept is discussed further elsewhere in this volume [7]. Initial steps have been taken to bring patients' experience, culture, and values into the core of clinical diagnosis through the Person-centered Integrative Diagnostic model and its practical application in the GLADP-VR. Further work on these developments is ongoing.

The theoretical considerations and approaches reviewed throughout this chapter can guide the process of comprehensive clinical assessment, diagnosis, and treatment collaboration. Ultimately, person-centered psychiatry aims to build on an understanding of experience to allow patients and clinicians to co-construct an approach to symptoms and suffering that leads to effective strategies for healing and recovery.

Appendix: Guidelines for Cultural Assessment[1]

The following questions can be used to explore aspects of illness experience and values in context. Not all questions are relevant to any given patient. The topics included and order of inquiry should be adapted to the clinical context to flow naturally from the patient's concerns and priorities. Additional questions should be devised for clarification and elaboration of key areas. Questions about identity, background, and social context should be introduced by explaining their clinical relevance to the patient so that they are not perceived as intrusive or irrelevant.

[1]Adapted from Kirmayer et al. [41] and from Mezzich et al. [49].

Cultural Identity of the Individual

Ethnic or Cultural Reference Group:

1. Where are you and your parents from?
2. What is your ancestry? What background, groups, or nations are you mainly affiliated with?
3. How close, connected, or committed do you feel to each of these cultural groups?
4. Are there any differences in the background of your mother and father; of you and your spouse?

Language:

1. What languages did you speak growing up?
2. What languages do you know (e.g., can speak or read)?
3. What languages do you speak at home?
4. Which language do you use in your community?
5. Which language do you prefer to use in your health care or when discussing personal issues?

For migrants, Involvement with Culture of Origin:

1. What is your original cultural background, ancestry, or country of origin?
2. How close do you feel to your original culture?
3. In what ways do you keep in touch and participate in your culture of origin?
4. Do you use the language of that culture?
5. How strongly does it affect you if that cultural group is praised or criticized in the media?
6. Do you share the values (politics, religion, etc.) of that culture?
7. Do you celebrate that culture's holidays?
8. Do you eat the foods typical of that culture?
9. Do you follow the newspapers, magazines, TV, radio, or Internet from that culture?
10. How closely do you follow the news or events related to your ethnic group?
11. What do you miss about the culture or community you came from?
12. Are there aspects of that culture or community that you are relieved to have left?

Involvement with Culture of Resettlement:

1. What is the culture or community to which you have moved?
2. How close do you feel to this new culture or community?
3. Do you use the language of this culture or community?

4. How strongly does it affect you if this cultural group or community is praised or criticized in the media?
5. Do you share the values (politics, religion, etc.) of this culture or community?
6. Do you celebrate holidays of this culture or community?
7. Do you eat the foods typical of this culture or community?
8. Do you follow the newspapers, magazines, TV, radio, or Internet from this culture or community?
9. What things about the current neighborhood, community, or culture you live in are most difficult for you and which do you like the most?
10. What are the main differences between the place you came from and the place you live in now?

Cultural Explanations of the Individual's Illness and Help-Seeking Experience

1. What happened around the time you got sick (your problems, symptoms, illness, etc. began)? How did others respond?
2. Have you ever had anything like this behavior or difficulty? Has anyone you know ever had the same type of problem?
3. What do you call the problem you have in your own language or to others in your family or community?
4. How do you describe this problem to health care providers?
5. How serious is this problem?
6. How has this problem affected your life?
7. What do you find most difficult about this problem?
8. What do you think are the causes of this problem?
9. What do others in your family think about this problem?
10. Who have you consulted to get help for the problems you have?
11. Have you consulted any other sources of help for this problem? (Any traditional healers or community helpers?)
12. What kind of treatment do you want?
13. What do you hope the treatment will do for you?
14. Do you have any concerns about this treatment?

Cultural Factors Related to Psychosocial Environment and Functioning

On Stressors:

1. What stressful (difficult, challenging) situations or events have played a role in your illness?
2. How are these stresses or events affecting your life and family?
3. What do others in your community think about the stresses you have experienced?

4. How are these stressful experiences or events generally viewed in your culture?
5. How difficult would it be for you to reveal or discuss your symptoms or illness in your community?

On Supports:

1. Is there someone you trust and can talk to about personal matters?
2. What other sources of emotional support can you rely on?
3. What are your main sources of support—for information, finances, help with everyday tasks, emotional support, or help in dealing with symptoms or illness?
4. What role do your family, friends, and community play in your life?
5. What role do work, school, and other pastimes play in your life?
6. What role does religion and spirituality play in your life?

On Functioning:

1. How do your illness or symptoms affect your ability to take care of yourself?
2. How do your illness or symptoms affect your ability to work?
3. How do your illness or symptoms affect your interactions and relationships with your family?
4. How do your illness or symptoms affect your life and social relations in general?
5. What do others in your community think about these difficulties you have been having?
6. How are these difficulties viewed in your culture?

Cultural Elements of the Relationship Between the Individual and the Clinician

Assessing the clinician-patient relationship involves participant-observation and self-reflection on the part of the clinician, which can be guided by the following questions:

1. What are the salient features of the clinician's own ancestry, identity, and cultural reference groups vis-à-vis this patient?
2. How do these facets of identity influence the clinician's perception of the patient?
3. How does the patient perceive the clinician?
4. How do intercultural differences influence trust, communication, and rapport between clinician and patient?
5. How do intercultural differences influence the elicitation of symptoms and the understanding of their significance?
6. How do similarities between clinician and patient blur or mask other sources of social difference or evidence of psychopathology?

7. How do intercultural differences influence the determination of whether a behavior is normal or pathological?
8. How do intercultural differences influence the negotiation of diagnosis, treatment objectives, and the delivery of care?

References

1. Abettan C. The current dialogue between phenomenology and psychiatry: a problematic misunderstanding. Med Health Care Philos. 2015;1–8.
2. Adeponle AB, Whitley R, Kirmayer LJ. Cultural contexts and constructions of recovery. In: Rudnick A, editor. Recovery of people with mental illness: philosophical and related perspectives. New York: Oxford University Press; 2012. p. 109–32.
3. Andreasen NC. DSM and the death of phenomenology in America: an example of unintended consequences. Schizophr Bull. 2007;33(1):108–12.
4. Asociación Psiquiátrica de América Latina, Sección de Diagnóstico y Clasificación. Guía Latinoamericana de Diagnóstico Psiquiátrico, Version revisada (GLADP-VR). Lima: Asociación Psiquiátrica de América Latina; 2012.
5. Berrios GE, Marková IS. Toward a new epistemology of psychiatry. In: Kirmayer LJ, Lemelson R, Cummings CA, editors. Re-visioning psychiatry: cultural phenomenology, critical neuroscience, and global mental health. New York: Cambridge University Press; 2015.
6. Biehl JG, Good B, Kleinman A. Subjectivity: ethnographic investigations. Berkeley: University of California Press; 2007.
7. Botbol M, Lecic-Tosevski D. Subjectivity, intersubjectivity and psychological functioning. In: Mezzich JE, Botbol M, Christodoulou GN, Cloninger CR, Salloum IM, editors. Person centered psychiatry. Heidelberg: Springer (in press).
8. Broome MR, Harland R, Owen GS, Stringaris A, editors. The Maudsley reader in phenomenological psychiatry. Cambridge: Cambridge University Press; 2013.
9. Choudhury S, McKinney KA, Kirmayer LJ. "Learning how to deal with feelings differently": psychotropic medications as vehicles of socialization in adolescence. Soc Sci Med. 2015.
10. Corin E. The thickness of being: intentional worlds, strategies of identity and experience among schizophrenics. Psychiatry. 1998;61(2):133–46.
11. Corin E, Lauzon G. From symptoms to phenomena: the articulation of experience in schizophrenia. J Phenomenological Psychol. 1994;25(1):3–50.
12. Crepaz-Keay D, Fulford KWM, Van Staden CW. Putting both a person and people first: interdependence, values-based practice and African Batho Pele as resources for co-production in mental health. In: Sadler JZ, Van Staden CW, Fulford KWM, editors. Oxford handbook of psychiatric ethics. Oxford: Oxford University Press; 2015. p. 60–87.
13. Csordas TJ. Cultural phenomenology and psychiatric illness. In: Kirmayer LJ, Lemelson R, Cummings CA, editors. Re-visioning psychiatry: cultural phenomenology, critical neuroscience, and global mental health. New York: Cambridge University Press; 2015. p. 117–40.
14. Desjarlais R, Throop JC. Phenomenological approaches in anthropology. Annu Rev Anthropol. 2011;40:87–102.
15. Eisenberg L. The physician as interpreter: ascribing meaning to the illness experience. Compr Psychiatry. 1981;22(3):239–48.
16. Fuchs T. Subjectivity and intersubjectivity in psychiatric diagnosis. Psychopathology. 2010;43(4):268–74.
17. Fulford KWM. Moral theory and medical practice. Cambridge: Cambridge University Press; 1989.

18. Fulford KWM. Values in psychiatric diagnosis: developments in policy, training and research. Psychopathology. 2005;38(4):171–6.
19. Fulford KWM, Christodoulou GN, Stein DJ. Values and ethics: perspectives on psychiatry for the person. Int J Pers Centered Med. 2011;1:131–3.
20. Fulford KWM, Van Staden CW. Values-based practice: topsy-turvy take home messages from ordinary language philosophy. In: Fulford KWM, Davies M, Graham G, Sadler JZ, Stanghellini G, Gipps R, Thornton T, editors. Oxford handbook of philosophy and psychiatry. Oxford: Oxford University Press; 2013. p. 383–410.
21. Gibbs RW. Embodiment and cognitive science. New York: Cambridge University Press; 2006.
22. Good BJ. Medicine, rationality, and experience: an anthropological perspective. Cambridge: Cambridge University Press; 1994.
23. Good M-JD, Brodwin PE, Good BJ, Kleinman A, editors. Pain as a human experience: an anthropological perspective. Berkeley: University of California Press; 1992.
24. Groleau D, Kirmayer LJ. Sociosomatic theory in Vietnamese immigrants' narratives of distress. Anthropol Med. 2004;11(2):117–33.
25. Groleau D, D'Souza NA, Bélanger E. Integrating the illness meaning and experience of patients: the McGill illness narrative interview schedule as a PCM clinical communication tool. Int J Pers Centered Med. 2013;3(2):140–6.
26. Groleau D, Young A, Kirmayer LJ. The McGill illness narrative interview (MINI): an interview schedule to elicit meanings and modes of reasoning related to illness experience. Transcul Psychiatry. 2006;43(4):671–91.
27. Hamkins S. The art of narrative psychiatry. Oxford: Oxford University Press; 2014.
28. Hollan D. The relevance of person-centered ethnography to cross-cultural psychiatry. Transcult Psychiatry. 1997;34(2):219–34.
29. Jaspers K. General psychopathology. Baltimore: Johns Hopkins University Press; 1997.
30. Jenkins JJ, Barrett RJ, editors. Schizophrenia, culture and subjectivity: the edge of experience. New York: Cambridge University Press; 2004.
31. Jylhä M. What is self-rated health and why does it predict mortality? Towards a unified conceptual model. Soc Sci Med. 2009;69:307–16.
32. Kahneman D. Thinking, fast and slow. New York: Macmillan; 2011.
33. Kirmayer LJ. Mind and body as metaphors: hidden values in biomedicine. In: Lock M, Gordon D, editors. Biomedicine examined. Dordrecht: Kluwer; 1988. p. 57–92.
34. Kirmayer LJ. The body's insistence on meaning: metaphor as presentation and representation in illness experience. Med Anthropol Q. 1992;6(4):323–46.
35. Kirmayer LJ. Broken narratives: clinical encounters and the poetics of illness experience. In: Mattingly C, Garro L, editors. Narrative and the cultural construction of illness and healing. Berkeley: University of California Press; 2000. p. 153–80.
36. Kirmayer LJ. Celan's poetics of alterity: lyric and the understanding of illness experience in medical ethics. Monash Bioeth Rev. 2007;26(4):21–35.
37. Kirmayer LJ. Psychotherapy and the cultural concept of the person. Transcult Psychiatry. 2007;44(2):232–57.
38. Kirmayer LJ. Culture and the metaphoric mediation of pain. Transcult Psychiatry. 2008;45 (2):318–38.
39. Kirmayer LJ. Re-visioning psychiatry: toward an ecology of mind in health and illness. In: Kirmayer LJ, Lemelson R, Cummings CA, editors. Re-visioning psychiatry: Cultural phenomenology, critical neuroscience, and global mental health. New York: Cambridge University Press; 2015. p. 622–60.
40. Kirmayer LJ. Empathy and alterity in psychiatry. In: Kirmayer LJ, Lemelson R, Cummings CA, editors. Re-visioning psychiatry: cultural phenomenology, critical neuroscience, and global mental health. New York: Cambridge University Press; 2015. p. 141–67.

41. Kirmayer LJ, Guzder J, Rousseau C, editors. Cultural consultation: encountering the other in mental health care. New York: Springer; 2014.
42. Kleinman A. Experience and its moral modes: Culture, human conditions, and disorder. In: Peterson GB, editor. The tanner lectures on human values, vol. 20. Salt Lake City: University of Utah Press; 1999. p. 357–420.
43. Kleinman A, Das V, Lock MM, editors. Social suffering. Berkeley: University of California Press; 1997.
44. Leventhal H, Breland JY, Mora PA, Leventhal EA. Lay representations of illness and treatment: a framework for action. In: Steptoe A, editor. Handbook of behavioral medicine. New York: Springer; 2010. p. 137–54.
45. Leventhal H, Weinman J, Leventhal EA, Phillips LA. Health psychology: the search for pathways between behavior and health. Annu Rev Psychol. 2008;59:477–505.
46. Lewis-Fernández R, Aggarwal NK, Hinton L, Hinton DE, Kirmayer LJ, editors. DSM-5 handbook on the cultural formulation interview. Washington, DC: American Psychiatric Publishing Inc.; 2015.
47. Liu JS, Mezzich JE, Zapata-Vega MI, Ruiperez MA, Yoon G. Development and validation of the Chinese version of the multicultural quality of life index (MQLI-Ch). Cult Med Psychiatry. 2008;32(1):123–34.
48. Luhrmann TM. Subjectivity. Anthropol Theory. 2006;6(3):345–61.
49. Mezzich JE, Caracci G, Fabrega H, Kirmayer LJ. Cultural formulation guidelines. Transcult Psychiatry. 2009;46(3):383–405.
50. Mezzich JE, Cohen NL, Ruiperez MA, Banzato CEM, Zapata-Vega MI. The multicultural quality of life index: presentation and validation. J Eval Clin Pract 2011;17:357–64.
51. Mezzich JE, Kirmayer LJ, Kleinman A, Fabrega H Jr, Parron DL, Good BJ, Lin KM, Manson SM. The place of culture in DSM-IV. J Nerv Ment Dis. 1999;187(8):457–64.
52. Mezzich JE, Kleinman A, Fabrega H, Parron DL, editors. Culture and psychiatric diagnosis: a DSM-IV perspective. Washington, DC: American Psychiatric Publishing; 1996.
53. Mezzich JE, Ruiperez MA, Perez C, Yoon G, Liu J, Mahmud S. The Spanish version of the quality of life index: presentation and validation. J Nerv Ment Dis. 2000;188(5):301–5.
54. Mezzich JE, Salloum IM, Cloninger CR, Salvador-Carulla L, Kirmayer LJ, Banzato CEM, Walcraft J, Botbol M. Person-centered integrative diagnosis: conceptual basis and structural model. Can J Psychiatry. 2010;55(11):701–8.
55. Mezzich JE, Otero A, Saavedra JE, Salloum IM. The GLADP-VR person-centered diagnostic formulation: background, concepts, and structure. Int J Pers Centered Med. 2013;3:228–42.
56. Mora PA, DiBonaventura MD, Idler E, Leventhal EA, Leventhal H. Psychological factors influencing self-assessments of health: toward an understanding of the mechanisms underlying how people rate their own health. Ann Behav Med. 2008;36(3):292–303.
57. Moss-Morris R, Weinman J, Petrie K, Horne R, Cameron L, Buick D. The revised illness perception questionnaire (IPQ-R). Psychol Health. 2002;17(1):1–16.
58. Northoff G. How the self is altered in psychiatric disorders: a neurophenomenal approach. In: Kirmayer LJ, Lemelson R, Cummings CA, editors. Re-visioning psychiatry: cultural phenomenology, critical neuroscience, and global mental health. New York: Cambridge University Press; 2015.
59. Parnas J. Philosophical and phenomenological perspectives on psychosis. In: Waters F, Massoud S, editors. The assessment of psychosis: a reference book. New York: Routledge; 2015. p. 17–43.
60. Parnas J, Gallagher S. Phenomenology and the interpretation of psychopathological experience. In: Kirmayer LJ, Lemelson R, Cummings CA, editors. Re-visioning psychiatry: cultural phenomenology, critical neuroscience, and global mental health. New York: Cambridge University Press; 2015.
61. Parnas J, Moller P, Kircher T, Thalbitzer J, Jansson L, Handest P, Zahavi D. EASE: examination of anomalous self-experience. Psychopathology. 2005;38(5):236–58.

62. Petrie KJ, Jago LA, Devcich DA. The role of illness perceptions in patients with medical conditions. Curr Opin Psychiatry. 2007;20(2):163–7.
63. Ramstead MJ. Naturalizing what? Varieties of naturalism and transcendental phenomenology. Phenomenol Cogn Sci. 2014;1–43.
64. Rashed MA, Du Plessis RR, Van Staden CW. Culture and Mental Health. Psychology: themes and variations. Cengage: South African Edition. Boston; 2015. p. 486–505.
65. Ratcliffe M. Experiences of depression: a study in phenomenology. Oxford: Oxford University Press; 2014.
66. Rumsfeld JS, Alexander KP, Goff DC, Graham MM, Ho PM, Masoudi FA, Zerwic JJ. Cardiovascular health: the importance of measuring patient-reported health status a scientific statement from the American Heart Association. Circulation. 2013;127(22):2233–49.
67. Ruiz-Casares M, Guzder J, Rousseau C, Kirmayer LJ. Cultural roots of well-being and resilience in child mental health. In: Ben Arieh A, Frones I, Casas F, Korbin J, editors. Handbook of child well-being. New York: Springer; 2014. p. 2379–2407.
68. Ryder A, Chentsova-Dutton YE. Cultural clinical psychology: from cultural scripts to contextualized treatments. In: Kirmayer LJ, Lemelson R, Cummings CA, editors. Re-visioning psychiatry: cultural phenomenology, critical neuroscience, and global mental health. New York: Cambridge University Press; 2015.
69. Sackett DL, Straus SE, Scott Richardson W, Rosenberg W, Haynes RB. Evidence-based medicine: how to practice and teach EBM. 2nd ed. Edinburgh and London: Churchill Livingstone; 2000.
70. Saint Arnault D, Shimabukuro S. The clinical ethnographic interview: a user-friendly guide to the cultural formulation of distress and help seeking. Transcult Psychiatry. 2012;49(2):302–22. doi:10.1177/1363461511425877.
71. Stanghellini G, Fuchs T, editors. One century of Karl Jaspers' general psychopathology. Oxford: Oxford University Press; 2013.
72. Van Staden CW. Diagnostic explanation and diagnostic understanding in psychiatry. Curr Opin Psychiatry. 2003;16:667–72.
73. Van Staden CW. The need for trained eyes to see facts and values in psychiatric diagnosis. World Psychiatry. 2005;4:94.
74. Van Staden CW. Mind, brain and person: reviewing psychiatry's constituency. S Afr Psychiatry Rev. 2006;9:93–8.
75. Van Staden CW. African approaches to an enriched ethics of person-centred practice. Int J Pers Centred Med. 2011;1(1):14–7.
76. Van Staden CW. Desirable objects of evaluation for measuring person-centered medicine: conceptual considerations drawing on African insights. Int J Pers Centered Med. 2013;3:187–90.
77. Van Staden CW, Coetzee K. Conceptual relations between loneliness and culture. Curr Opin Psychiatry. 2010;23:524–9.
78. Van Staden CW, Fulford KWM. Hypotheses, neuroscience and real persons: the theme of the 10th international conference on philosophy, psychiatry and psychology. S Afr J Psychiatry. 2007;13:68–71.
79. Van Staden CW, Fulford KWM. The Indaba in African values-based practice: respecting diversity of values without ethical relativism or individual liberalism. In: Sadler JZ, Van Staden CW, Fulford KWM, editors. Oxford handbook of psychiatric ethics. Oxford: Oxford University Press; 2015. p. 295–318.
80. Weiss M. Explanatory model interview catalogue (EMIC): framework for comparative study of illness. Transcult Psychiatry. 1997;34(2):235–63.
81. WHOQOL. The world health organization quality of life assessment (WHOQOL): development and general psychometric properties. Soc Sci Med. 1998;46(12):1569–85.
82. WHOQOL, SRPB Group. A cross-cultural study of spirituality, religion, and personal beliefs as components of quality of life. Soc Sci Med. 2006;62(6):1486–97.

83. Weinman J, Petrie KJ, Moss-Morris R, Horne R. The illness perception questionnaire: a new method for assessing the cognitive representation of illness. Psychol Health. 1996;11(3): 431–45.
84. Yoon G, Mezzich JE, Ruiperez M, Zapata-Vega M, Shin S-K, Liu J. Multicultural quality of life index, Korean version. J Immigr Minor Health. 2008;10:73–80.

Categories, Dimensions, and Narratives for Person-Centered Diagnostic Assessment

15

Michel Botbol, MD, Claudio E.M. Banzato, MD, PhD
and Luis Salvador-Carulla, MD, PhD

15.1 Introduction

Classifications are multipurpose tools. They have to serve different and sometimes conflicting objectives: healthcare management as much as doctor–patient relation, collective and individual needs, research, and clinical practice.

At the same time, every classification has to deal with multiple epistemological constraints. Even if we can consider with Levi-Strauss [17] that "any classification is better than chaos," the classifier's Holy Grail is to find a classification corresponding to the natural order of things: that is to say, to establish between the classes it defines, connections corresponding to the real relations between the things it classifies. If a classification does not give us knowledge about the things themselves, it gives us knowledge about the relations between these things [10]. This quest, is particularly difficult in psychiatry where the relations between things (the "disorders") remains elusive as knowledge about the complex pathophysiological

M. Botbol, MD (✉)
Professor of Child and Adolescent Psychiatry, University of Western Brittany, Brest, France; Service Universitaire de Psychiatrie Infanto Juvénile, CHU de Brest, Hôpital de Bohars, Bohars 29820, France
e-mail: michel.botbol@orange.fr

C.E.M. Banzato, MD, PhD
Associate Professor, Department of Psychiatry, Medical School, University of Campinas-UNICAMP, Campinas, Brazil
e-mail: claudio@lexxa.com.br

L. Salvador-Carulla, MD, PhD
Professor of Disability and Mental Health, Faculty of Health Sciences, University of Sydney, Sydney, Australia

J.E. Mezzich et al. (eds.), *Person Centered Psychiatry*,
DOI 10.1007/978-3-319-39724-5_15

mechanisms behind the symptoms and the syndromes is still lacking. It may be helpful to draw on the illuminating distinction made by Hacking [12] between constellations and nebula. In constellations, the constitutive objects are put together not because of their real physical relation but because of the figures they draw in the sky, whereas in nebula they "form natural groups" where they are united by physical causes. The choice of characters on which a classification is based is then essential: between the things and their classifications there is a theory determining the way in which we define, describe, and classify things [14]: this is particularly problematic in psychiatry where there are many competing (and often not explicit) theories about the very nature of its object.

As is well recognized, DSM-III attempted to resolve these constraints through a categorical model intended to be minimally inferential ("atheoretical" as it put it). But the price to pay was very high: in order to remain as descriptive and objective as possible (that is, there is an implicit observational theory at play), key aspects such as subjectivity and psychodynamics were ruled out. Regarding demarcatory issues, a cautious stance was adopted: "*there is no assumption that each category of mental disorder is a completely discrete entity with absolute boundaries dividing it from other mental disorders or from no mental disorders*" [1]. However, many promptly forgot this statement and, following the dominant biomedical paradigm, "naturalization" of the disorder's categories became widespread among most DSM users both in research and clinic. Driven by scientific high hopes, many psychiatrists and mental health stakeholders bridged the gap between disease and disorder, transforming a provisional descriptive construct into a natural thing [5]. By so doing they ignored Spinoza's warning [27]: "the constellation of dog does not bark." This reductionist disorder-centered perspective neglected all subjective dimensions of the disorder and therefore the person of the patient, "letting us with half a science" [28] and a nosography not well adapted to clinical practice. The gains obtained with such strategy were far more modest than expected: "*the goal of validating these syndromes and discovering common etiologies has remained elusive. Despite many proposed candidates, not one laboratory marker has been found to be specific in identifying any of the DSM defined syndromes. Epidemiologic and clinical studies have shown extremely high rates of comorbidities among the disorders undermining the hypothesis that the syndromes represent distinct etiologies*" [17].

Globally, the DSM III, IV [2], and 5 nosographical perspective raises two types of criticism:

The first type could be considered internal and is well illustrated by Widiger and Samuel in their 2005 paper [30]. These authors showed that the frustration we have discussed above should bring back to the forefront the long-standing issue questioning "whether mental disorders are discrete clinical conditions or arbitrary distinctions along dimension of functioning" [13]. Widiger and Samuel consider that two issues, "endemic to the diagnostic manual," underpin this frustrating outcome: excessive diagnostic co-occurrence and irresolvable boundary disputes [30]. Following a discussion of researchers that address "whether mental disorders are accurately or optimally classified categorically or dimensionally," they conclude advocating a dimensional mental disorder approach.

The second type of criticisms is external and well illustrated by the movement that has developed around the concept of person-centeredness in psychiatry and in medicine more generally. As stated by its proponents [23] in their paper in the Canadian Journal of Psychiatry, "*one of the prominent endeavors within the broad paradigmatic health development outlined [by person centered psychiatry] is the design of Person-centered Integrative Diagnosis (PID). This diagnostic model articulates science and humanism to obtain a diagnosis of the person (of the totality of the person's health, both ill and positive aspects), by the person (with clinicians extending themselves as full human beings), for the person (assisting the fulfillment of the person's health aspirations and life project), and with the person (in respectful and empowering relationship with the person who consults). This broader and deeper notion of diagnosis goes beyond the more restricted concepts of nosological and differential diagnoses.*"

To achieve this goal, the person-centered integrative diagnosis model is based on "three keys": (a) to cover both ill health and positive health domains along three levels: health status, experience of health, and contributors to health, (b) to implement a co-construction of the diagnostic process involving clinicians, patients and families and, last but not least, (c) to use pluralistic descriptive procedures (categories, dimensions, and narratives).

This paper will address specifically this last issue: why this pluralistic descriptive procedure is necessary? and how should it be able to contribute to the person-centered model in medicine in general and in psychiatry in particular?

15.2 Categories

Categories have been widely considered the nosography gold standard, at least from a biomedical point of view. They are seen as easier to use [11] and good enough to convey, in a clear and simple manner, a great amount of useful clinical information [30]. To do so they have, however, to reduce the number and the specificity of the criteria on which they are based. To maintain their utility and their simplicity they have, moreover, to neglect the conceptual differences between those criteria that are in fact dimensional (that is to say those criteria that are considered present when the value observed in this dimension surpasses a given threshold in a continuum between normal and pathological, i.e., in somatic medicine vascular hypertension or hyperglycemia and, in psychiatry, i.e., hyperactivity or psychomotor slowing in mood disorders, etc.) and those that are not (i.e. in somatic medicine the presence of cancerous cells or in psychiatry, delusional psychotic phenomena). It is likely that the weight of what they are then neglecting is different according to the type of criteria. The relative importance of each type of criteria in the definition of a category will seemingly influence the fact that "a disorder" would be category like (rather than dimension like) when "this disorder," is characterized by a "within-category homogeneity and between-category qualitative differences" [9].

This may explain why numerous empirical studies have shown that some disorders (especially the personality disorders) are better classified by a dimensional classification than by a categorical one [25].

Because it is broader and takes into account positive health aspects, the context of the patient and his experience of his health status, a person-centered approach adds to the complexity of the object to consider (the totality of the person in his context) the weight of the continuous aspects (the dimension-like aspects) in the classification of this person's health status. A categorical approach may however be useful to define subtype (even if their criteria are mainly based on dimensions) when needed or to include discrete data provided by standardized instruments used to assess these dimensions. This approach is of course well adapted to assess objective factors following the medical traditional clinical model, but it can be easily extended to subjective factors as long as enough space is given to the patient narratives to allow their assessment through standardized instruments or through the clinician empathy and narratives.

The way these categorical approaches will be finally classified is another important issue. Algorithms are of course a useful way to encompass multiple symptoms (or dimensions) in a syndromic approach. Considered by the DSM-III, DSM-IV, and DSM-5 teams to increase validity and accuracy, they have been thoroughly criticized for their reductionism and their non specificity. On this point, Linden and Muschalla are clear: "The core problem with algorithms is that they can be no more valid as the symptoms they are based upon. If the assessment of symptoms is invalid, the conclusion derived from these symptoms will also be invalid. From a clinical perspective, the impression is that many "diagnoses" which are based on standardized interviews and algorithms may be useful for research but not reflect clinical entities" [20].

These criticisms seem to be particularly convincing in their claims for the benefits of the dimensional criteria and the importance of the need to ensure a proper consideration of the subjective aspects of the person's situation. In a person-centered approach, a prototypical approach to categorization [6, 31] would be preferable because it might help to better articulate the several dimensions that are to be included in the person-centered diagnostic process. However, here again, one has to be aware that, implicitly or explicitly, prototypes are metaphors, and as such, are based on the narratives of clinician, taking into account the narratives of the patient and of his carers [7].

15.3 Dimensions

The use of dimensions should be preferred when there is a "within category heterogeneity and between category quantitative difference" [9] that is to say when the differences between the individuals are less important than the differences between normal and pathological or between disorders. A dimensional approach is then likely to be more individualized and less disorder centered. It may be, therefore, more compatible with a person-centered approach because it allows for a more individualized appraisal of the patient's characteristics, as long as they can be assessed in a continuum. Subjective dimensions involved in the patient's health situation can meet this condition, and can be taken into account by the diagnostic process if this process gives enough space to their recognition and finds an adequate methodology to assess them. This means that, if a dimensional approach may be more adapted to approach the subjective dimensions in the patient's health, it does not, in itself, warrant person-centeredness because person-centered care requires the fulfillment of at least two other conditions:

- To give enough attention to the patient's narratives, to his positive health aspects, and to his context so that it can inform the physician narratives and interact with him to build up a dimensional assessment of the patient's health situation, including its subjective aspects.
- To integrate all the assessed dimensions, including the subjective ones, into a holistic appraisal of the person.

Categorical and dimensional approaches can be combined to generate ordinal classification modeling to psychiatric diagnosis that may incorporate severity levels into the classification system. These models have been applied to the assessment of mental health areas and can be also used in psychiatric classification.

15.4 Narratives

As we have seen, both categorical and dimensional approaches can be useful in a person-centered approach in medicine in general and in psychiatry in particular. Instruments such as the "Day Reconstruction Method" provides an example of the standardization and cultural differences in diaries of positive and negative affects in different countries [4]. However, these procedures can become person-centered if and only if they take a full account of the subjective aspect of the patient's health status.

For instance, the person-centered integrative diagnosis (PID) model [23] is based on the previous *International Guidelines for Diagnostic Assessment* (*IGDA*) [21] and constructed on the results *of* a series of focus groups (involving psychiatrists, health professionals and other health stakeholders as patients, families, and advocates) and of a survey realized by a global network of national classification [26]. One of the main findings of this systematic work is that the patients' perception, values, and experiences of illness and health are key components of their health status and can be provided only if dimensions and narratives (idiosyncratic formulations) are added to traditional descriptive procedures. For this reason, a PID matrix included in the diagnostic process affords a new and specific level corresponding to the patient's *Experience of Health* with the aim to take into account the patient's health-related individual and cultural values and experiences, approached through a guided narrative procedure, built upon the worldwide experience of the Cultural Formulation [22].

The person's illness narrative [16] and account of health and resilience offer the clinician a clear picture of issues and priorities that can organize and guide clinical intervention [15]. For this reason, the PID model incorporates as assessment recommendations, the use of pluralistic descriptive procedures [23].

To understand this domain and to allow its practical applicability the physician has to access the patient's conscious and unconscious feelings and representations. To achieve this goal, the physician cannot rely only on what he observes of the patient behavior or physical condition. He has also to listen to what the patient says. Though this is certainly crucial, it may be insufficient if the patient does not have clear access to his own conscious feelings, or cannot express them directly. In these cases one needs to take into account some of his less conscious psychic life. Empathy is the only tool to access the patient's subjectivity in these situations. Defined as the feeling induced in others (the physician, the carers…) by the contact with the patient through verbal and behavioral interactions, empathy is the only way to go behind the screen of the visible if the physician allows himself to give meaning to his empathic subjective feelings; in other words, empathy gives way to the patient's subjectivity if the physician gives enough space and value, not only to the patient's narratives but also to his own narratives. The empathy implied by this process is not a plain Mirror Empathy, but rather a Narrative Empathy using the therapist's representations and affects to approach and understand the patient's health situation beyond what he shows and says. This Narrative Empathy uses the idiosyncratic sensitivity of each of the persons in the patient's environment and, among them, the carers, and the treating team members who in constant interaction with the patient will naturally amplify different aspects of the patient's subjective life. As part of this person-centered perspective the physician and the team members subjectivity is not seen as a negative side effect of the patient-professional relation; it is rather a key asset in person-centered diagnostic and therapeutical processes, provided that this subjectivity is properly analyzed and controlled by the professionals themselves. Here what is meant is that health professionals should be properly trained to use their feelings and representations as valuable factors in the diagnostic process and as important contributors to care, in a person-centered perspective.

15.5 Conclusions

The practical implementation of *Pluralistic Descriptive Procedures* within the PID model implies a full change of mental health assessment, particularly because of its incorporation of narratives, personal experiences and positive health components such as resilience and quality of life [23]. Narratives have been used extensively in qualitative research where they have been considered a most valuable source of information [8], and calls have been recently made for a more extensive use of patients' narratives and narrative theory in psychiatry [19]. However, the development of a set of metaphors for quantitative analysis, and its use in routine practice or to generate evidence-informed care poses many challenges to psychiatric evaluation. The use of Semantic Web Knowledge techniques [29] in the analysis of narratives may allow extensive review of severely mentally ill patients personal experiences taking into account not only the ill aspects of health status but also positive accounts of recovery [24]. From this perspective, the development of *narrative banks* of health experiences could be proposed to contribute to a better understanding of positive and negative aspects of health and may also contribute to improved diagnosis and treatment planning based on personal preferences and experiences.

Person-centered diagnosis is a critical component of Person-centered medicine in general and Person-centered Psychiatry in particular. Both categorical and dimensional approaches can contribute to person-centered diagnosis. However, incorporation of narrative is necessary to allow these approaches to become fully person-centered. Improving the analysis and use of narratives is therefore a crucial issue for the advancement of the field.

References

1. American Psychiatric Association. DSM-IV TR. Washington, DC: American Psychiatric Association; 2000.
2. American Psychiatric Association. DSM-5. Washington, DC: American Psychiatric Association; 2013.
3. Appleyard J. Diagnostic procedure in pediatrics, presented at the Fourth Geneva Conference on Person Centered Medicine, International College of Person Centered Medicine; 2011.
4. Ayuso-Mateos JL, Miret M, Caballero FF, Olaya B, Haro JM, Kowal P, Chatterji S. Multi-country evaluation of affective experience: validation of an abbreviated version of the day reconstruction method in seven countries. PLoS One. 2013;8(4):e61534.
5. Banzato CEM, Mezzich JE, Berganza CE. Philosophical and methodological foundations of psychiatric diagnosis psychopathology, vol. 38; 2005.
6. Banzato CEM. Critical evaluation of current diagnostic systems. Indian J Psychiatry. 2008;50 (3):155–7.
7. Botbol M. Person-centered child and adolescent psychiatric care. Int J Integr Care. 2010;10 (Suppl):e028.
8. Charon R. Narrative medicine: honoring the stories of illness. New York: Oxford University Press; 2006.
9. De Boeck P, Wilson M, Acton GS. A conceptual and psychometric framework for distinguishing categories and dimensions. Psychol Rev. 2005;112(1):129–58.
10. Duhem P. *La Théorie physique, son objet, sa structure*, Chevalier et Rivière, Paris, 1906, reedition. Vrin, Paris; 1981.
11. Frances AJ, First MB. & Pincus HA (1995). DSM IV guidebook. Washington DC: American Psychiatric Press
12. Hacking I. A tradition of natural kinds. Philos Stud. 1991;61(1–2):109–26.
13. Kendell RC. The role of diagnosis in psychiatry. Oxford, England: Blackwell Scientific Publications; 1975.
14. Kirsch M. La connaissance des choses: définition, description, classification. Philopsis e-edition; 2008.

15. Kirmayer LJ. Broken narratives: clinical encounters and the poetics of illness experience. In: Mattingly C, Garro L, editors. Narrative and the cultural construction of illness and healing. Berkeley: University of California Press; 2000. p. 153–80.
16. Kleinman A. Illness narratives: suffering, healing and the human condition. New York: Basic Books; 1989.
17. Kupfer DJ, First MB, Regier DE. Introduction. In: Kupfer DJ, First MB, Regier DE, editors. A research agenda for DSM-V. Washington, D.C: American Psychiatric Association; 2002.
18. Levi-Strauss C. Tristes tropiques. Paris: Plon; 1955.
19. Lewis B. Taking a narrative turn in psychiatry. The Lancet. 2014;383(9911):22–3.
20. Linden M, Muschalla B. Standardized diagnostic interviews, criteria, and algorithms for mental disorders: garbage in, garbage out. Eur Arch Psychiatry Clin Neurosci. 2012.
21. Mezzich JE, Berganza CE, von Cranach M, Jorge MR, Kastrup MC. Murthy RC, Okasha A, Pull C, Sartorius N, Skodol AE, Zaudig M. Essentials of the WPA International Guidelines for Diagnostic Assessment (IGDA). Br J Psychiatry. 2003;182(Suppl. 45).
22. Mezzich JE, Caracci G, Fabrega H Jr, Kirmayer LJ. Cultural formulation guidelines. Transcult Psychiatry. 2009;46(3):383–405.
23. Mezzich JE, Salloum I, Cloninger R, Salvado-Carulla L, Kirmayer L, Banzato CEM, Wallcraft J, Botbol M. Person-centred integrative diagnosis: conceptual bases and structural model. Can J Psychiatry. 2010;55(11):701–8.
24. Roberts GA. Narrative and severe mental illness: what place do stories have in an evidence-based world? Adv Psychiatr Treat. 2000;6:432–41.
25. Ruscio J, Ruscio AM. Categories and dimensions advancing psychological science through the study of latent structure. Curr Dir Psychol Sci. 2008;17(3):203–7.
26. Salloum IM, Mezzich JE. Conceptual appraisal of the person-centered Integrative Diagnosis Model. Int J Pers Cent Med. 2011;1:39–42.
27. Spinoza B. L'Ethique, Folio Essai, Paris, 1ère édition, 1677; 1994.
28. Strauss JS. Diagnosis and reality: a noun is a terrible thing to waste. Psychopathology. 2005;38:189–91.
29. Tao C, Wei WQ, Solbrig HR, Savova G, Chute CG. CNTRO: a semantic web ontology for temporal relation inferencing in clinical narratives. AMIA Annu Symp Proced. 2010:787–91.
30. Widiger TA, Samuel DA. Diagnostic categories and dimensions? A question for the diagnostic and statistical manual of mental disorders—fifth edition. J Abnorm Psychol. 2005;4:494–504.
31. World Psychiatry. Forum: advantages and disadvantages of a prototype-matching. World Psychiatry. 2012;11(1):16–31.

Part III
Person Centered Care Approaches

Interdisciplinary Team Approach to Clinical Care

16

Tesfamicael Ghebrehiwet PhD, Maria Ammon PhD, Ilse Burbiel PhD and Michel Botbol MD

16.1 Introduction

The concept of health integrates a complex and holistic system involving biological, psychological, physical, cultural, socioeconomic, and environmental factors interacting with each other. Addressing complex problems including health problems requires the use of diverse information and skill set that cannot be provided by one profession. As Rowe [31] indicated health problems are broad and complex and need to be looked at from an interdisciplinary approach.

The interdisciplinary team approach is widely recognized as an important organizational factor in providing quality patient care. This approach is supported by a growing research evidence that demonstrates that team functioning is asso-

T. Ghebrehiwet PhD (✉)
Former Consultant, Nursing and Health Policy, International Council of Nurses;
Board Director, International College of Person-Centered Medicine, Calgary, Canada
e-mail: tesfa@shaw.ca

M. Ammon PhD
Psychotherapist and Psychoanalyst, President of the German Academy for Psychoanalysis (DAP) and Secretary General of the World Association for Dynamic Psychiatry (WADP), Berlin, Germany

I. Burbiel PhD
Psychotherapist and Psychoanalyst, Governor of the German Branch of WADP and Member of the World Psychiatric Association Psychoanalysis Section, Geneva, Switzerland

M. Botbol MD
Professor of Child and Adolescent Psychiatry, University of Western Brittany, Board Member of the International College of Person-Centered Medicine, Brest, France

J.E. Mezzich et al. (eds.), *Person Centered Psychiatry*,
DOI 10.1007/978-3-319-39724-5_16

ciated with better patient outcomes, cost savings, reduced hospitalization, improved service provision, and enhanced patient and staff satisfaction.

Research evidence suggests that these benefits occur because well-functioning teams make good decisions, cope effectively with complex tasks, and are able to coordinate their interventions and expertise. However, despite the growing awareness of potential benefits, many heath care organizations lack effective teamwork, with negative consequences on patient outcomes. The barriers to team approach have been attributed to several factors including lack of interprofessional education, professional hierarchy, frequent changes in caregivers due to shift work and patient transfers that make coordination and teamwork complicated.

This chapter highlights the interdisciplinary team approach in health care including definition, effectiveness in terms of patient outcomes, cost savings, and patient and provider satisfactions.

16.2 Definitions: What to Call the Team

The word “team” is often used as a catchword to mean different types of teams that can range from two people to more than 10; could have members of the same discipline or of different disciplines; and comprise specialists or generalists. A health team can be described as a group of health providers with diverse skills and different responsibilities but with common objectives related to patient outcomes and cost of health care [8].

Despite the seemingly clear definition of a team, several terms are often used interchangeably to refer to health care teams resulting in lack of clarity and miscommunication. These include: multidisciplinary, interdisciplinary, collaborative, Interprofessional, cross-disciplinary, polydisciplinary, and transdisciplinary. Despite this terminological jungle, health administrators, and health care provides assume and they understand each other when they may be referring to different concepts of teams Drinka and Clark [15].

After much pondering about which term to use, Drinka and Clark, argue that the term *interdisciplinary* seems more appropriate for its inclusiveness and it has been in use for a long time. In line with this argument, the health care team that the authors refer to in this chapter are interdisciplinary health teams. According to the free encyclopedia Wikipedia [40] “interdisciplinarity” is defined as “the use of approaches, ways of thinking, or at least methods of different disciplines.” In contrast to “multi-disciplinarity,” which represents the weakest form of cooperation with regard to content in subject-transcending work [41], “interdisciplinarity” is regarded as methodological, terminological, or conceptional exchange and integration between the disciplines, developing an uniform conceptual frame and working on common strategies for solving problems. What is at stake is a frame of work that allows for interactive and reciprocal activities as opposed to working side-by-side. For the interdisciplinarity and its integration, eclecticism is a possible component to integrate clinical methods of different sources. Eclecticism is the weakest form of cooperation between the various disciplines.

According to Küchenhoff [27], the prerequisites for an effective integration process are the ability to cooperate, curiosity, knowledge of and respect for the perspectives of the other participants, competence, not claiming methodological omnipotence, and the refraining from participating in "religious wars" within the profession. The metatheory requested by him should relate the different methods to each other and bring them into a structural interrelation. In addition, it should reveal what effect is performed by which elements on the whole structure. A common language has to be found, a language that is creative, innovative, and motional.

To go further in this line, let us define multidisciplinary and interdisciplinary health teams with the intention to show the difference and clarity of these terms.

In multidisciplinary teams: Health professionals from diverse backgrounds share information and consult each other in planning care. However, members identify with their discipline more than the team. In contrast, in interdisciplinary teams, health professionals work collaboratively to define and achieve commonly defined goals. Members have strong team identity, mutual respect, and view their actions as interwoven. Roles change based on client needs. A working definition of interdisciplinary health team is provided by Drinka and Clark [15]:

> An interdisciplinary health team integrates a group of individuals with diverse training and backgrounds who work together as an identified unit or system. Team members consistently collaborate to solve patient problems that are too complex to be solved by one discipline or many disciplines in sequence. …An interdisciplinary health team creates formal and informal structures that encourage collaborative problem solving. Team members determine the team's mission and common goals; work interdependently to define and treat patient problems; and learn to accept and capitalise on disciplinary differences, differential power and overlapping roles. …They share leadership that is appropriate to the presenting problem and promote the use of differences for confrontation and collaboration. They also use differences of opinion and problems to evaluate the team's work and its development (page 6).

At the core of the interdisciplinary team approach is the person who has health problems and who should be an active partner in care. The provision of quality patient care requires an identifiable team structure and functioning.

16.3 Interdisciplinary Team Formation and Team Functioning

The shift from the traditional biomedical view of the human body to a biopsychosocial approach has resulted in greater understanding of the complex relationships between health, illness, and disease. This holistic view of the complexity of the multiple dimensions of illness and disease requires the involvement of professionals with varied skills and knowledge working in interdisciplinary teams to provide quality patient care [9]. However, the growing trend toward specialization in the health professions may lead to a narrow understanding of interdisciplinary team comprising professionals with the same basic training but with a speciality such as internists, psychiatrists, and endocrinologists that may lead to fragmentation of care.

In its broad sense, the term interdisciplinary refers to an interprofessional perspective that includes physicians, nurses, occupational therapists, social workers, and other health-related professionals. The interdisciplinary team approach may help in preventing fragmentation of care due to specialization as patients who receive care from a team can benefit from the perspectives of different professionals with wider skills [37].

Historically, health care delivery was hierarchical and dominated by physicians. However, the current trend shows a shift to broader and inclusive teams of professionals. A more recent development shows that the concept of health team has been broadened to include the perspectives of patients giving rise to the notion of person-centered medicine. According to Ammon, the criterion for interdisciplinarity and its method integration should be the human being, together with an understanding for illnesses and also for constructive, creative development opportunities. Thus, Ammon recommends a holistic approach in clinical care that integrates the findings of different branches of science but also aspects of diverse schools. All this is put under a central principle, the holistically formulated image of man. A model for interdisciplinarity and integration should be measured by the benefit for the person, i.e., to understand them better and to develop better healing methods [3]. The theoretical model should never be systemized or inflexible according to Ammon. It should be an open system with the possibility of change and constant integration processes.

To integrate different disciplines in clinical care it needs to have a theoretical concept as a basis to rely on. The central theoretical basic conceptions of the interdisciplinary methods—integrative approach of Dynamic Psychiatry are: in the first place the concept of social energy, furthermore the personality structure model in connection with the identity concept [2].

For the person-centered care, this means the involvement of the whole team into the treatment process, including nurses, psychotherapeutically trained psychiatrists, doctors and psychologists, social-workers, milieu therapists, therapists for the expressive therapies, as well as the administration and kitchen personnel into treatment as parts of the social-energetic field.

Interdisciplinary team approach for person-centered clinical care implies,

1. that all people and professions involved in the interdisciplinary healing process cooperate in the various designated groups on the basis of a commonly shared holistic image of man, and, derived from it, a model of personality and a common understanding of health, illness, healing, and development.
2. Since, the goal of dynamic-psychiatric treatment is to open up patients by emotionally corrective and new group dynamic experiences so that they will regain their health, it is important that the total hospital, as well as its different team and patients groups are structured and dynamized as spaces for con-

structive social-energetic exchange processes as much as possible. It is therefore the daily task of the leader group and of the team to reflect and regulate both conscious and unconscious group dynamics that develop within and between the various groups, including the dynamics of the 'plenary group' [1]. A real interdisciplinary approach is always open for development and further integrative possibilities which will be necessary for the treatment of patients.

The use of teams in health care delivery is driven by a number of factors including demographic changes with an aging population, health system restructuring and reorganization, cost containment, and the increasing complexity of health care knowledge and work [20]. In the current complex landscape of health care systems with rapid growth in information that is required to solve problems, no single health professional can have all the knowledge or skills to provide the continuum of services needed. Because of the increasing complexity and scope of patient problems including presence of multiple diseases or comorbid conditions presenting to the health care environment, patient care needs to combine the efforts of physicians of different disciplines, skilled nursing professionals, and other health care professionals, as solving these problems are beyond the scope of expertise and training of any one provider [36].

The diagnosis and treatment of disease as well as health promotion and disease prevention require the expertise of different health professionals engaged in collaborative work. That is why an interdisciplinary health team is needed to provide quality health care that is accessible and cost-effective. Team approach enables health professionals with diverse skills to view clients and their families as whole persons, and in this regard it is compatible with person-centered medicine.

A key tenet of interdisciplinary team work is communication between the different members on continuous basis. High quality communication, mutual respect, trust, and active participation by all team members often result in stronger team identity, reduction in status differential and hierarchy, increased responsiveness to job demands, higher job satisfaction, and better staff retention [38]. Similarly, an organizational culture that institutionalizes consistent and effective communication leads to low staff turnover, better clinical outcomes, shorter hospital stay, and higher quality of care [35]. Gittel [18] observed that interdisciplinary teams that successfully manage their differences through well designed and maintained communication are more likely to demonstrate continual high performance and achieve positive patient outcomes.

Another important tenet of team work is team leadership. Successful team leadership acknowledges the need for team members to contribute and collaborate in a positive manner. Skills in team building and team functioning are fundamental to the success of the interdisciplinary health team in setting common goals and in achieving positive patient outcomes.

Effective leaders facilitate the team's environment so that members feel that their perspectives are welcomed and appreciated, their expertise is trusted, expectations are clear, accountability and excellence are the norm, and there are common goals [33].

Team leadership means that the leader and the members must be willing to share team leadership responsibilities and be aware of group dynamics in order to work with professionals that have widely diverse skills, values, and interests [29].

16.4 Interdisciplinary Team Approach and Person-Centeredness

Psychological dimensions and subjectivity are crucial components of person-centered cares [11]. It challenges the ideal of objectivity which is a crucial component of disorder-centered medicine: in its attempt to approach this ideal, this disorder-centered medicine neglects the subjective aspects and the complexity of the person, adopting a perspective in which reductionism is not only a methodological tool but also a theoretical assumption (see Botbol et al.: Categories, dimensions and Narratives for person-centered diagnostic assessment, in this book). However, person-centered psychiatry's ideal is not antiscientific when tackling the issue of subjectivity: on the contrary, one of its main objective is to find a non-metaphysic way to integrate subjectivity (including spirituality) as a key component of psychiatry and medicine. The naturalistic observation of what health professionals do in clinical settings, shows that empathy is an essential tool to understand the patient state of mind and subjective feelings. Defined as the affect induced in the professional by the relation with a patient through what he says or does, empathy appears then as a first methodological step to go behind the screen of the visible: an holistic way to approach the patient's subjectivity as an holistic dimension, through the mirroring of the patient's feeling.

However, this mirroring function is not sufficient to access the patient's subjective life and to understand his personal needs and his psychic problematic. To be able to access these aspects, essential in a person-centered perspective, the professional has to resort to a second methodological step: metaphorization and narratives to give meaning to these mirroring feelings. Patients' Narratives are indeed the best way for him to trigger the professional's empathy as long as the latter gives enough attention to them. But the professional's auto-narratives are of equal importance because they are the best way for him to recognize and give meaning to the empathic affects induced in him by the contact with the patient. This second step is then required to shift from mirror empathy (which, following [6], we think preferable to call sympathy) to a metaphorizing empathy where the professional mirrors the patient without giving up on the recognition of his irreducible otherness. Team work becomes then a necessary third methodological step to limit the risk that the integration of the professional's subjectivity in the diagnostic and therapeutic process would lead to their scholastic or projective interpretations. In this work, the team uses the idiosyncratic sensitivity of its members to amplify various aspects of the patient's subjective life and put it into more or less common narratives. In this perspective, team members subjectivity is not considered an adverse side effect of the therapeutic relation but an important tool for diagnostic and care, given that the team members are adequately trained to use their affects and representations as central dimensions of their team work, in close interaction with the patient and his carers.

16.5 Effectiveness of Interdisciplinary Health Care Team

There is a growing body of research literature that demonstrates the effectiveness of team approach to patients, providers, and organizations. After an extensive review of the literature on health care team effectiveness, Lemieux-Charles and McGuire [30], and Bosch et al. [10] found that there is some evidence that shows interdisciplinary team care which can lead to better clinical outcomes and patient satisfaction. For example, studies that examined geriatric teams reported higher functional status, better mental health, decreased dependence, and decreased mortality [13, 26]. Patient satisfaction and health-related quality of life were higher when care was provided by interdisciplinary health teams [13]. Similarly, studies of teams in critical care reported increased survival to discharge and decreased readmission to critical care [4]: fewer adverse events, lower mortality rates after surgery, and shorter length of hospital stay [5]. Care provided by a team in a primary care setting resulted in improvements in symptoms of depression, but resulted in increased cost [21].

Overall, a review of the research evidence shows interdisciplinary team care which can lead to better clinical outcomes and patient and staff satisfaction as well as cost savings than traditional care that did not use a team approach. These include:

- Increased survival to hospital discharge and decreased readmission to critical care [4].
- Fewer adverse events, lower mortality rates after surgery, and shorter hospital stays [5].
- Higher patient satisfaction and health-related quality of life [13].
- Higher patient and staff satisfaction [13, 17].
- Cost-effectiveness and cost savings [19].
- Reduced hospitalization [32].
- Improved service provision [25].

To sum up, the research shows that team functioning is associated with better patient outcomes, cost savings, reduced hospitalization, improved service provision, as well as increased patient and provider satisfaction. The provider satisfaction is associated with lower staff turnover [17].

Organizational support and resources influence team functioning and higher functioning teams achieve better patient outcomes [12]. These outcomes occur because well-functioning teams make quality decisions, cope effectively with complex tasks, and are able to coordinate their interventions and expertise [19].

However, despite the growing literature on the benefits of team approach to care, many heath care organizations lack effective teamwork, with negative consequences on patient outcomes. The barriers to team approach have been attributed to several factors including professional hierarchy frequent changes in caregivers due to shift work and patient transfers that make coordination and teamwork complicated [34]. At the same time, health professionals tend to resist to a team-based care model because of poor organizational support, system-wide barriers such as fragmentation in reimbursement for health care services, regulatory restrictions, and the education of health professionals which takes place in silos [24, 28].

16.6 Interprofessional Education (IPE) for Team Work

The World Health Organization, WHO [42] identifies IPE as the process by which a group of more than two profession-specific students from health-related occupations with different educational backgrounds learn together during certain periods of their education with interaction as an important goal. Governments around the world are looking for innovative solutions to ensure the appropriate supply, mix, and distribution of the health workforce. One of the most promising solutions can be found in interprofessional collaboration [42].

Interdisciplinary team approach is the hallmark of positive outcomes for the health of patients, families, and communities. However, a number of reports affirm team formation and team functioning do not come naturally to health professionals and require a paradigm shift in educational programs [7, 22]. As Frenk et al. [16] have affirmed, the excessive focus on hospital-based education that is segregated into professional silos does not prepare health professionals for team work, and for leadership skills in the twenty-first century health services.

In general, most health care organizations and health profession educational institutions devote little or no time and resources to promote interdisciplinary functioning [15]. In fact, the different health profession training programs take place in different buildings, and in different colleges or schools often within the same campus. Often similar courses are taught separately for the different health professions, adding to the silo approach of educational institutions [15].

As shown in Table 16.1, a WHO environmental scan of interprofessional education practices in 42 countries with 396 respondents showed generally low levels of IPE among different health professionals.

Table 16.1 Types of learners who received IPE at their institutions

Health Professional	% Reporting IPE
Community health workers	4.3
Doctors	10.2
Nurses	16.0
Social workers	9.3
Pharmacists	7.7
Physiotherapists	10.1

Adapted from Framework for Action on Interprofessional Education and Collaborative Practice: WHO [42]. http://www.who.int/hrh/nursing_midwifery/en/.

As a result, there is a lacuna in the education of health profession in relation to team formation and team functioning. As Lee [29] has noted, the dominant model of health profession education does not emphasize collaboration, shared team decision making, or shared team leadership. Most health professionals tend to be trained to function in silos and they may have difficulty to function in interdisciplinary teams with negative consequences on patient care.

Despite their clinical expertise, health professionals are often hampered to provide quality care due to lack of effective team work and collaboration. As the Institute of Medicine [23] reported a lack of interprofessional collaboration as one of the most often cited reasons for medical errors. In contrast effective interprofessional collaboration is linked with better patient care outcomes [39].

While acknowledging the value of team-based models of care, Jansen [24] raises doubts about implementation because, among other things, of the lack of interprofessional education of health professionals. Jansen argues that investments in health professionals must be made in terms of system support and interprofessional education if the notion of interdisciplinary team approach is to be implemented. For example, educational institutions must provide interdisciplinary team-based learning opportunities including knowledge of collaborative practice, participation in team decision making and an appreciation of the values and competencies of other professionals.

To this end, the Department of Health of the United Kingdom [14], the US Institute of Medicine [23], and the World Health Organization [42] continue to advocate for educational programs for health professionals to include opportunities for working in interdisciplinary teams.

16.7 Conclusions

The literature on team approach to health care is vast and an exhaustive review is beyond the scope of this chapter. However, a comprehensive review showed the benefits of team approach to patients, organizations, and health professionals. The type and diversity of clinical expertise involved in team decision making largely accounts for improvements in patient care and organizational effectiveness. Collaboration, conflict resolution, participation, and cohesion are most likely to influence staff satisfaction and perceived team effectiveness. Quality and outcome of care was better when care was provided by teams compared to traditional care where this model of care is lacking. Organizations also benefit in terms of cost savings and system efficiency when team care is implemented. Team care improves patient and staff satisfaction resulting in lower staff turnover. However, despite the benefits and value of team-based care there is reluctance on the part of organizations and health professionals to shift to this model because of a number of barriers and challenges.

The implications for practice include the need for providing teams with organizational support, resources such as development guidelines; access to training and team building; and opportunities for interprofessional education.

References

1. Ammon M. Dynamische Psychiatrie—ein integratives theoretisches und praktisches multidisziplinäres Behandlungskonzept. Dynamische Psychiatrie/Dynamic Psychiatry. 2014;262(263):89–107.
2. Ammon G. Entwurf eines Dynamisch- Psychiatrischen Ich-Struktur-Konzepts—Zur Integration von funktional-struktureller Ich-Psychologie und Narzißmus-Theorie. In: Ammon G, editor. Handbuch der Dynamischen Psychiatrie I. Munich: Reinhardt; 1979. p. 95–159.
3. Ammon G. Metodenintegration aus der Sicht der Dynamischen Psychiatrie. 39–40 In: Ammon G, Editor *Handbuch der Dynamischen Psychiatrie 2*. Munich: Reinhardt; 1982. p. 25–48.
4. Ball C, Kirby M, Williams S. Effect of the critical care outreach team on patient survival to discharge from hospital and readmission to critical care: non-randomised population based study. Br Med J. 2003;327:1014–8.
5. Bellomo RD, Goldsmith S, Uchino J, Buckmaster G, Hart H, et al. Prospective controlled trial of effect of medical emergency team on postoperative morbidity and mortality rates. Crit Care Med. 2004;32(4):916–21.
6. Berthoz A. Une théorie spatiale de la difference entre la sympathie et les processus de l'empathie. In: Botbol M, Garret N, editors. A. Besse: L'empathie au Carrefour des sciences et de la clinique. Doin, Paris; 2014.
7. Bhutta A, Cohen J, Crisp N, Evans T, Fineberg H, et al. Education of health professionals for the 21st century: a global independent Commission. The Lancet. 2010;375(9721):1137–8.
8. Blackmore G. Diagnosing and improving functioning in interdisciplinary health care teams. The Health Care Manager. 2012;31(3):197–205.
9. Boon HS, Mior SA, Barnsley J, Ashbury FD, Haig R. The difference between integration and collaboration in patient care: results from key informant interview working in multiprofessional health care team. J Manipulative Physiol Ther. 2009;32(9):715–22.
10. Bosch J, Faber MJ, Cruijsberg J, Voerman GE, Leatherman S, et al. Review artcile: effectiveness of patient care teams and the role of clinical expertise and coordination: a literature review. Med Care Res Rev. 2009;66:5S.
11. Botbol M, Garret-Gloanec N, Besse A. Empathy et Clinique integrative. In: Botbol M, Garret-Gloanec N, Besse A, editors. L'Empathie au Carrefour des Sciences et de la Clinique. Paris: Doin; 2014.
12. Bower P, Campbell S, Bojke C, Sibbald B. Team structure, team climate and the quality of care in primary care: an observational study. Quality and Safety in Health Care. 2003;12 (4):273–9.
13. Cohen HJ, Feussner JR, Weinberger M, Carnes M, Hamdy RC, Hsieh F, Phibbs C, Lavori P. A controlled trial of inpatient and outpatient geriatric evaluation and management. N Engl J Med. 2002;346(12):905–12.
14. Department of Health, United Kingdom. A Health Service for all the talents: developing the NHS workforce. London: Department of Health; 2000.
15. Drinka TJK, Clark PG. Health care teamwork: interdisciplinary practice and teaching. Connecticut: Auburn House; 2000.
16. Frenk J, et al. Health professionals for a new century: transforming education to strengthen health systems in an interdependent world. The Lancet. 2010;376:1923–58.

17. Galletta M, Portoghese I, Battistelli A, Leiter MP. The roles of unit leadership an nurse-physcian collaboration on nursing turnover intention. Adv Nurs. 2013;69(8):1771–84.
18. Gittel J. High performance healthcare: using the power of relationships to achieve quality, efficiency and resilience. New York, N.Y: McGraw-Hill; 2009.
19. Grumbach K, Bodenheimer T. Can health care teams improve primary care practice? Jama-Journal of the American Medical Association. 2004;291(10):1246–51.
20. Hainemann GD. Teams in health care settings. In Heinemann GD, Zeisss AM, editor. Team performance in health care. New York: Kluwer; 2002 p. 3–18.
21. Hedrick SC, Chaney EF, Felker B, Liu CF, Hasenberg N, et al. Effectiveness of collaborative care depression treatment in veterans' affairs primary care. J Gen Intern Med. 2003;18:9–16.
22. Institute of Medicine. The Future of Nursing Leadership. Advancing Health: Washington, D. C., National Academy Press; 2011.
23. Institute of Medicine. Health professions education: A bridge to quality. Washington: D.C., National Aacademy Press; 2003.
24. Jansen L. Collaborative and Interdisciplinary Health Care Teams: Ready or Not? J Prof Nurs. 2008;24(4):218–27.
25. Jansson A, Isacsson A, Lindholm LH. Organisation of healthcare teams and the population's contact with primary care. Scandinavian Journal of Health Care. 1992;10:257–65.
26. Kaplan GA, Willims JA, Daly B, Abraham K. A randomised controlled trial of comprehensive geriatric assessment and multidisciplinary intervention after discharge of elderly from the emergency department – The Deed II Study. J Am Geriatr Soc. 2004;52:1417–23.
27. Küchenhoff J. Der integrative Prozess in der psychotherapie: methodenvielfalt—synergismus —integration. Schweizer Archiv für Neurologie und Psychiatrie. 2009;160(1):12–9.
28. Landman N, Aannestad LK, Smoldt RK, Cortese DA. Teamwork in Health Care. Nurs Admin Q. 2014;36(3):198–205.
29. Lee T. Turning doctors into leaders. Harvard Business Review, 2010. p.50–58.
30. Lemieux-Charles L, McGuire WL. What do we know about health care team effectiveness? a review of the literature. Med Care Res Rev. 2006;63:263–300.
31. Rowe J. Approaching interdisciplinary research. In Kessel F, Rosenfield P, Anderson N, editors. Explaining the boundaries of health and social science: case studies in interdisciplinary innovation. New York, N.Y.: Oxford University Press; 2003. p. 3–9.
32. Sommers LS, Marton KI, Barbaccia JC, Randolph J. Physician, nurse and social worker collaboration in primary health care for chronically ill seniors. Arch Intern Med. 2000;160:1825–33.
33. Spreier S, Fontaine M, Malloy R. Leadership run amok. The destructive potential of overachievers. Harvard Business Review, 2006. p.73–82.
34. Storch JL. Division of Labour in health care: Pragmatics and ethics. Humane Medicine. 1994;10(4):262–9.
35. Suchman A, Sluyter D, Williamson P. Leading change in healthcare: transforming organisations using complexity, positive psychology and relationship-centred care. London, England: Radcliffe Publishing; 2011.
36. University of Washington. Interdisciplinary team issues. 1998. http://depts.washington.edu/bioethx/topics/team.html Accessed 15 Jan 2015.
37. Wagner EH. The role of patient care teams in chronic disease management. British Medical Jouranl. 2000;320:569–72.
38. Weiss D, Tilin F, Morgan M. The interprofessional health care team: leadership and development. Burlington, MA.: Jones & Bartlett Learning; 2014.
39. Wheelan SA, Burchill CN, Tilin F. The link between teamwork and patients' outcomes in intensive care units. Am J Crit Care. 2003;12:527–34.
40. Wikipedia. 2014. Interdisziplinarität. n.d. https://en.wikipedia.org/wiki/Interdisciplinarity.

41. Wikipedia. 2013. Multidisziplinarität. n.d. https://de.wikipedia.org/wiki/Multidisziplinarit%C3%83_%C2%A4t.
42. World Health Organization: Health Professions Network Nursing and Midwifery Office within the Department of Human Resources for Health. Framework for Action on Interprofessional Education & Collaborative Practice. WHO HRH/HPN/10.3. Geneva: World Health Organization. 2010. http://www.who.int/hrh/en/.

Person-Centred Prevention in Psychiatry

17

Nikos G. Christodoulou MBBS, PhD, MRCPsych,
Dusica Lecic-Tosevski MD, PhD
and Roy Abraham Kallivayalil MD, DPM, MAMS

17.1 Introduction

Medicine is characterised by an unsurprising paradox: whereas its ultimate aim is health, its development is driven by disease. An important consequence of this is that, in the majority of cases, the conceptual basis of available healthcare options is geared towards tackling disease. This phenomenon further extends into regional management of resources and overall national and international policies. The nosocentric approach has given rise to remarkable discoveries and outcomes in terms of tackling diseases, but has come short of achieving science's potential for prevention and health promotion. Equally, focusing on disease has resulted in medical practice often forgetting the person involved, despite clinical reality consistently reminding us that the person is central. This apparent void in research, education, clinical practice and policy represents an opportunity for development. Preventive psychiatry and person-centred medicine

N.G. Christodoulou MBBS, PhD, MRCPsych (✉)
Honorary Assistant Professor in Psychiatry, University of Nottingham and
Consultant Liaison Psychiatrist, Nottingham, UK; Department of Psychological Medicine,
Queen's Medical Centre, B Floor, Nottingham NG7 2UH, UK
e-mail: Nikos.Christodoulou@nhs.net

D. Lecic-Tosevski MD, PhD
Professor of Psychiatry, School of Medicine, Serbian Academy of Sciences and Arts,
University of Belgrade, Belgrade, Serbia

R.A. Kallivayalil MD, DPM, MAMS
Vice-Principal, Professor and Head, Department of Psychiatry,
Pushpagiri Institute of Medical Sciences, Tiruvalla 689 101, Kerala, India;
Secretary General, World Psychiatric Association, Geneva, Switzerland

J.E. Mezzich et al. (eds.), *Person Centered Psychiatry*,
DOI 10.1007/978-3-319-39724-5_17

are two approaches that have naturally emerged to cover that gap, and together provide a synergy to suggest a paradigm shift away from nosocentric approaches [6].

Person-centred psychiatry and preventive psychiatry share a substantial theoretical and practical interface. This interface is substantial enough for the two concepts to combine in clinical practice into an indistinguishable amalgam. The main implication of introducing person-centred prevention as an important shift to current practice is that the current nosocentric mentality may be complemented by a more effective and cost-effective preventive, person-centred approach. In addition to improving diagnostic and therapeutic outcomes, this shift promotes empowerment, holism and autonomy, and importantly expands implementation beyond the narrow remit of medicine to include the whole population. Due to the complexity of a personalised preventive approach, theoretical application guidelines are meaningless. Instead, in this chapter, we provide a small collection of pivotal case studies to demonstrate the practical synergy of person-centred and preventive psychiatry.

17.2 Conceptual Confluence of Person-Centred Medicine and Preventive Psychiatry

Preventive medicine, consisting of all measures that focus on preventing illness as opposed to just treating it, is not exactly what it says on the tin. According to the American College of Preventive Medicine, "(Preventive Medicine) … focuses on the health of individuals, communities, and defined populations. Its goal is to protect, promote, and maintain health and well-being and to prevent disease, disability, and death" (www.acpm.org). It is evident that illness prevention and health promotion are both included in the notion of "preventive" medicine, and that is not surprising, as there is a practically indistinguishable relationship between the two. The main difference is that, while promotion is concerned with the determinants of health, prevention focuses on the causes of disease [4, 7]. The WHO on the other hand defines health as "a complete state of physical, mental and social well-being, and not merely the absence of disease or infirmity" (www.who.int), worded in a way that suggests that preventing illness is *necessary* in order to achieve health. But this is also not accurate, as exemplified best in the case of psychiatry; For instance, it is possible for a person with a severe mental illness to have positive mental health (e.g. resilience, mental capital, autonomy and empowerment, positive relationships, a positive outlook etc.). Conversely, it is also possible not to have a diagnosed mental illness but still have poor (negative) mental health factors (e.g. isolation, disempowerment, poor psychological awareness, etc.). Therefore, it becomes clear that health and illness (and by extension health promotion and illness prevention) are not linearly related concepts, but can rather be visualised as existing on a Cartesian field simultaneously and even partly independently [16].

Person-centred medicine (PCM) is a dynamic medical ethos which re-focuses medical practice on the person. PCM embodies the archetypal focus of medicine on the person, in line with Hippocratic wisdom ("It is more important to know what person has a disease, than to know what disease a person has"). It may even be argued that attaching the epithet "person-centred" to "Medicine" is, in fact, a pleonasm. Nevertheless, the articulation of a clear and consistent movement serves to establish person-centredness as a pivotal ethos in medicine. This is important as very few paradigms of pragmatic implementation of person-centredness are evident at present, and even fewer stretch beyond a superficial mention.

Preventive psychiatry (mental illness prevention and mental health promotion) employs a host of strategies towards preventing mental illness, but also towards promoting health for both people who are at risk of developing mental illness and those who are mentally ill. Thus, preventive psychiatry applies to all people, at all times and at every stage of life. While illness prevention and health promotion serve two conceptually different purposes, in practice attainable goals are reached through an interlacing of the two. For example, building up family bonds serves both towards improving someone's quality of life and towards improving their psychological resilience against adversity. One major conceptual difference between prevention and promotion is that, while illness prevention is predominantly nosocentric (disease-centred), health promotion is predominantly hygeiocentric (health-centred). An important caveat applies here in that the practical interlacing of the two attenuates that conceptual divide, thus making health promotion partly nosocentric and illness prevention partly hygeiocentric, in their own right.

On the other hand, PCM is by definition person-centred. Its remit includes a holistic approach towards the person, including personal, cultural, spiritual and existential approaches among others. The PCM approach is analytical, providing comprehensive theoretical understanding of the person, whereas Preventive Medicine is pragmatically less exhaustive as it is inherently aimed at a practical goal; namely prevention and promotion. PCM comprehensively deals with the totality of a person's existence and needs, including objective and subjective understanding, internal (the patient-person) or external (the therapist-person, the family, the person's circumstances, etc.) views, and adapts diagnosis and therapy accordingly [1]. Inherent of course is the notion that considerations may belong to the past, current, future or be diachronical. In their latter temporal quality, PCM considerations feed into those of prevention and promotion. In some ways therefore, preventive medicine can be seen as one of the practical arms of PCM. This does not imply that PCM is impractical; on the contrary, it is necessary for application to occur. In fact, PCM is necessary for preventive medicine to be even possible, therefore in some ways PCM and preventive medicine are complementary through their differences, because they are necessary for each other. For instance, in approaching a person's needs for prevention and promotion one *has to* take into account person-centred factors. Similarly, as stated above, a PCM approach would not be complete without a temporal consideration and, practically, future planning. As both health and illness characterise a person, PCM deals with both simultaneously and without much differentiation. In that way, not only does it automatically include preventive medicine (i.e. health promotion and illness prevention), but also automatically and effortlessly combines the two in practice. This is far from a trivial achievement, as those who work with prevention and promotion at heart will be able to attest.

Hence, even though conceptually the approach of preventive medicine is different to that of PCM, in practice they have a very similar and complementary remit.

17.3 Practical Implementation

Person-centred medicine and preventive psychiatry share a substantial conceptual, but also a practical interface [2, 3].

The only way to apply preventive psychiatry properly is through a holistic approach to a person's life, and through a profound understanding of the personal and interpersonal needs of that particular individual and their circumstances. While this is most obviously true about health promotion, it is equally relevant to illness prevention. Considerations in preventive psychiatry go beyond the strict boundaries of the bio-psychosocial model and include elements pertaining to the remit of person-centred medicine. This is a necessity, as mental illness prevention requires a multi-faceted and highly flexible and individualised approach. As this approach is the only way for preventive psychiatry to be effective, preventive psychiatry needs to be intrinsically holistic and person-centred.

But preventive psychiatry and PCM share both application remits and implementation problems. As discussed above, their grossly overlapping conceptual bases often translate to indistinguishable practical implementation (for instance, refer to the Early Intervention case study below). This renders the two synergistic and presents with important opportunities beyond clinical application in, among others, service development, dissemination and education.

Starting from the latter point, educational activities can be shared, enhanced and mutually supported between PCM and preventive psychiatry. For instance, the holism that characterises both approaches may be taught in conjunction rather than independently. An important example of this is the opportunity to develop educational curricula based on the two approaches [4, 7]. In this way, not only will PCM and preventive psychiatry be demystified, but the concept of holistic medicine will become more readily associated with these approaches. Another example of educational synergy involves service development in the sense that policy-makers and healthcare managers may be more effectively informed—and convinced—on principles shared by PCM and preventive psychiatry rather than in isolation. Using common communication and publication channels can lead to the amplification of the dissemination of knowledge, skills and attitudes in both fields. Beyond common education and dissemination, fulfilling similar needs offers opportunities for both common service development and service ethos development. Using the Early Intervention paradigm again, person-centredness may form part of management in conjunction with preventive psychiatry. In fact, it would be fair to argue that this is already taking place by default, but in addition may be a labelling opportunity.

Perhaps the most rewarding exercise when considering preventive psychiatry and PCM is to compare the difficulties encountered by either field and identify common grounds for intervention and resolution of problems. An interesting common characteristic of both PCM and preventive psychiatry is that they are misunderstood.

There is good reason for the above, as in an evidence-based era it is hard to argue for the development of nebulously defined and broadly applied approaches. Both PCM and preventive psychiatry may defend against this argument by suggesting that the intended benefits are so obvious that defy proof, and therefore, refusal to implement these approaches would constitute intentional non-beneficence. However, even this argument can be countered by a relativity question (perhaps another, equally obvious, approach is more effective and cost-effective?), which further necessitates the need for research-produced evidence.

The latter is made difficult in both PCM and preventive medicine by the fact that their intended direct and collateral effects are multifaceted and longitudinal [5]. This makes it very difficult to attribute specific causality and effectiveness of any PCM or preventive intervention on an overall longitudinal outcome. Preventive psychiatry was faced with this criticism two decades ago, and in response produced some evidence on shorter, specific and well-circumscribed cases, not necessarily on overall outcomes. Such shorter case studies of the cost-effectiveness of prevention and promotion-based interventions has yielded very positive results suggesting financial benefits as well as health benefits, in some cases from year one of the investment [17]. As a result, these snippets of evidence represent indicators for cost-effectiveness that have been convincing enough for major policy makers to adopt preventive psychiatry in their programmes [10, 24].

One interesting advantage of applying PCM and preventive psychiatry synergistically is that their remits may be mutually expanded. For instance, a person-centred preventive effect renders post-preventive person-centred care obsolete, and on the other hand the need for secondary and tertiary prevention may decrease following person-centred care.

Pragmatically, PCM and preventive psychiatry are currently being practiced under different approaches. A prominent example is the "Recovery" movement which incorporates some elements of person-centredness and others of preventive psychiatry. For instance, through the concept of empowerment and their personal journey, people with mental illness, their carers and mental health professionals formulate a person-centred understanding of the situation. Similarly, as the name "Recovery" implies, a secondary/tertiary prevention and a mental health promotion processes are involved. As useful as they may be, such movements have significant drawbacks. In the case of Recovery, for instance, the mere assumption that someone is "recovering" implies that an insult has already taken place in the past, and therefore emphasis on primary prevention is weak, at least conceptually. Additionally, focusing on recovering from an illness makes this movement intrinsically nosocentric, thus attenuating its person-centred character. Overall, it is important to encourage affiliated movements which indeed strengthen person-centred practice and support prevention and promotion, but it is also important to keep the person-centred movement as a strong point of reference.

17.4 Case Studies

The practical interplay between preventive and person-centred components can be very complex and at the same time blatantly obvious, as in some ways it represents expected practice. Discussing the theoretical underpinnings of such an interplay can never reflect the potential for practical applicability in specific cases. It may therefore be more easily understood through indicative examples. Here we offer three such case studies.

17.4.1 Early Intervention

Early intervention refers to the intention by services to get involved in a person's care as soon as possible in the course of their illness. It is most commonly applied in the case of psychosis, but also in mood disorders and substance misuse, among others. Unless especially set-up, early intervention services offer secondary and tertiary prevention. They also offer health promotion interventions and supportive interventions for family and other important areas of a young person's life (e.g. school, work, etc.). As expected, in order for early intervention to be effective, a holistic spectrum of factors affecting a young person's life need to be addressed simultaneously, including biological, psychological and social factors. In addition, all relevant considerations must be made and planned within the cultural, spiritual and existential context that defines each particular person. It transpires that a necessary prerequisite for such an undertaking to have any meaningful reflection is for any measure to be informed by the person concerned and be concordant with their personal circumstances.

Diagnosis in early intervention in psychosis is dependent on the recognition of prodromal symptoms, which are sometimes difficult to differentiate from adolescent turbulence. Such a differentiation is crucial towards achieving early and effective limitation of the duration of untreated psychosis (DUP), the toxic period between first symptoms and the beginning of treatment, which has a strong bearing on prognosis [20]. Increasing the accuracy and speed of diagnosis depends exactly on being able to relate any symptoms to the array of complex personal and environmental factors that compose a young person's world. A person-centred diagnostic approach is indicated for tackling that level of complexity, a feat which is often beyond the capabilities of a conventional service. Using a person-centred perspective allows for accurate diagnostic synthesis and greatly potentiates early intervention services. Successful diagnostic manuals have been devised which combine practicality with person-centredness, for instance the Revised Version of the Latin American Guide of Psychiatric Diagnosis (GLADP-VR), which has been recently published by the Latin American Psychiatric Association [21].

By adopting a person-centred approach, preventive and health promotional interventions will not only serve to avert illness and enhance health, but will also establish themselves in a long-lasting, ego-syntonic way with the person.

Ego-syntonic because measures will match a person's life (and not vice versa), and long-lasting because such measures will therefore likely continue beyond the time of therapy. These two characteristics (long-lasting, ego-syntonic) are the absolutely crucial contributions of person-centredness in the case of early intervention in psychosis, where two of the most frequent problems encountered are loss of continuity and reduced insight. Therefore, from a practical and clinical perspective, person-centred thinking and practice is not only compatible with preventive practice in early intervention, but it fulfils an important missing role that improves its long-term effectiveness [3].

17.4.2 Personality Disorders

Personality disorders are entities entwined more than other mental illnesses with PCM. Early recognition and diagnostics of these multiple faces disorders [18] as well as an understanding of their multifactorial origin are necessary for prevention and mental health promotion.

There are significant problems in prevention and treatment of personality disorders, which are surrounded with pessimism and controversy. Many clinicians believe that these disorders are untreatable, and that individuals with personality disorders have little capacity for change. Not surprisingly, they remain sceptical about the prospects of their prevention, with many reasons causing it. Personality disorders develop early, their symptoms are ego-syntonic, and defences primitive and alloplastic, their psychopathological architectonics is stable. These highly demanding patients confront psychiatrists with limitation of their art, give little gratification and endanger therapists' narcissism, so that many therapists avoid treating them.

Some clinicians identify personality disorders with the antisocial personality or psychopathy and state that these patients pose dilemma for physicians and society. The dominant view that there is a frequent failure to achieve cure has divided the medical and legal communities, as well as society in general. However, some experts believe that funds should be committed for more research and special facilities for treatment of psychopathic patients [9]. These patients have children who grow up, and through a transgenerational transmission might create a vicious circle of aggression and violence, which are becoming prominent in contemporary society [19].

There is no doubt that mental health professionals should do their best to prevent personality disorders. And, whilst the innate temperament cannot be changed, understanding factors that influence development of personality disorders (genetic risks, predisposing and precipitating factors) or leave a child resilient in response to childhood trauma (protective factors) might help prevention and treatment. Mental health professionals have challenging roles to play in preventing malignant memories of traumatic experiences and subduing their pernicious effects as well as examining the chain of interactions among environment, personality and behaviour initiated by early trauma.

The role of childhood trauma in development of personality disorders was indicated as crucial by numerous studies. Most violent adolescents and adult persons with personality disorders have been abused and emotionally deprived and undernourished as children [22]. Childrearing that includes a great deal of punishment, criticism, and humiliation paves the way for later delinquent and even criminal behaviour [11].

Strategies to reduce precipitating and increase protective factors in a child are necessary. It is important to acquire knowledge of the factors which protect children from psychiatric illness, which could be learnt from the so-called "invulnerable children" [23]. The identification of high-risk groups at an early stage before delivery and the intervention at that stage should be a target of the primary care.

High-quality parenting and early intervention can play a critical role in the development of healthy personality as well as in facing environmental adversities during the "magic years" of childhood. Therefore, there is a need for a worldwide parenting education and preventive programmes, which would enable parents to see their own role as a paramount, their own action able to bring changes for the better in their children's behaviour, and an awareness of the family's strengths rather than weaknesses.

Treatment and prevention of personality disorders are difficult and slow, but should not be neglected because of their high public health significance. They should be multidimensional, continuous, multimodal and eclectic, and part of extensive community programmes. There is a need for carefully planned outpatient and inpatient treatment, as well as for assertive programmes, and psychoeducational interventions for families of personality disorders. PCM movement advocating an integrated approach to mental health and mental disorders as well as a revival of the ancient Hippocratic wisdom is the most relevant for the science of well-being [8].

17.4.3 Suicide Prevention

Suicide has become an important public health problem world over. Not only psychiatrists and psychologists, but also sociologists, NGOs, the media, religious leaders and politicians have come up with opinions highlighting their own viewpoints. Scientific studies are limited in the field of suicidology in many parts of the world. The limited data available show that the profile and pattern are different in western and eastern countries [12].

WHO defines suicide as a deliberate act of self harm with fatal outcome and suicide attempt as an injury with varying degrees of lethal intent. Suicide is a complex problem with biological, psychological, social, spiritual, economic, political and philosophical underpinnings. Are suicides really preventable? If they are, what should be the appropriate strategy based on available scientific evidence? Are strategies used in developed world appropriate in developing countries?

Person-centred preventive strategies have a paramount place in suicide prevention- and they are relevant in all parts of the world. Behaviour that risk injury to self is a ubiquitous feature of human behaviour. Understanding this complex behaviour requires inquiry from different angles and disciplines ranging from biology and medicine to economics and philosophy. Suicidal behaviour and its determinants varies across different cultures, ethnic and age groups, and from one period in history to another. Multidisciplinary and cross disciplinary approaches may give us better insight into the causes and practical preventive strategies. The different pieces of this difficult jigsaw puzzle may ultimately fall in place to give us a better picture, at a time when we are able to put the findings of scientific studies from different disciplines together [15].

Abnormalities in serotonin transporter, sensitivity to frustrations, low levels of 5-hydroxy indole acetic acid in spinal fluid, impulsivity, limited coping abilities, high levels of steroid hormones, inadequate problem solving abilities, guilt, depression, aggression turned inside, economic recession, falling price of cash crops, the role of alcohol and psychoactive substances, the availability of methods, media influence, egoism and anomie, erosion of value systems and support systems and change from joint family system to nuclear family—all these factors may finally fit into this evolving complex picture.

17.4.3.1 Suicide Prevention: A Person-Centred Approach

Suicide can be seen as a major public health problem of our times. It is one among the 10 leading causes of death. More than a million people die of suicide every year in the world. It is the third major cause of 'Life Years Lost', next only to heart disease and cancer. The highest risk for suicide is among the adolescents and old people. People who are divorced, separated or living singly also show a high incidence. The high suicide rates in young people is strikingly high in many South Asian countries. Most of them commit suicide, on an impulse. Hence suicide prevention strategies aimed at these vulnerable groups become very important.

It is well known that the large majority of people who commit suicide do so due to emotional and mental problems. Depression is the single biggest cause for suicide. Getting them professional help, thus remains crucial. In South Asia we have several instances when even medical personnel have not referred people with severe depression for psychiatric help. This may be due to stigma or because of deficient medical training or because of inability to properly communicate a diagnosis of mental illness to patients [14]. Many doctors may not like to take up the responsibility of communicating unpleasant truths. This happens mainly because of lack of awareness of the importance of person-centred care [13]. Family members should also share an equal blame. Often they allow the depressed person to suffer in silence, without getting him or her psychiatric help. Another leading cause for suicide is alcoholism and drug addiction. All these may end up in suicides, thus ending valuable and productive lives.

17.4.3.2 Person-Centred Prevention: Dispelling Myths About Suicide

There are certain myths about suicide, especially in many Asian countries.

Myth No 1: "Those who speak about suicide will never do so". In fact, the truth is exactly the opposite. Most people who commit suicide, would have communicated their intent to someone very close to them. The person usually tells this to some significant person in his life.

Myth No 2: "If someone has decided to end his life, no one can stop him". This is also untrue. Most people do not want to die- they simply want an end to their suffering. Only, they are considering suicide as the option. If help arrives, or proper treatment is given, this perception will immediately disappear and the life can be saved.

Myth No 3: "If you enquire about suicide, you are going to plant this idea in his mind". In fact when you enquire, the person entertaining suicidal ideas would have felt better understood. He/she would have known, not everything is lost and there is still joy in the world.

17.4.3.3 Media and Suicide

There is a tendency in the media to sensationalise and glorify suicides. Media may also give undue prominence to suicide. This has to be stopped. Sensationalising and glorifying suicide, will tempt young persons to model the victim and achieve glory or fame. The media must exercise utmost restraint. Suicide news should never be a front page story. One sided stories highlighting the character strengths of the suicide victim should not be given. If reported, it should be factual, mentioning his strengths as well as weaknesses, so that suicide is not seen as the act of the strong minded.

Public awareness of suicide and attempted suicide is very important. Most often, such people would be suffering from depression or personality problems. If we know this, we can treat them and help them. Person-centred care encourages the fight against the stigma associated with suicide, by seeing it as not as an act against society but as the cry of a sick person. Engaging the family members of the suicide victims with compassion and sensitivity and respecting their privacy is very important. Suicide Prevention Clinics, Crisis Intervention Centres and telephonic help lines are very useful. NGOs, educationalists, religious leaders and public activists have an important responsibility in spreading proper awareness about suicide prevention strategies. They are best successful in saving lives when working with person-centred approaches.

17.5 Conclusions

PCM is a new approach to the field of psychiatry and preventive psychiatry is an important aspect of psychiatric practice. Both focus on the person holistically in illness and in health. Both conceptually and in practice reiterate each other and at points complete and complement each other. This becomes obvious whenever the clinical need arises, and it is impressive to re-discover that they operate as a caring instinct. In such cases, the synergy between the two is instantaneous and consistent, but it is important to articulate a clear account of their relationship for reasons of quality assurance and conceptual completeness. Finally, the onus for both remains the generation of enough evidence so that policy-makers adopt their collective principles and support their implementation.

References

1. Botbol M. Conclusion generale. Du manifeste au subjectif: ce qu'est la medicine de la personne. In: Kipman SD, editor. Médecine de la personne: un manifeste collectif qui s'adresse aux médecins, soignants, malades et décideurs. Paris: Wolters Kluwer; 2012. p. 317–26.
2. Christodoulou GN, Christodoulou NG. Mental health promotion: concept and practice. Int J Pers Cent Med. 2012;2(1):24–8.
3. Christodoulou GN, Christodoulou NG. Early intervention in psychiatry. Early Interv Psychiatry. 2007;1(1):7–8.
4. Christodoulou GN, Jenkins R, Tsipas V, Christodoulou NG, Lecic-Tosevski D, Mezzich JE. Mental health promotion: a conceptual review and guidance. Eur Psychiatr Rev. 2011;4(1): 9–13.
5. Christodoulou NG. General prevention research and person centered medicine. Int J Pers Cent Med. 2013;3(2):133–6.
6. Christodoulou NG, Ramalho R. Changement de paradigme d'une medicine preventive centree sur la maladie a une medicine preventive centree sur la personne. In: Kipman SD, editor. Médecine de la personne: un manifeste collectif qui s'adresse aux médecins, soignants, malades et décideurs. Paris: Wolters Kluwer; 2012. p. 47–54.
7. Christodoulou NG, Ramalho R, Larsson M, Karpenko O. Person-centred medicine and professional development. Int J Pers Cent Med. 2011;1(3):581–4.
8. Cloninger CR. The science of well-being: an integrated approach to mental health and its disorders. World Psychiatry. 2006;5:71–6.
9. Davis-Barron S. Psychopathic patients pose dilemma for physicians and society. CMAJ. 1995;152(8):1314–7.
10. European Parliament Resolution of 19 February 2009 on Mental Health. P6 TA[2009]0063. Available at http://www.europarl.europa.eu.
11. Fink B. Violence and parenting education. In: Christodoulou GN, Lecic-Tosevski D, Kontaxakis V, editors. Issues of preventive psychiatry. Basel: Karger; 1999. p. 30–8.
12. Kallivayalil RA. Suicide, attempted suicide & suicide prevention. Kerala Med J. 2010;10 (3):97–9.
13. Kallivayalil RA. The importance of psychiatry in undergraduate medical education in India. Ind J Psychiatry. 2012;54(3):208–16.
14. Kallivayalil RA, Kumar PNS. Education in person-centered medicine: Indian perspectives. Int J Pers Cent Med. 2012;2(2):155–8.
15. Kallivayalil RA, Punnoose VP. Editorial in suicide prevention—a handbook for community gatekeepers. Kottayam: National Alliance for Mental Health; 2009.
16. Keyes CL. The mental health continuum: from languishing to flourishing in life. J Health Soc Behav. 2002; 43(2):207–22.
17. Knapp M, McDaid D, Parsonage M, editors. Mental health promotion and mental illness prevention: the economic case. London: Department of Health; 2011.
18. Lecic Tosevski D. Many faces of personality disorders. In: Kittas C, Lykouras E, Papadimitriou G, editors. Honorary volume in honor of Professor George N. Christodoulou. Betamedarts: University of Athen; 2011. p. 200–206.
19. Lecic-Tosevski D, Draganic Gajic S, Pejovic Milovancevic M, Popovic Deusic S, Christodoulou N, Botbol M. Child is father of the man—child abuse and development of future psychopathology. Psychiatriki. 2014;25(3):26–31.

20. Lieberman JA, Perkins D, Belger A, Chakos M, Jarskog F, Boteva K, et al. The early stages of schizophrenia: speculations on pathogenesis, pathophysiology, and therapeutic approaches. Biol Psychiatry. 2001;50:884–97.
21. Mezzich JE, Otero EA, Saavedra EJ, Salloum MI. The GLADP-VR person-centered diagnostic formulation: background, concepts, and structure. Int J Pers Cent Med. 2013;3 (3):131–3.
22. Mitkovic Voncina M, Lecic Tosevski D, Pejovic Milovancevic M, Popovic Deusic S. Linking child maltreatment history with child abuse potential: relative roles of maltreatment types. Arch Biol Sci. 2014;66(4):1681–7.
23. Rutter M. Psychosocial resilience and protective mechanisms. Am J Orthopsychiatry. 1987;57:316–31.
24. World Health Organization. Summary report: prevention of mental disorders - effective interventions and policy options. Geneva: World Health Organization; 2004.

Person-Centered Psychopharmacotherapy

18

Miro Jakovljević MD and Mohammed T. Abou-Saleh MD, PhD

18.1 Introduction

Psychopharmacotherapy, today, is a fascinating field that can be viewed in many different ways with different consequences. It is argued to be scientific, rational, and objective, very much evidence-based, and often the fundamental form of treatment for all major mental disorders. However, current psychopharmacotherapy is commonly criticized to be just a symptomatic treatment, related mainly to placebo response, and even reflect an inappropriate medicalization of life problems. There are those who view it as a means of controlling people and their minds by society. Unfortunately, there are also the people who think psychopharmacotherapy is a dark art and an expression of toxic psychiatry. With the 1990s Decade of Brain the field of pharmacopsychiatry has expanded hugely, introducing controversial concepts and treatment paradigms, creating both new problems and opportunities. The availability of a significant number of effective and well tolerated psychopharmaceuticals has increased opportunities for successful treatment of many mental disorders with much better treatment outcome including full recovery. However, there is a huge gap between possibilities for achieving high treatment effectiveness and poor results in clinical practice: the gap between efficacy and effectiveness as pharmacotherapy is optimally effective in a whole system of care. Stigmatization and widespread pessimism with low therapeutic expectations, institutionalized in many ways contribute significantly to poorer treatment outcome. Psychiatric patients have been commonly told that "they could not be cured or obtain full

M. Jakovljević MD (✉)
Professor of Psychiatry, Department of Psychiatry, University Hospital Centre Zagreb, School of Medicine, University of Zagreb, Kispaticeva 12, 10000 Zagreb, Croatia
e-mail: jakovljevic.miro@yahoo.com

M.T. Abou-Saleh MD, PhD
Professor of Psychiatry, St George's Medical School, University of London, London, UK

J.E. Mezzich et al. (eds.), *Person Centered Psychiatry*,
DOI 10.1007/978-3-319-39724-5_18

recovery and that they would have to take mental health medications whole life." Rational psychopharmacotherapy is often equated with the therapeutic action of medicines in mental disorders in exclusively biological terms. Patients are commonly treated just as biological organisms that respond neurochemically to medications, but not also as subjects who respond to the meaning that those medications and mental disorders have [27]. Conventional psychopharmacology paradigms focusing just on a disease perspective and a "one size fits all" treatment are often regarded as inadequate and disjunctive [22, 26]. Simply treating a psychiatric condition as only a brain disorder, without treating the whole person, is increasingly considered detrimental. Additionally, advances in the genomics and pharmacogenomics of mental disorders provide promise for more personalized and effective approaches to treatment [14].

The good news is that there is a trend for developing a personalized, complex systems approaches which integrate many diverse inputs and perspectives into a unique network [20, 21]. Changing the prevalent treatment philosophy may be a critical step toward overcoming what some view as "therapeutic stagnation in psychiatry" and providing better treatment effectiveness and efficiency for patients benefit. A "paradigm shift" is needed from the mechanistic, formalistic, and reducionistic way of thinking to contextualized and systemic thinking with new treatment approaches individualizing and personalizing psychopharmacotherapy in a creative manner. The concept of person-centered psychopharmacotherapy is a major advance in clinical practice and bridge the gap by increasing treatment effectiveness and efficiency.

18.2 Person-Centered Psychopharmacotherapy: Definition and Fundamental Principles

> It is more important to know what kind of a patient has a disease than what kind of a disease a patient has (William Osler)

The term person-centered psychopharmacotherapy may have different conceptions for mental health practitioners. From our perspective the concept of person-centered psychopharmacotherapy refers to an art, science, and practice of mental health drug treatment based on medicine of person of Paul Tournier [7] and person-centered psychiatry [4, 25], transdisciplinary integrative psychiatry [15, 19] and creative psychopharmacology [3, 20, 21], the fifth discipline learning organization (see [33]), and positive psychology [30, 32]. Person-centered psychopharmacotherapy is not a competitor to traditional, evidence-based psychopharmacotherapy (see Table 18.1); they are a complementary duality, as intimately connected as brain and soul [24]. While the psychiatrist is an expert with specialized knowledge about drug treatments, the patient is the expert on his or her life, and the best evaluator of the treatment outcome. Patients always bring into treatment unique characteristics related to their vulnerability, resilience, and potential for personal growth. Disease has to be treated,

Table 18.1 Comparison of traditional and person-centered psychopharmacotherapy [24]

Traditional psychopharmacotherapy
–Standardized, based on knowledge and research, impersonal and dismissive of individuality
–Epidemiological and more scientific (modern science)
–Based on linear and mechanistic thinking and deductive logic
–Self-determination of patients reduced
–Patients' compliance is expected or requested
–Only psychiatrists have access to information (e.g., drug treatment plans, assessments, records, etc.)
Doctors know the best
–Focus is on pathology (disease or illness), weakness and disadvantages
–Symptoms, dysfunctions, disabilities, deficits drive treatment
–Patients are more objects of treatment
–Clinical (symptomatic and functional) remission/recovery is valued
–Drug treatment is defined by treatment guideline
–Avoidance of risk ("Primum non nocere"). Protection of patient and community
–Evidence-based practice
Person-centered psychopharmacotherapy
–Pluralistic, based on wisdom, research and practice, personal and respective of individuality
–Individualistic and more humanistic (postmodern science)
–Based on lateral thinking, imagination and inductive logic
–Self-determination of patients is promoted
–Alliance is much more than compliance. Patients' active participation and personal mastery is essential
–Patients and their families have also access to the information. Doctors and patients together know the best. Shared decisions
–Patients are best experts on their life
–Focus on self-actualization, health and quality of life, strengths and advantages
–Therapeutic goals drive treatment
–Patients are more subjects, active participants and stars of treatment
–In addition to clinical and personal recovery is valued
–Drug treatment is rooted in creative and systematic thinking
–Responsible risk taking and personal growth. Avoid risk, whenever is possible
–In addition to evidence-, value- and narrative-based practice

but the needs of the suffering person have also to be met, helped with and healed. So, person-centered psychopharmacotherapy is a part of personal recovery-oriented treatment. Treatment that focuses only on symptoms elimination and decreasing illness may be like the tail wagging the dog. Patients need to learn specific skills of positive psychology: how to have more positive thinking and emotions, more creativity and engagement, more gratitude, love and life fulfillment, more accomplishment, and better human relations [32].

Person-centered psychopharmacotherapy draws on biological perspectives of the person [6] and includes always an individualized approach because each patient is a unique individual comprised of body, mind, and soul. Sensitivity to different medications varies from one individual to another. Genetics, personal history, particularly drug history, and comorbidity may significantly influence an individual's response to pharmacological treatment. Major brain pathways are specified in genome, but personalized connections are uniquely fashioned by, and consequently reflect, socially mediated experience in the world [11]. Furthermore, human behavior is not the passive consequence of genes or gene–environment interactions; rather human beings shape their environment and influence the expression of their own genome by their self-aware actualization of their personal life narrative within the broad constraints of the rich innate endowment of human beings. Gene expression is a dynamic adaptive process. Individuals shape and are shaped by the changing expression of their genomes [5]. The human genome can be viewed more as a basic design that can be actively modified to enhance human potential by a self-aware person, rather than as a fixed antecedent determinant of human behavior. Psychobiological treatment of any of the systems of human learning may be helpful in optimizing the well-being of a person [6].

The field of pharmacogenetics and epigenetics is a rapidly evolving science investigating the genotype as a possible reason for good, poor or no responding to drugs as well as for deleterious side effects. Although this field heralds great promise for individualized patient healthcare, there are only a few reliable markers in clinical practice. When starting with psychopharmacotherapy, it is important to choose medicines that (1) can treat comorbid conditions present, (2) have no a particular side effect, (3) do not complicate a medical condition, (4) have no a negative interactions with another medicines indicated, (5) have side-effect that may be to the patient's benefit, (6) are preferred by the patient, (7) have been effective in a close relatives of the patient, and (8) are affordable for the patient [10]. Each patient should get highly specific and individually adjusted drug treatment in given circumstances [18]. Generally speaking, the optimal treatment regime, in terms of drug selection, dosage, duration, effectiveness (efficacy and tolerability) should be taylor-made for the individual and person-centered. In support of this approach, applied psychometrics have been considered as a discipline focusing on pharmacopsychology rather than psychopharmacology as illustrated by the pharmacopsychometric triangle illustrating the measurements of wanted and unwanted effects of pharmacotherapeutic drugs as well as health-related quality of life [2].

Psychopharmacotherapy is a context-dependent practice because different contexts at many levels reflect the contribution and meaning of biological variables in different ways. It is an important fact that "the genome operate within the context of the cell, the cell within the context of the body, the body within the context of the self, the self within the context of the society, the society within the context of the cosmos" [5]. The close interconnectedness of the spirit, mind, brain, endocrine, and immune systems suggests a self-aware "operating and healing system" of human beings, which works silently in the background regulating and coordinating all living processes. Mental health medications can produce changes at different levels, and vice versa their effects can be under influence within different contexts. Culture, community, and different treatment contexts can affect treatment outcome. That is the reason that person-centered psychopharmacotherapy is firmly associated with creating a favorable treatment context which promotes therapeutic alliance and partnership. Person-centered psychopharmacotherapy is a transculturally sensitive practice, too.

The psychology of taking mental health medications is very complex. Patients are always subjects who give sense and respond more or less actively to meanings that disease, illness, and treatment have for them and their physicians. Hence, each treatment is associated with placebo (latin word "I shall please") or nocebo (latin word "I shall harm") response which can significantly modify the overall treatment outcome. These phenomena are universal and of great importance for psychopharmacotherapy and medicine in general. Person-centered psychopharmacotherapy is placebo-response increasing and nocebo-response decreasing-oriented practice.

Person-centered psychopharmacotherapy is patients' creativity-enhancing treatment [22]. Creative thinking helps them see an opportunity in every adversity. Research confirmed that creative activities can have a healing and protective effect on mental health and resilience by promoting self-expression, boosting the immune system, and reducing distress. Psychiatric medications may alter, preserve, foster, or damage creativity of patients in ways that significantly influence quality of life and personal recovery. Patients often discontinue medication complaining on creativity diminution and cognitive impairments caused by drug treatment. Creativity asserts life, frees the human spirit, improves self-esteem, motivation, self-actualization, and achievement and so helps conquer mental disorders. The possible effects of mental health medications on patients' creativity are an essential component of a proper medication treatment choice.

18.3 Creating Favorable Treatment Context Is Fundamental

Homo homini remedium est

In addition to the optimal treatment regime in terms of drug selection and dosage, creating specific favorable treatment contexts for each patient is an essential part of person-centered psychopharmacotherapy. The term context refers to the particular setting, such as time, place, and people present, that gives meaning to all events and activities during treatment. The fact is that in addition to physical world, we also live in the world of ideas, symbols, and meanings. Certain actions are possible or positive in one context, whereas they are negative or not allowed in some other context. Nothing is either good or bad in itself and nothing has meaning only in itself, including mental health drugs application. Information or an event has always to be understood in the context so that the meaning we derive from any experience depends on the frame we apply. Many of the concepts of mental health, wellness, and illness as well as the use of psychiatric medications are often mysterious for patients and their families and filled with myths, misconceptions, prejudice, and fears [20]. The patient's beliefs concerning the origin of symptoms and mental health medicines action may contribute positively (placebo) or negatively (nocebo) to drug treatment response. In addition to their pharmacodynamic mechanisms, mental health medications work also on account of meanings, expectations, and relationships. Hence, treatment effectiveness depends on (1) what psychiatrists and patients believe how medications work, (2) quality of a physician–patient relationship including rapport (mutual trust and respect) and patient's confidence in the psychiatry as a whole, (3) characteristics of the treatment (color, shape, smell, taste and name of medications, method and place of application, etc.); (4) communication and emotional expressiveness within the patient's family, (5) respecting patients' human rights. Always we should have in mind that "pharmakon," which means both "remedy" and "poison" is closely related to "pharmakos," which means "scapegoat" and to "pharmakeus," "magician" or "sorcerer" [9, 29]. Positive beliefs and good human relations may be "ariston pharmakon," "most effective remedy," whereas negative and wrong beliefs as well as bad human relations may be scapegoating. When beliefs are an expression of hubris, they can become more dangerous poison than any pharmakon. The creation of favorable treatment context and creative collaboration with patient and her or his family may significantly improve treatment outcome increasing treatment adherence, enhancing placebo, and decreasing nocebo response.

The creation of favorable therapeutic context is significantly associated with active participation of patients and their commitment to treatment. The purpose of psychopharmacotherapy is to empower the patients to control their disease, to obtain full personal recovery, and to regain control over their life. However, taking medications only is often not enough for full treatment success. Psychopharmacotherapy as a sole form of treatment may carry the wrong message that patients do not have to change their life style and do not have to learn any new skills, they just have to receive their medication on time because the only problem is in brain chemistry. Psychopharmacotherapy is one essential external support, alongside a whole range of other type of resilience-promoting supports, skills, and strengths. The goals of medication treatment are not only to decrease illness and prevent relapse, but also to improve neuroplasticity and help patients learn new ways of thinking, emotional response and behavior to get more love, freedom, power, joy, and sense of life. Creation of the favorable treatment context is based on the human rights FREDA (fairness, respect, equality, dignity, autonomy) concept [8], shared decision model, shared vision of treatment goals, and shared learning with patients (see [33]). Learning in this context does not mean getting more information, but expanding the ability to produce the results truly wanted [33] in psychiatric treatment. Improving personal mastery, involving self-care and self-management of patients goes beyond competence and skills, as well as beyond spiritual unfolding or opening, it means living life from a creative as opposed to reactive viewpoint [33]. Creative collaboration with patients and their families include building the shared treatment goals as well as the pictures of their future that foster their genuine commitment and enrollment more than simple compliance. Alliance is much more than compliance. A shared vision is the first step in allowing people who mistrusted each other to begin to work together [33]. Motivational interviewing with matching, pacing, and leading techniques is an essential step in establishing a creative treatment context because it helps the patients to articulate personally meaningful goals, while taking medications may facilitate achieving their goals. Being able to set and pursue personal goals provides much of the motivation for better cooperation and active participation in treatment. As patients develop more personal mastery over their symptoms, they become able to better master over their lives and to realize their own vision of recovery.

18.4 Personal Recovery Focused Psychopharmacotherapy

Treat the disease, heal the illness [12]

The concept of person-centered psychopharmacotherapy supports a shift from impersonal disease model and demoralizing prognostic skepticism toward optimism and personal recovery broadening treatment goals beyond symptom reduction and elimination. Due to the present psychopharmacological arsenal, achieving personal recovery has become a real strategic goal. Recovery orientation has become a guiding principle in many countries, while recovery-oriented services promote a new culture of care and therapeutic relationships [1]. Mental disorders are usually associated with negative or auto-destructive sense of self or loss of a sense of self, loss of power, including agency, choice and personal values, loss of meaning, such as through loss of valued social roles, loss of hope, leading to giving up withdrawal [34]. Some patients complain of spirit breaking interactions with mental health professionals engendering feeling of being disrespected, discouraged, and hopeless [34]. Lack of hope has detrimental consequences in terms of nonadherence with treatment and prevalence of nocebo responses. Creating and fostering hope, meaning, personal responsibility, spirit of optimism, and commitment can significantly contribute to overall positive response to pharmacotherapy, but in the other way round drug treatment can contribute to creation and fostering hope, meaning, personal responsibility, spirit of optimism, and commitment. Hope, which includes perceived external resources, perceived internal resources, and positive expectations, is recognized as the starting point for personal recovery. Patients with high hope are more likely to cope successfully with future adversity. Personal recovery involves a journey from disengagement to engagement, from surviving to living and growing, it has many routes and each patient's journey is unique with taking back control over own life and finding hope for a better future [34]. Love (attachment, connecting, belonging), freedom (choice, independence, autonomy), power (learning, achievement, control), joy (fun, play, pleasure, enjoyment), and purpose (meaning, sense of life) are important components of personal recovery. Loss of a sense of self which is replaced by a role or identity as a mental patient, loss of power and freedom, including agency, choice and personal values, loss of meaning, such as through loss of valued social roles and loss of hope, leading to giving up and withdrawal are crucial targets of personal recovery-oriented treatment [34]. Developing a positive identity, framing the 'mental illness', self-managing the mental illness, developing valued social roles, putting into practice more love and meaning are important tasks of personal recovery-oriented treatment.

Recognizing or finding meaning in life is fundamental issue for everybody, with or without mental disorder, and it is associated with making sense of experience and generating a story. The story is a natural framework for a very different conclusion about how we live and what we do; and what is the meaning of everything. Personal recovery is associated with the cognitive rebuilding of a viable assumptive world view which integrates the realms of vulnerability, resilience, meaning, and self-esteem in order to create a better new life story. The message is this: psychopharmacotherapy may help setting the stage for beneficial changes and personal growth. In other words, personal recovery is related to the potential for spiritual and psychological growth: that means that episodes of mental disorders, although clearly distressing and disabling, may be also developmental and educative experiences. Patients who want to live more healthily can reformulate their inner values and deep beliefs, shift their identities and develop a dominant positive life-oriented illness perspective instead a disease-oriented illness perspective. In addition to disease demotion, treatment should be oriented to wellness promotion.

Personal recovery is related to working toward better mental health, regardless of the presence of mental disorders. It is closely associated with stress-coping skills, self-care, and self-management [34]. Self-care refers to the practice of activities that patients initiate and perform on their own behalf in maintaining life, health, and well-being; whereas self-management refers to activities which patients perform to live well with mental disorder managing illness and utilizing resources. A normal life can be achieved through various self-management strategies focusing on life perspective ("increase wellness, decrease illness concept"). When patients learn to live with mental disorders, they strive to reconstruct life as normal. They are "actively engaged in working away from Floundering (through hope-supporting relationships) and Languishing (by developing positive identity), and toward Struggling (through framing and self-managing mental illness), and Flourishing (by developing valued social roles)" [34]. Stress-coping and problem-solving skills, self-management, and self-care in addition to psychopharmacotherapy may significantly influence therapeutic outcome, leading to better functional ability, life satisfaction, fewer symptoms, and fewer complications.

18.5 Patients Should Be Active Participants in Their Pharmacotherapy

There are many different reasons why patients take or refuse to take mental health medications. Besides the wish for resolving symptoms, patients may decide to take medications to please the spouse, to save their marriage, to keep their children satisfied, to save their job, to please clinician, because someone else (a friend, relative or celebrity) they respect has already tried medication and found it helpful, to prove that medications are not effective, to help in a lawsuit, claim for disability or child custody, to satisfy the courts or the law [10]. Although nonadherence with medication occurs throughout medicine, there are several issues that make it very challenging in psychiatry. The majority of patients who are resistant to treatment, have relapsed or rehospitalized are intentionally or unintentionally nonadherent, completely or to some degree. Nonadherence with mental health medicines has been usually associated with the notion of the so-called "difficult to treat" patients including the lack of insight patients, the minimal contact patients, the negative drug attitude patients, the patients preoccupied with side effects and negative expectations from drug treatment, the suspicious and paranoid patients, the patients who need to be in charge, the misinformation overloaded patients, the nocebo responders, etc. (see [10, 13, 23]).

Active participation of patients in their treatment is an essential part of person-centered psychopharmacotherapy. Patients are not only carrier of symptoms, disease, or illness, they are primarily human beings, persons, and personalities with their power, autonomy, needs, values, and desires purpose of life. Shared decisions and shared vision of therapeutic goals made in collaboration and alliance when patients assume that they are respected and valued as a person will facilitate patients' commitment to treatment goals and continued improvement. According to philosophy of person-centered psychopharmacotherapy patients should be stars of treatment, not a stage for medication trials and errors. Patients should be educated by their psychiatrists regarding optimistic and realistic expectations for the effectiveness of medication therapy and achieving personal recovery. Motivational interview, psychoeducation and informed consent should help patients to experience possible choice of treatment as his/her good choice. Helping patients decide to try mental health medicines and stay on them is an important goal of therapeutic contract.

18.6 Conclusions

With available mental health medications, it is possible to achieve a more positive impact and better treatment outcome by individualizing and personalizing treatments in a more creative and rational manner. According to many experts, impersonal and technical psychopharmacotherapy is generally insufficient for complete recovery. Person-centered psychopharmacotherapy recognizes that the healing process is more than chemical equilibration related to mental health drugs and their bioavailability in the blood and brain. Framing a positive therapeutic context in which mental health medicines are prescribed and used by patients who are stars of treatment is an essential component. Attention to promoting healthy life styles, general well-being, social integration, and spirituality are very important elements of holistic and integrating treatment that enhances favorable drug response, and vice versa psychopharmacotherapy supports better mental and social integration, self-directedness, cooperativeness, and spirituality. An integrative and holistic person-centered approach involves simultaneous and synergistic application of mental health medications, psychological, interpersonal, and family interventions in the context of well-being oriented treatment and life coaching.

References

1. Amering M. Recovery—reshaping our clinical and scientific responsibilities. Psychiatria Danubina. 2012;24(suppl 3):291–7.
2. Bech P. Applied psychometrics in clinical psychiatry: the pharmacopsychometric triangle. Acta Psychiatr Scand. 2009;120:400–9.
3. Bernstein JG. Drug therapy in psychiatry. 3rd ed. Maryland: Mosby; 1995.
4. Christodoulou G, Fulford B, Mezzich JE. Psychiatry for the person and its conceptual bases. Int Psychiatry. 2008;5:1–3.
5. Cloninger CR. Feeling good: the science of well-being. Oxford: Oxford University Press, 2004.
6. Cloninger CR, Abou-Saleh MT, Mrazek DA, Moeller HJ. Biological perspectives on psychiatry for the person. Int J Pers-Cent Med. 2011;1:137–9.
7. Cox J, Campbell AV, Fullford BKWM, editors. Medicine of the person—faith, science and values in health care provision. London: Jessica Kingsley Publishers; 2007.
8. Curtice MJ, Exworthy T. FREDA: a human rights-based approach to healthcare. The Psychiatrist. 2010;34:150–6.
9. Derrida J. Dissemination. Chicago: University of Chicago Press; 1982.
10. Doran CM. Prescribing mental health medication—the practitioner's guide. London: Routledge; 2003.
11. Eisenberg L. The social construction of the human brain. Am J Psychiatry. 1995;152:1563–75.
12. Freeman MP. Rewriting the self: history, memory, narrative. Routledge; 1993.
13. Haddad PM, Brain C, Scott J. Nonadherence with antipsychotic medication in schizophrenia: challenges and management strategies. Patient Related Outcome Measures. 2014;5:43–62.
14. Hamilton SP. The promise of psychiatric pharmacogenomics. Biol Psychiatry. 2015;77:29–35.
15. Jakovljević M. Transdisciplinary holistic integrative psychiatry—a wishfull thinking or reality? Psychiatria Danubina. 2008;20:341–8.
16. Jakovljević M. The side-effects of psychopharmacotherapy: conceptual, explanatory, ethical and moral issues—creative psychopharmacology instead of toxic psychiatry. Psychiatria Danubina. 2009;21:86–90.
17. Jakovljević M. Psychopharmacotherapy and comorbidity: conceptual and epistemological issues, dilemmas and controversies. Psychiatria Danubina. 2009;21:333–40.
18. Jakovljević M, Reiner Z, Milicic D, Crncevic Z. Comorbidity, multimorbidity and personalized psychosomatic medicine: epigenetics rolling on the horizon. Psychiatria Danubina. 2010;22:184–9.
19. Jakovljević M. Conceptual cacophony or different parts of a complex puzzle of mental disorders: transdisciplinary holistic integrative perspective. Psychiatria Danubina. 2011;23:232–6.

20. Jakovljević M. How to increase treatment effectiveness and efficiency in psychiatry: creative psychopharmacotherapy—part 1: definition, fundamental principles and higher effectiveness polipharmacy. Psychiatria Danubina. 2013;25:269–73.
21. Jakovljević M. How to increase treatment effectiveness and efficiency in psychiatry: creative psychopharmacotherapy—part 2: creating favourable treatment context and fostering patients' creativity. Psychiatria Danubina. 2013;25:274–9.
22. Jakovljević M. Creativity, mental disorders and their treatment: recovery-oriented psychopharmacotherapy. Psychiatria Danubina. 2013;25:311–5.
23. Jakovljević M. The placebo-nocebo response: controversies and challenges from clinical and research perspective. Eur Neuropsychopharmacol. 2014;24:333–41.
24. Jakovljević M. Person-centered psychopharmacotherapy: what is it?—each patient is a unique, responsive and responsible subject. Psychiatria Danubina. 2015;27(suppl 1):s28–33.
25. Mezzich JE. The dialogal basis of our profession: psychiatry with the person. World Psychiatry 2007;6:129–130.
26. Mezzich JE, Salloum IM. Clinical complexity and person-centered integrative diagnosis. World Psychiatry. 2008;7:1–2.
27. Mintz DL. Teaching the prescriber's role: the psychology of psychopharmacology. Acad Psychiatry. 2005;29:187–94.
28. Moneta GB. Positive psychology: a critical introduction. New York: Palgrave Macmillan; 2014.
29. Pakman M. A systemic frame for mental health practices. In: Prosky PS, Keith DV, editors. Family therapy as an alternative to medication—an appraisal of pharmaland. New York: Brunner-Routledge; 2003.
30. Seligman MEP. Learned optimism. 2nd ed. New York: Pocket Books (Simon and Schuster); 1998.
31. Seligman MEP, Csikszentmihalyi M. Positive psychology. An introduction. Am Psychol. 2000;55:5–14.
32. Seligman MEP. Flourish—a visionary new understanding of happiness and well-being. New York: Free Press; 2012.
33. Senge PM. The fifth discipline—the art and practice of the learning organisation. London: Random House; 2006.
34. Slade M. Personal recovery and mental illness—a guide for mental health professionals. Cambridge: Cambridge University Press; 2011.

Person-Centered Psychotherapy 19

C. Robert Cloninger, MD, PhD and Kevin M. Cloninger, PhD

19.1 What Is Person-Centered Therapeutics?

Person-centered therapeutics (PCT) is the branch of person-centered medicine (PCM) concerned with the promotion of positive health and the treatment of disease. The health of a person has three major aspects—the body (soma), the mind (analytical thinking), and the soul (psyche, involving seeking meaning through humanism, creativity, and freedom of will). Therefore, PCT must address physical, mental, and social–existential aspects of health in order to promote and maintain well-being and treat disease. From an existential perspective, PCM does not use spiritual interventions; rather, we use physical, mental, and social interventions in PCM to encourage a person to be a free and responsible agent determining his or her own development of well-being, thereby respecting the person's freedom of will. This person-centered approach makes it possible to promote integration and balance among all three aspects of being without being reductionist or dogmatic.

PCT is partly described by its use of an interpersonal alliance and humanistic dialogue to orchestrate lifestyle change and other procedures as needed to heal illness, prevent disease, and promote health [75]. However, PCT depends on more than the working alliance being person-centered. The effectiveness of PCT also depends heavily on the integration of physical, mental, and spiritual interventions to active dynamic change in the level of well-being, as will be described in some detail later. Hence we suggest here that the effectiveness of PCT depends on the three major characteristics: (1) use of a person-centered working alliance, which is the

C.R. Cloninger, MD, PhD (✉)
Department of Psychiatry, Washington University School of Medicine,
Campus Box 8134, 660 South Euclid Avenue, St. Louis, MO 63110, USA
e-mail: crcloninger44@gmail.com

K.M. Cloninger, PhD
President, Anthropedia Foundation, St. Louis, Missouri, USA

J.E. Mezzich et al. (eds.), *Person Centered Psychiatry*,
DOI 10.1007/978-3-319-39724-5_19

physical component critical for PCT efficacy; (2) the assessment of personality structure and function to promote self-awareness and a developmental perspective on health in a person's creative life narrative, which is the mental component critical for PCT efficacy; and (3) the integration of evidence-based physical, mental, and social interventions, which synergistically activate the mechanisms underlying the maintenance and promotion of well-being. These three characteristics of PCT will be considered individually and then jointly.

19.2 Benefits of a Person-Centered Working Alliance

Randomized controlled trials of treatments in the context of a person-centered working alliance have lower dropout, relapse, and recurrence rates than other treatment approaches [20, 21]. For therapeutics to be effectively person-centered, it must involve an awareness and respect for the whole person, whose health is certainly more than his or her symptoms of illness and past medical history [79]. The unique experiences, goals, and values of each person are assessed and treated in a person-centered therapeutic alliance, which optimally seeks to promote complete physical, mental, social, cultural, and spiritual well-being. PCT addresses the needs *of* the person (of the totality of the person's health, both ill and positive aspects), and is engaged *by* the person (with clinicians extending themselves as full human beings), *for* the person (assisting the fulfillment of the person's health aspirations and life project), and *with* the person (in a respectful and empowering relationship with the person who consults) [54].

The conditions that promote well-being and recovery from illness involve a set of common features of health that include hope, empathy, and respect for one's self and others [1]. These common characteristics of well-being emerge from a self-transcendent outlook on life with a sense of participation in the boundless unity of all things or inseparable connectedness with nature and other people [3, 19]. Self-transcendent outlooks and values are typical of healthy and creative people in all human cultures [67]. An outlook of separation predisposes a person to feelings of fear, alienation, and individual pride or shame, thereby predisposing to dissatisfaction with life and ill health.

Person-centered care promotes health by providing the experience of an outlook of unity in the therapeutic alliance, which can later be generalized beyond the alliance. An outlook of unity fosters well-being by activation of a synergistic spiral of increasing self-directedness, cooperativeness, and self-transcendence [19–21, 30–32]. Only about 15 % of the variance in treatment outcome is attributable to specific techniques of different psychotherapeutic schools whereas about 85 % of the variance in psychotherapy outcomes is explained by common factors shared by different approaches [47, 50, 51]. What is attributed to the strong placebo effects observed in most drug or psychotherapy trials is substantially determined by common psychosocial factors, which can be as large or larger than putatively specific treatments [51].

The common factors in all treatments include the patient's characteristics, the therapist's qualities of respect (i.e., prizing, unconditional positive regard, acceptance, trust), empathic understanding, and genuineness (i.e., realness, authenticity), and the quality of the therapeutic alliance between them (shared goals, emotional engagement, and exchange) [14, 18]. These common factors are characteristic of all truly healthy interpersonal relationships [73], and are important for maintenance and recovery of all aspects of well-being, whether physical, mental, or spiritual [12, 13, 22]. Claims of the evidence for the specificity of particular techniques for specific disorders are rarely justified because of inadequate assessment of these common factors [47]. Nevertheless, in research under the auspices of the Anthropedia Foundation, we have found it is essential to go beyond a simple common factor approach to assess and understand the mechanisms by which a person changes as a dynamic multistep process involving a spiral of synergistic changes in functioning, plasticity, and virtue [16, 20, 21, 24–26, 62, 70].

In other words, a clinician's effectiveness in treatment depends substantially on his or her *attitude* toward—and *understanding* of—the patient. The interpersonal attitudes of respect, genuineness, and empathic understanding are crucial for the development of well-being [20, 21, 63]. When physicians rely only on symptom-based diagnosis and treat patients without respectful exchange in dialogue, there are usually high rates of dropout and noncompliance with treatment prescriptions, as well as high rates of burnout in the physician and stigma in the patient [20, 21]. A person-centered working alliance is a crucial component of effective PCT, but it is only one of the three essential components.

19.3 Benefits of a Developmental Perspective

An understanding of how a person's habits, goals, and values predispose them to diseases is crucial to motivating a person to take charge of promoting their health and preventing disease. Even people who were not considering changing their personality or lifestyle can learn to recognize the connections between their personality, their activities, and the physical, mental, and social problems they experience [27, 58].

In order to increase in well-being, a person must give up some of the temporary advantages that keep a person stuck in a maladaptive or suboptimal rut within the overall potential of their fitness landscape. Such relative stability of particular configurations of a complex adaptive system is illustrated in Fig. 19.1. As shown in Fig. 19.1, in the process of increasing from lower to higher well-being, things get worse before they get better. For example, a drug addict may resist giving up their addiction because of the transient pleasure or relief of suffering they experience when they use drugs, even though their life and health are being destroyed by their addiction. In order to change their lifestyle, they must clearly recognize the advantages of a different way of living and must have hope and confidence that they can succeed. In other words, a person's self-directedness (i.e., being resourceful, purposeful, and responsible) and self-efficacy (i.e., confidence that a person will

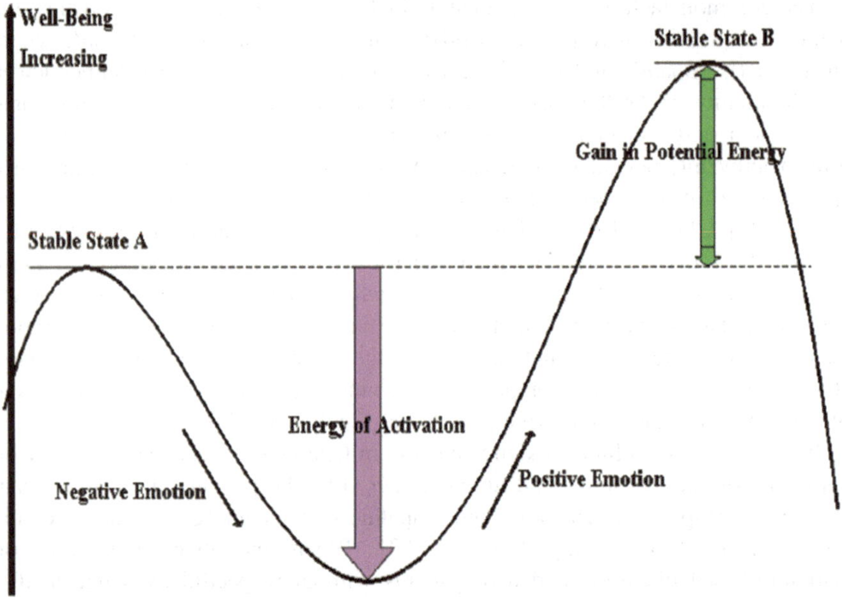

Fig. 19.1 The nonlinear dynamics of well-being

succeed in changing their behaviors) are strong predictors of success in lifestyle change and recovery from illness in both medical disorders (e.g., heart disease, chronic lung disease, diabetes) [4, 12, 17] and psychiatric disorders (e.g., eating disorders, addictions, depression) [2, 11, 64]. People can be motivated to change their life in healthy ways, such as learning to relax and self-regulate stress, exercise regularly, and eat a healthy diet, if they understand and experience the value in doing so personally [17], whether their initial intention to do so was weak or nonexistent [4, 58]. Such change in lifestyle is essential to prevent or reduce the complications of chronic diseases [23].

Unfortunately, most contemporary medical treatment is focused on relief of acute symptoms of illness rather than the promotion of health and well-being [32, 80]. As a result, contemporary medical practice is ineffective in the prevention and management of chronic diseases, which are common and complex in their etiology and treatment. Dropout, relapse, and recurrence rates are also high even for acute illness when treatments are not directed toward promotion of well-being [20, 21]. Furthermore, impersonal approaches to therapeutics have failed to increase the average level of physical, emotional, or social well-being in the general population despite substantial advances in technical capacities and health care expenditure [19, 54]. Treatments directed at acute symptoms of illness, rather than its causes, result in temporary relief, frequent relapse and recurrence, and no lasting improvement in public health [20, 21].

Together a person-centered working alliance and awakening the motivation to change one's life as a valued developmental commitment are substantial predictors of change, particularly in people who previously had weak intentions for change. However, if a person has a strong intention to change, there is still much variability in outcome that is not predicted by the working alliance and/or strength of intention [35]. Good intentions, even with a supportive working alliance, are insufficient to account for who will and who will not succeed in improving their health and well-being, as people all learn when they assess how well they did in keeping resolutions at New Years.

We learned clearly from longitudinal studies of personality development that it is difficult to understand the sufficient conditions for predicting who will change [19, 30]. Most people do not change even when they are intellectually aware that it would be beneficial to do so [49], a consequence of the nonlinear dynamics of well-being depicted in Fig. 19.1. What is the energy of activation that allows well-being to increase is depicted in Fig. 19.1?. What provides the power and energy that allows some people to develop toward greater well-being while others remain stuck in suboptimal ruts of ill health in which they are short-lived, unhappy, and unfulfilled? No one wants to be unhealthy or miserable so what keeps them from changing their life for the better?

We suggest that the energy of activation comes from increasing in awareness and enlarging consciousness, which in turn establish a positive feedback cycle of increasing plasticity, virtue, and healthier functioning. This is illustrated in Fig. 19.2, which provides a general description of complex adaptive pathway to well-being. This pathway of interactive components is also called the motor of well-being because it operates as the driving force to maintain and promote health in each moment [24–26].

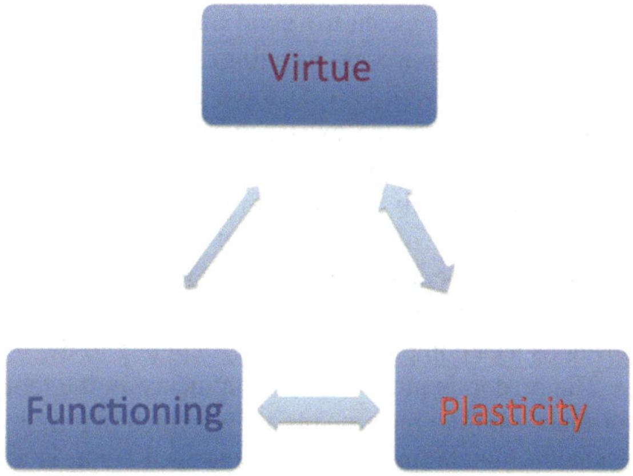

Fig. 19.2 The motor of well-being: reciprocal interactions among plasticity, virtue, and functioning

19.4 Benefits of Integrative Therapy

The first major clue that helped us recognize the conditions needed for growth in well-being came from the current public dissatisfaction with current medical practice, which is often impersonal, specialized to focus on individual organs or diseases, and reduces the patient to someone who is passive except for having to follow the directions of the doctor prescribing medications and procedures.

The inadequacies of impersonal therapeutics have led to a widespread and growing interest in alternative therapies that are more personal, participatory, and holistic. Evidence-based treatments used by adults for medical conditions are highly diverse, including physical exercise, diet, sleep hygiene, deep breathing exercises, muscular relaxation, social engagement, narrative therapy, and meditation [8, 15, 69]. Such self-regulatory and alternative treatments produce results that are often indistinguishable from more conventional allopathic interventions, suggesting that a common mechanism is being influenced by complementary pathways [74]. Success in self-regulation from repeated practice in one type of situation, such as exercises to monitor and improve posture, monitor mood, or monitor and record eating, consistently leads to greater self-control (i.e., willpower and freedom of will) in other unpracticed situations, again suggesting a common underlying mechanism, or a synergistic set of mechanisms of well-being [6, 7, 56].

A *second major clue* about the sufficient conditions for activating growth in well-being came from the facts that personality profiles predict all aspects of well-being (physical, mental, social, and spiritual) [31, 32]. Likewise, all aspects of well-being vary together when a population is stressed by violence or social inequity [61]. Thus the three aspects of well-being interact synergistically to promote health so the neglect of any one of them impedes the healthy development of the whole person [24–26]. This suggested that the components of well-being are inseparable because they are activated by a common motor in which plasticity (i.e., the capacity for adaptive change), virtue (i.e., self-transcendent values that regulate passions and guide conduct as a means to a good and wholesome life), and healthy functioning (i.e., fulfillment of purpose and meaning) are synergistic mechanisms [24–26]. However, as mentioned previously, we adopt an existential perspective for all persons in PCM. That is, we respect the existence of each person as a free and responsible agent cultivating his or her own development through personal acts of will.

Without plasticity, a person is unwilling or unable to change. Without virtue, a person is unaware of what goals and values lead to life satisfaction. Without effective functioning, a person fails to fulfill even the best of their intentions. Each of these components of well-being exerts influences each of the others, so well-being develops as a complex adaptive system due to the reciprocal interactions [19].

The predominant direction of influence in the motor of well-being (Fig. 19.2) is for functioning to increase plasticity, which in turn influences virtue, and then virtue enhances functioning, so the way to well-being is a virtuous cycle of growth. The interactions operate, but more weakly, in the other directions. That is, practicing a particular way of functioning facilitates the development of plasticity for such behavior, whereas plasticity has its predominant effect mediated by virtue, rather than directly on functioning. Increasing plasticity provides the freedom and flexibility for a person to recognize more effective opportunities for healthy functioning, so plasticity increases virtuous as a means to the good life. Recognition of what is good and wholesome guides a person's conduct so that he or she can function in a healthier way. In other words, in order to grow in well-being, it is necessary to simultaneously cultivate the willingness and ability to change, evaluate, and regulate what behaviors lead to what we value, and to function in ways consistent with our goals and values.

Consequently, all the components of well-being depend on the development of character [31, 32]. Character is what we make of ourselves intentionally and is measured in terms of our goals and values, which allow us to regulate our irrational emotional drives (i.e., temperament) [28, 29]. Without character strengths, a person is limited in responsibility, empathy, and freedom of will, functioning as a slave to fears, excessive desires, vanity, and/or shame.

It is useful to consider some specific examples of physical, mental, and social components of well-being to better illustrate the functioning of the motor of well-being. Since growth in well-being is a developmental process, it is convenient to take examples that have been described in prior theoretical and empirical work on personality development from another perspective to see how we can enrich our understanding of them as a complex adaptive system (see Table 19.1). Remember that each of the components of the motor of well-being (Fig. 19.2) also has physical, mental, and social subcomponents and these interact in all possible combinations, giving nine subcomponents. It is beyond the scope of this paper to discuss all nine subcomponents of plasticity, of virtue, and of functioning, but the three that are fully physical, mental, and social–existential are described briefly in Table 19.1 to illustrate the scope of PCT.

It is well recognized that stage theories of psychological development like those of Freud [37] and Erikson [78] are not really linear, so there is a clear need for their refinement as nonlinear dynamic systems [19, 46, 68]. Table 19.1 provides a description of nine of the twenty-seven subcomponents of the motor of well-being. It describes sets of interacting subcomponents (a component of plasticity, a component of virtue, and a component of functioning).

Table 19.1 Dynamic elements of physical, mental, and spiritual components of well-being (adapted from Erikson and Vailliant's empirical descriptions)

Aspect of well-being	Plasticity	Virtue	Function
Physical	Vigor versus frailty/fatigue	Industry versus apathy	Competence versus inferiority
Mental	Conflict resolution versus poor executive attention	Fairness versus injustice	Intimacy versus isolation
Social–existential	Free will versus entrenchment	Wisdom versus control	Creativity versus tradition

Vigor, industry, and competence interact with each other to contribute to physical well-being. Conflict resolution, fairness, and intimacy interact to contribute to mental well-being. Freedom of will, wisdom, and creativity interact to contribute to spiritual well-being. Note that competence, intimacy, and creativity are components of healthy functioning, much as described in longitudinal studies of the development of psychosocial functioning [68, 78]. Competence is success in accomplishing adaptive skills needed in daily life, as is prominent in what Freud called the latency period of 6–11 years of age. Intimacy is the social intelligence to be empathic and self-accepting to enable a person to form lasting intimate relationships and social alliances with others; this requires responsible and principled actions as well as empathy and sharing, as normally develops in early adulthood. Creativity involves original, adaptive, and beneficial innovation rather than being entrenched in traditional and conventional ways of functioning [27, 71].

Industry, fairness/justice, and wisdom are related virtues (i.e., self-transcendent values). Industry refers to the aspect of virtue that leads to satisfaction and cheerfulness connected with working hard and being diligent. Fairness or justice is the aspect of virtue that finds satisfaction with consideration of the dignity of others, which motivates equitable treatment of all people. Wisdom is consciousness of freedom of will, which motivates the realization of that freedom in the creative advance of civilization as a harmonious conscious component of the universal unity of being as a whole. This form of wisdom could be called holiness and is distinguished from prudence, which is practical wisdom.

The corresponding plasticities (i.e., capacities for adaptive change) are vigor, conflict resolution (executive attention), and freedom of will. It is important to distinguish these components in a systematic way because they require different interventions. Furthermore, people differ in their profile of strengths and weaknesses for these components that promote well-being, so a person-centered intervention must take these differences into account. Average effects of interventions are likely to be weak and inconsistent when the unique profiles of plasticities, virtues, and functioning of each person are not taken into account.

19.5 Empirical Evidence About Activating the Motor of Well-Being

Evidence-based treatments used by adults for medical conditions are highly diverse, including physical exercise, diet, sleep hygiene, deep breathing exercises, muscular relaxation, guided imagery, and meditation [8, 9, 15, 69]. Diverse therapeutic techniques influence health and personality development in ways that are largely indistinguishable from one another or from effective allopathic treatments, suggesting that there is a final common pathway to well-being [74].

Evidence-based interventions may be physical–behavioral (e.g., diet, regular physical exercise, deep breathing exercises, heart-rate-variability biofeedback, behavioral conditioning), emotional–cognitive (e.g., emotional self-regulation, nonviolent emotional communication, empathy training, attention training, mindfulness-based cognitive therapy), or social–existential (e.g., social engagement, narrative therapy, meditation). When applied separately such interventions have weak and inconsistent effects, but when combined together in an appropriately coordinated way, they interact synergistically to produce strong and consistent improvements [27].

It is beyond the scope of this paper to detail all the evidence for all the components of the motor of well-being. It is sufficient here to consider one component in detail as an illustrative example. We will take the first component in Table 19.1 as our example—the plasticity vigor, which is described as fatigue or fatigability in states of ill-being (i.e., when there is a lack of vigor). Vigor is a major component of physical vitality and is measured as the presence of strength, enthusiasm, and energy. If a person is highly vigorous, he or she feels full of energy and ready to work with enthusiasm and strength, whereas if vigor is low, they complain of fatigue, lack of enthusiasm, and low exercise tolerance [5]. The plasticity of low vigor is also described as the syndrome of "frailty," i.e., a vulnerability to adverse outcomes associated with being weak, fatigued, and fragile from dysfunction in multiple physiological systems [38, 39]. There are many randomized controlled trials using reliable measures of vigor and frailty that have evaluated a wide range of interventions to promote vigor and vitality along with reducing frailty and fatigue (see Table 19.2), which is a common adverse feature of many common chronic disease states, such as cancer, cardiovascular disease, chronic lung disease, diabetes, arthritis, and depression.

Empirical research shows that there are diverse treatments that reduce fatigue and promote vigor, but that the individual interventions have inconsistent benefits and overall weak effects sizes (0.2–0.3) [9]. The evidence-supported treatments for this individual physical plasticity are once again ternary in range (see Table 19.2).

Table 19.2 Evidence-supported treatments for physical, mental, and spiritual components of the plasticity vigor (versus frailty)

Type of intervention	Interventions for vigor versus frailty	Supporting evidence
Physical–behavioral	Physical exercise	USDHHS [77], Giannuzzi et al. [41], Strong et al. [72], O'Connor and Puetz [59], Martinson et al. [53], Marks and Landaira [52]
	Nutrition education	Boyle et al. [10] and Nigg et al. [58]
	Sleep hygiene	Bower [9], Finnegan-John et al. [34] and Jain et al. [45]
Emotional–cognitive	Stress reduction	Kangas et al. [48]
	Cognitive therapy	Bower [9] and Montgomery et al. [55]
	Mind–body awareness	Horton [44], Trombetti et al. [76] and Bower [9]
Social–existential	Social engagement	Sabbath et al. [66] and Naylor et al. [57]
	Narrative therapy	Goncalves and Stiles [42, 43]
	Meditation	Perez-De-Albeniz and Holmes [60] and Fjorback et al. [36]

The effective treatments include physical–behavioral interventions (e.g., sleep hygiene, nutrition education, and regular physical exercise), as would be expected for physical vigor. In addition, effective treatments include emotional–cognitive interventions, such as stress reduction, cognitive behavioral therapy with and without mindfulness, and exercises to promote mind–body awareness and coordination using combinations of music and dance. The effective means to promote vigor also include social–existential interventions, including social engagement, narrative therapy to find more meaning in activities, and meditation, which has psychological, social, and physiological benefits (see Table 19.2).

For example, consider the treatment of a 49-year-old women presenting with a chief complaint of chronic fatigue for the past 6 months. Described herself as usually a high-functioning person until the past year, when unrefreshing sleep, fatigue, headaches, and pain in her head, stomach, and back began to interfere with her work and other daily activities. Personality assessment revealed that she had a cautious temperament (i.e., very high Harm Avoidance, low Novelty Seeking, and high Reward Dependence), so she had difficulty dealing with rejection and was easily stressed. She was also high in Persistence (i.e., she was a perfectionist), and low in Self-directedness and average in Cooperativeness and Self-transcendence. This personality profile is typical of individuals with somatizing disorders, such as Chronic Fatigue Syndrome and/or Fibromyalgia [33, 40]. The personality profile suggested that the patient was vulnerable to stress from rejection and tended to become socially isolated, anxious, and depressed, and then to slip into a cycle of increasing social isolation, poor sleep, fatigue, and bodily distress. She had high standards for herself and tended to be harshly critical of her mistakes, particularly when she did not perform to the level of her unreasonably high expectations of herself. In order to improve the patient's well-being, we discussed her goals, which include reducing the symptoms of her chronic fatigue syndrome, and also helping her to increase in self-directedness and positive emotions. To do this we discussed the relationship of her somatic symptoms to her personality, particularly her tendency toward social isolation as a result of her rejection sensitivity. We also discussed that the possibility of her becoming better able to regulate her emotions and cultivate greater self-directedness. To promote self-directedness, she decided to start well-being coaching to encourage her to exercise regularly to gain in vigor and to experience the self-confidence that comes from setting and accomplishing SMART goals [24–27]. She acquired skills in relaxation and mindfulness, additional evidence-based interventions for vigor (Table 19.2). Her understanding of herself was promoted through humanistic dialogue, and she began to gain self-confidence so that she could be more socially engaged in community activities. After several months of coaching, she was actively engaged in daily social and physical activities in addition to having a regular mindfulness practice, thereby addressing her physical, mental, and social needs in ways that were meaningful to her in an existential sense. Her chronic fatigue remitted as she cultivated a healthy, happy, and meaningful narrative for her life.

These observations illustrate the structure of the interdependent components of the developmental pathway to well-being. Physical activity, cognitive therapy, or social engagement alone would be insufficient to permit the example of our patient with CFS develop a happy life. It was all three types of interventions acting in synergy that promoted her well-being.

19.6 Conclusions

The promotion of well-being must usually begin by a person recognizing what brings them health and lasting satisfaction, or they would not be motivated to change. Dialogue about a person's self-description of their personality traits allows reflection and contemplation of any discrepancy between how to live well and how a person is currently living. Humanistic dialogue is the foundation for developing shared goals in a therapeutic alliance that will lead to well-being [65, 75, 80]. Dialogue about the way the components of personality interact to produce illness or health is what makes the therapeutic encounter truly person-centered and often initiates a process of rapid spontaneous change [80]. Such reflection on the relations between personality and health automatically activates synergy among a person's way of functioning, plasticity, and virtue, as we have initially described elsewhere [24–26].

Most people have a spontaneous need to be self-actualizing, that is, to become a fully functioning human being [19, 63, 65]. However, different people may be receptive and responsive to different treatments depending on their genetics, life experiences, personality, and current resources, and circumstances. The evidence-based treatments used by adults for medical conditions are highly diverse, including physical exercise, diet, sleep hygiene, deep breathing exercises, muscular relaxation, social engagement, narrative therapy, and meditation. Such alternative treatments produce results that are often indistinguishable from one another and from more conventional allopathic interventions when they are effective, suggesting that operation of a synergistic set of mechanisms, or that a common mechanism is being influenced by complementary pathways. However, different people often respond to different treatments, so that the average responses to evidence-based treatments do not tell us how to treat any particular person who comes to a physician, mental health counselor, or coach for help.

What a person needs and wants to change must be tailored skillfully to their individual needs using PCT [32, 54]. Each person must be respected as a free and responsible agent who cultivates his or her own path of development with the guidance they seek, no more and hopefully no less. As a result, effective PCT is based on describing and understanding the personalities of the people involved in any therapeutic encounter as soon as possible while preserving the continuity of a person's identity with respect and compassion.

Person-centered care promotes a feeling of connectedness with an interpersonal outlook of unity, which in turn promotes attitudes of hope, empathy, and respect. Such shifts in outlook facilitate the development of healthier functioning, plasticity, and virtue, which appear to be the common set of self-actualizing mechanisms that consistently promote well-being.

References

1. Amering M, Schmolke M. Recovery in mental health. New York: Wiley; 2009.
2. Anderson CB, Joyce PR, Carter FA, McIntosh VV, Bulik CM. The effect of cognitive-behavioral therapy for bulimia nervosa on temperament and character as measured by the temperament and character inventory. Compr Psychiatry. 2002;43(3):182–8.
3. Anthropedia F. Know yourself. 2011, from http://anthropedia.org (2009).
4. Bandura A. Health promotion by social cognitive means. Health Educ Behav. 2004;31 (2):143–64.
5. Bann CM, Kobau R, Lewis MA, Zack MM, Luncheon C, Thompson WW. Development and psychometric evaluation of the public health surveillance well-being scale. Qual Life Res. 2012;21(6):1031–43.
6. Baumeister RF, Bauer IM, Lloyd SA. Choice, free will, and religion. Psychol Relig Spirit. 2010;2(2):67–82.
7. Baumeister RF, Gailliot M, DeWall CN, Oaten M. Self-regulation and personality: how interventions increase regulatory success, and how depletion moderates the effects of traits on behavior. J Pers. 2006;74(6):1773–801.
8. Bertisch SM, Wee CC, Phillips RS, McCarthy EP. Alternative mind-body therapies used by adults with medical conditions. J Psychosom Res. 2009;66(6):511–9.
9. Bower JE. Cancer-related fatigue–mechanisms, risk factors, and treatments. Nat Rev Clin Oncol. 2014;11(10):597–609.
10. Boyle RG, O'Connor PJ, Pronk NP, Tan A. Stages of change for physical activity, diet, and smoking among HMO members with chronic conditions. Am J Health Promot. 1998;12 (3):170–5.
11. Bulik CM, Sullivan PF, Fear JL, Pickering A. Outcome of anorexia nervosa: eating attitudes, personality, and parental bonding. Int J Eat Disord. 2000;28(2):139–47.
12. Burns JW, Evon D. Common and specific process factors in cardiac rehabilitation: independent and interactive effects of the working alliance and self-efficacy. Health Psychol. 2007;26(6):684–92.
13. Burns JW, Glenn B, Bruehl S, Harden RN, Lofland K. Cognitive factors influence outcome following multidisciplinary chronic pain treatment: a replication and extension of a cross-lagged panel analysis. Behav Res Ther. 2003;41(10):1163–82.
14. Castonguay LG, Goldfried MR, Wiser S, Raue PJ, Hayes AM. Predicting the effect of cognitive therapy for depression: a study of unique and common factors. J Consult Clin Psychol. 1996;64(3):497–504.
15. Chiesa A, Serretti A. A systematic review of neurobiological and clinical features of mindfulness meditations. Psychol Med. 2009; 1–14.
16. Cicchetti D. Resilience under conditions of extreme stress: a multilevel perspective. World Psychiatry. 2010;9(3):145–54.
17. Clark NM, Dodge JA. Exploring self-efficacy as a predictor of disease management. Health Educ Behav. 1999;26(1):72–89.
18. Clarkson P. The psychotherapeutic relationship. In: Clarkson P, Pokorny M, editors. Handbook of psychotherapy. London: Routledge; 1994. p. 28–48.
19. Cloninger CR. Feeling good: the science of well-being. New York: Oxford University Press; 2004.
20. Cloninger CR. The science of well being: an integrated approach to mental health and its disorders. Psychiatr Danub. 2006;18(3–4):218–24.
21. Cloninger CR. The science of well-being: an integrated approach to mental health and its disorders. World Psychiatry. 2006;5(2):71–6.
22. Cloninger CR. Spirituality and the science of feeling good. South Med J. 2007;100(7):740–3.
23. Cloninger CR. Person-centered health promotion in chronic disease. Int J Pers-Cent Med. 2013;3(1):5–12.

24. Cloninger CR, Cloninger KM (2011) Development of instruments and evaluative procedures on contributors to health and illness. Int J Pers-Cent Med 1(1), (in press, this volume).
25. Cloninger CR, Cloninger KM. Development of instruments and evaluative procedures on contributors to illness and health. Int J Pers-Cent Med. 2011;1(3):446–55.
26. Cloninger CR, Cloninger KM. Person-centered Therapeutics. Int J Pers-Cent Med. 2011;1 (1):43–52.
27. Cloninger CR, Cloninger KM. People create health: Effective health promotion is a creative process. Int J Pers-Cent Med. 2013;3(2):114–22.
28. Cloninger CR, Keady B, Lester N, Kedia S, Cloninger KM. Empirical measurement of Plato's model of the human psyche: validation by the neuroscience of personality. In: Stoyanov D, editor. Towards a new philosophy of mental health: perspectives from neuroscience and humanities. Cambridge: Cambridge Scholars Publishing; 2015. p. 128–155.
29. Cloninger CR, Svrakic DM, Przybeck TR. A psychobiological model of temperament and character. Arch Gen Psychiatry. 1993;50(12):975–90.
30. Cloninger CR, Svrakic NM, Svrakic DM. Role of personality self-organization in development of mental order and disorder. Dev Psychopathol. 1997;9(4):881–906.
31. Cloninger CR, Zohar AH. Personality and the perception of health and happiness. J Affect Disord. 2011;128(1–2):24–32.
32. Cloninger CR, Zohar AH, Cloninger KM. Promotion of well-being in person-centered mental health care. Focus. 2010;8(2):165–79.
33. Conrad R, Schilling G, Bausch C, Nadstawek J, Wartenberg HC, Wegener I, Geiser F, Imbierowicz K, Liedtke R. Temperament and character personality profiles and personality disorders in chronic pain patients. Pain. 2007;133(1–3):197–209.
34. Finnegan-John J, Molassiotis A, Richardson A, Ream E. A systematic review of complementary and alternative medicine interventions for the management of cancer-related fatigue. Integr Cancer Ther. 2013;12(4):276–90.
35. Fishbein M, Hennessy M, Yzer M, Douglas J. Can we explain why some people do and some people do not act on their intentions? Psychol Health Med. 2003;8(1):3–18.
36. Fjorback LO, Arendt M, Ornbol E, Walach H, Rehfeld E, Schroder A, Fink P. Mindfulness therapy for somatization disorder and functional somatic syndromes: randomized trial with one-year follow-up. J Psychosom Res. 2013;74(1):31–40.
37. Freud S. Standard edition of the complete psychological works. London: Hogarth Press; 1966.
38. Fried LP, Tangen CM, Walston J, Newman AB, Hirsch C, Gottdiener J, Seeman T, Tracy R, Kop WJ, Burke G, McBurnie MA, Cardiovascular Health Study Collaborative Research. Frailty in older adults: evidence for a phenotype. J Gerontol A Biol Sci Med Sci. 2001;56(3): M146–56.
39. Fried LP, Xue QL, Cappola AR, Ferrucci L, Chaves P, Varadhan R, Guralnik JM, Leng SX, Semba RD, Walston JD, Blaum CS, Bandeen-Roche K. Nonlinear multisystem physiological dysregulation associated with frailty in older women: implications for etiology and treatment. J Gerontol A Biol Sci Med Sci. 2009;64(10):1049–57.
40. Fukuda S, Kuratsune H, Tajima S, Takashima S, Yamagutchi K, Nishizawa Y, Watanabe Y. Premorbid personality in chronic fatigue syndrome as determined by the temperament and character inventory. Compr Psychiatry. 2010;51(1):78–85.
41. Giannuzzi P, Mezzani A, Saner H, Bjornstad H, Fioretti P, Mendes M, Cohen-Solal A, Dugmore L, Hambrecht R, Hellemans I, McGee H, Perk J, Vanhees L, Veress G. Physical activity for primary and secondary prevention. Position paper of the working group on cardiac rehabilitation and exercise physiology of the european society of cardiology. Eur J Cardiovasc Prev Rehabil. 2003;10(5):319–27.
42. Goncalves MM, Ribeiro AP, Silva JR, Mendes I, Sousa I. Narrative innovations predict symptom improvement: studying innovative moments in narrative therapy of depression. Psychother Res; 2015; 1–11.
43. Goncalves MM, Stiles WB. Narrative and psychotherapy: introduction to the special section. Psychother Res. 2011;21(1):1–3.

44. Horton MM. The effect of stepping as a group music therapy intervention on group cohesion and positive oral statements of African-American female adolescents attending an educational treatment center. Florida State University Electronic Theses, Treatises and Dissertations. Tallahassee, Florida, Florida State University Library. http://diginole.lib.fsu.edu/etd (2005).
45. Jain S, Boyd C, Fiorentino L, Khorsan R, Crawford C. Are there efficacious treatments for treating the fatigue-sleep disturbance-depression symptom cluster in breast cancer patients? A rapid evidence assessment of the literature (REAL((c))). Breast Cancer (Dove Med Press). 2015;7:267–91.
46. Josefsson K, Jokela M, Cloninger CR, Hintsanen M, Salo J, Hintsa T, Pulkki-Raback L, Keltikangas-Jarvinen L. Maturity and change in personality: developmental trends of temperament and character in adulthood. Dev Psychopathol. 2013;25(3):713–27.
47. Joyce AS, Wolfaardt U, Sribney C, Aylwin AS. Psychotherapy research at the start of the 21st century: the persistence of the art versus science controversy. Can J Psychiatry. 2006;51 (13):797–809.
48. Kangas M, Bovbjerg DH, Montgomery GH. Cancer-related fatigue: a systematic and meta-analytic review of non-pharmacological therapies for cancer patients. Psychol Bull. 2008;134(5):700–41.
49. Kobau R, Sniezek J, Zack MM, Lucas RE, Adam B. Well-being assessment: an evaluation of well-being scales for public health and population estimates of well-being among US adults. Appl Psychol: Health Well-Being. 2010;2(3):272–97.
50. Lambert MJ. Bergin and Garfield's handbook of psychotherapy and behavior change. New York: Wiley; 2003.
51. Lambert MJ. Early response in psychotherapy: further evidence for the importance of common factors rather than "placebo effects". J Clin Psychol. 2005;61(7):855–69.
52. Marks R, Landaira M. Musical exercise: a novel strategy for advancing healthy aging. Healthy Aging Res. 2015;4:31.
53. Martinson BC, Sherwood NE, Crain AL, Hayes MG, King AC, Pronk NP, O'Connor PJ. Maintaining physical activity among older adults: 24-month outcomes of the keep active minnesota randomized controlled trial. Prev Med. 2010;51(1):37–44.
54. Mezzich JE, Salloum IM, Cloninger CR, Salvador-Carulla L, Kirmayer LJ, Banzato CE, Wallcraft J, Botbol M. Person-centred integrative diagnosis: conceptual bases and structural model. Can J Psychiatry. 2010;55(11):701–8.
55. Montgomery GH, David D, Kangas M, Green S, Sucala M, Bovbjerg DH, Hallquist MN, Schnur JB. Randomized controlled trial of a cognitive-behavioral therapy plus hypnosis intervention to control fatigue in patients undergoing radiotherapy for breast cancer. J Clin Oncol. 2014;32(6):557–63.
56. Muraven M, Baumeister RF, Tice DM. Longitudinal improvement of self-regulation through practice: building self-control strength through repeated exercise. J Soc Psychol. 1999;139 (4):446–57.
57. Naylor E, Penev PD, Orbeta L, Janssen I, Ortiz R, Colecchia EF, Keng M, Finkel S, Zee PC. Daily social and physical activity increases slow-wave sleep and daytime neuropsychological performance in the elderly. Sleep. 2000;23(1):87–95.
58. Nigg CR, Burbank PM, Padula C, Dufresne R, Rossi JS, Velicer WF, Laforge RG, Prochaska JO. Stages of change across ten health risk behaviors for older adults. Gerontologist. 1999;39(4):473–82.
59. O'Connor PJ, Puetz TW. Chronic physical activity and feelings of energy and fatigue. Med Sci Sports Exerc. 2005;37(2):299–305.
60. Perez-De-Albeniz A, Holmes J. Meditation: concepts, effects and uses in therapy. Int J Pyhotherapy. 2000;5(1):49–59.
61. Pickett K, Wilkinson R. The spirit level: why greater equality makes societies stronger. New York: Bloombury Press; 2009.
62. Prochaska JO, Velicer WF. The transtheoretical model of health behavior change. Am J Health Promotion. 1997;12(1):38–48.

63. Rogers CR. A way of being. Boston: Houghton Mifflin; 1995.
64. Rowe S, Jordan J, McIntosh V, Carter F, Frampton C, Bulik C, Joyce P. Dimensional measures of personality as a predictor of outcome at 5-year follow-up in women with bulimia nervosa. Psychiatry Res. 2010;185(3):414–20.
65. Ryan RM, Deci EL. On happiness and human potentials: a review of research on hedonic and eudaimonic well-being. Annu Rev Psychol. 2001;52:141–66.
66. Sabbath EL, Matz-Costa C, Rowe JW, Leclerc A, Zins M, Goldberg M, Berkman LF. Social predictors of active life engagement: a time-use study of young-old french adults. Res Aging. 2015.
67. Schwartz S. Universals in the content and structure of values: theoretical advances and empirical tests in 20 countries. In: Zanna M, editor. Advances in experimental social psychology, vol. 25. Orlando: Academic Press; 1992. p. 1–65.
68. Schwartz SJ. The evolution of Eriksonian and Neo-Eriksonian theory and research: a review and integration. Identity: Int J Theor Res. 2001;1(1):7–58.
69. Servan-Schreiber D. Healing without Freud or Prozac. London: Rodale International; 2005.
70. Sexton TL, Ridley CR, Kleiner AJ. Beyond common factors: multilevel-process models of therapeutic change in marriage and family therapy. J Marital Fam Ther. 2004;30(2):131–49.
71. Sternberg RJ, editor. The nature of creativity. Cambridge: Cambridge University Press; 1988.
72. Strong WB, Malina RM, Blimkie CJ, Daniels SR, Dishman RK, Gutin B, Hergenroeder AC, Must A, Nixon PA, Pivarnik JM, Rowland T, Trost S, Trudeau F. Evidence based physical activity for school-age youth. J Pediatr. 2005;146(6):732–7.
73. Strupp HH, Hadley SW. Specific vs nonspecific factors in psychotherapy. A controlled study of outcome. Arch Gen Psychiatry. 1979;36(10):1125–36.
74. Targ EF, Levine EG. The efficacy of a mind-body-spirit group for women with breast cancer: a randomized controlled trial. Gen Hosp Psychiatry. 2002;24(4):238–48.
75. Tournier P. The best of Paul Tournier: Guilt & Grace, the meaning of persons, the person Reborn, to understand each other. New York: Iverson-Norman; 1977.
76. Trombetti A, Hars M, Herrmann FR, Kressig RW, Ferrari S, Rizzoli R. Effect of music-based multitask training on gait, balance, and fall risk in elderly people: a randomized controlled trial. Arch Intern Med. 2011;171(6):525–33.
77. USDHHS. Physical activity and health: a report of the surgeon general. U.S. Department of Health and Human Services. Atlanta: US Public Health Service; 1996.
78. Vailliant GE, Milofsky E. Natural history of male psychologial health: IX. Empirial evidence for Erikson's model of the life cycle. Am J Psychiatry. 1980;137:1348–59.
79. WHO. Definition of health: preamble to the constitution of the World Health Organization. New York: World Health Organization; 1946.
80. Wong K, Cloninger CR. A person-centered approach to clinical practice. Focus. 2010;8 (2):199–215.

Person-Centered Sociotherapy

20

Barbara Probst, PhD, LCSW

20.1 Introduction: The Role of Sociotherapy

The term "sociotherapy" refers to interventions that emphasize modification of the environment, including improvement in interpersonal relationships, as a means of alleviating distress and facilitating wellbeing. Sociotherapy focuses on the social dimension of human experience rather than the biological or psychological. While it is impossible to isolate these dimensions since each affects and is affected by the others, one or another dimension often dominates in clinical practice depending on individual training and preference, agency mission, historical era, and prevailing paradigm.

In the contemporary US, a biological approach is rapidly gaining ground, dominating both research funding and reimbursement for services; an endeavor is even underway, funded by the National Institute of Mental Health, to identify the neurobiological underpinnings of mental disorder "from genes to neural circuits," with the aim of developing a more "scientific" way to explain and categorize human dysfunction (http://www.nimh.nih.gov/research-priorities/rdoc/index.shtml). In previous eras, the psychological dimension has been central. Beginning with Freud and continuing for much of the twentieth century, the roots of dysfunction were believed to lie in internal conflict or early traumatic experience. It was not a matter of brain, but of psyche. The mechanism of change was in the individual whose personal insight and intrapsychic efforts were the keys to enhanced wellbeing.

In contrast, social work has traditionally highlighted the role of environment—the complex interaction of culture, social networks, relationships, and socioeconomic position. In her seminal book *Social Diagnosis* (1917), Richmond [20], often

B. Probst, PhD, LCSW (✉)
Smith College, School for Social Work, Lilly Hall, Northampton, MA 01063, USA
e-mail: bprobst@smith.edu

J.E. Mezzich et al. (eds.), *Person Centered Psychiatry*,
DOI 10.1007/978-3-319-39724-5_20

cited as the founder of social work, emphasized the need to understand people within their environments and to intervene at points of interface. A split soon arose in the profession, with some viewing human suffering as stemming from internal difficulty, indicating psychological intervention, and others viewing it as stemming from problems in living, indicating ecological intervention.

In a radical departure from the community reformist approach of Jane Addams and other social work pioneers, Mary Jarrett, in her 1919 speech to the National Conference of Social Work, proposed that *internal* factors were just as legitimate a focus of social work as *external* ones. The idea was quickly embraced by many social workers eager for the enhanced status that seemed to accompany a psychological orientation. These new psychiatric methods seemed more advanced since "even when caseworkers were able to successfully manipulate their clients' environments, their clients frequently continued to remain unhappy and maladjusted" [1, p. 90]. Freudian theory seemed to provide the missing answer. Richmond's formulation that growth occurs through adjustment *between* person and environment was rapidly eclipsed by psychoanalytic theory that emphasized forces *within* the psyche, shifting social work's focus away from its historic person-in-environment framework [14]. Environmental manipulation was replaced by exploration of the unconscious.

In the decades that followed, internal processes became the focus of work, and it was not unusual for a social work client to receive no environmental intervention at all. Hollis and Woods [13] even advised that, for many, intervening in the environment would be counter-productive of psychotherapeutic aims. "Environmental manipulation practiced unnecessarily can undermine treatment and can have a negative effect upon the client's self-esteem and autonomy" [1, p. 95]. Improving the environment would, in other words, simply mask the underlying psychopathology and deprive an individual of the opportunity for the internal change that was actually needed.

In a similar way, the current emphasis on neurobiology—the idea that defective "wiring" or neurotransmission is the cause of mental disorder—has deflected attention away from the role of context in the genesis of disorder. For many social workers, this represents a disturbing movement to trivialize the impact of trauma, abuse, oppression, and the benefits that can ensue from changes in a person's environment. As Kirk [15] comments, the biomedical paradigm "directly diminishes the importance of the social environment as both contributing cause and element of treatment" (p. 10).

It is not a matter of deciding which dimension is most critical—as if there were a fundamental competition among paradigms—so much as it is a matter of ensuring that *no* important dimension is omitted; the relative significance of biological, psychological, and sociological factors varies from individual to individual, and all need to be considered. That is the rationale behind multiaxial systems of assessment such as the one utilized in the third and fourth editions of the *Diagnostic and Statistical Manual of Mental Disorders (DSM)* prior to its abandonment in *DSM-5* [18]. Unfortunately, it is the social aspect that is most often overlooked when developing interventions. Perhaps that is because it seems easier (and less expensive) to offer psychotherapy and pharmacology than it is to change a person's environment.

Sociotherapy focuses on life context and social relationships as the agents of change, rather than directly addressing internal conflict, erroneous cognitions, or maladaptive emotional responses. Instead of beginning with internal change, assumed to eventually manifest as improved external functioning, the direction of influence is reversed. A person's daily living environment is both the arena and the instrument of intervention. "Sociotherapy differs from psychotherapy in the sense that sociotherapy therapeutically uses the milieu… as a model that confronts a patient with his 'outside world.' This is the opposite of confronting a patient with his 'inside world' during psychotherapy" [21, p. 101].

20.2 Theoretical Basis: Person-in-Environment

Sociotherapy principles strongly echo the notion of person-in-environment that has been the hallmark of social work's approach to alleviating human suffering [9, 17].

> The person-in-environment approach views the individual and his or her multiple environments as a dynamic, interactive system, in which each component simultaneously affects and is affected by the other. It views the individual and his or her environments as forming an ecosystem, consisting of the individual, all the systems with which the individual has reciprocal relationships, the wider environment in which the individual acts, and all the mutual interrelationships that occur between the individual and the various subsystems [27, p. 65].

"Human behavior and the social environment" is, in fact, the first course social work students take, introducing the core principles of mutual interaction between people and their environments and the need to intervene at multiple levels. The professional definition adopted by the International Federation of Social Workers reflects this orientation. "Utilizing theories of human behavior and social systems, social work intervenes at the points where people interact with their environments" [12, p. 411]. The idea of multiple environments is key, since each person exists within concentric, overlapping, and sometimes incompatible contexts, each with norms, roles, and patterns of interaction.

"The person-in-situation perspective has underpinned social work practice since its inception, and it has served us well. There is not a contemporary theory of personality that does not take the effects of the social environment into account" [11, pp. 11–12]. It is the defining base from which the profession has steadily evolved [14], the "conceptual umbrella" beneath which all clinical social work takes place [17]. As far back as 1976, the Registry of Clinical Social Workers clearly stated: "Clinicians must understand that their clients' personal problems often reflect broader social realities and not only their intrapsychic and relational dynamics" [10, p. 18]. For this reason, social workers are careful to note that what is called "mental" disorder may, in fact, be the result of environmental stress (hardship, trauma, cumulative disadvantage) that exceeds an individual's capacity to cope; it may even be a "normal" response to an abnormal environment. Since the cause of dysfunction is (at least partly) environmental, intervention also needs to be (at least partly) environmental. That might mean expanding access to resources in the person's family and community, and/or reducing harmful influences.

The idea that human development and behavior are shaped by multiple, nested, and interacting environments was first articulated by developmental psychologist Bronfenbrenner [2, 3] whose ecological systems theory has been applied across professional domains from psychology to education. Bronfenbrenner proposed five layers of environment, each embedded in the next: the first four represent increasingly inclusive levels of socio-cultural influence; the fifth represents the evolution of these systems over time and is reflected in differences between historical cohorts. Similarly, Germain and Gitterman [8], architects of the person-in-environment perspective in social work, conceptualized environment as interwoven layers of social and physical context. From this perspective, all problems, even if related to internal disorder, exist and need to be viewed in transactional or adaptive terms; the onus for change, like the source of a problem, does not rest solely on the client's psyche. Identity is social identity, and finding one's place through socialization and affiliation is an essential part of healthy development.

At the same time, the ecological approach is not a practice model and does not offer any guidelines for clinical decisions [17, 10]. A perspective rather than a theory, it does not provide an explanatory model for *why* or *how* person and environment affect each other [25]—a set of mechanisms or pathways through which specific elements of the environment affect specific aspects of human functioning and development. "Although the ecological and systems perspectives have helped social workers orient themselves to environmental factors influencing clients' lives, the abstract nature of these perspectives may fail to promote practitioners' understanding of the precise activities and experiences required for change to occur" [5, p. 68].

Interestingly, Bronfenbrenner proposed a research agenda more than three decades ago to investigate the impact of specific ecological elements on human behavior. He proposed a series of "rigorously designed experiments, both naturalistic and contrived"—i.e., by random assignment to experimental groups or by studying naturally occurring groups that differed along dimensions of interest—to explore the diverse relationships between person and environment. "Systematic contrast between two or more environmental systems or their structural components, with a careful attempt to control other sources of influence" [2, p. 517] could, he believed, illuminate the role of environmental elements in both normal and disordered development.

Bronfenbrenner's agenda was never carried out. Clearly, there are ethical and practical difficulties in trying to isolate features of the environment in order to test hypotheses. Establishing theoretical connections is complicated further by the fact that different causes can lead to the same effect. As Wakefield [26] pointed out, a symptom can be a result of a "true" mental dysfunction in the neurobiological sense or an attempt to cope with an adverse environment. The only way to establish causality would be, as Bronfenbrenner implies, to undertake a prospective controlled experiment. Alternatively, causality could be inferred retrospectively by comparing the results of interventions based on different mechanisms of change. If, for example, the depressive symptoms of homebound seniors who received sociotherapy improved significantly more than the symptoms of an equivalent group who received cognitive psychotherapy, it might be inferred that social isolation was a more significant contributor to their depression than erroneous thinking.

Logical as this sounds, it is a bit misleading. To say that social isolation was the "cause" of depression because social contact—its inverse—is the "cure" would be like declaring that because aspirin relieves a headache, the headache must have been caused by a lack of aspirin. The causal chain cannot be established retrospectively. In addition, there may be mediating factors. For example, the source of depression might not lie in social isolation itself but in its effect on areas of the brain associated with sound, touch, and other sensory stimuli.

Wilkins [28] argues that sociotherapy can mitigate or even prevent the effects of negative environmental conditions that lead to emotional distress and impaired mental health. Certainly, the likelihood of mental disorder tends to be higher for those who have experienced deficient or dysfunctional environmental conditions such as abuse, neglect, poverty, or oppression. Wilkins also points to a decline in community and mutual support, with a corresponding reduction in the sense of affiliation, participation, and care for the wellbeing of the group. To reduce the risk of mental disorder, the process needs to be reversed.

Sociotherapy makes sense as a general strategy, although how *specific* interventions are selected remains unclear. It is one thing to say that intervening into the environment is helpful. It is another to demonstrate through what channels or mechanisms it is helpful. The question is not whether a client's living situation and relationships are important. Scarcely anyone would argue nowadays for de-contextualized treatment based entirely on introspective talk. Rather, the question is *why* and *how* ecological factors contribute to a theory of change. Without a coherent theoretical or empirical basis linking elements of the social environment to aspects of individual dysfunction and their amelioration, the rationale for sociotherapy can be challenged as being more of a value position than an empirically grounded treatment.

20.3 Theoretical Basis: Social Identity and Social Relationships

Belonging and relating appear to be fundamental human needs; when absent or distorted, suffering results. The research of Bowlby, Ainsworth, and others who have studied attachment in infant development confirms this idea; recent scholarship, such as the work of Louis Cozolino on social neuroscience and the biology of attachment, offers additional support. So too, popular literature proclaims that human beings are "hard wired" for connection; the profound damage to the Rumanian orphans who were left alone in their cribs, never cuddled or spoken to, is further testimony of what happens when human connection is absent.

The relational dimension of environment has several intertwined aspects. There is the amount, quality, and consistency of social engagement and support; the degree to which social roles are thwarted, fulfilled, mutually enriching or, on the contrary, a source of conflict; and the patterns of interaction and communication that signal which groups a person belongs to and thereby contribute to social identity. Social identity, once adopted, is enacted through performance of social roles and engagement in socially structured relationships. Crossing boundaries, breaking tabus, isolating oneself, or failing to meet social expectations violate social identity, often with negative consequences. The loss of important social roles (though unemployment, the death of loved ones, "aging out," or macro events such as political conquest) can be a source of profound distress. Failure to fulfill social roles in healthy, productive ways can also be a source of distress—to the person, to others, and to the community. In fact, the P.I.E. or person-in-environment system of classification [29] uses the concept of social role functioning as the basis for formulating the source and nature of an individual's dysfunction.

Conversely, strong social networks, positive interactions, and social support have been identified as predictors of health and wellbeing. A theoretical understanding of how these elements contribute to positive outcome remains elusive, however, in part because they tend to be conflated and viewed as if they are products of the same underlying mechanism [6]. Challenging this assumption, Cohen maintains that different social variables influence health through different, independent pathways. He suggests three distinct social relationship variables—social integration, social support, and negative interaction—that influence health outcome through distinct mechanisms and offer specific targets for intervention. Similarly, Corcoran and Nichols-Casebolt [7] propose a "risk and resilience" ecological framework of specific risk and protective factors at micro, mezzo, and macro levels that can provide a scaffold for assessment and intervention. Unlike Cohen, they emphasize the interactional and cumulative effect of these elements, rather than considering each in isolation. Risks and protective factors, they maintain, "interact to determine an individual's ability to function adaptively despite stressful life events" (p. 212), each risk factor exacerbating the others, and each protective factor increasing the likelihood of other protective factors.

20.4 Principles of Sociotherapy

As a general modality, sociotherapy is person-centered, culturally sensitive, holistic, individualized, and egalitarian. A sociotherapist does not do something *to* the client, but works *with* the client through mutual encounter and recognition of shared humanity. The relationship between therapist and client is cooperative, collaborative, cocreated, and co-experienced [28].

Sociotherapy principles mesh well with the principles of person-centered psychiatry and person- centered health care. Sociotherapy is holistic, relational, dynamic, and complex, responsive to the changing needs of multiple interconnected systems across micro, mezzo, and macro levels. Its ethics also mesh well with the Social Work Code of Ethics. As Salvador-Carulla et al. [24] note, person-centered psychiatry is based on "a bio-psycho-socio-cultural understanding of health … guided by the ethical principle of respect for the autonomy, dignity, and responsibility of each person" (p. 110). Both disciplines embrace collaboration, empowerment, context, and nonlinearity. In this holistic vision of mental-physical-spiritual-relational wellbeing, strength and resilience are just as important as disorder and dysfunction.

Like all person-centered approaches to care, sociotherapy's core principles include democracy, non-directivity, equality, a focus on reality, and an orientation to building a positive future. Based on these principles, Richter et al. [21] propose humanist guidelines for developing and implementing a community-wide sociotherapy project:

- Full communication so all participants can take part in decisions from an informed basis.
- Shared leadership with collective power and responsibility.
- Continuation of discussion until consensus is reached that includes people at all levels.
- Social learning by social interaction in the here-and-now.

The Society for the Furtherance of Sociotherapy offers additional principles on which sociotherapy is based (http://www.pantarhei.org/literat/uksoc01.htm):

- A holistic vision of mankind in which each human being is seen as a somatic, psychic, social, and spiritual unity.
- A view of the individual as an autonomously functioning creature and, simultaneously, a socially interdependent creature.
- Belief that human development occurs through contact with others. Thus, malfunctioning social systems can create serious obstacles to healthy development and wellbeing.
- Acquisition of social skills in vivo through a recovery-based environment. This can be an important therapeutic instrument through which clients acquire needed skills that can be transported into other settings.
- Recognition that sometimes a person cannot function within a social system that is not, in itself, unhealthy. When this occurs, one person can create a situation in which none of the members the system can function properly. Intervention must thus occur at the level of both individual and group.

20.5 Sociotherapeutic Methods for Individuals, Groups, and Communities

A holistic, interactive approach that engages people in situ, sociotherapy can be utilized at micro, mezzo, and macro levels to address the needs of individuals, groups, and entire communities. At the individual level, strategies range from changing the physical living conditions (e.g., getting rid of clutter) to fostering engagement in activities to develop a latent interest or bolster social skills. A sociotherapist in a nursing home, for example, might try to induce an introverted resident to take part in social activities, with participation in games and conversation serving as both a tool for intervention and a way to monitor the effects of the intervention. Sociotherapy has been used in rehabilitation programs for individuals with severe mental illness and their families; interventions for people with co-occurring substance use disorder and mental illness; residential and family-centered dementia care; projects to promote resilience in at-risk youth; and family-based substance abuse treatment.

Group sociotherapy can be organized around common interests or concerns such as parenting or bereavement. It can also take place through social networking sites and internet support groups; this may especially be useful for the homebound or elderly, providing a means of interaction across geographic distance for extended family members and individuals with similar challenges. Intervention can also be at the level of the entire community as residents develop and carry out programs to improve neighborhood safety, marshal resources, strengthen social networks, and augment the community's ability to withstand or rebound from stress [23]. One such endeavor is the Rwandan Community Based Sociotherapy Program [21]. The program uses a context- and participant-driven group therapy approach, bringing community members together for weekly sessions conducted by trained local leaders to facilitate psychological healing, interpersonal reconciliation, and social cohesion (http://www.sociotherapy.org/). Sociotherapy has also been applied a wide range of community-based programs in the arena of public health, as summarized by McLeroy et al. [16] in their typology based on the notion of community as setting, target, agent, and/or resource for change.

Sociotherapy need not be vast in scope, however. Saleebey [23] points to "the power of small" found in the "immediate, proximal, often small environments where people play out much of their lives" (p. 7). Small changes can be powerful. In the "broken windows" theory, first articulated by Kelling and Wilson in 1982, windows broken and left broken send a message to neighborhood youth that no one cares—so why should they? In this context, the impetus to vandalism and crime does not come from intrapsychic features but from "particular and often seemingly inconsequential features of the ambient environment" [23, p. 10]. The way to decrease crime is to repair the windows, clean up the graffiti, and change the proximal environment in small concrete ways that signal pride and care rather than shame and indifference.

Cohen [6] offers several additional suggestions. First, he recommends intervention in natural social networks that can provide a vehicle for sustaining as well as initiating change. Second, he suggests increasing the potency of social support within existing networks by improving individual social skills and building stronger ties to other network members. Third, he recommends strategies to directly reduce negative interactions. He notes that researchers need to "identify the characteristics of those who benefit most and least from social integration and support interventions" (p. 682).

Wilkins goes even further, urging not only activities to increase social connectedness but also an active inner practice of forgiveness, gratitude, compassion, and kindness based on awareness of interdependent human connection. Forgiveness, he says, "reduces hurt, anger, stress, anxiety, and depression and … is good for the heart, as it reduced blood pressure and improves circulation" (p. 247). He cites the increase in oxytocin during person-centered encounters, which reduces blood pressure, facilitates healing of wounds, and prevents damage to the cardiovascular system (p. 247). There is, in fact, strong empirical support for the notion of bio-psycho-social wholeness. The health benefits of Mindfulness-Based Stress Reduction have been well documented, as have the benefits of Forgiveness Therapy practiced with families of people completing suicide, terminally ill patients, and survivors of trauma such as incest or domestic violence.

Sociotherapy can also be preventive. Strategies to promote positive social interaction and mutuality can be implemented *before* problems arise. Wilkins [28] notes, by way of comparison, that efforts to promote good nutrition and sanitary living conditions have saved more lives than the reparative efforts of heart and brain surgeons. Applying the same principle, he urges policy efforts to promote the societal conditions that can prevent the need for extensive (and expensive) reparative interventions.

20.6 Empirical Basis: What Is the Evidence?

Overall, the literature on sociotherapy consists of descriptive reports about specific programs (e.g., [21]) or generic articles on its principles and benefits (e.g., [28, 6]). Empirical studies that demonstrate actual relationships and pathways are scant, and thus the research basis for person-in-environment—the explanatory construct on which sociotherapy is based—remains elusive. Salvador-Carulla et al. [24] make an eloquent plea for studies that can generate evidence for the various domains of person-centered care, diagnostic models, and clinical interventions, yet this remains more of a research agenda than a research achievement.

One reason for this difficulty is that ecological and sociotherapeutic concepts tend to be used in flexible, nonspecific ways [22], lending credence to Wakefield's [25] view that person-in-environment is simply too broad and vague a notion to be prescriptive.

> This flexibility constitutes one of the construct's most important beneficial attributes, or most serious limitations ... Either the perspective is so ingrained in social work practice that there is no need to name it, or that it is much less a guiding perspective than the profession may claim or believe [22, p. 64].

Several studies have explored professional attitudes toward using environment as a treatment modality, although that is not the same as exploring the modality's effectiveness. Weiss-Gal [27], for example, compared the extent to which environment was part of Israeli social workers' professional ideology with the degree to which they actually used an environmental approach in their practice. Their findings pointed to a significant disparity: although person-in-environment was strongly reflected in respondents' stated views of the goals and activities of their profession, it was scarcely evident in their work. In Buchbinder et al.'s [4] study, social workers were asked how they understood a "psychosocial approach" and how that affected their practice. Using the metaphor of figure-and-ground to represent a shifting focus along a continuum, the authors note: "At one extreme are those who view the psycho as the figure and the social as a blurred ground or as an instrument to bring the psycho to completion. At the other extreme are those who view the social as the figure and the psychological as the ground" (p. 537).

In Probst's [19] study of how clinical social workers understand the notion of environment, participants embraced a broad definition spanning diverse elements from political climate and the culture of poverty to life stressors, relational support or isolation, situational triggers and ruptures, and the overall effects of culture, geography, and community. Notions of environment included proximal elements such as family, school/work, and peers as well as large-scale enduring factors such as ethnicity and socioeconomic class.

Participants identified three benefits of using a person-in-environment approach, all of which resonate with the principles of person-centered healthcare [24]. First, viewing a person in context brought a fuller, deeper understanding of how distress had arisen, what was maintaining it, what tools and supports might be available, and what the problem meant to the client as an individual rather than a member of a category. Second, environment provided an alternative lens for conceptualizing a client's problem; struggle or dysfunction might be a legitimate reaction to a pathology-inducing context, rather than the result of internal disorder. Third, changing the environment might be an important part of the treatment. For most participants, environment played a more central role in assessment than in intervention. While information about environment contributed directly to understanding the nature and meaning of a client's problem, it shifted to the background during the treatment process, providing a *context* for change but not a *mechanism* for change.

20.7 Implications and Future Directions

Interventions that take place "in the world," rather than "in the therapist's office," have always been an important part of clinical work. There are countless avenues: play therapy for young children; peer mentoring and leadership programs for disaffected teens; dance, music, and art therapy for people whose natural form of expression is not verbal; occupational, recreational, and animal-assisted therapy for people who need to engage through their bodies, to name just a few. What these examples have in common is the principle that intervening *externally* can affect *internal* wellbeing, rather than assuming that change must first take place inside.

Sometimes both are needed. A strength of sociotherapy lies in its capacity for integration into *any* clinical practice. It may be most effective, in fact, as part of an integrated effort that also addresses psychological factors like cognition, affect tolerance, and flexibility of coping strategies. This view of sociotherapy as complement rather than replacement for other treatments challenges the more "traditional" view of sociotherapy as "any treatment emphasizing modification of the environment and improvement in interpersonal relationships *rather than* intrapsychic factors" (http://medical-dictionary.thefreedictionary.com/sociotherapy, italics mine). The use of the phrase *rather than* implies that the clinician must select one *or* the other avenue of change, and that the two approaches can or should be separated for both research and treatment.

As discussed above, it would be difficult to set up a randomized controlled trial (RCT) to isolate and measure the independent effects of a sociotherapy intervention on, for example, persons experiencing social anxiety. Such a design would require that one group receive supportive or insight-based individual psychotherapy, while another group receives sociotherapy through a program such as structured social engagement. Yet it is a false design, based on a false dichotomy. Clients bring material from their lives to psychotherapists, who often make suggestions about actions they might take in their outer lives. Similarly, any sociotherapy involving interpersonal relationships or environmental change is bound to affect thoughts, perceptions, and emotions.

It is not a matter of environment *or* psyche, as implied by the words "rather than," but of varied emphasis along a continuum. On one end, social policy advocates focus almost entirely on the environment, believing that improvement in external conditions will lead to improvement in the quality of individual lives. Psychoanalysis, on the other hand, focuses almost entirely on internal factors, believing that self-awareness and resolution of conflict will lead to change in behavior. Between these two poles is a continuum of approaches that draw on both psychotherapy *and* sociotherapy.

An unanswered question is how sociotherapy "works," assuming that it does. Treatment that includes outreach into an individual's living situation and relationships clearly resonates with person-centered values, but what is the evidence for its effectiveness? As noted above, demonstrating efficacy through an RCT is unrealistic, yet theoretical plausibility may offer an alternative approach. It is possible, for instance, that after a sociotherapy intervention such as arranging a family reunion or taking long-delayed art lessons, depressive symptoms might abate. But why? One possibility is that the reunion or art lessons do not address the mental health condition directly but, rather, affect an intermediary agent such as hope or shame, which in turn affects the depression. Thus, the effect of sociotherapy may pass through a mediating link, in the same way that exercise elevates mood through the release of endorphins.

It is also possible that sociotherapy does not affect the mental health condition at all, directly or indirectly, but instead adds something to the totality of the person's life and experience, causing the depression to take up "less space;" as a result, there is less internal preoccupation, less time and energy allocated to negative experience. By offering an exception to the dominant narrative of unworthiness or hopelessness, as in Michael White's narrative therapy or the "Black Swan" proposition, sociotherapy breaks the stronghold of depressive habits.

Further research is needed to understand the variables that can affect the outcome of sociotherapeutic approaches such as the timing, scope, and duration of the intervention in relation to individual factors, such as culture and gender roles, as well as sociotherapy's place within a more comprehensive person-centered model of care. Many avenues of fruitful inquiry lie ahead.

20.8 In Conclusion

As noted above, the contextualized perspective of sociotherapy need not be seen as a stand-alone approach but, rather, as a valuable addition to *any* model of clinical practice. Viewing sociotherapy in this way—i.e., as a nonexclusive complement, rather than a competitor or substitute for psychotherapy—can help to resolve the false dichotomy of internal versus external mechanisms of change and locate sociotherapy solidly within person-centered models of healthcare.

References

1. Alperin RM, Hollman BC. The social worker as psychoanalyst. Clin Soc Work J. 1992;20 (1):89–98.
2. Bronfenbrenner U. Toward an experimental ecology of human development. Am Psychol. 1977;32(7):513–31.
3. Bronfenbrenner U. The ecology of human development. Cambridge, MA: Harvard University Press; 1979.
4. Buchbinder E, Eisikovits Z, Karnieli-Miller O. Social workers' perceptions of the balance between the psychological and the social. Soc Serv Rev. 2004;78(4):531–52.
5. Cameron M, Keenan EK. The common factors model: implications for transtheoretical clinical social work. Soc Work. 2010;55(1):63–73.
6. Cohen S. Social relationships and health. Am Psychol. 2004;59(8):676–84.
7. Corcoran J, Nichols-Casebolt A. Risk and resilience ecological framework for assessment and goal formulation. Child Adolesc Soc Work J. 2004;21(3):211–35.

8. Germain CB, Gitterman A. The life model of social work practice. New York: Columbia University Press; 1980.
9. Germain CB. Chapter two: technological advances. In: Rosenblatt A, Waldfogel D, editors. Handbook of clinical social work. Jossey-Bass; 1983. p. 26–57.
10. Goldstein E. Social work education and clinical learning: yesterday, today and tomorrow. Clin Soc Work J. 2007;35:15–23.
11. Goldstein E. The relationship between social work and psychoanalysis: the future impact of social workers. Clin Soc Work J. 2009;37:7–13.
12. Hare I. Defining social work for the 21st century. Int Soc Work. 2004;47(3):407–24.
13. Hollis F, Woods ME. Casework: a psychoscial therapy. 3rd ed. New York: Random House; 1981.
14. Janchill MP. Systems concepts in casework theory and practice. Soc Casework. 1969;74–82.
15. Kirk SA, editor. Mental disorders in the social environment: critical perspectives. New York: Columbia University Press; 2005.
16. McLeroy KR, Norton BL, Kegler MC, Burdine JN, Sumaya CV. Community-based interventions. Am J Public Health. 2003;93(4):529–33.
17. Meyer CH. The search for coherence. In: Meyer CH, editor. Clinical social work in the eco-systems perspective. New York: Columbia University Press; 1983. p. 5–34.
18. Probst B. The life and death of axis IV: caught in the quest for a theory of mental disorder. Res Soc Work Pract. 2014;24(1):123–31.
19. Probst B. Living with and living within: visions of "environment" in contemporary social work. Qual Soc Work. 2012. doi:10.1177/1473325012455086).
20. Richmond M. Social diagnosis. New York: Russell Sage Foundation; 1917.
21. Richters A, Dekker C, Scholte WF. Community-based sociotherapy in Byumba. Rwanda Interv. 2008;6(2):100–16.
22. Rogge ME, Cox ME. The person-in-environment perspective in social work journals: a computer-assisted content analysis. J Soc Serv Res. 2001;28(2):47–68.
23. Saleebey D. The power of place: another look at the environment. Fam Soc. 2004;85(1):7–16.
24. Salvador-Carulla L, Cloninger CR, Thornicroft A, Mezzich JE. Background, structure, and priorities of the 2013 Geneva declaration on person-centered health research. Int J Pers-Cent Med. 2013;3(2):109–13.
25. Wakefield JC. Does social work need the eco-systems perspective? Soc Serv Rev. 1996;1–30 (March).
26. Wakefield JC. Disorders versus problems of living in DSM: rethinking social work's relationship to psychiatry. In: Kirk SA, editor. Mental disorders in the social environment: critical perspectives. Columbia University Press; 2005.
27. Weiss-Gal I. The person-in-environment approach: professional ideology and practice of social workers in Israel. Soc Work. 2008;53(1):5–75.
28. Wilkins P. Person-centred sociotherapy: applying person-centred attitudes, principles and practices to social situations, groups and society as a whole. Hellenic J Psychol. 2012;9:240–54.
29. Williams J, Karls JM, Wandrei K. The Person-in-Environment (PIE) system for describing problems of social functioning. Hosp Commun Psychiatry. 1989;40(11):1125–7.

Person-Centered Psychiatric Rehabilitation

21

Marianne Farkas ScD, William Anthony PhD, Roger Montenegro MD and Elena Gayvoronskaya MD, PhD

21.1 Introduction

The mental health field has accepted psychiatric rehabilitation as one of the preferred methods for helping individuals with serious psychiatric disabilities [53, 4, 20]. Nevertheless, it remains less clearly understood or effectively practiced in part due to

This article is based in part on work that was supported, in part by the HHS—National Institute of Disability, Independent Living and Rehabilitation Research (within ACL), and Substance Abuse Administration, Center for Mental Health Services RRTC on Individuals with Serious Psychiatric Disabilities 1979–2015. The contents of this chapter do not necessarily represent the policy of NIDILRR, ACL, SAMHSA, HHS, nor imply endorsement by the US Federal Government.

M. Farkas ScD (✉)
Professor, Center for Psychiatric Rehabilitation, Boston University,
940 Commonwealth Ave. West, Boston, MA 02215, USA
e-mail: mfarkas@bu.edu

W. Anthony PhD
Professor Emeritus, Center for Psychiatric Rehabilitation, Boston University,
Boston, USA

E. Gayvoronskaya MD, PhD
Assistant Professor of Psychiatry, N. N. Burdenko State Medical University,
Voronezh, Russia

R. Montenegro MD
President, Fundacion Contener, Buenos Aires, Argentina

R. Montenegro MD
Former Secretary of Education, World Psychiatric Association, Geneva, Switzerland

R. Montenegro MD
Former Director, Institute of Post Graduate Education, Association of Argentinian
Psychiatrists, Buenos Aires, Argentina

J.E. Mezzich et al. (eds.), *Person Centered Psychiatry*,
DOI 10.1007/978-3-319-39724-5_21

the fact that many types of mental health practitioners, including psychiatric rehabilitation practitioners, deliver psychiatric rehabilitation. In addition, relevant research and conceptual articles appear in a wide range of professional journals. The term "psychosocial interventions" and "psychiatric rehabilitation" have come mistakenly to be used interchangeably, a confusion which has led some researchers to complain that there is no consistent method to categorize psychosocial treatment [12]. The broad disabilities associated with mental illnesses cannot be addressed with a single focused intervention alone. Psychiatric rehabilitation is a field, not just a series of unique interventions or program models. It has a defined set of values, techniques, program practices, and relevant outcomes developed over the past thirty years (e.g. [4, 16, 46]). In [70], the World Health Organization developed a Consensus statement on the definition "Psychosocial rehabilitation is a process that facilitates the opportunity for individuals … to reach their optimal level of independent functioning in the community. It implies both improving individuals; competencies and introducing environmental changes in order to create a life of the best quality possible for people who have experienced a mental disorder, who have an impairment of their mental capacity which produces a certain level of disability … stressing individuals' choices on how to live successfully in the community." (pg2). "Psychosocial" rehabilitation or "Psychiatric rehabilitation" as a field and a service within a comprehensive mental health system, is delivered with the overall purpose of contributing to an individual's recovery and since its inception has incorporated "person centeredness" as a fundamental principle [16, 1]. While the actual development of person-centered psychiatric rehabilitation (PCPR) may have differed somewhat across different countries, most understand its philosophy, values, and overall techniques similarly [53]. PCPR is the process of basing the provider–person relationship on the individual's vision of their own recovery and promoting their capacity to reach their rehabilitation goals within that vision. This chapter will describe the context for PCPR and the basic principles and practices associated with it.

21.2 For Whom is PCPR Designed?

First and foremost, PCPR was designed to serve *people with* psychiatric disabilities. Using the term "people with …," also known as "Person First" language, focuses PCPR helping individuals with many characteristics, talents, strengths, and interests—and who also have serious mental illnesses, regain valued roles in society. PCPR traditionally serves primarily individuals with serious psychiatric disability. Various definitions of serious psychiatric disability share common elements: a diagnosis of mental illness, prolonged duration, with functional or role incapacity [7, 34]. Whether the target population is defined using medical, rehabilitation, mental health, or empirically derived criteria, all definitions coalesce around the description of a disability that persist over a period of time (usually two or more years), with resulting functional impairment, that substantially limits one or more major life activities [28]. For example, some outcome studies have demonstrated that impairment in school or work functioning is a persistent problem for those experiencing serious mental illnesses, either presaging the onset of the psychiatric disability [33, 38] or present at the time of first diagnosis [62, 50].

Within the group with these characteristics, are many subgroups: people across different points in the life span, people with co-occurring conditions (e.g. substance abuse and mental illnesses), people who are homeless, and those from a wide range of cultural and ethnic backgrounds [4, 10]. As such, those who can use PCPR services cross diagnostic and demographic categories.

21.3 Recovery and PCPR

The context for individuals with serious mental illnesses has changed considerably over the past forty years. Whereas, keeping people out of the long-term psychiatric hospital was considered to be the highest goal of mental health services even up to 1990's [2, 19], the advent of the notion of recovery changed the focus of mental health service systems in the United States [47, 58, 59] as well as many other countries such as England, Scotland, New Zealand, Canada (e.g. [22, 36, 55]). The empirical basis for recovery for individuals with serious mental illnesses, was first established during the 1970–1980's (e.g. [63]), but remarkably did not really impact the field until the 1990's. Longitudinal studies carried out between 1972 and 1987 in different countries, had remarkably similar outcomes. One-half–two-thirds of people with serious mental illnesses, predominantly schizophrenia, showed marked improvement in terms of variables ranging from symptom reduction to no current signs and symptoms of any mental illness, no current use of medication, working, relating well to family, and being integrated into their community [30, 31]. These early findings were confirmed by a later WHO longitudinal study [32], collecting data in a fifteen year and twenty-five year follow-up period with fourteen culturally diverse cohorts, in countries ranging from India, China, Japan, to Poland, Netherlands, Ireland, Britain, and the U.S. While the results showed heterogeneity of outcomes, the authors concluded that a significant proportion of those diagnosed with psychoses showed favorable long-term outcomes consistent with those of the earlier studies [30, 31, 32].

Typically, therefore, recovery outcomes have included multidimensional variables ranging from an increase in physical health and wellbeing to gaining or regaining valued social roles, as well as reducing symptoms [18]. In addition to objective outcomes such as increased success functioning in a range of life roles (e.g. worker, student, wife, softball team member, etc.), equally important are subjective outcomes such as an increased sense of self-worth and empowerment. These types of outcomes are most central to a person's recovery from mental illness. The most cited definition of recovery concludes that recovery is "… a deeply personal, unique process of changing one's attitudes, values, feelings, goals, skills and/or roles. It is a way of living a satisfying, hopeful, and contributing life even with limitations caused by the illness. Recovery involves the development of new meaning and purpose in one's life as one grows beyond the catastrophic effects of mental illness" [2].

In the current emphasis on recovery oriented services, implementing the process of PCPR has achieved greater prominence because PCPR's outcomes go beyond simply supporting adaptation or survival in the community. PCPR can and does promote a vision of recovery or the achievement of a meaningful life [14, 15], through its emphasis on gaining or regaining valued roles. The process of PCPR is designed to help people *be successful and satisfied in the living, working, learning, and social environments of their choice* [4, 5]. Rehabilitation operates at the intersection between the individual, an individual's personal network, and the wider social context [6]. Rehabilitation, of any kind (i.e., physical, psychiatric, social, etc.) is ecological ("person-environment fit") and specifically targets improving role performance. The term "psychiatric rehabilitation" reflects the focus of this field on *people with psychiatric disabilities* and *their improved abilities within their specific preferred role* in the "real" world, using the development of skills and supports as its primary types of interventions [4, 5]. Without a process committed to supporting chosen roles and settings, functioning may be improved, but the individual's vision of a meaningful life may still not be achieved. Rehabilitation, therefore, works with social relationships, work, leisure, family life, higher education, and other student pursuits, using interventions that focus on increasing competencies or skills and providing environmental supports, rather than focusing on symptoms and pathology. It does not deny that symptoms and pathology exist, nor the importance of intervening to reduce these, however, its own expertise targets the International Classification of Impairment, Disability, and Handicap (ICIDH) dimensions of activity, participation, and environment [68], rather than health. In 2003, having concluded that the mental health system was in fact nonfunctional, U.S. President George W. Bush's New Freedom Commission on Mental Health [47] envisioned a future "*when everyone with a mental illness will recover* and is helped *to live, work, learn, and participate fully in their communities*" strikingly consistent with the role related outcomes emphasized by PCPR.

21.4 Basic Recovery Values that Guide PCPR

PCPR is a *recovery facilitating* process rather than simply a method of organizing staff service delivery. As such, the underlying values that drive a recovery promoting service are integrated into the process of PCPR. While there are many values cited as important to recovery, at least four are universally recognized as critical: *person orientation, person involvement, self-determination, and hope* [15]. These four values together reflect the "person centered" aspect of 'person centered' psychiatric rehabilitation.

Person Orientation—Accounts written by individuals with serious psychiatric disabilities, describe both how appreciative people are when providers express interest in their strengths and talents and how damaging it is when providers reduce people to the list of symptoms they have or the label they carry [11, 67]. PCPR expresses the importance of the value of "person orientation" or seeing the person holistically, in that it focuses its assessments of physical, emotional, and intellectual functioning and support on both strengths and deficits. Individuals go through a process of identifying their own vision of a recovered life with a specific role that they hope to achieve within it. Their interests shape their perspective on what role they prefer (e.g. part time worker, college student, tenant, mother with children) and that role determines which skills and supports are evaluated.

Person Involvement—The fundamental basis for psychiatric rehabilitation interventions is a commitment to an equal partnership between the provider and the individual receiving services. Research data suggest that outcomes are better for people who have an opportunity for meaningful involvement in the planning and delivery of their services [39]. In recovery oriented services, people with psychiatric disabilities are partners in the delivery of interventions that promote their recovery. They bring their expertise about their own recovery process to the table, while providers bring expertise about interventions. In PCPR, providers use the expertise of the people being served to decide which components of the PCPR process to deliver, to decide on goals and types of interventions used. The entire process is based on the perspective of the person with the disability, with provider skills such as reflective or active listening, forming the core provider competency needed to create equal footing in the partnership. Providers function as coaches and teachers in PCPR rather than as the experts whose role is to solve problems. As such they teach, coach, and consult to the person with the psychiatric disability about what s/he needs to know to be able to choose, get, and keep the valued role s/he wants to achieve.

Choice or Self-Determination—Self-determination and self-choice is the cornerstone of the process designed to promote an individual's journey to achieving their own vision of a meaningful life. The opportunity to choose one's long-term goals, the methods to be used to get to those goals, and the individuals or providers who will assist in the process, are all components of a service acknowledging this value. PCPR helps individuals determine where and in what role they want to live, learn, work, or socialize. Beginning rehabilitation with this process helps to establish the individual'*s hopes* for a future, rather than beginning with an assessment of strengths and deficits and then determining a goal that "fits." Starting with a choice empowers individuals with serious mental illnesses to take control of their rehabilitation and ensures that the goals of rehabilitation are indeed related to their own vision of their recovery. When individuals being served do not have much experience making important choices in their lives, PCPR helps to arrange opportunities for people to experience different options and then helps them to clarify what they learned was important in these options, rather than taking over and making the choice for the person. Putting the individual receiving services at the center of care and supporting that person's autonomy is seen as a basic underlying premise for the provision of modern healthcare in general [29, 56]. In mental health services, taking part in decision-making processes have shown a positive impact on the individual's capability to reflect on old habits in more constructive ways as well as to improve psychosocial functioning [41]. Promoting self-determination and choice does not mean that practitioners have no right to share their opinions and thoughts in the PCPR process. As Anthony [3] points out, while there are times when an individual may have difficulty being the 'captain of his ship,' the onus is on the PCPR practitioner to explain *why* the person cannot make their own choice in the moment, rather than operating on the *assumption* that the person cannot do so. While there is evidence that has shown that offering choice and shared decision making is more effective than traditional authoritarian approaches to treatment [48], the issue of providing choice is less based on empiricism and is important more as a question of empowering individuals to regain control over their lives, their rights and citizenship in society [20].

Hope—Hope is the basis for a willingness to change. Having someone believe in a person, even when s/he do not believe in him or herself, has been identified by individuals with serious mental illnesses as the critical ingredient in their recovery [11]. While research has consistently shown that professionals do no better than random chance in predicting success [4], some staff believe that the people they serve are "too sick" to recover and that the data on recovery surely refers to types of clients other than the ones they serve. For example, many mental health professionals believe that work is too stressful [40, 50], despite abundant evidence to the contrary [37]. Unfortunately, these providers contribute to the fear of going to work by focusing on deficits and chronicity, and using professional coercion [49], which can demoralize and distress even the most resilient person [13]. PCPR increases hope by first focusing on the roles that reflect the person's aspirations—rather than beginning by assessing their limitations and then finding something that fits. This insistence on a process that helps individuals consider options and choose a role and setting they prefer, communicates to the person that their dreams are valid and that the process of PCPR involves helping them to figure out what skills and resources they have or do not have in relation to achieving their goal. Some individuals of course have lost their hope, in the years they have spent struggling with the illness, the accompanying poverty, loss of relationships and opportunities. PCPR acknowledges these negative realities and uses a systematic approach to help the person understand where they are currently in relation to considering their future.

21.5 The Process: Values Plus Techniques

PCPR as a process attempts to help people determine the living, education, work, and social roles they want to reach over the subsequent 6–24 months. Roles chosen within a period of two years are likely to be concrete enough to motivate the person, (as compared to long term goals which are closer to a vision than a goal) and far away enough that the person has improved the opportunity to achieve them. For example, a goal might be "I intend to live in an apartment with a roommate, in the Falmouth district of the city by July of 2017." Some people are not prepared to even consider setting a goal. Techniques of assessing and developing readiness for rehabilitation [9, 17] are designed to identify factors that provide obstacles considering change, with techniques designed to inspire that hope. Some of these factors include a lack of satisfaction or success in the person's current situation (greater dissatisfaction leading to greater willingness to consider a new situation); a perception by the individual that change may be possible, bring positive results, and is manageable for the person to do; a level of awareness about options and an awareness of personal values and interests. For those who *are* prepared to set a goal, providers facilitate the individual's self-determination by helping the person to develop the ability to select a role and setting, which they wish to reach or improve on. For those with little experience in making important choices in their lives, PCPR arranges for the person to experience a variety of options in order to promote their ability to identify their criteria for making a choose. Such activities are then followed by engaging the person in a systematic method of problem solving [8].

After setting a "role goal," provider assistance is focused on helping people to identify what they need and what they know how to do well (skills), and what they have or need to have (support or support resources) in order to achieve these goals. The relationship in which this occurs emphasizes an equal partnership, a holistic perspective and hopefulness. For example, the person in the previous goal example might have the intellectual skill of "Organizing my belongings" (a skill important when living with a roommate in a small apartment) but not have the emotional skill of "Resolving conflicts" (a skill equally important to living with a roommate). Functional assessment, or the evaluation of physical, emotional, and intellectual skill strengths and deficits are only done in relation to the demands of the preferred role, rather than being a generic checklist of skills that anyone might need to do anything (e.g. budgeting, transportation, grooming)—but that might not be helpful to the specific goal. For example, the Falmouth region of the city might not require transportation skills if everything the person needs is within walking distance. The roommate chosen to live in the apartment might not care about the person's grooming. Budgeting might only be important to the extent to which the person can pay rent—budgeting for other items may make no difference. In this way, assessments are kept specific to the goal that has been selected by the person and are tailored to be manageable for the precise demands of a specific environment. Therefore, people are helped to develop those unique skills and/or supports intended to help them to become successful and satisfied in the specific roles they have selected. Individuals are thus either taught to perform skills they do not have or supported in overcoming obstacles to using the skills they have, but do not perform sufficiently well to be successful and satisfied in the selected role. Support needs are met by either linking people to resources they might not have or helping to modify existing resources so that they can provide more support. PCPR includes both techniques to help the person make changes in their environment *and* techniques that help to modify the environment around the person (e.g. facilitating changes in laws, attitudes to people with psychiatric disabilities that create barriers to the person's achievement of their chosen valued role). In simpler terms, the PCPR process helps people determine their own goals and then obtain the skills and environmental support necessary to achieve them [4].

PCPR, as described here, has been studied in empirical studies conducted in the United States [51, 52, 57] and in a few studies conducted in European countries [27, 61, 64]. More recent studies have also confirmed the efficacy of this approach. For example, a two-year follow-up study conducted in Sweden followed a group of 71 clients across a county in Sweden where they were receiving psychiatric rehabilitation services. Of these 71 clients, 49 were still being followed at the end of two years. Results indicated that 65 % of the clients reported that they had mainly or almost completely achieved their self-formulated rehabilitation goals at the two-year follow-up. There were significant differences with regard to health, empowerment, quality of life, and psychosocial functioning for those who reported that they had mainly/completely achieved their self-formulated rehabilitation goals compared to those who reported that they only had to a small extent or not at all reached their goals [60].

From the perspective of the person for whom the service is intended, person-oriented psychiatric rehabilitation helps people choose their goals, obtain, and/or maintain them, depending on their needs and willingness [5]. This client view of the process has been called "Choose-Get-Keep." A qualitative study [35] conducted on the experience of the person being served in the two-year follow-up study focused on a subset of 10 participants who had been in services continuously for 24 months and were over 18 years of age. Participants responded to open-ended questions and were encouraged to describe their experiences in their own words. The analysis of the clients' experiences resulted in three categories: increased self-understanding, getting new perspectives, and being in a trusting relationship, which can be seen as important part of a sense of being connected to oneself and others. The clients' expressed experiences of the PCPR approach as an opportunity to recognize and verbalize their individual goals. The findings show that clients often do not recognize or are not able to verbalize their personal goals before having been given the possibility to reflect on their thoughts in collaboration with a trusted person. The participants' experiences of being respected as equal individuals and the importance of getting the necessary resources and insights to be able to make decisions and set goals according to individual preferences was a strong theme throughout the interviews. The approach is described by the interviewees as engaging the person by regularly giving them the opportunity to get their perspective reflected and to be able to participate in decision making regarding their own rehabilitation.

21.6 Developments Within Psychiatry

While the recovery movement and PCPR has become part of overall service delivery in mental health systems in many countries, particular developments within psychiatry have strengthened its dissemination internationally. As Mezzich et al. [43] point out, developments in medicine have currently begun to shift from an emphasis on disease to a focus on the person. As a result, Person-Centered Medicine is aimed at promoting health and wellbeing for the total person, incorporating their biological, social, psychological, cultural, and spiritual dimensions. Paralleling the international movements in recovery and rehabilitation [14, 15], international consensus around Person-Centered Medicine [42], includes the perspective that the individual is the expert on his/her own life, implementing his/her own 'life project.' Person-Centered Medicine considers not only ill health but also positive health, pays much attention to strengths and protective factors and promotes wellbeing and wellness in the process of recovery [45, 66]. This comprehensive view of the person has led, for example, to the development of the Person-Centered Integrated Diagnostic Model, which proposes a focus on the whole person in context, as the center and goal of clinical care and public health, encouraging a more flexible and conversational style of communication in health care [54].

In Eastern Europe, health has been described as the person's subjective experience of successful adaptation to their personal environment, based on their mental and physical capacity [21]. A person's functioning is viewed to be the balance between their adaptation and their lack of adaptation. "Disadaptation" leads to *functional failures* in one or more domains: biological, psychological, social (behavioral), and spiritual. Developments based on the notion of adaptation and disadaptation and a focus on strengths and protective factors have broadened the work of Person-Centered Medicine to include the development of rehabilitation processes for individuals with various mental and somatic disorders such as dementia, stroke, and traumatic brain injury, children with special needs, chronic pain, adult learning disabilities, maternity, anxiety and depressive disorders, and age-related changes. These processes are increasingly using techniques beyond the usual verbal or behavioral interventions, to incorporate elements such as dance and the healing environment of sensory rooms with additional external therapeutic stimuli aimed at strengthening the effectiveness of the more common rehabilitation interventions [24, 25, 26]. Interventions such as the Expressive Therapies, help to integrate support for individuals by expanding the focus of interventions to include ways of reaching the person through comprehensive avenues—intellectual, emotional, and their physical expression [23].

As early as 2002, the WHO reported on the alarming impact of mental illnesses around the world, including as a result of stigma and discrimination [69]. In Latin America, the focus on Person-Centered Psychiatry has come to also include a focus on social justice issues such as stigma and discrimination—a topic of great importance globally. An Argentinian organization, for example, "Fundacion Contener" was created to protect the rights of individuals with mental illnesses and to fight stigma and discrimination, believing that "Revolutions take place when the so-called 'problem people' become people who solve their own problems." This organization joined others in the Buenos Aires Declaration of 2014 on Person-Centered Medicine [44, 65] to affirm the need to: focus research, advocacy, funding of mental health services (at least to the level of funding for physical health), toward the integration of persons with mental health disorders into society, providing opportunities for occupational rehabilitation, diminishing stigma and discrimination, and safeguarding the human rights including individuals with mental illnesses.

21.7 Conclusion

Recent international developments in Medicine support PCPR and the importance of recovery for individuals with serious mental illnesses. The generalization of PCPR to populations other than individuals with serious mental illnesses or psychiatric disabilities provides more evidence of the importance of the basic ideas of this approach. Person-centered psychiatric rehabilitation is an approach to helping individuals with serious psychiatric disabilities, among other issues, to choose, get, and keep their preferred role in society. Using a wide variety of tools and possible perspectives and strategies to increase activity and participation or disability and handicap, it contributes to the person's recovery journey, helping the individual move toward a unique vision of a meaningful life.

References

1. Anthony WA. The principles of psychiatric rehabilitation. Baltimore: University Park Press; 1979.
2. Anthony WA. Recovery from mental illness: the guiding vision of the mental health service system in the 1990s. Psychosoc Rehabil J. 1993;16(4):11–23.
3. Anthony WAA. Shared decision making, self-determination and psychiatric rehabilitation. Psychiatr Rehabil J. 2010;34(2):87–8.
4. Anthony WA, Cohen MR, Farkas M, Gagne C. Psychiatric rehabilitation. 2nd ed. Boston: Boston University, Center for Psychiatric Rehabilitation; 2002.
5. Anthony WAA, Farkas M. The essential guide to psychiatric rehabilitation. Boston: Center For Psychiatric Rehabilitation. 2011. http://www.bu.edu/cpr/products/books/titles.
6. Barbato A. Psychosocial rehabilitation and severe mental disorders: a public health approach. World Psychiatry. 2006;5:162–3.
7. Center for Disease Control. Serious mental illness in the adult household population. Adv Data. 1992;218.
8. Cohen MR, Farkas M, Cohen B, Unger K. Establishing an overall rehabilitation goal: psychiatric rehabilitation trainer technology. Boston, MA: Center for Psychiatric Rehabilitation; 1992.
9. Cohen MR, Forbess R, Farkas M. Developing readiness for rehabilitation: psychiatric rehabilitation trainer series. Boston, MA: Center for Psychiatric Rehabilitation at Boston University; 2000.
10. Corrigan PW, Morris SB, Michaels PJ, Rafacz JD, Rusch N. Challenging the public stigma of mental illness: a meta-analysis of outcome studies. Psychiatr Serv. 2012;63(10):963–973.
11. Deegan P. Spirit breaking: when the helping professions hurt. Humanist Psychol. 1990;18:301–13.
12. Dixon LB, Dickerson F, Bellack AS, Bennett ME, Dickinson D, Goldberg RW, Kreyenbuhl J. The 2009 PORT psychosocial treatment recommendations and summary statements. Schizophr Bull. 2010;36:48–70.
13. Drake RE, Bond GR. The future of supported employment for people with severe mental illness. Psychiatr Rehabil J. 2008;31(4):367–76.
14. Farkas M. Identifying psychiatric rehabilitation interventions: an evidence and values based practice (commentary). World Psychiatry. 2006;5(3):6–7.
15. Farkas M. The vision of recovery today: what it is and what it means for services. World Psychiatry. 2007;6(2):1–7.

16. Farkas M, Anthony WA, editors. Psychiatric rehabilitation programs: putting theory into practice. Baltimore, MD: Johns Hopkins University Press; 1989.
17. Farkas M, Cohen MR, McNamara S, Nemec PB, Cohen BF. Assessing readiness for rehabilitation: psychiatric rehabilitation trainer series. Boston, MA: Center for Psychiatric Rehabilitation at Boston University; 2000.
18. Farkas M, Gagne C, Anthony WA, Chamberlin J. Implementing recovery oriented evidence based programs: identifying the critical dimensions. Commun Ment Health J. 2005;41(2):141–58.
19. Farkas M. Introduction to psychiatric/psychosocial rehabilitation (PSR): history and foundations. Curr Psychiatry Rev. 2013;9:177–187.
20. Farkas M, Anthony WAA. Psychiatric rehabilitation interventions: a review. Int Rev Psychiatry. 2010;22(2):114–129.
21. Garbuzov V. Conception of instincts and psychosomatic pathology. St. Petersburg: SOTIS; 1999.
22. Gawaith L, Abrams P. Long journey to recovery for Kiwi consumers: recent developments in mental health policy and practice. Aust Psychol. 2006;41:140–8.
23. Gayvoronskaya E, Shapovalov D. Integrative dance/movement psychotherapy and the aging process. Body, Mov Dance Psychother. 2010;5(2):185–96.
24. Gayvoronskaya E. State-of-art capabilities of rehabilitation of patients with mental disorders—different aspects. XVII World Congress of the World Association of Dynamic Psychiatry. Multidisciplinary approach to and treatment of mental disorders: myth or reality? St. Petersburg, 14–17 May 2014; p. 17.
25. Gayvoronskaya E. Sensory Correction of Anxiety and Depressive Disorders. XVII World Congress of the World Association for Dynamic Psychiatry. Multidisciplinary Approach to and treatment of mental disorders: myth or reality? St. Petersburg, 14–17 May 2014; p. 18.
26. Gayvoronskaya E, Gurko O. Sensory correction of psychosomatic desadaptation in the age-related aspect. Traditions and Innovations in Psychiatry. WPA Regional Meeting, St. Petersburg, 10–12 June 2010; p. 233–234.
27. Gigantesco A, Vittorielli M, Pioli R, Falloon IRH, Rossi G G, et al. The VADO approach in psychiatric rehabilitation: a randomized controlled trial. Psychiatr Serv. 2006;57:1778–83.
28. Goldman HH, Gattozzi AA, Taube CA. Defining and counting the chronically mentally ill. Hosp Commun Psychiatry. 1981;32:21–7.
29. Grol R. Improving the quality of medical care. Building bridges among professional pride, payer profit, and patient satisfaction. J Am Med Assoc. 2001;286:2578–85.
30. Harding CM. An examination of the complexities in the measurement of recovery in severe psychiatric disorders. In: Ancill RJ, Holliday D, MacEwan GW, editors. Schizophrenia: exporing the spectrum of psychosis. Chichester: J. Wiley & Sons; 1994. p. 153–69.
31. Harding CM, Zhaniser JH. Empirical correction of seven myths about schizophrenia with implications for treatment. Acta Psychiatrica Scandinavica. 1994;90(Suppl 384):140–6.
32. Harrison G, Hopper K, Craig T, Laska E, Siegal C, Wanderling J, et al. Recovery from psychotic illness: a 15-and 25-year international follow-up study. Br J Psychiatry. 2001;178:506–17.
33. Harvey PD, Green MF, Keefe RS, Velligan DI. Cognitive functioning in schizophrenia: a consensus statement on its role in the definition and evaluation of effective treatments for the illness. J Clin Psychiatry. 2004;65:361–72.
34. Jans L, Stoddard S, Kraus L. Chartbook on mental health and disability. Washington, D. C.: US Department of Education, National Institute on Disability and Rehabilitation Research; 2004.
35. Jormfeldt H, Svensson B, Hanssen L, Svedberg P. Clients' experiences of the Boston psychiatric rehabilitation approach: a qualitative study. Int J Stud Health Well Being. 2014;9. doi:10.3402/qhw.v9.22916 (online 8 Apr 2014).
36. Kirby MJ, Keon WJ. Out of the shadows at last: highlights and recommendations. Final Report of the Standing Senate Committee on Social Affairs. Science and Technology. Government of Canada: Ottawa; 2006.

37. Kukla M, Bond GR, Xie H. A prospective investigation of work and nonvocational outcomes in adults with severe mental illness. J Nerv Ment Dis. 2012;200:214–22.
38. MacCabe JH, Wicks S, Löfving S, David AS, Berndtsson Å, Gustafsson JE, Dalman C. Decline in cognitive performance between ages 13 and 18 years and the risk for psychosis in adulthood: a Swedish longitudinal cohort study in males. J Am Med Assoc Psychiatry. 2013;70:261–70. doi:10.1001/2013.jamapsychiatry.43.
39. Majumder RK, Walls RT, Fullmer SL. Rehabilitation client involvement in employment decisions. Rehabil Couns Bull. 1998;42:162–73.
40. Marwaha S, Balachandra S, Johnson S. Clinicians' attitudes to the employment of people with psychosis. Soc Psychiatry Psychiatr Epidemiol. 2008;44:349–60. doi:10.1007/s00127-008-0447-5.
41. McCann TV, Clark E. Advancing self-determination with young adults who have schizophrenia. J Psychiatr Ment Health Nurs. 2004;11:12–20.
42. Mezzich JE. The Geneva conferences and the emergence of the international network of person-centered medicine. J Eval Clin Pract. 2011;2011(17):333–6.
43. Mezzich JE, Botbol M, Salloum IM. Mental health and person centered medicine. Int J Pers Cente Med. 2015;5:1–8.
44. Mezzich JE, Montenegro R. A report: second international congress on person centered medicine. Int J Pers Cente Med. 2014;4(4):257–61.
45. Mezzich JE, Snaedal J, Van Weel C, Heath I. Conceptual explorations in person-centered medicine. Int J Integr Care. 2010;10 (Supplement).
46. Pratt C, Gill K, Barrett N, Roberts M. Psychiatric rehabilitation. San Diego, CA: Academic Press (Elsevier Inc); 2014.
47. President's New Freedom Commission on Mental Health. Achieving the promise: transforming mental health care in America. Final report: DHHS Pub. No. SMA-03-3832 Rockville, MD; 2003.
48. Priebe S, McCabe R, Bullenkamp J, Hansson L, Lauber C, Martinez-Leal R. Structured patient-clinician communication and 1-year outcome in community mental healthcare: cluster randomised controlled trial. Br J Psychiatry. 2007;191:420–6.
49. Rapp CA, Goscha RJ. The strengths model: case management with people with psychiatric disabilities. 2nd ed. New York: Oxford University Press; 2006.
50. Rinaldi M, Perkins R, Glynn E, Montibeller T, Clenaghan M, Rutherford J. Individual placement and support: from research to practice. Adv Psychiatr Treat. 2008;13:50–60.
51. Rogers E, Anthony W, Farkas M. The choose-get-keep model of psychiatric rehabilitation: a synopsis of recent studies. Rehabil Psychol. 2006;51(3):247–56.
52. Rogers E, Anthony WA, Lyass A, Penk WE. A randomized clinical trial of vocational rehabilitation for people with psychiatric disabilities. Rehabil Couns Bull. 2006;49(3):143–56.
53. Rossler W. Psychiatric rehabilitation today: an overview. World Psychiatry. 2006;5(3):151–7.
54. Salloum IM, Mezzich JE. Conceptual appraisal of the person centered integrative diagnostic model. Int J Pers Cente Med. 2011;1:39–42.
55. Scottish Government. Mental health Strategy for Scotland 2012–2015. Published August 2012. Accessed 9 July 2015. http://www.gov.scot/Publications/2012/08/9714, ISBN 978-1 78045-995-0.
56. Sensky T. Withdrawal of life sustaining treatment. Br Med J. 2002;325:175–6.
57. Shern DL, Tsemberis S, Anthony W, Lovell AM, Richmond L, Felton CJ, et al. Serving street—dwelling individuals with psychiatric disabilities: outcomes of a psychiatric rehabilitation clinical trial. Am J Public Health. 2000;90:1873–8.
58. Substance Abuse, Mental Health Services Administration (SAMHSA). Leading the change 2.0: advancing the behavioral health of the nation 2015–2018. HHS Pub No. (PEP14-1. LeadCHANGE-2) Rockville MD, Substance Abuse, Mental Health Services Administration; 2014.
59. Substance Abuse, Mental Health Services Administration (SAMHSA). Operationalizing recovery oriented systems. Expert Panel Report, 17 Aug 2012. Center for Mental Health

Services and Center for Substance Abuse Treatment. Accessed 10 July 2015. http://www.samhsa.gov/sites/default/files/expert-panel-05222012.pdf.
60. Svedburg P, Svensson B, Hanssen L, Jormfeldt H. A 2-year follow-up study of people with severe mental illness involved in psychosocial rehabilitation. Nordic Psychiatry. 2014;68 (6):401–8.
61. Swildens W, Van Busschbach JT, Michon H, Kroon H, Koeter WJM, Wiersma D, et al. Effectively working on rehabilitation goals: 24-month outcome of a randomized controlled trial of the Boston psychiatric rehabilitation approach. Can J Psychiatry. 2011;56(12):751–60.
62. Turner N, Browne S, Clarke M, Gervin M, Larkin C, Waddington JL, O'Callaghan E. Employment status amongst those with psychosis at first presentation. Soc Psychiatry Psychiatr Epidemiol. 2009;44:863–9. doi:10.1007/s00127-009-0008-6.
63. Turner JC, Wallcraft J. The recovery vision for mental health services British perspective. Psychiatr Rehabil J. 2002;25:245–54.
64. Van Busschbach J, Wiersma D. Does rehabilitation meet the needs of care and improve the quality of life of patients with schizophrenia or other chronic mental disorders? Commun Ment Health J. 2002;38(1):61–70.
65. Wagner P, Perales A, Armas R, Codas O, de los Santos R, Elio-Calvo D, et al. Latin American bases and perspectives on person centered medicine and health. Int J Pers Cente Med. 2014; 4 (4):220–227. Available at http://www.ijpcm.org/index.php/IJPCM/article/view/494. Date accessed 24 July 2015. doi:http://dx.doi.org/10.5750/ijpcm.v4i4.494.
66. Wallcraft J, Gayvoronskaya E, Salloum I. Strengths and protective factors in person-centered integrative diagnosis. Int J Pers Cente Med. 2012;2(2):193–5.
67. Weingarten R. Despair, learned helplessness and recovery. Innov Res. 1994;3:5–7.
68. World Health Organization. International classification of impairments, disabilities and handicaps. Geneva: World Health Organization; 2001.
69. World Health Organization. Mental Health Global Action Programme: MH GAP. MH/NMH/MSD 02.1. Geneva: World Health Organization; 2002.
70. World Health Organization. Psychosocial rehabilitation: a consensus statement. Division of Mental Health and Prevention of Substance Abuse. WHO/MNH/MND/96-2. Geneva: World Health Organization; 1997.

Person-Centered Mental Health Promotion and Public Health Perspectives

22

George N. Christodoulou MD, PhD, Wolfgang Rutz MD, PhD, Helen Herrman MD, Nikos G. Christodoulou MD, PhD and Margit Schmolke PhD

22.1 Introduction

Prevention of illness and Promotion of health have been popular concepts since ancient times. It is noteworthy that the ancient Greeks worshipped primarily Hygieia (the goddess of Preventive Medicine) and secondarily Panacea (the goddess of therapeutic medicine) as exemplified in the Hippocratic Oath where Hygieia is mentioned first and Panacea follows [25]. In later times, the focus changed toward therapeutic medicine but more recently we have seen a revival of attention to preventive medicine and health promotion.

G.N. Christodoulou MD, PhD (✉)
Hellenic Psychiatric Association, 11 Papadiamantopoulou Street, 11528 Athens, Greece;
Emeritus Professor of Psychiatry, University of Athens, Athens, Greece
e-mail: profgchristodoulou@gmail.com

W. Rutz MD, PhD
Professor of Social Psychiatry, University of Coburg, Coburg, Germany;
Senior Consultant, International and Public Mental Health, Stockholm, Sweden

H. Herrman MD
Professor of Psychiatry, The National Center of Excellence in Youth Mental Health and the University of Melbourne, Melbourne,, Australia; President-elect, World Psychiatric Association, Geneva, Switzerland

N.G. Christodoulou MD, PhD
Clinical Assistant Professor of Psychiatry, University of Nottingham, Nottingham, UK;
Consultant Psychiatrist, Nottingham General Hospital, Nottingham, UK

M. Schmolke PhD
Psychologist, Psychoanalyst and Director of the Munich Training and Research Institute of the German Academy of Psychoanalysis, Munich, Germany

J.E. Mezzich et al. (eds.), *Person Centered Psychiatry*,
DOI 10.1007/978-3-319-39724-5_22

Health promotion is associated with general, mainly socioeconomic measures, not necessarily linked with the health sector, with public health measures and on an individual level with the implementation of concepts and actions like positive health, empowerment, resilience, self-help, holism, recovery, salutogenesis, etc. that focus on reinforcing the capacity of the individual to remain healthy and create health. Within this framework the person-centered approach and the people-centered approach occupy a cardinal position [16].

The conceptual confluence of Person-centered Medicine and Preventive Psychiatry (mental illness prevention and mental health promotion) has been examined in detail elsewhere in this volume [18].

There are many similarities between illness **prevention** and health **promotion** but there is a basic difference and this is that the key target in prevention is **illness** whilst the key target in promotion is **health**. Prevention's aim is to avoid illness whilst the aim of promotion is to enhance health.

22.2 Health

A conceptual review of health reveals that this concept is not as clear as would be expected and so are the ways to advance it.

In ancient Greece, before the fifth century BC, health was considered as a divine gift and illness as punishment. It was Hippocrates (c 460–377 BC) who reversed this conception and advocated medical reasons as responsible for even the "sacred disease" (epilepsy). Such a formulation required a lot of courage at that time.

The concept of health was originally associated with soundness of the body [21]. The inclusion of "wellbeing" is a more recent addition and has been criticized on the basis of its corresponding more to happiness than health [45]. Yet, this definition is more consonant with the concept of mental health promotion and positive mental health and as such it is most welcome, specially by the mental health community.

The WHO definition of Health is the most typical paradigm of inclusion of wellbeing in the concept of health ("health is a state of complete, physical mental and social wellbeing and not merely the absence of disease or infirmity") [51]. It is important to note that although this definition appeared as early as 1948 yet it is very up to date and in line with the modern ideas of what health should stand for.

As expected, there have been many criticisms and one of the valid ones is that the word "complete" "makes it unlikely that anyone would be healthy for a reasonable period of time" [4].

Among the other definitions of health, reported in detail elsewhere [15] the Australian Aboriginal concept of health is noteworthy because it incorporates the social dimension ("health does not refer solely to the physical wellbeing of the individual but also to the social, emotional, spiritual and cultural wellbeing of the whole community") [36].

22.3 Mental Health

There are various definitions of mental health. The statistical criterion and the nosological criterion are no longer valid and it is generally believed that absence of mental illness is not a sufficient criterion to define mental health.

Mental health has been conceptualized as a positive emotion (affect), such as feelings of happiness; as a personality trait inclusive of the psychological resources of self-esteem and mastery; and as resilience, which is the capacity to cope with adversity [30].

Positive mental health has been defined as "a state of well-being in which the individual realizes his or her own abilities, can cope with the normal stresses of life, can work productively and fruitfully and is able to make a contribution to his or her community" (cited in [24]).

Wellbeing, salutogenic factors, resilience (coping with adversity), and quality of life are all components of positive mental health. Quality of life is defined by the WHO as "an individual's perception of his/her position in life in the context of the culture and value systems in which he/she lives and in relation to the goals, expectations, standards and concerns" [55]. Recovery (reinforcing the strengths of a person even if this person suffers from serious psychopathology) is an important part of positive mental health. Mental capital (the cognitive and emotional resources of a person) [7] is a useful concept that can help in the evaluation and promotion of positive mental health.

22.4 Health Promotion

Health promotion is defined as action and advocacy to address the full range of potentially modifiable determinants of health [52].

22.4.1 Antecedents of Health Promotion from a Person-Centered Perspective

As pointed out by Schmolke [46] Aaron Antonovsky's concept of Salutogenesis [3] may be considered as an antecedent of health promotion. Salutogenesis is a concept closely related to the person-centered perspective. More specifically, the search for the total history of the person and not just his/her illness and the emphasis on active adaptation to one's environment are practices very much akin to those advocated by the person-centered perspective.

Yet another antecedent of health promotion that is also linked with person-centered mental health is the concept of alliance with the patient's healthy Ego parts advocated by Günter Ammon's [1] Dynamic Psychiatry. Strengthening the healthy aspects in patients and integrating positive health into clinical psychiatry are important elements in dynamic psychiatry as well as in person-centered psychiatry.

22.4.2 Mental Health Promotion

Mental health promotion covers a variety of strategies aimed at having a positive effect on mental health. Among them are the encouragement of individual resources and skills as well as improvements in the socioeconomic environment [53].

22.4.3 Targets

Three target areas have been identified with reference to mental health promotion, the following:

- ***Personal target area***
  Ability to deal with one's internal psychological world, like thoughts, feelings, resilience, etc. [31].
- ***Social target area***
  Ability to deal with the social environment [10, 35].
- ***Environmental target area***
  Ability to deal with and help in creating healthy communities [35].

Any action that is taken to protect and promote mental health or any action not taken for this purpose but resulting in it can be part of mental health promotion [10].

Socio-political activities, such as reduction of unemployment (especially in view of its association with suicide), improvement of schooling, reduction of discrimination, prevention of conflicts, and effective management of economic crises are indeed measures that serve mental health promotion and such is also the case with the protection of civil, economic, social, political and cultural rights of the people. Mental health promotion is also strongly associated with concepts like "recovery," "sense of hope," "empowerment," "social inclusion," and "resilience."

Peace and social justice have also been seen as targets of mental health promotion [54]. Under this light, the initiatives of the task forces on Disasters and Violence of the World Psychiatric Association in conjunction with the Hellenic Psychiatric Association that have resulted in the production of antiwar statements by the Lebanese and the Israeli Psychiatric Associations with the agreement of the Palestinian Psychiatric Association [14] have served health promotion. Is this in essence a political action? Partly, yes. Yet, from the mental health perspective it is mental health promotion that is basically served and in view of the grave mental health consequences of war, actions aiming at termination of war conflicts everywhere in the world should be categorized among the broad targets of mental health promotion.

On an individual basis but also within a public health framework, mental health promotion should be exercised in a **holistic manner**. Psyche and soma go hand in hand. They interact, cross-talk and depend on each other, forming an integral psychosomatic entity. Persons with physical illness have a greater risk of experiencing depression and people with depression are prone to developing cardiovascular illness, diabetes, cancer and respiratory illness (these four illness categories leading to 60 % of premature deaths [58]). So, improving physical health helps mental health promotion and improving mental health promotes physical health.

Reduction of **stigma and discrimination** certainly promotes mental health but efforts toward this aim should be carried out in a thoughtful way. Preaching does not help. It is through paradigm, general nondiscrimination measures and integration of stigmatized groups in the society that this can be done more effectively. The same stands for the stigmatization of psychiatrists and other mental health professionals who often share stigma with their patients in spite of evidence that doctors who select psychiatry as a specialty have more stable personalities compared to their medical counterparts [11, 32].

Mental health promotion is very much in line with the person-centered perspective that places the person of the patient at the center of healthcare. This approach advocates the importance of practicing medicine and psychiatry ***of, for, by,*** and ***with*** the person [33] but also "***through***" the person, in view of the importance of a good interpersonal relationship in treatment, prevention, and promotion. As pointed out elsewhere in this volume [18] the person as a concept is recognized not only in the singular but also in the plural (i.e., people in society). Therefore, mental health promotion addressed to the public is also very much related to the person-centered perspective.

22.4.4 The Target Population

The whole population is in need of mental health promotion. Yet, one needs to prioritize certain groups not only because of the limited available funds and because evaluation of the efficacy of mental health promotion of the whole population is difficult to achieve but also because the person-centered perspective is better served in this way.

Which are the target groups?

22.4.5 Children and Adolescents

School children and adolescents form a vulnerable group in need of care for their mental health.

Academic challenges, peer pressure (including bullying and experimentation with drugs) the developmental need to differentiate the adolescents' behavior and attitude from those of their parents' and other challenges consistent with their developmental phase contribute to the shaping of their personalities, a process that is decisive for their mental health now and in the future.

Additionally, the onset of mental illness and especially of schizophrenic psychopathology often occurs during adolescence and it is important to advance mental health during this period in one's life.

22.4.6 Old People

In the years to come, old people will increase manifold [22]. Special promotional attention should therefore be provided to this group.

Old age is paradoxical because it represents a natural developmental period in one's life and yet this development is in a negative direction, as it is characterized by a variety of losses (emotional, cognitive and social).

Preparation for this period is a *sine qua non* mental health promotion necessity, especially for people who have to discontinue their work routine. Hobbies may be important for some people, church and social support for others, family ties for the lucky ones but it is important to understand that all these alternatives are determined by availability as well as by personal preferences and people should not be pushed into them in a procrustean way.

Mental health goes hand in hand with physical health and the same stands for mental and physical health promotion. Care for physical health, including physical activity, is important. If the latter is carried out in a group setting it serves the target of retaining social ties or even promoting the creation of new ties (although this is difficult in old age, especially with reference to people with rigid or "rigified" personalities).

Cognitive exercises like mental arithmetic may be helpful and (temporarily) effective in improving cognitive function.

As a general rule, activities associated with intact memory function, sexual, or athletic performance and aesthetic appearance should not be encouraged. Frustration, depression, ridicule, and a variety of narcissistic blows should be expected in these cases.

Retirement is usually considered as a negative life event although in some cases it may be welcomed. Irrespective of positive or negative charge, however, it is an important life event, creating a new atmosphere and may produce a lot of stress especially if it is associated with other life events—financial problems, somatic illness of self, or a family member and especially with a life event of cardinal importance, like loss of one's partner.

22.4.7 Women

Mental health problems in women are prevalent and determined by many factors including structural factors and circumstances of day-to-day life, and by gender-based risks. They are associated with significant disability and reduced quality of life and capacity to participate. The burden and determinants of mental ill-health in women differ consistently from those experienced by men. Non-psychotic 'common mental disorders', for example, depressive, anxiety, adjustment, and somatoform disorders, are more prevalent among women than men [23].

Overall, in all countries, women are more likely than men to be poor and less able to influence personal or household financial decision-making. They are more likely to experience violence and coercion from an intimate partner or other family member. Women are also less likely to have access to the protective factors of full participation in education, paid employment and political decision-making [19]. Girls and women face discrimination in many settings. These include female feticide, preference for male children leading to lower survival and worse nutritional status and health in young girls, female genital mutilation, no or limited education for females, restrictions on income generating activities, and adolescent marriage [29]. Gender disparities in opportunities, responsibilities, and roles throughout the life course have consequences for all aspects of health, including mental health [23].

Violence against women and children and its consequences for mental health is probably the most pressing priority for women's mental health. Violence damages the capacity to respond to stress and predisposes to mental and physical illnesses [40]. Exposure to childhood sexual abuse is a risk factor for mental health problems later in life. Gender-based violence occurs in all societies but especially in cultures in which women have low status, their roles are restricted and their rights are not respected. Violence in intimate relationships is experienced much more commonly by women than by men and is a clear predictor of depression, anxiety, suicidal ideas and substance abuse [23]. This violence is associated with perinatal mental health problems as well as other mental health and health problems.

Perinatal mental disorders are highly prevalent worldwide, and depression is the most common and best recognized of these. These disorders cause suffering and economic and social problems for women and their families and communities. The growing recognition of the salience of these problems for countries of all types is described in a recent Lancet series on this topic [26]. These conditions are associated with increased risk of adverse health and development outcomes for children especially in socioeconomically disadvantaged populations and low-income countries. In some countries for instance infant stunting and underweight are associated with depression in mothers. However, these adverse consequences are not inevitable. The most important strategies to address these problems include: assessment of the local community needs and the social determinants of the mental health of young mothers including emotional, physical, and sexual violence perpetrated by an intimate partner [26].

Empowerment of women is important in various parts of the world in which this has yet to be achieved. Financial and emotional dependence as well as restrictions in education are important factors that limit their choices in life and have an impact on their mental health [37].

Women's education and empowerment in turn way lead to better mental health prospects in women [28, 34].

A cross-sectoral response to mental health promotion in women is crucial, especially for those facing adversity in low and lower middle income countries. Addressing social causes of mental health problems through the realization of girls' and women's human rights to education, nutrition, health care, equal social, and economic participation, safety, individual autonomy, and freedom from discrimination is an essential first step. In the health sector, gender-sensitive and evidence-informed strategies for prevention, early intervention and treatment are required. Gender-informed clinical and public health research is needed to provide local evidence and monitor and evaluate interventions. Research and advocacy for these strategies by mental health workers can be powerful sources of empowerment for women [23].

22.4.8 Men

Especially in Eastern European countries, it is men that seem to have suffered most prominently during the heavy societal transition of the last decade. This transition has resulted not only in depression, aggression, violence, high numbers of suicide, self-destructive life styles, homicides, and accidents, but also in somatic pathology like cardio and cerebrovascular morbidity and mortality [43]. Men are in need of gender-specific, individualized, and person-centered approaches because they often adopt noncompliance and non-help-seeking behavior patterns.

Suicidality in men has been dealt with extensively by Rutz and Rihmer [44] and the need for understanding, communication, and social interaction between genders as strong health promotion actions is underlined.

22.4.9 Migrants

Mental health promotion in this high-risk group of people is of great importance, especially when migration is forced as is the case with migration occurring as a consequence of war in one's country of origin [8]. Of special importance is the group of people who have failed to adjust to their new environment and have to return to their country of origin.

Value changes, the secularized questioning of religious and moral values and value migration together with identity losses are among the main factors that burden immigrants [43].

22.4.10 Lesbian, Gay, Bisexual, and Transgender Individuals (LGBT Group)

Stigma and discrimination are particularly pronounced in this group and this may produce a variety of stresses that contribute to psychopathology. Taking suicidal ideation and actual suicide as an example, we note that individuals who belong to the sexual minorities have three times higher rates than those of heterosexual subjects [41]. This calls for mental health promotion, especially in view of the fact that LGBT people may not seek professional help fearing that their sexual identity will be revealed. Additionally, there is lack of mental health professionals who have been trained in treatment and health promotion of LGBT persons. The resistances and psychodynamics of heterosexual therapists constitute handicaps and LGBT therapists are perhaps preferable.

22.4.11 Other Categories

Other categories of people needing person and people-centered mental health promotion efforts are the victims of natural and man-made disasters [18] persons with job insecurity and debts, people in situations where there are inbalances between responsibility and influence leading to defects in participation [43] people who are overworked [57] and people who suffer during economic crises and are at risk of developing depression and exacerbation of preexisting psychopathology, or even just experiencing normal and adaptive but also painful sadness [17].

22.5 Health Resources

Health resources like optimism, resilience, coping competences, social support or access to health care may serve as "resistance resources" [2] against stressful events.

However, some resources with originally positive function for the person may either promote or restrain health [49] depending on the circumstances and the recipient. For example social support may have a negative effect on well-being and health if it is provided to a person with low self-esteem [47]. It is therefore important to provide person-centered and individually tailored care.

22.6 Mental Health Promotion Initiatives

As is the case in Prevention, in Mental Health Promotion also, interventions can be categorized in **Universal** (pertaining to the whole population) **Selected** (targeted to vulnerable groups) and **Indicated** (addressed to high-risk groups or persons).

The aim of promotion is to improve the ability of people to function well, adapt to new circumstances (that are new or are perceived as new), manage to relate to people (and thus function well in family and social settings) and succeed in deriving pleasure from life.

Interventions range from social and community interventions (that usually require collaboration with government or community authorities) to individual-level interventions (aiming at change of attitudes toward more healthy living) [9, 11, 12].

Kalra et al. [28] have summarized the suggested ways forward as follows: Identifying and setting priorities, improving the social ties, developing healthy habits and lifestyle, increasing mental health education and awareness, respecting cultural diversity, implementing school mental health programs.

Within the above framework it is important to first identify the needs of the population and set priorities [27]. Citizen participation should be encouraged. Non-profit organizations and advocacy groups (like the World Federation for Mental Health and other organizations) have an important role to play. The use of celebrities as brand ambassadors has been helpful in some cultures.

Social ties and strengthening of the social capital are important in mental health promotion. Family, friends, social clubs, special interest and mutual support groups etc. may serve as shock-absorbers against stressful situations arising from significant life events but even against minor stresses of everyday life. This is particularly true when it refers to ethnically congruent groups in multi-ethnic societies.

It is interesting that a National Jewish Population survey (2000–2001) has shown that social ties were associated with better self-rated health [48].

Is lifestyle important in health promotion? Yes, if lifestyle involves use of drugs and alcohol, risk-taking behavior, unhealthy habits like overeating, armchair TV immobility, or defensive avoidance of social interaction it can play a very negative role. On the contrary, if lifestyle involves physical activity, building social capital through group recreational activities and promoting spirituality one is likely to benefit. However, it should be stressed again that all these activities should be tailored to satisfy the needs and preferences of each individual. The idea should be to cope with life stresses—not create new ones by forcing people to be involved in activities they dislike.

Increasing mental health literacy and awareness can be an important part of mental health promotion. Collaboration with media (TV, radio, and newspapers) and mental health education of journalists is of value in these cases. Use of the internet for health promotion purposes is proving to be more and more popular.

A paradigmatic program of mental health promotion along these lines, aiming at increasing mental health awareness of not only journalists but also educators, judges, police and army officers, general practitioners, priests, etc. has been carried out at Athens University Department of Psychiatry in collaboration with the Hellenic Psychiatric Association and the Society of Preventive Psychiatry [50]. The program lasted 18 months and was based on the "radiation" effect (training of trainers). It was continued for several years after its original implementation.

A successful example of campaigns to increase mental health awareness is the Defend Depression Campaign of the Royal College of Psychiatrists and the Royal College of General Practitioners from 1992 to 1996 [38]. In view of the low level of mental health awareness in the general public, efforts like these are worth pursuing. A transient improvement of depressive symptoms has been observed following a mental health literacy intervention in older adults [56].

Collaboration of mental health providers with school authorities in mental health programs has given positive results [20] and in some schools (e.g., Athens College in Greece) there are permanent positions of psychologists for screening, follow up, advice and counseling. Training adolescents in coping strategies to effectively deal with stress can be very helpful in the long run.

In dealing with all the above it is important to respect cultural diversity. Even countries which up to recently existed within a "pure" cultural and religious framework have started developing into multiethnic and multicultural countries due to globalization and migration. This calls for special, urgent, and intensive mental health promotion strategies, aiming at provision of equitable and dignified services to all people in need of help but especially those who are discriminated upon and are consequently more vulnerable to the development of psychopathology.

22.6.1 Effectiveness and Sustainability

Mental health promotion projects, as is the case with all interventions in Medicine and Psychiatry, must prove their effectiveness. The Taskforce on Evidence of the European Commission Mental Health Working Party [27] has stated that evidence of effectiveness is a condition for making a case for investment in mental health.

In mental health promotion programs, sustainability of the programs, e.g., continued availability of resources, is essential. This is one of the most valuable recommendations made in the Summary Report of the WHO [54].

22.7 Public Health Perspective

As mentioned earlier, the person-centered perspective in mental health is applicable not only in the singular but also in the plural as people-centered perspective. Under this light, Public Health has a very important role to play in Person-centered Mental Health Promotion. Furthermore, as explained earlier, mental health promotion is not so much the result of the work of mental health professionals but more so the consequence of general measures. Under this perspective, the involvement of public health in person-centered mental health promotion is not only legitimate but also strongly recommended.

Individual health is interrelated with public health as exemplified by the relationship of societal stress and premature mortality [42]. Therefore, the aggregate level is very important in promoting person-centered health.

It has been argued that the relevance of people-centered mental health promotion is particularly marked in societies in transition (e.g., in some societies in Eastern Europe) where stress-related morbidity and mortality due to depression, suicide, violence, abuse, homicide, risk-taking lifestyles, etc. has been observed [42].

Political action is a neglected area in mental health promotion and mental health professionals are very reluctant to point out to decision-makers the value of, for example, investment in mental health.

The interdisciplinary perspective and the involvement of service users and carers are important in shaping a useful strategy in people-centered mental health promotion.

22.8 Mental Health Promotion Guidance

A basic principle to follow with reference to guidance is to decide to whom the guidance is addressed. The socioeconomic situation in each country, the degree of mental health development, the mental health literacy and the priorities in each country are among the parameters to be taken into consideration.

A point to remember is that mental health promotion is not the business of mental health professionals only, but "everybody's" business [24]. Direct professional interventions are probably of lesser importance than general political, administrative, social, educational and cultural interventions that can affect mental health indirectly as a "side benefit." For example, promotion of mental hygiene or encouragement of children of immigrants to go to school can have an important indirect benefit.

Guidance should be based on evidence. As pointed out earlier, without evidence of effectiveness it is difficult to make a case for investment in mental health [27].

Informed decision-making processes for the implementation of mental health promotion can be facilitated by relevant literature (e.g., a booklet produced by the European Commission Mental Health Working Party [27], a review by Christodoulou et al. [15]) and advice on how mental health promotion programs must be implemented for the best outcome is provided by Barry and Jenkins [5].

A World Health Organization report [24] has identified certain areas in which there is evidence that mental health promotion programs are effective. These include preschool psychosocial interventions, empowerment of women (access to education) support for the elderly, support for vulnerable groups (minorities, prisoners, indigenous people, migrants, people affected by conflicts and disasters) mental health promotion in schools and at work, in prisons, orphanages and hospitals, community development programs and debt management and financial exclusion programs. Most of the published evidence is derived from high-income countries. Evidence for the scaling up and sustainability of mental health promotion interventions in low- and middle-income countries needs to be strengthened. Mental health in scarce-resource settings has received more attention in the new millennium, with special notice of the health-promoting effects of broader development interventions [39]. A systematic review of the effectiveness of mental health promotion interventions for young people in low-and middle-income countries was conducted recently [6]. Interventions promoting the mental health of young people can be implemented effectively in school and community settings with moderate to strong evidence of their impact on both positive and negative mental health outcomes. There is a paucity of evidence relating to interventions for younger children in primary schools in these countries.

Sustainability of programs, like continued availability of resources is stressed in the above reports. Such is also the case with reference to all mental health-related activities. Sometimes it is preferable to refrain from initiating a program if the diachronic component (mainly financial consistency) can not be guaranteed [13].

22.9 Concluding Remarks

Person-centered mental health promotion programs are particularly relevant in our current transitional times that are characterized by uniformity and globalization, dehumanization, profit maximalization, consumerism, and social behavior reminiscent of borderline personality dysfunction.

The aim of our efforts should be to transfer the person-centered humanistic, holistic and dignity-promoting approach into mental health promotion salutogenic strategies that will promote the mental health of not only the persons who suffer from mental illness but also those who are more vulnerable to stress and other nosogenic factors and are therefore more prone to develop mental illness.

Collaboration with the Government authorities in trying to achieve this is essential and the language that should be used is the one that politicians understand, namely cost/effectiveness. There is, fortunately, increasing evidence indicating that mental health treatment, prevention and promotion in the long-run are cost/effective. It is our duty as mental health professionals and advocates to bring this evidence to the attention of decision-makers and the public.

References

1. Ammon G. Schizophrenie. In: Ammon G, editor. Handbuch der Dynamischen Psychiatrie, Band 1, München, Ernst Reinhardt; 1979.
2. Antonovsky A. Unraveling the mystery of health. How people manage stress and stay well. San Francisco: Jossey-Bass; 1987.
3. Antonovsky A. The salutogenetic model as theory to guide health promotion. Health Promot Int. 1996;2:11–8.
4. Awofeso N. Re-defining "Health". Commentary on editorial by Üstün and Jacob. Bull World Health Organ. 2005. Available at www.who.int/bulletin/bulletin_board/83/ustun11051/en/. 2010;83:802.
5. Barry M, Jenkins R. Implementing mental health promotion. London: Elsevier; 2007. p. 1–355.
6. Barry MM, Clarke AL, Jenkins R, Patel V. A systematic review of the effectiveness of mental health promotion interventions for young people in low and middle income countries. BMC Public Health 2013, 13:835.
7. Beddington J, Cooper L, Field J, et al. The mental wealth of nations. Nature. 2008;455:1057–60.

8. Bhugra D, Gupta S. Migration and mental health. 1st ed. New York: Cambridge University Press; 2011.
9. Christodoulou GN. Aspects of preventive psychiatry. Basel: Karger; 1981.
10. Christodoulou GN, Kontaxakis VP. Topics in preventive psychiatry. Basel: Karger; 1994.
11. Christodoulou GN, Lykouras LP, Mountokalakis T, Voulgari A, Stefanis CN. Personality characteristics of psychiatric trainees. In: Christodoulou GN, Kontaxakis VP, editors. Topics in preventive psychiatry. Basel: Karger; 1994. p. 137–42.
12. Christodoulou GN, Lecic-Tosevski D, Kontaxakis VP. Issues in preventive psychiatry. Basel: Karger; 1999.
13. Christodoulou GN. Psychiatric reform revisited. World Psychiatry. 2009;8:121–2.
14. Christodoulou GN, Ploumpidis D, Christodoulou N, Anagnostopoulos D. Mental health profile of Greece. Int Psychiatry. 2010;7:64–7.
15. Christodoulou GN, Jenkins R, Tsipas V, Christodoulou NG, Lecic-Tosevski D, Mezzich JE. Mental health promotion—a conceptual review and guidance. European Psychiatr Rev. 2011;4:9–14.
16. Christodoulou GN, Christodoulou NG. Mental health promotion: concept and practice. Int J Pers-cente Med. 2012;2:24–8.
17. Christodoulou NG, Christodoulou GN. Financial crises: impact on mental health and suggested responses. Psychother Psychosom. 2013;82:279–84.
18. Christodoulou GN, Mezzich JE, Christodoulou NG, Lecic-Tosevski D. Disasters: mental health context and responses. Cambridge Scholars Publishing (in press); 2016.
19. CSDH. Closing the gap in a generation: health equity through action on the social determinants of health. Final report of the commission on social determinants of health. Geneva: World Health Organization; 2008.
20. DeSocio J, Stember L, Schrinsky J. Teaching children about mental health and illness: a school nurse health education program. J Sch Nurs. 2006;22:81–6.
21. Dolfman M. The concept of health: an historic and analytic examination. J Sch Health. 1973;43:491–7.
22. Fillit HM, Butler RN, O'Connell AW, Albert MS, Birren JE, Cotman CW, et al. Achieving and maintaining cognitive vitality with aging. Mayo Clin Proc. 2002;77:681–96.
23. Fisher J, Herrman H, Cabral de Mello M, Chandra P. Women's mental health. In: Patel V, Minas H, Cohen A, Prince M, editors. Global mental health. USA, New York: Oxford University Press; 2013. p. 354–84.
24. Herrman H, Saxena S, Moodie R, editors. Promoting mental health: concepts, emerging evidence, practice. A report from the World Health Organization Department of Mental Health and Substance Abuse in collaboration with the Victorian Health Promotion Foundation (VicHealth) and the University of Melbourne. Geneva: WHO; 2005.
25. Hippocrates. The Hippocratic Oath. Translated by Michael North, National Library of Medicine. In: Christodoulou GN, Ploumpidis DN, Karavatos A, editors. Anthology of greek psychiatric texts. Athens: Beta Publishers; 2011. p. 3–4.
26. Howard LM, Piot P, Stein A. No health without perinatal mental health. Lancet. 2014;384:1723–4.
27. Jané-Llopis E, Katschnig H, McDaid D, Wahlbeck K. Commissioning, interpreting and making use of evidence on mental health promotion and mental disorder prevention: an everyday primer. Lisbon. 2007.
28. Kalra G, Christodoulou GN, Jenkins R, Tsipas V, Christodoulou NG, Lecic-Tosevski D, Mezzich J, Bhugra D. Mental health promotion: guidance and strategies. European Psychiatry. 2012;27:81–6.
29. Kastrup M, Niaz U. The impact of culture on women's mental health. In: Chandra PS, Herrman H, Fisher J, Kastrup M, Niaz U, Rondón MB, et al., editors. Contemporary topics in women's mental health: global perspectives in a changing society. John Wiley & Sons Ltd: Chichester, West Sussex; 2009. p. 463–84.

30. Kovess-Masfety V, Murray M, Gureje O. Evolution of our understanding of positive mental health. In: Herrman H, Saxena S, Moodie R, editors. Promoting mental health: concepts, emerging evidence, practice. Geneva: WHO; 2005. p. 35–46.
31. Lahtinen E, et al. Framework for promoting mental health in Europe. Hamina, (STAKES). Finland: National Research and Development Centre for Welfare and Health, Ministry of Social Affairs and Health; 1999.
32. Lecic-Tosevski D, Pejovic-Milovancevic M, Tenjovic L, Draganic-Gajic S, Christodoulou GN. Personality characteristics of psychiatric trainees. Psychother Psychosom. 2005;74(2): 129–30.
33. Mezzich JE. Psychiatry for the person: articulating medicine's science and humanism. World Psychiatry. 2007;6:65–7.
34. Mrazek P, Haggerty R. Reducing risks of mental disorder: frontiers for preventive intervention research. Washington: National Academy Press; 1994.
35. Naidoo J, Wills J. Health promotion: foundations for practice. Edinburgh: Harcourt Publishers; 2000.
36. National Health and Medical Research Council. Promoting the health of indigenous Australians. A review of infrastructure support for Aboriginal and Torres Strait Islander health advancement. Final report and recommendations, vol. 2(4). Canberra: NHMRC; 1996.
37. Niaz U, Hassan S. Culture and mental health of women in South-East Asia. World Psychiatry. 2006;5:118–20.
38. Paykel ES, Hart D, Priest RG. Changes in public attitudes to depression during the defeat depression campaign. Br J Psychiatry. 1998;173:519–22.
39. Petersen I, Bhana A, Flisher AJ, Swartz L, Richter L, editors. Promoting mental health in scarce-resource contexts: emerging evidence and practice. South Africa: HSRC Press; 2010.
40. Rondon M. Priority issues in women's mental health. World Psychiatry. 2013;12:275–6.
41. Rotheram-Borus M, Reid H, Rosario M, Van Rossen R, Gills R. Prevalence, course and predictors of multiple problem behaviors among gay and bisexual male adolescents. Dev Psychol. 1995;31:75–85.
42. Rutz W, Richmer Z. Suicidality in men—practical issues, challenges, solutions. J Men's Health Gender. 2007;4:393–401.
43. Rutz W. Reflections on public health: principles for a person-centered promotion of mental and physical health. Intern. J. Pers-cente Med. 2011;1:435–9.
44. Rutz W. Person-centered public health promotion: an overview and a plea. Int J Pers-cente Med. 2012;2:306–9.
45. Saracci R. The World Health Organization needs to reconsider its definition of health. BMJ. 1997;314:1409–10.
46. Schmolke M. Health promotion and multi-modal research perspectives. Dyn Psychiatry. 2003;36:254–71.
47. Schulte-Cloos C, Baisch A. Lebenskraft-Ressourcen im Umgang mit Belastungen und was Helfer dazu meinen. Verhaltenstherapie und Psychozoziale Praxis. 1996;28:421–40.
48. Simkin DR. Adolescent substance use disorders and comorbidity. Pediatr Clin North Am. 2002;49:463–77.
49. Straus F, Höfer R. Kohärenzgefühl soziale Ressourcen und Gesundheit. In: Wydler H, Kolip P, Abel T, editors. Salutogenese und Kohärenzgefühl. Grundlagen, Empirie und Praxis eines gesundheitswissenschaftlichen Konzepts. Weinheim: Juventa; 2000. p. 115–128.
50. Vassiliadou MS. Athens mental health promotion programme. In: Saxena Shekhar, Garrison Preston, editors. Mental health promotion. Case studies from Countries: WHO; 2004. p. 41–3.
51. Walker JG, Mackinnon AJ, Batterham P, Jorm AF, Hickie I, McCarthy A, et al. Mental health literacy, folic acid and vitamin B12, and physical activity for the prevention of depression in older adults: randomized controlled trial. Br J Psychiatry. 2010;197:45–54.
52. Warr P. A conceptual framework for the study of work and mental health. Work & Stress. 1994;8:84–97.

53. WHO. Preamble to the Constitution of the WHO (entered into force on 7 April 1948), vol. 2. Geneva: WHO; 1948. p. 100.
54. WHO. Health promotion glossary. Geneva: World Health Organization; 1998.
55. WHO. Strengthening mental health promotion. 1999. Fact Sheet No 220, April 1999, revised Nov. 2001.
56. WHO. Promoting mental health: concepts, emerging evidence, practice, summary report. Geneva; 2004.
57. WHOQOL Group. The World Health Organization Quality of Life Assessment (WHOQOL): position paper from the World Health Organization. Soc Sci Med. 1995;41:1403–9.
58. World Federation for Mental Health. World Mental Health Day (Mental Health and Chronic Physical Illness); 2010. Available at: www.wfmh.org.

Part IV
Person-Centered Care for People with Specific Mental Conditions

Dementia

23

Dawn J. Brooker, PhD and Jon Snaedal, MD

23.1 The Challenge of Dementia

It is estimated that there are 35.6 million people living with dementia worldwide. This is set to increase to 65.7 million by 2030 and 115.4 million by 2050. Nearly two-thirds live in low and middle income countries, where the biggest increases will occur during this time period [65]. In the UK, the number of people with dementia is estimated to be 820,000, with a cost to services of £23 billion per annum. This is more than costs for cancer (£12 billion per year) and heart disease (£8 billion per year) combined [2].

We describe dementia as being present when a person is experiencing significant changes in their cognitive functioning, for example changes in memory, finding words, recognising objects, carrying out practical tasks or making considered judgements. For a person to have dementia more than one of these problems needs to be present and they have to be sufficiently severe to have an impact of the person's life. The underlying cause of these changes is one of a number of processes that affect the health of the person's brain. There are many causes of dementia, with the most common being Alzheimer's Type Dementia, Vascular Dementia, Dementia with Lewy Bodies; Parkinson's Dementia and Fronto-temporal dementias. The disease course varies according to sub-type and concomitant health status but in general there is a slow progressive decline in cognition and functioning over a period of years through to the point where individuals are unable to survive without a very high level of personal support.

D.J. Brooker, PhD (✉)
Professor, Association for Dementia Studies, University of Worcester, St Johns Campus, Worcester WR2 6AJ, UK
e-mail: d.brooker@worc.ac.uk

J. Snaedal, MD
Professor of Geriatric Medicine, Landspitali University Hospital, Reykjavik, Iceland

J.E. Mezzich et al. (eds.), *Person Centered Psychiatry*,
DOI 10.1007/978-3-319-39724-5_23

Maintaining good physical health and well-being for people with dementia is also a challenge. When someone has the label of dementia, there is a tendency for family carers, care staff and professionals to attribute any increase in confused behaviour to the dementia. However, people with dementia are also much more susceptible to acute confusional states and delirium arising from physical health problems such as urinary or chest infections, constipation, hormonal imbalances, dehydration, malnutrition, overmedication and sedation. This is compounded further by the fact that many people with dementia will not be able to give an accurate account of their symptoms because of their memory and communication difficulties.

Pharmacological treatments have been used to try to improve the functioning of the person with dementia, or to reduce distressing symptoms. This is an area of pharmacology which has changed rapidly over the past few years and it continues to change. Currently, there is no pharmacological treatment that can convincingly alter the course of the underlying disease processes.

Behavioural and Psychological Symptoms of Dementia (BPSD) is a term that is used to describe many of the common problems that people living with dementia face. Anxiety, depressed mood, vocalisations, hallucinations, restlessness, delusions, agitation, wandering, sexual disinhibition and hoarding are cited under this heading. These are the types of behaviour listed on the Neuro Psychiatric Inventory (NPI) and sometimes also called neuropsychiatric symptoms, challenging behaviours or distress behaviours.

These problems are seen as secondary and arising out of the cognitive impairments in memory, language, perception and planning that are the primary signs of dementia [59]. The term is contentious in some circles as it can give the impression that these are an inevitable consequence of dementia. Nonetheless, it is these symptoms that often trigger admission to care homes and hospital and are highly distressing for people living with dementia, their families and the staff who support them. These are the problems that often lead to people being prescribed anti-psychotic medication or being physically restrained or sedated.

The use of pharmacological treatments such as anti-psychotics to treat BPSD is contentious. Anti-psychotics were developed for treating severe mental illness such as schizophrenia and most have very little evidence to support their use in dementia but in spite of that, we have seen extensive use of this medication in treating BPSD symptoms. Excess sedation, falls, symptoms like Parkinson's disease and an increased risk of stroke may all occur as side effects of these medications. There has been so much concern about these that both clinicians and professional groups have called for a dramatic reduction in their use in dementia care [3, 7].

Although BPSD is common there is no suggestion that there is a single underlying cause for this syndrome [48]. For example, there can be a multiplicity of reasons why someone with dementia might exhibit aggressive behaviour or agitation. Agitation may be a reaction to pain caused by an underlying physical problem; poor communication on the part of care staff; or a misperception caused by the person's cognitive impairment. It could even involve all three of these causes. In order to understand why these problems occur, or to ensure we deliver services in a way that makes their manifestation unlikely, we need to see the person and their life as a whole. We need to understand the importance of underlying causes on an individual basis [27].

The majority of BPSD's are the result of untreated delirium, untreated pain, lack of understanding of cognitive capacity, poor nutrition and hydration, poor communication, lack of knowledge about the person's history, poor general care, boredom and unmet emotional needs. Many of these problems occur through lack of understanding of what it is like to be a person living with dementia. This understanding does not happen automatically. There is often a gap in the experience between those living with dementia and those providing care and support. This gap widens as the dementia progresses. Professionals seek to "manage" behaviour without really understanding why it is occurring.

This is the arena in which skilled care really counts and really makes a difference. By understanding why the behaviour is occurring and by providing supportive interactions where people are met with warmth, inclusion, respect and empathy people will feel less confused, and more relaxed, socially confident and joyful. This will directly reverse or decrease BPSD. This does not mean that the dementia has gone away BUT it does mean that the person feels less like they are losing their mind.

23.2 Tom Kitwood, Personhood and Person-Centred Approaches in Dementia Care

It has been over 20 years since the late Professor Tom Kitwood first used the term person-centred approaches in relation to the long-term care for people living with dementia. In an attempt to move away from a reductionist medical model, the term was first used to bring together ideas and ways of working that emphasised communication and relationships. The term was intended to be a direct reference to Rogerian psychotherapy with its emphasis on authentic contact and communication. Kitwood's work was part of the ground swell of psychosocial approaches to dementia care that came into being during the 1980s and 1990s. Writing throughout this period, Kitwood published a continuous stream of articles in prominent journals during the 1980s and 1990s [35, 36, 37, 38, 39, 40, 41, 42, 43, 46]. He brought these ideas together in his most well-known book *Dementia reconsidered: The person comes first* [44]. For a critical analysis the reader is directed to Baldwin and Capstick [5].

Kitwood focussed on the maintenance of personhood as being central to person-centred care. He defined personhood as:

> A standing or status that is bestowed upon one human being, by others, in the context of relationship and social being. It implies recognition, respect and trust [44, p. 8].

Kitwood identified the primary outcome of person-centred care for people with dementia as maintaining their personhood in the face of declining mental powers. There is an assumption here that people with dementia have the capacity to experience relative well-being and ill-being and that their behaviour has meaning. According to Kitwood, high levels of challenging behaviour, distress or apathy occur more commonly in care situations that are not supportive of personhood. In care environments that are supportive of personhood, we expect to see a greater preponderance of well-being and social confidence. Kitwood's view of person-centred care for people with dementia was that it took place in the context of relationships. His theorised that as verbal abilities are lost, the importance of warm, accepting human contact through non-verbal channels become even more important than before. With the onset of dementia individuals are very vulnerable to their psychological defences being radically attacked and broken down. As the sense of self breaks down, it becomes increasingly important that the sense of self is held within the relationships that the person with dementia experiences. These relationships are a key part of the social psychological milieu. He described personhood as being undermined when individual needs and rights are not considered, when powerful negative emotions are ignored or invalidated and when increasing isolation from human relationships occurs.

Kitwood described the various common ways that he had observed personhood being undermined in care settings, coining the phrase *Malignant Social Psychology (MSP)* as an umbrella term. MSP includes episodes where people are intimidated, outpaced, not responded to, infantilised, labelled, disparaged, blamed, manipulated, invalidated, disempowered, overpowered, disrupted, objectified, stigmatised, ignored, banished and mocked. Kitwood was at pains to say that episodes of MSP are very rarely done with any malicious intent. Rather, episodes of MSP become interwoven into the care culture.

New staff members learn how to communicate with people with dementia from existing staff. If the staff communication style is one that is characterised by the infantilisation and outpacing of people with dementia, then the new member of staff is likely to follow their lead. The malignancy in MSP is that it eats away at the personhood of those being cared for and it also spreads from one member of staff to another very quickly. Kitwood also described what a positive social psychology might look like for people with dementia. Much can be done to ensure that the social milieu is generally supportive of the needs of people with dementia. If personhood is undermined by MSP then it should also be possible to describe the sorts of everyday interactions that would promote the maintenance of personhood. He used the term *Positive Person Work* to describe ten different forms of interaction that would maintain personhood. These included recognition, negotiation, collaboration, play, timalation (engagement through the senses), celebration, relaxation, validation, holding and facilitation.

Kitwood and colleagues developed dementia care mapping (DCM) [45] as an observational tool that has been used in formal dementia care settings such as hospital wards, care homes and day care facilities since 1991. Kitwood described DCM as:

> a serious attempt to take the standpoint of the person with dementia, using a combination of empathy and observational skill [44] p 4

The DCM tool is only available by undertaking a course delivered by licensed trainers using standardised training methods and has been through a number of iterations [16]. DCM has been translated into many languages and training in DCM adheres to international quality standards [9].

23.3 From Person-Centred Care to Citizenship

Since Kitwood's early writing there has been a significant change in how people with dementia are treated in their relation to being active agents in their own lives. The right to be aware of diagnosis and treatment options has come to the forefront [15]. The recognition that the voice of the person with dementia needs to be heard directly in shaping and developing services, has become an accepted way of working [1]. More and more direct accounts of what it is like to live with dementia are available [17] and public figures who have been diagnosed with dementia are talking about their experiences. Self-advocacy groups are becoming more prominent in the Alzheimer charities. It is still relatively novel to see the rights of people with dementia expressed in terms of citizenship and as active agents in their own right. However, this is now starting to emerge in a number of countries worldwide [32]. Even in long-term care facilities, where people have significant cognitive impairments, their voice is now frequently heard in qualitative research reflecting directly on their perspective [31]. Citizenship tends to be linked with individuals acting in their own right which may not be strictly helpful as a model in severe dementia. Nonetheless, the recognition of sociological factors in how people with dementia are viewed in society is important to consider [8].

23.4 The VIPS Framework for Person-Centred Dementia Care

In the years since Kitwood first described it, person-centred dementia care practice has come to mean different things to different people in different contexts and in different countries. The concepts in person-centred care are not easy to articulate in a straightforward manner [50]. In an earlier review of definitions of person-centred care [11] it was noted that PCC was being interpreted as meaning individualised care, and the emphasis on relationships that Kitwood promoted has been lost. Recent analysis of policy documents revealed that the narrative about person-centredness at this level often emphasised a consumerist as opposed to a psychosocial approach [57]. Indeed, the concept of relationship centred care has emerged as a counter to this emphasis on the individual [56].

The VIPS definition of person-centred care was an attempt to synthesise these different threads of person-centred care whilst maintaining the sophistication of Kitwood's original work. Put simply, the VIPS definition of person-centred care encompasses:

V A **value** base that asserts the absolute value of all human lives
I An **individualised** approach, recognising uniqueness
P Understanding the world from the **perspective** of the person living with dementia
S Promotion of a positive **social psychology** in which the person living with dementia can experience relative well-being.

This can be summarised in the equation PCC (person-centred care) = V + I + P + S.

This equation does not give a pre-eminence of any element over another, just that they are all contributory. The VIPS definition was used in the English NICE/SCIE Guideline on Dementia [55] which defined the principles of person-centred care as asserting:

- The human value of people with dementia, regardless of age or cognitive impairment, and those who care for them;
- The individuality of people with dementia, with their unique personality and life experiences among the influences on their response to the dementia;
- The importance of the perspective of the person with dementia;
- The importance of relationships and interactions with others to the person with dementia, and their potential for promoting well-being.

The VIPS elements can be used as guiding principles for health care practitioners to reflect on their interactions with people with dementia and their families. Reflective questions include:

- Does my behaviour and the manner in which I am communicating with this person show that I respect, value, and honour them?
- Am I treating this person as a unique individual with a history and a wide range of strengths and needs?
- Am I making a serious attempt to see my actions from the perspective of the person I am trying to help? How might my actions be interpreted by this person?
- Does my behaviour and interactions help this person to feel socially confident and that they are not alone?

These principles apply in every situation where direct communication occurs. They apply when we are undertaking any health or social care intervention, such as giving someone an injection, helping them to use the toilet, assisting them to complete an advanced care plan or running a reminiscence group. It is not the task that is person-centred but the way in which that task is done that can make it person-centred or not.

This definition was used as the structure for the evidence base for good practice in person-centred care dementia care [12]. This provided a set of concrete indicators that care providers could bench mark their services against. Pilot indicators were reviewed by around 50 care providers and service user organisations worldwide to arrive at a detailed description of what a person-centred care provider should have in place. This list of 24 indicators is grouped around the four elements of the definition set out above has become known as the VIPS framework [13]. It has been taken up by many English speaking care providers and the concepts have been translated into German, Japanese, Spanish and Norwegian.

The 24 indicators set out below provide a checklist that care providers can use as a benchmark to assess the person-centredness of their service.

V—Does this service actively show that we value and respect for the experiences of people with dementia and their families?

1. Is the service actively welcoming to people with dementia and their families?
2. Is the service valuing of good quality direct care for people with dementia and their families? Do we have a management ethos that fosters the best direct care?
3. Are staff empowered to act in the best interests of people with dementia and their families? Do we have a management ethos that empowers staff to act in this way?
4. Is the workforce skilled in person-centred dementia care at all levels from frontline to leaders?
5. Generally are the physical and social service environments designed to be easy for people with dementia and their families to use?
6. Does the service know about and act upon the needs and concerns of people with dementia and their families?

I—Are systems in place to enable staff to get to know the person, to provide continuity of care and to ensure the person feels like a unique individual?

1. Do staff know each person's strengths and needs across physical, social and psychological domains?
2. Are staff alert to changes in these strengths and needs over time?
3. Do staff know what personal possessions and relationships that are important to each person to help them feel calm?
4. Do staff know each person's likes and dislikes and preferred everyday routines and are these utilised in everyday care?
5. Do staff know each person's history and key stories and are these utilised in every-day care?
6. Do staff know how to engage each person in enjoyable activities?

P—Do we take time to understand the Perspective of the person with dementia and their family?

1. Do staff check out preferences, consent and opinions using verbal and non-verbal means?
2. Can staff empathise with how each person is feeling and show this in their everyday care?

3. Do staff regularly ensure that the physical environment is as comfortable as possible for each person?
4. Are staff vigilant about physical health needs that the person may not be able to tell them about directly?
5. If the person is showing "challenging behaviour" do staff try to understand why and what the person may be trying to communicate?
6. Do staff treat the rights of the individual with dementia as important as the rights of other people?

S—Are we providing a Supportive Social Psychology to enable the person with dementia to feel socially confident and that they are not alone?

1. Do staff help the person feel included and not "talked across"?
2. Do staff treat each person respectfully and not use a "telling-off" tone or derogatory labels to describe people?
3. Do staff come across as warm and caring and not cold and indifferent?
4. Do people know that staff take their fears seriously and that they won't be left alone for long periods in emotional distress?
5. Do staff help people to be active in their own care and activity as far as possible and not just do things to people without communicating with them?
6. Do staff facilitate to help the person keep important relationships and make sure that they stay in touch with people and activities they value?

Person-centred care requires sign-up to working in this way across the whole care provider organisation if it is to be sustained over any length of time. Particular elements require leadership at different levels.

Valuing; requires leadership from those responsible for leading the organisation at a senior level.

Individual Care; requires leadership particularly from those responsible for setting care standards and procedures within the organisation.

Perspectives and Social Environment; requires leadership for those responsible for the day-to-day management and direct provision of care.

This framework enables care providers to break down the complexities of person-centred care into achievable steps. We have used it as part of our education courses for developing specialist practice in dementia care with over a 1000 participants to date. Initially, course participants rate their service on each of the 24 indicators (using a simple scale of Excellent, Good, OK, Needs more work) in order to provide a profile of where they are doing well and what they need to improve upon. We then ask them to discuss this assessment with a variety of staff working at different levels within the organisation and with service users and carers where possible. Out of these discussions the managers and leaders learn a lot about the person-centredness of their organisation. As part of the education programme we then ask them to choose one or two areas that they have the ability and resources to work on to improve the quality of person-centred care. The framework has worked very well and led to sustained changes in practice.

The VIPS framework also underpins the Care fit for VIPS website. This is a free website www.carefitforvips.co.uk initially aimed at decreasing anti-psychotic use in care homes. Versions are also available for domiciliary care, day care and housing. It is also widely used by hospital and health staff. The website carries pages on each indicator where the provider is asked a series of questions to assess their performance on each indicator. There are then pages providing a Plan, Do, Study, Act action planning cycle for any area that requires a quality improvement plan. In order to assist with quality improvements there is an extensive web links to books, articles, training resources, you tube clips linked to each indicator. These are regularly updated as new resources are identified. All resources are vetted to make sure they are of reasonable quality and person centred. Feedback and re-visits to the website pay testament to its practical application.

The VIPS framework has been adopted as a means of internally benchmarking the person-centredness of practice within a number of service settings, particularly within the care home sector. Baker [4] describes utilising VIPS as an organising principal for an internal quality improvement programme (PEARL) in a large "for-profit" care homes provider in the UK. In Norway, Rosvik and colleagues have developed the VIPS Practice Model as a means of improving quality of care for care homes residents [61, 60]. Mork Rokstad et al. [54] examined the impact of the VIPS Practice Model and DCM when compared to usual dementia education sessions. Nursing home residents who were cared for by teams using the VIPS practice model showed significantly less depressive symptoms over time. Those who were cared for using the DCM method reported significantly improved quality of life.

In the US, [58] utilised the VIPS framework to develop a series of workshops on improving communication skills of care workers in a large for-profit long-term care facility. Using a pre-post evaluation the course participants reported improved attitudes and skills as a result of the workshops.

23.5 Evidence Base for Person-Centred Dementia Care

Developing an evidence base within such a complex area of endeavour as person-centred dementia care is not an easy task. The maintenance of valued relationships is an important factor in providing care that is person centred. Interventions that improve the maintenance of family relationships can be seen as part of person-centred approaches. Family caregiver intervention programmes have considerable potential to improve the quality of life of family caregivers and people with dementia. In particular, good coping skills and adequate support appear to mediate the impact on family caregivers of dementia-related problems. Family support interventions which have been shown to demonstrate positive outcomes appear to a number of key features, including on-going support and continuity of care for the family member throughout their care-giving journey; a focus on providing emotional support; they help the family develop coping strategies over time and the importance that the intervention are delivered by skilled and knowledgeable practitioners [10, 52, 64].

There is a strong track record in clinical psychology for using a functional or behavioural analysis approach to understand why people are experiencing the sorts of problems described as challenging [53]. Functional analysis-based interventions are sometimes called the ABC approach because they begin with a very clear description of the target behaviour (B); the events that lead up to it (A—the antecedents) and what happens as a result (C—the consequences). Functional analysis takes behavioural analysis to a much more sophisticated level in recognising that the relationship between antecedents, behaviours and consequences is often nonlinear and complex [29].

There is also a growing evidence that the provision of general person-centred care has an important role in minimising the likelihood of distress behaviours or BPSD occurring. A small number of randomised control trials have shown that simple individualised psychosocial interventions can decrease agitation in people with dementia living in care homes [21]. Engaging people in appropriate activity has also been demonstrated to improve quality of life and decreases BPSD [20]. The CALM-AD Trial [6] showed positive outcomes utilising a brief intervention comprising of social interaction, personalised music or removal of environmental triggers as a means of alleviating clinically significant agitation. Personalised activities utilising i-pads and new technologies are starting to appear, e.g. [49].

How we ensure that these ways of working become part of everyday practice is an area that requires further research. Providing care in a humanistic and person-centred way is a challenge where frontline care staff often feel under-valued. Consequences for staff can be demoralisation, burnout and stress, lower work satisfaction or job clarity, lower psychological well-being and high workforce turnover [22]. Staff burnout has been shown to be associated with less willingness to help residents, low optimism and negative emotional responses to their behaviour [63]. High levels staff turnover, staff shortages and poorly trained staff exacerbated feelings of depression in care home residents [19].

There is evidence to suggest that staff groups who have received training and on-going support in delivering person-centred care show positive outcomes [18, 23, 24, 26] and that beliefs about the personhood of people with dementia influence staff behaviour [56]. Studies have also reported that person-centred interventions lead to decreased job stress and strain as well as increased personal and professional satisfaction [30, 51]. Educational programmes utilising drama and creative approaches can improve empathy and quality of care [47]. A series of research studies in developing and evaluating a whole organisation approach called the Enriched Opportunities Programme [14] has demonstrated positive outcomes on quality of life, incidence of depressive symptoms and social inclusion for people with dementia. Understanding the culture of care and what aspects impact on the provision of person-centredness shows the interconnectedness of relationships between those in receipt of care, those who work in care and those who manage and direct care [33, 34].

23.6 From Evidence to Guidelines

The next natural step after a period of evidence-based reports and local projects is to integrate the approach into regional or national guidelines. In 2010, the Swedish National Board of Health and Welfare published its first national guidelines for care of individuals with a dementia disorder [62]. The guidelines address 16 different domains of care with the concept of person-centeredness as the underlying philosophy. They include operational criteria with recommendations for care practice on a 10 points priority scale, the strength of each based on the level of evidence. Person-centred care in these guidelines is described as: focusing on the person more than the disease or its symptoms; respecting the personal understanding of reality as perceived by the person with dementia; personalising care activities and decisions to the person's past, present and emerging life history; and preferences to the largest extent possible. Following the publication of the guidelines, a survey on the effect of implementation was conducted in 24 small scale units for demented individuals with totally 200 residents [25]. The primary endpoints were intervention effects on person-centeredness of care and the environment and the secondary endpoints were staff strain and stress of conscience. The intervention resulted in significantly higher scores on person-centeredness of care at follow up 12 months later and the facilities were rated as being more hospitable. A significant reduction of staff stress conscience was also found, which suggests that staff could provide the care and activities they wanted to provide after the intervention. The results indicate that intervention in person-centred care based on national guidelines, consisting of knowledge translation, generation and dissemination was an effective strategy.

23.7 Conclusions

Kitwood challenged us to see the PERSON with dementia first, rather than the DEMENTIA first and the person second. If we are to put this into practice we need to be mindful of our communication with people with dementia and the assumptions that we make about them. Since his initial theories in person-centred dementia care, much has been achieved in practice to ensure that we see the person behind the disease label and recognise them as full citizens. Whilst much of what constitutes person-centred care appears to have a moral and ethical imperative, the challenge remains to ensure that person-centredness occurs as part of everyday health care practice.

Acknowledgements Thanks to Heather Yemm at the Association for Dementia Studies for assistance in the preparation of this manuscript.

References

1. Allen K. Communication and consultation; exploring ways for staff to involve people with dementia in developing services. Bristol: The Policy Press; 2001.
2. Alzheimer's Research Trust. Dementia 2010: the economic burden of dementia and associated research funding in the United Kingdom. Health Economics Research Centre, University of Oxford for the Alzheimer's Research Trust. 2010.
3. Alzheimer's Society. Optimising treatment and care for people with behavioural and psychological symptoms of dementia. London: Alzheimer's Society; 2011.
4. Baker C. Developing excellent care for people with dementia living in care homes. London: Jessica Kingsley; 2014.
5. Baldwin C, Capstick A. Tom Kitwood on dementia: a reader and critical commentary. Berkshire: Open University Press; 2007.
6. Ballard C, Brown R, Fossey J, Douglas S, Bradley P, Hancock J, James IA, Juszczak E, Bentham P, Burns A, Lindesay J, Jacoby R, O'Brien J, Bullock R, Johnson T, Holmes C, Howard R. Brief psychosocial therapy for the treatment of agitation in alzheimer disease (the CALM-AD trial). Am J Geriatr Psychiatry. 2009;17(9):726–33.
7. Banerjee S. The use of anti-psychotic medication for people with dementia: a time for action. London: Dept Health; 2009.
8. Bartlett R, O'Connor D. From personhood to citizenship: broadening the lens for dementia practice and research. J Aging Stud. 2007;21(2):107–18.
9. British Standards Institute. PAS 800:2010 use of dementia care mapping for person-centred care in a care provider organization—guide. London: BSI; 2010.
10. Brodaty H, Green A, Koschera A. Meta-analysis of psychosocial interventions for caregivers of people with dementia. J Am Geriatr Soc. 2003;51(5):657–64.
11. Brooker D. What is person-centred care for people with dementia? Rev Clin Gerontol. 2004;13:212–22.
12. Brooker D. Person-centred dementia care: making services better. London: Jessica Kingsley; 2007.
13. Brooker D. Good practice inside. In: Dening T, Milne A, editors. Mental health and care homes. Oxford: Oxford University Press; 2011.
14. Brooker D, Argyle E, Clancy D, Scally A. Enriched opportunities programme: a cluster randomised controlled trial of a new approach to living with dementia and other mental health issues in extra care housing schemes and villages. Aging Men Health. 2011;15(8):1008–17.
15. Brooker D, La Fontaine J, Evans S, Bray J, Saad K. Public health guidance to facilitate timely diagnosis of dementia: alzheimer's cooperative valuation in Europe (ALCOVE) recommendations. Int J Geriatr Psychiatry. 2014;29:682–93.
16. Brooker DJ. Dementia care mapping. In: Abou-Saleh MM, Katona CLE, Kumar A, editors. Principles and practice of geriatric psychiatry. 3rd ed. Chichester: Wiley;ISBN; 9780470747230.
17. Bryden Christine. Dancing with dementia: my story of living positively with dementia. London: Jessica Kingsley; 2005.
18. Chenoweth L, King MT, Jeon Y-H, Brodaty H, Stein-Parbury J, Norman R, Haas M, Luscombe G. Caring for aged dementia care resident study (CADRES) of person-centred care, dementia-care mapping, and usual care in dementia: a cluster-randomised trial. Lancet/Neurol. 2009;8:317–25.
19. Choi NG, Ransom S, Wyllie R. Depression in older nursing home residents: the influence of nursing home environmental stressors, coping, and acceptance of group and individual therapy. Aging Ment Health. 2008;12(5):536–47.
20. Cohen-Mansfield J, Dakheel-Ali M, Marx MS. Engagement in persons with dementia: the concept and its measurement. Am J Geriatr Psychiatry. 2009;17(4):299–307.

21. Cohen-Mansfield J, Libin A, Marx MS. Nonpharmacological treatment of agitation: a controlled trial of systematic individualized intervention. J Gerontol Series A: Biol Sci Med Sci. 2007;62(8):908–16.
22. Cole RP, Scott S, Skelton-Robinson M. The effect of challenging behaviour, and staff support, on the psychological wellbeing of staff working with older adults. Aging Ment Health. 2000;4 (4):359–65.
23. Commission for Social Care Inspection—CSCI. See me, not just the dementia: understanding peoples' experiences of living in a care home. London: CSCI; 2008.
24. Deudon A, Maubourguet N, Gervais X, Leone E, Brocker P, Carcaillon L, Riff S, Lavallart B, Robert PH. Non-pharmacological management of behavioural symptoms in nursing homes. Int J Geriatr Psychiatry. 2009;24(12):1386–95.
25. Edvardsson D, Sandman PO, Borell L. Implementing national guidelines for person-centered care of people with dementia in residential aged care: effects on perceived person-centeredness, staff strain and stress of conscience. Int Psychogeriatr. 2014;26(7):1171–79.
26. Fossey J, Ballard C, Juszczak E, James I, Alder N, Jacoby R, Howard R. Effect of enhanced psychosocial care on antipsychotic use in nursing home residents with severe dementia: cluster randomised trial. Br Med J. 2006;332:756–61.
27. Fujii M, Ishizuka S, Azumi M, Sasaki H. Hypothesis of behavioral and psychological symptoms of dementia. Psychogeriatrics. 2010;10(3):113–6.
28. Hunter PV, Hadjistavropoulos T, Smythe WE, Malloy DC, Kaasalainen S, Williams J. The personhood in dementia questionnaire (PDQ): establishing an association between beliefs about personhood and health providers' approaches to person-centred care. J Aging Stud. 2014;27(3):276–287.
29. James IA. Understanding behaviour in dementia that challenges; A Guide to Assessment and Treatment. London: Jessica Kingsley; 2011.
30. Jeon YH, et al. Staff outcomes from the caring for aged dementia care resident study (CADRES): a cluster randomised trial. Int J Nurs Stud. 2012;49:508–18.
31. Kaufmann EG, Engel SA. Dementia and well-being: a conceptual framework based on Tom Kitwood's model of needs dementia. Published online 19 June 2014. doi:10.1177/1471301214539690.
32. Kelly F, Innes A. Human rights, citizenship and dementia care nursing. Int J Older People Nurs. 2013;8(1):61–70.
33. Killett A, Burns D, Kelly F, Brooker DJ, Bowes A, La Fontaine J, Latham I, Wilson M, O'Neill M. Digging deep: how organisational culture affects care home residents' experiences. Ageing Soc. 2014;. doi:10.1017/S0144686X14001299.
34. Kirkley C, Bamford C, Poole M, Arksey H, Hughes J, Bond J. The impact of organisational culture on the delivery of person-centred care in services providing respite care and short breaks for people with dementia. Health Soc Care Commun. 2011;19(4):438–48.
35. Kitwood T. Dementia and its pathology: in brain, mind or society? Free Assoc. 1987;8:81–93.
36. Kitwood T. Explaining senile dementia: the limits of neuropathological research. Free Assoc Press. 1987;10:117–38.
37. Kitwood T. The technical, the personal, and the framing of dementia. Soc Behav. 1988;3:161–79.
38. Kitwood T. Brain, mind and dementia: with particular reference to alzheimer's disease. Ageing Soc. 1989;9(1):1–15.
39. Kitwood T. The dialects of dementia: with particular reference to alzheimers's disease. Ageing Soc. 1990;10(2):177–96.
40. Kitwood T. Understanding senile dementia: a psychobiographical approach. Free Assoc. 1990;19:60–76.
41. Kitwood T. Quality assurance in dementia care. Geriatr Med. 1992;22:34–8.
42. Kitwood T. Person and process in dementia. Int J Geriatr Psychiatry. 1993;8:541–5.
43. Kitwood T. Towards a theory of dementia care: the interpersonal process. Ageing Soc. 1993;13:51–67.

44. Kitwood T. Dementia reconsidered: the person comes first. Buckingham: Open University Press; 1997.
45. Kitwood T, Bredin K. A new approach to the evaluation of dementia care. J Adv Health Nurs Care. 1992;1(5):41–60.
46. Kitwood T. A dialectical framework for dementia. In: Woods RT, et al editors. Handbook of clinical psychology of ageing, 1995. p. 267–82.
47. Kontos PC, Mitchell JG, Mistry B, Ballon B. Using drama to improve person-centred dementia care. Int J Older People Nurs. 2010;5(2):159–68.
48. Lawlor B. Managing behavioural and psychological symptoms in dementia. Br J Psychiatry. 2002;181:463–5.
49. Leng FY, Yeo D, George S, Barr C. Comparison of iPad applications with traditional activities using person-centred care approach: impact on well-being for persons with dementia. Dementia. 2014;13(2):1–9.
50. Li J, Porock D. Resident outcomes of person-centered care in long-term care: a narrative review of interventional research. Int J Nurs Stud. Available online 18 Apr 2014. ISSN 0020-7489, http://dx.doi.org/10.1016/j.ijnurstu.2014.04.003.
51. McKeown J, Clarke A, Ingleton C, Ryan T, Repper J. The use of life story work with people with dementia to enhance person-centred care. Int J Older People Nurs. 2010;5:148–58.
52. Mittleman M, Brodaty H, Wallen A, Burns A. A three-country randomized controlled trial of a psychosocial intervention for caregivers combined with pharmacological treatment for patients with Alzheimer disease: effects on caregiver depression. Am J Geriatr Psychiatry. 2008;16 (11):893–904.
53. Moniz-Cook ED, De Vugt M, Verhey F, James I. Functional analysis-based interventions for challenging behaviour in dementia. Cochrane Database of Systematic Reviews. 2008;1. Art. No. CD006929.
54. Mork Rokstad AM, Røsvik J, Kirkevold O, Selbaek G, Saltyte Benth J, Engedal K. The effect of person-centred dementia care to prevent agitation and other neuropsychiatric symptoms and enhance quality of life in nursing home patients: a 10-month randomized controlled trial. Dementia Geriatr Cogn Dis. 2013;36:340–53.
55. NICE-SCIE (National Institute for Health and Clinical Excellence—Social Care Institute for Excellence). Dementia: A NICE-SCIE guideline on supporting people with dementia and their carers in health and social care. National clinical practice guideline number 42; 2007.
56. Nolan M, Ryan T, Enderby P, Reid D. Towards a more inclusive vision of dementia care practice and research. Dementia. 2002;1(2):193–211.
57. O'Dwyer C. Official conceptualizations of person-centered care: which person counts? J Aging Stud. 2013;27(3):233–42.
58. Passalacqua SA, Harwood J. VIPS communication skills training for paraprofessional dementia caregivers: an intervention to increase person-centered dementia care. Clin Gerontol. 2012;35(5):425–45.
59. Robert PH, Verhey FR, Byrne EJ, Hurt C, De Deyn PP, Nobili F, Riello R, Rodriguez G, Frisoni GB, Tsolaki M, Kyriazopoulou N, Bullock RA, Burns A, Vellas B. Grouping for behavioral and psychological symptoms in dementia: clinical and biological aspects consensus paper of the European alzheimer disease consortium. Eur Psychiatry. 2005;20(7):490–6.
60. Rosvik J, Brooker DJ, Mjorud M, Kirkevold O. What is person-centred care in dementia? Clinical review into practice: the development of the VIPS practice model. Rev Clin Gerontol. 2013;23:155–63.
61. Rosvik J, Kirkevold M, Engedal K, Brooker DJ, Kirkevold O. A model for using the VIPS framework for person-centred care for persons with dementia in nursing homes: a qualitative evaluative study. Int J Older Peoples Nurs. 2011;6:227–36.
62. The Swedish National Board of Health and Welfare. Nationella riktlinjer för vård och omsorg vid demenssjukdom 2010: stöd för styrning och ledning. Stockholm: Socialstyrelsen; 2010.

63. Todd SJ, Watts SC. Staff responses to challenging behaviour shown by people with dementia: an application of an attributional-emotional model of helping behaviour. Aging Ment Health. 2005;9(1):71–81.
64. Ulstein I, Sandvik L, Wyller T, Engedal K. A one-year randomized controlled psychosocial intervention study among family carers of dementia patients—effects on patients and carers. Dementia Geriatr Cogn Dis. 2007;24(6):469–75.
65. Wimo A, Prince M. World alzheimer report 2010: the global economic impact of dementia, Alzheimer's Disease International. 2010.

Substance Use Disorders

24

Mohammed T. Abou-Saleh MD, PhD, Ralph E. Tarter PhD
and Ihsan M. Salloum MD, MPH

24.1 Introduction

The *Diagnostic and Statistical Manual* of *Mental Disorders* developed under the aegis of the American Psychiatric Association (DSM-5), and the *International Classification of Diseases* spearheaded by the World Health Organization (ICD-10) are the two taxonomic systems most frequently employed to formulate diagnosis of substance use disorder (SUD). Similarities between the two systems outweigh their differences; however, the DSM-5 emphasizes psychosocial impairment whereas the ICD stresses the physical dependence aspects of SUD. In contrast to both taxonomies, person-centered integrative diagnosis (PID) [39] advances a person-centered health diagnosis of people experiencing SUD that additionally incorporates positive aspects of health, psychological well-being, and interpersonal relationships so as to provide a balanced comprehensive characterization of the individual. PID, therefore, aligns closely with the World Health Organization's definition of health as "*a state of complete physical, mental and social well-being and not merely the absence of disease or infirmity*" [47].

M.T. Abou-Saleh MD, PhD (✉)
St George's School of Medicine, University of London, London, UK
e-mail: mabousal@gmail.com

R.E. Tarter PhD
Professor, Center for Education and Drug Abuse Research, School of Pharmacy, University of Pittsburgh, Pittsburgh, PA, USA

I.M. Salloum MD, MPH
Professor of Psychiatry, University of Miami School of Medicine, Miami, FL, USA;
Chair, Section on Classification, Diagnostic Assessment and Nomenclature, World Psychiatric Association, Geneva, Switzerland

J.E. Mezzich et al. (eds.), *Person Centered Psychiatry*,
DOI 10.1007/978-3-319-39724-5_24

The ubiquitous feature of SUD is persistent consumption of alcohol, drugs, or euphoria-inducing chemicals (e.g., solvents), despite the hazard to health and/or impaired performance of social roles. Self-injurious consumption, denoting *substance misuse*, results from the interplay of three factors: (1) toxic and addictive properties of the particular substance, (2) biobehavioral disposition of the individual, and (3) characteristics of the social environment, including prevailing drug regulatory policies, laws and mores. Considering the fact that drugs having the potential for misuse directly cause more than 70 medical diseases [2], complemented by findings from the Global Burden of Disease Study showing that mental disorders account for approximately 22.9 years of life with disability, it is a high priority to design, make available, and implement effective evidence-based prevention and treatment.

24.2 Characteristics of Abusable Drugs

Toxicity and addiction liability vary widely between substances. For example, any amount of tobacco consumption is hazardous, whereas moderate consumption of alcohol poses little, if any, risk to health. Indeed, regular consumption of moderate quantity of red wine has been shown to promote health. Moreover, the large majority of regular tobacco users, in contrast to a minority of regular alcohol users, develop dependence. Thus, health and social service providers need to be cognizant of the properties of each substance consumed by the individual with respect to the potential to cause disease and physical dependence.

A main intervention task, therefore, involves harm reduction; that is, substituting where possible the currently used dangerous drug with a less hazardous substance. For example, a first step in treatment of nicotine dependence may begin with transitioning the person from tobacco products, thereby avoiding consuming carcinogens, to gum or patch. However, the ever-expanding pharmacopeia is a major obstacle to intervention. Habitual consumption of unregulated versions of legal drugs (e.g., powder preparations of caffeine and alcohol, e-cigarettes), designer drugs (e.g., "synthetic" cannabis), prescription medicines (e.g., stimulant, analgesic and anxiolytic medications), and so-called nutrition and performance supplements may lead to misuse and cause organ-system injury. One obvious consequence of the expansion in number of readily available abusable drugs is more opportunity for regular consumption, and accordingly, heightened risk for adverse events such as overdose, traumatic injury, and suicide.

Intervention usually focuses on the particular substance associated with misuse or dependence. Treatment frequently is confined, for example, to specifically tobacco cessation. It is also noteworthy that individuals are tacitly appraised according to the particular drug dependence. For example, a person dependent on cocaine is viewed more negatively than a person who is dependent on alcohol. Thus, eliminating stigmatization according to type of drug dependence is an important priority, especially since empirical research has shown that all substances having abuse potential are strongly interrelated along a continuous interval scale.

Legal substances are located toward the lower (left) end, whereas illegal "hard" drugs are located toward the more severe (right) end [24]. In effect, all abusable substances project onto one dimension denoting their severity, thereby explaining why (1) the typical pattern of consumption is polysubstance abuse, (2) substance substitution occurs when a preferred drug is not available, and (3) consumption of substances having different or even opposite (e.g., alcohol and nicotine) pharmacological properties is commonplace. Biochemical and metabolic differences between substances notwithstanding, they all impact on frontal-mesolimbic circuitry integral to emotion regulation, behavior control and reinforcement [44]. Paralleling these findings, the various of SUDs are indicators of a unidimensional interval scale. Thus, rather than distinct categories, the different SUDs are actually variants of one disorder [24]. SUDs consequent to using legal drugs are located in the left end of the continuum, whereas SUDs resulting from consumption of hard illegal drugs are located in the right end of the continuum. Aligning with these psychometric findings, it has been shown that almost one hundred percent of the genetic contribution to etiology is common to all SUDs [18, 19, 42].

Substances having the potential for misuse, viewed from an economic perspective, are commodities. Forces impacting supply and demand determine the size of the substance using market reflected as consumption prevalence. To protect public safety, national and local jurisdictions determine whether the possession and consumption of a particular commodity should be classified as legal or illegal, and if legal, the chronological age when consumption is sanctioned. These laws change over time. For example, in 1960, an 18-year old in the U.S. could drink alcohol legally (but not vote), whereas the opposite is currently the case. Currently, the legal status of cannabis is in flux. Historically, the most concerted attempts to lower consumption prevalence have been directed at reducing the supply or availability of abusable substances. These efforts have largely emphasized formulating new laws and vigorous enforcement through the judicial system, including interdiction along drug distribution routes, prosecution of individuals for possession and selling contraband drugs, and impeding access (e.g., eliminating cigarette dispensing machines). Attempts to lower prevalence by reducing demand have largely involved taxation. This policy strategy carries the risk, however, of shifting consumption to cheaper and potentially more dangerous substances.

Health and social services professions align with demand reduction to avert onset of consumption (prevention) or terminate misuse (treatment). Reducing motivation for consumption requires, however, surmounting-entrenched social behavior and attitudes. Notably, person-centered psychiatry applied to SUD emphasizes the importance of leveraging cultural and ethnic traditions and rituals and secular folkways (e.g., "happy hour") to potentiate fidelity to and impact of interventions aimed at lowering motivation for substance consumption.

24.3 Characteristics of Individuals Prone to Substance Misuse/SUD

Individuals markedly differ with respect to the predisposition to develop substance misuse/SUD and clinical presentation. The most ubiquitous childhood characteristic presaging SUD is suboptimal socialization that is accompanied in varying degree by externalizing behavior disorders. The cardinal feature of low socialization, namely indifference to mores and laws, is often a transient manifestation of adolescent rebellion. Nevertheless, it is disconcertingly common. For example, approximately half the population of students in the U.S. smoked marijuana at least one time prior to graduation from high school [17]. Using illegal drugs is also common among adults. It is estimated that 149 million people worldwide in 2009 used an illicit drug, including at least 125 million users of cannabis and 15 million users of opioids, amphetamines, or cocaine (Degenhardt L, et al PMID 23993281). In addition, individuals with poor capacity to modulate emotions, including internalizing psychiatric disorders, have a strong propensity for substance use [16]. It is noteworthy that externalizing (e.g., behavior undercontrol) and internalizing (e.g., anxiety) disturbances are strongly correlated. Together they comprise a unidimensional trait indicating poor psychological self-regulation [28], which is the most salient feature of transmissible (intergenerational) risk for SUD [43], as well as predicts all SUD categories in adults [37] and in children who manifest SUD in adulthood [21].

24.4 Characteristics of the Environment

The family is the child's most proximal environment. Notably, children having biological parents who do not have SUD but are raised by adoptive parents who do have SUD are at elevated risk to develop SUD [33]. Thus, even in the absence of genetic vulnerability, quality of the family environment influences risk for developing SUD. The peer environment is another important influence. Substance use typically begins with an offer of alcohol or a drug from a friend and most often in a party setting. Furthermore, the neighborhood is a critically important factor. Dealing in illegal drugs, high density of retail alcohol and tobacco outlets, and tolerance of social deviancy are more commonplace in disadvantaged neighborhoods where abandoned or boarded-up buildings provide seclusion for substance use.

In summary, substance misuse/SUD results from the interaction of (1) drug toxicity/pharmacology, (2) psychological disposition, and (3) environmental context. The manifold variables spanning these three domains are configured uniquely within each individual. The singular composition of factors influencing SUD risk and severity underscores the importance of an intervention model anchored to around human individuality.

24.5 Rationale for Person-Centered Approach for Preventing and Treating Substance Misuse/SUD

Enormous strides beginning in the latter half of the nineteenth century were made in prevention (e.g., vaccination, water fluoridation, and sanitation) and treatment (e.g., antibiotics) of infectious diseases. These interventions have low cost and are so robust that biological and psychological differences between individuals have little, if any, bearing on effectiveness. Their effectiveness has imbued, however, a nomothetic mindset in which all individuals manifesting a particular disorder benefit from the same treatment.

The nomothetic approach is not likely to be effective for prevention or treatment of psychiatric disorders. Wide variation in therapeutic response obtained from a particular medication or behavioral intervention argues against deploying the same intervention ("one size fits all") for all individuals. Nomothetic interventions are especially not appropriate for substance misuse/SUD due to vast heterogeneity in both predisposing liability for the disorder and severity and pattern of clinical presentation. It is well-recognized, for example, that SUD usually manifests in conjunction with other SUDs as well as other axis I and axis II psychiatric disorders. Myriad variations in clinical presentation thus do not allow placing an individual in a discrete category requiring a particular recommended intervention. The etiology of SUD also varies between individuals. Substance misuse may emanate, for example, from a need to alleviate pain, lower affective distress, or enhance performance. Furthermore, the composition of factors influencing the trajectory to substance misuse/SUD is distinct in each person. Hence, effective intervention requires an individualized (i.e., *idiographic*) person-centered strategy.

Person-centered psychiatry aligns with the U.S. National Institute of Health *Roadmap.* The core principle specifies that effective intervention is contingent on targeting the factors integral to etiology and maintenance of the disorder [48]. This requirement is, however, challenging for substance misuse/SUD because all of the salient characteristics are commonly also present in other medical and psychiatric disorders. For example, low propensity for physical exercise is common in substance misusing adolescents [4, 26, 36]. Low motivation for exercise is also associated with obesity and depression. Commensurate with the person-centered perspective, a main task, therefore, involves delineating the factors to substance misuse/SUD. Toward this goal, effective prevention or treatment hinge on obtaining a comprehensive *Life History Narrative*.

24.6 Elucidating Etiology of Substance Misuse/SUD from the Life History Narrative

The life history narrative delineates the individual's etiological trajectory to substance misuse/SUD taking into account the properties of the drug(s), psychological makeup, and environmental context within an ontogenetic framework. Furthermore, the life history narrative captures information about the factors that may have buffered risk for, and severity of, the substance misuse. In this fashion, the person's assets and resources can be leveraged to potentiate intervention effectiveness. Considering that 70 % of SUD cases are manifest before 30 years of age; which is within 5 years after completing neuromaturation, an ontogenetic framework is indispensable for obtaining a comprehensive understanding of the etiology and progression to substance misuse/SUD.

Family History. It is well known that SUD frequently runs in families. Intergenerational continuity of SUD, termed *transmissibility*, denotes the combined influence of parental genetic and childrearing factors on risk for and severity of substance misuse/SUD. Research has shown, for instance, that over 40 % of variance associated with development of cannabis use disorder relates to factors that are transmissible across generations [13]. Approximately, half the population of children of SUD parents similarly develops SUD. Children of SUD parents have elevated rates of attention deficit hyperactivity disorder (ADHD) and conduct disorder compared to the general population. These later disorders share significant genetic risk with SUD and frequently presage SUD. Children of SUD parents are also commonly reared in an adverse home environment where parenting is deficient, ineffective, or abusive. Furthermore, SUD parents frequently have co-occurring criminality, psychiatric disorder or medical disability that negatively impact children. In addition, quality of social assimilation by immigrant families influences the propensity for and problems resulting from substance use. Lastly, the extent the family participates in religious, ethnic, and cultural traditions is closely related to the child's acquisition of values and beliefs required to desist substance consumption in secular society where alcohol and drugs are omnipresent. Understanding parental psychiatric history and family environment is thus crucial for elucidating intergenerational vulnerability for substance misuse/SUD.

Fetal Development. Women who do not plan pregnancy are often unprepared for and/or disinterested in childrearing. In this circumstance, maternal investment in the health of the fetus is weak. Accordingly, there is little incentive to adhere to health behaviors resulting in the fetus experiencing teratogenic injury caused by abusable drugs and their metabolites, environmental toxins, poor nutrition, stress hormones, and infections. These adversities during prenatal development also potentially modify gene activity (epigenesist) to exacerbate the vulnerability for psychiatric and medical disorders, including substance abuse. Although it is not possible to retroactively ameliorate the impact of these adversities, documenting their presence is nevertheless important in order to characterize the quality of parental investment in the child's welfare. Smoking cigarettes, for example, begins earlier among youths whose mothers smoked during pregnancy. The neurological sequelae of prenatal drug exposure are most prominently reflected as a lesion in frontal cortex subserving emotion and behavior regulation. Moreover, neurobehavior disturbances associated with SUD risk have been frequently documented in children whose mothers misused alcohol or other drugs during pregnancy.

Infancy. It has been long known that secure emotional attachment of the infant to the caregiver is essential for the child's long-term mental health and social adjustment. Substance misuse/SUD in youths and adults has been traced to insecure attachment of the baby to the caregiver [8]. Forging secure attachment is contingent, however, on affective synergy between the caregiver and baby. Psychiatric disorder, poor coping skills, preoccupation with substance use, physical and intellectual disability, and low parenting competencies are common examples of caregiver limitations that hamper the mother's capacity to bond with the baby. The child's characteristics also strongly influence the prospect of establishing secure attachment. For example, neonatal abstinence syndrome may persist for up to a month after birth in babies whose mothers regularly used illicit or prescribed opioids during pregnancy. Symptoms such as irritability, gastrointestinal distress, extended wakefulness, and persistent intense crying are stressful to parents and thus hamper caregiving motivation, especially if the caregiver has psychiatric or medical disability. These latter characteristics are also often present in an otherwise healthy baby (i.e., "colic"). The dysregulated infant is thus faced with the adaptational challenge of managing persistent stress where the caregiver is indifferent to or cannot reliably provide the extra required caregiving.

Childhood. Poor physiological and emotion regulation during infancy often segues to difficult temperament in toddlerhood. Overtly expressed emotion dysregulation and behavior undercontrol, and temperament disturbances in children as young as 3 years of age elevate risk for developing SUD in adulthood [3, 14]. Temperament disturbances during toddlerhood also commonly segue to disruptive behavior in middle childhood which potentiates conflict with parents and other adults along with rejection by normative behaving children. Friendships are thus confined to similarly disruptive and socially marginalized peers, thereby facilitating opportunities for engaging in behaviors that violate mores and the law, including substance use.

Adolescence. Adolescence, roughly corresponding with the developmental period when sexual, physical, and intellectual maturation are completed, is featured by increasing assumption of adult social roles and activities such as working for pay, driving an automobile, and forming intimate relationships. Smoking tobacco or drinking alcohol may, therefore, be an expression of "adult" behavior, although illegal in most jurisdictions or a violation of cultural mores. Biological factors may also prompt onset of substance use. For example, secondary sex characteristics evinced at a young chronological age evoke a physical appearance of advanced maturity leading to inclusion in an older friendship cluster. Since substance use increases in tandem with chronological age during adolescence, affiliating with older youths amplifies the likelihood of substance use, especially if the youngster is psychologically dysregulated and/or poorly socialized [15]. It is important to note in this regard that first the use of an abusable substance during adolescence typically occurs in context of interactions with peers and, with exception of caffeine, is illegal or a violation of social mores. In effect, initiating substance use during adolescence involves a violation of societal norms even when consumption is tacitly accepted or tolerated by adults in the child's environment.

The quality of subjective experience consequent substance use also influences the probability of habitual consumption that in turn influences risk for SUD [12]. Furthermore, the adolescent period of development is marked by reward hypersensitivity [11], thereby potentiating the subjective experience obtained from substance use. Epidemiological research showing that cannabis use disorder has peak prevalence before 19 years of age illustrates the rapid progression from initial use that typically begins in adolescence to diagnosis [46].

Adulthood. SUD occurs before 30 years of age in over 70 % of individuals. These epidemiological findings concur with clinical research showing that substance misuse/SUD is an outcome of a heritable neurodevelopmental disturbance (see [40, 44, 45] for reviews). During childhood and adolescence, the disturbance is overtly evinced as poor emotion regulation and behavior undercontrol. In severe cases, these characteristics satisfy criteria for diagnosis of attention deficit hyperactivity disorder, conduct disorder, or oppositional defiant disorder that usually co-occur in various combinations. The core disorder of psychological dysregulation during adolescence and adulthood is often manifest as an axis II psychiatric disorder, particularly borderline personality disorder (more prevalent in females) and antisocial personality disorder (more prevalent in males) co-occurring with substance misuse/SUD.

After age 30, when neuromaturation is completed, substance use is typically a maladaptive attempt to alleviate stress. Many stressors in middle (e.g., divorce, unemployment) and late (e.g., widowhood, insomnia, pain) life induce emotional and physiological distress that may prompt substance use as a coping tactic. Substance misuse/SUD commonly also ensues following habitual consumption of prescription medications with or without medical supervision. The challenge for the clinician is to understand the client's motivation for substance consumption so that alternative coping strategies can be inculcated.

Summary. The life narrative delineates etiology so as to inform targets for prevention or treatment. Because manifold factors integral to etiology and maintenance of substance misuse/SUD are uniquely configured in each individual, intervention needs to be directed at ameliorating the factors particular to each person so as to lower motivation for consumption. This idiographic framework underpins the practice of person-centered psychiatry pertaining to SUD. In addition, effective intervention, as discussed below, is contingent on targeting the particular factors that sustain substance misuse specific to each individual.

24.7 Intervention Informed by Assessment of Current Problems

The presence of only two characteristics ("symptoms") in the DSM-5 taxonomy of SUD qualifies the person for diagnosis. Hence, hundreds of different symptom combinations can qualify a person for SUD. One result is the large heterogeneity of the clinical presentation, including individuals for the same disorder, even individuals having completely different symptom but the same diagnosis. Unlike other chronic non-communicable medical disorders, the diagnostic criteria for SUD do not require a necessary condition that must be present in all affected individuals. Moreover, it should be noted that the criteria do not inform intervention. Also, it should be noted that the symptoms comprising the criteria are not equal in terms of denoting severity of disturbance. Thus, classifying SUD as mild, moderate, or severe based on tabulating the number of symptoms may not accurately depict SUD severity. It is additionally important to note that substance misuse/SUD, even if it is the presenting problem, may not necessarily be the main or most severe problem. As discussed above, substance misuse is often secondary to stress-induced psychiatric (e.g., depression) or physiological (e.g., insomnia) disorder.

Designing a prevention or treatment intervention that is tailored to the individual requires: (1) identifying the spectrum of problems concurrent to substance use, (2) ranking the severity of the identified problems to prioritize urgency of interventions, (3) determining whether the manifest problems preceded or emerged consequent to substance misuse, and (4) specifying the person's assets and resources that can be leveraged to maximize intervention effectiveness. Before undertaking these tasks, it is essential, however, to determine whether substance misuse/SUD is indeed present, recognizing that many individuals who consume an abusable substance (caffeine, prescription medications, alcohol, etc.) do not exhibit a hazardous pattern of consumption.

Objectively determining whether a problem is present can be readily achieved using gender-specific versions of the *Quick Screen* derived from the Drug Use Screening Inventory (DUSI-DQS). This self-administered screen, taking about 3 min to complete, quantifies severity of substance involvement (Part A) and substance-related maladjustment (Part B) [22]. Percentile scores denote whether there is correspondence between level of substance involvement and severity of maladjustment. Available at no cost on the internet, the DQS is thus a practical and efficient tool for population screening or for routine assessment in clinical and social service settings. Importantly, there are several age-specific versions spanning adolescence to adulthood, thereby enabling longitudinal monitoring. Furthermore, concurrent and predictive validity of the DQS are established so that the scores automatically inform the clinician about the probability that the person currently has or will in the future qualify for SUD. Lastly, because the results summarize information provided by the individual, the DQS is a valuable tool for initiating a discussion with the client about the need for intervention.

Once the need for intervention is established, the next task involves delineating the spectrum of disturbances sustaining substance misuse. First, information needs to be obtained to characterize consumption behavior with respect to (1) frequency, quantity and type of regularly consumed substances, (2) pattern of simultaneous use of multiple substances, (3) beliefs held by the person about the risks and perceived benefits of substance consumption, (4) level of confidence to desist consumption, (5) usual social context of consumption, and (6) drug-induced positive (euphoria) and negative (relief from aversive state) reinforcement. Complementing documentation of substance use topology, magnitude of disturbances encompassing health, behavior, role performance, and interpersonal relationships also needs to be quantified. The Drug Use Screening Inventory (DUSI), self-administered on the Web (see http://www.yourhealthcheck.org/ecenter_research), measures problems severity in ten main domains: (1) physical dependence and associated symptoms of substance misuse, (2) mental health disturbances, (3) behavior disorder, (4) health problems, (5) family dysfunction, (6) education underperformance and maladjustment, (7) disruptive peer relationships, (8) work maladjustment, (9) suboptimal social skills, and (10) inadequate leisure and recreation. In addition, the DUSI's specialized subscales screen serious psychiatric and behavior disturbances, including attention deficit hyperactivity disorder, conduct disorder/antisocial personality, anxiety, depression, paranoia, and schizophrenia. Additional DUSI subscales screen for susceptibility to anger, social withdrawal, interpersonal aggression, suicide risk, and non-violent violations of the law. Lastly, the score on the 10-item Lie scale indicates whether the client is making an intentional effort at deception. The DUSI, available in multiple languages, can be completed in approximately 15 min using any device connected to the Web. Comprehension of the questions requires only a fifth grade reading level; however, a text to voice option is available if the respondent cannot read at this level.

All of the DUSI scales are scored on the same metric spanning 0–100 % severity. In this fashion, severity of problems can be ranked to prioritize interventions. Also, because the results are scored and profiled automatically after completing the 159-item inventory, the results are immediately available for discussion with the client. Furthermore, once the client is engaged in intervention, the software enables tracking and graphing changes in each problem. Assessments during after-care afford the opportunity to detect trends in problem severity and associated substance use severity so that timely intervention can be implemented prior to florid relapse. Finally, the DUSI's software efficiently aggregates data to (1) evaluate effectiveness of a treatment program, (2) measure effectiveness of service providers, (3) estimate prognosis for particular subgroups or subtypes of patients, and (4) conduct cost-effectiveness analyses.

24.8 Intervention for Substance Misuse/SUD

The discussion up to this juncture described the life narrative and multidimensional assessment to determine intervention needs and set priorities. In this fashion, objective evaluation, non-subjective clinical impression, constitutes the platform to initiate discussion with the client about the need to address substance misuse. Because all the information is provided by the client, evasiveness, and denial are avoided. Conversation can thus be directed at catalyzing the decision to initiate intervention. Toward this goal, [35] described a schema that involves a series of transitions from pre-contemplation for treatment to awareness of a need for treatment and subsequently an action plan to initiate rehabilitation. Assisted by the information provided by the client, the motivational interview, a widely used office-based intervention, catalyzes the client toward action.

The motivational interview is "*a collaborative, person-centered form of guiding to elicit and strengthen motivation for change*" [31]. Motivational interviewing is culturally neutral since it focuses on evoking from the client proactive motivation rather than imposing requirements to adhere to a prescriptive intervention. Four principles guide the motivational interview: (a) empathy, (b) develop discrepancy, (c) roll with resistance, and (d) support self-efficacy. Moreover, as collaboration between the clinician and client, intrinsic motivation is catalyzed by the person's resourcefulness to advance behavioral change.

Once the client is engaged and motivated to initiate change, the intervention program needs to be tailored to the specific factors that promoted and currently maintain substance misuse. Toward this goal, intervention should emphasize attaining recognizable progress early on so as to consolidate motivation for continued involvement in treatment. Pharmacotherapy should also be considered at the outset of treatment. Where possible, engagement with Alcoholics Anonymous (or Narcotics Anonymous) by the client and Al-Anon and Al-Ateen by other family members should be strongly encouraged. This self-help grassroots fellowship provides lifelong social support. In addition, informed by the DUSI profile, the intervention program may need to target problem areas requiring specialized professional skills (family therapy, cognitive behavior therapist, etc.). It is beyond the scope of this discussion to review the variety of methods for prevention and treatment of SUD; however, similar to all chronic medical disorders, a major challenge involves maintaining the client's adherence to the selected regimen.

24.9 A Person-Centered Approach to Addiction Treatment

A person-centered medicine approach to treatment is uniquely befitting for the optimal treatment of addictions: addictions particularly addiction to illegal drugs have for long been considered criminal, immoral, self-inflicted conditions, and importantly the most stigmatizing health conditions in all communities and cultures. In recent decades, addictions have been dignified by their recognitions as serious health conditions included under mental disorders in international classification systems and accumulating evidence for effective treatment and preventative interventions that now shape policy including issues of decriminalization and legalisations.

The disease perspective views compulsive use of substances symptomatic of the underlying pathology that at least in part has genetic basis. This perspective endorses a compassionate treatment since it regards addictive behavior is beyond the control of the individual. The 12–Step Recovery Movement was established on this disease model of addiction. Addictions are also considered maladaptive learned behavior—"problem behaviour that is clearly under the control of environmental, family, social, and or even cognitive contingencies" [41]. This problem behaviour is not viewed as a sinful, out of control or freely chosen but the addicted individual is instead seen as an "A victim of destructive learning conditions." This perspective employs learning strategies in treating the addictive behavior, including contingency management, modeling, social skills training, assertiveness training, behavioral self-control training, and overall relapse prevention skills training [26].

24.10 Motivational Interviewing: The Core Experience of Person-Centered Approach

There is preponderance of evidence that indicates that therapist and client factors are much more important than treatment approach [7]. Rogers was the first to articulate this distinction in his paper "the necessary and sufficient conditions of therapeutic personality change" stating that effective therapy is dependent upon the existence of six conditions. The first condition (client vulnerability) would appear to be a precondition for all effective therapy including addiction treatment; this demands engagement with the client and the establishment of a collaborative relationship. The other conditions are considered the core conditions and elaborate the therapist conditions that are critical for producing growth and change in clients: empathic understanding or accurate empathy; therapist congruence, genuineness, honesty and authenticity; and therapist unconditional positive regard, consistent acceptance, and none—possessive interpersonal caring and warmth [7, 38].

The introduction of the trans theoretical stage of change model was a major factor that influenced the transition from the harsh confrontational approach to a more respectful humane approach in addiction treatment in the late 1980s and early 1990s [35]. This model postulated the change process as a sequence of five stages through which people advance as they create, modify or stop behaviors.

People who make behavioral changes move from being unaware or unwilling to do anything about the problem to considering the possibility of change, then to becoming determined and prepared to make the change, and finally to taking action and sustaining or maintaining that change over time [5].

Since 1991 there has been an increased emphasis on using a person—centered approach in the treatment of addictive disorders [29] who defined motivational interviewing as "a goal—directive, client—centered counseling style for eliciting behavioural change by helping clients to explore and resolve ambivalence". Miller and Rodnick have recently updated the definition of motivational interviewing to "a collaborative, person—centered form of guiding to elicit and strengthen motivation for change close quote [31] and is by far the most widely used and research—person-centered approach for the treatment of addictions, with over 200 clinical trials demonstrating its effectiveness on it. Miller and Rose [32] state that "motivational interviewing is a psychotherapeutic method that is evidence—based through the brief, specifiable, applicable across a wide variety of problem areas, complementary to other active treatment methods and learnable by a broad range of helping professionals" [7].

The four guiding principles of motivational interviewing are considered far more important than any specific strategy or technique used in therapy: express empathy, develop discrepancy, roll with resistance, and support self—efficacy. These principles of motivational interviewing lead to a collaborative therapy process in which the client provides the content and the therapist guides the process. Motivation interviewing is also a culturally neutral style of relating to clients if the four guiding principles are followed since the focus is on evoking from the client what is already there rather than imposing something on clients: "motivational interviewing honors and respects the individual's autonomy to choose. It is a collaborative, not a prescriptive, approach, in which the counselor evokes the person's own intrinsic motivation and resources for change. Implicit is the belief that such motivation and resourcefulness within each individual and need to be evoked rather than imposed [7, 30].

24.11 Person-Centered Approach to Intervention Adherence

Intervention frequently requires accessing diverse and often disconnected health and social services to address multiple longstanding problems. Substance misuse may diminish the person's motivation and capacity to access and sustain engagement with diverse service delivery systems as well as other needed resources such as food security, safe housing, transportation, and child care. A one-to-one relationship with a dependable person who helps the client surmount health and social systems barriers while also providing supportive counseling augments the prognosis of patients with chronic non-communicable medical disorders. Termed, *patient navigation*, the client thus has a trusted readily available "go to" resource [10] to help engage in and sustain intervention The navigator is especially valuable for socioeconomically disadvantaged individuals who are often more inclined to (1) have distrust or fear of health and social services providers, (2) have difficulty keeping appointments due to child care, physical disability or lack of transportation, (3) have problems communicating in the required language, and (4) have low fiscal resources [9]. Patient Navigation is, therefore, an especially valuable intervention for the vulnerable populations by "*working with patients and other actors in both the social network of the organization itself and the community in which the organization resides*" [34, p. 518]. The one-to-one relationship between patient and navigator ideally realizes practice of person-centered psychiatry pertaining to substance misuse/SUD treatment.

24.12 International Context

24.12.1 The UK Experience

The National Treatment Agency of Substance Misuse provides a treatment framework and a process intended to support the move toward a consensus on the essential components of specialist substance misuse services and the importance of links with other health, social care, and criminal justice agencies. The guidance structure ranks substance misuse services in four tiers ranging from Tier 1 (non specialist services, including general psychiatric services) to Tier 4a (residential care specifically for substance misusers) and Tier 4b (highly specialized services unrelated to substance misuse such as forensic psychiatric services and specialist personality disorder services). The guidance also stipulates the development of integrated care pathways as the preferred method of applying care in a coordinated integrated way. Integrated care pathways provide a means of merging local referral and treatment protocols to define where and when a particular service user needs to be referred.

The Government Drug Strategy 2010 took a step toward lowering harm caused by drug misuse and more emphasis on recovery. Individuals do not take drugs in isolation from what is happening in the rest of their lives. The causes and drivers of drug and alcohol dependence are complex and personal and the solutions need to be holistic and centered around each individual, with the expectation that full recovery is possible and desirable.

The Strategy stipulated that recovery involves three overarching principles—well-being, citizenship, and freedom from dependence and it is an individual, person-centered journey, as opposed to an end stage, and one that will mean different things to different people "we must therefore, put the individual at the heart of any recovery system and commission a range of services at the local level to provide tailored packages of care and Support".

One of the best predictors of recovery being sustained is an individual's 'recovery capital': the resources necessary to start, and sustain recovery from drug and alcohol dependence. The "recovery capital's" resources are social, physical, human and cultural.

Marsden et al. [27] have recently introduced the Development of the Addiction Dimensions for Assessment and Personalized Treatment (ADAPT) which is designed to help clinicians tailor therapies and demonstrated that it is a valid instrument for substance use disorder treatment planning, clinical review and outcome evaluation.

The UK government commissioned a sector-wide consultation on the model of care to implement the Building Recovery in Communities aim of the Drug Strategy 2010. This highlighted widespread agreement for an integrated approach to treatment and recovery support.

The key messages from the treatment field are that an integrated recovery system should focus on the following: Collaborative working between al partners to commission services based on outcomes; prompt access to appropriate interventions for drug-dependent people, including offenders; high-quality treatment tat prepares service users for recovery while protecting communities; encouraging service users to successfully complete treatment without putting them at risk; links to support networks to sustain long-term recovery and reintegrate people back into society.

24.13 US Experience

In 2009, the National Council for Community Behavioral Healthcare issued Behavioral Health/Primary Care Integration and the Person-Centered Healthcare Home which summarized a bidirectional approach to delivering Mental Health (MH) and Substance Use (SU) services in primary care settings and primary care services in MH/SUD settings.

The 2009 paper suggested that the expanded scope of th4e PCMH with MH/SU capacity and stepped care could be reflected by renaming the patient-centered medical home as the person-centered healthcare home, signaling that MH/SU treatments are a central part of healthcare and that healthcare includes a focus on supporting a person's capacity to set goals for improved self-management, using the resources of the community and personal support systems.

Person-Centered Healthcare Homes provide:

1. Health screening and registry tracking in MH/SU settings as well as in primary care
2. Nurse practitioner or PCP in MH/SU treatment setting as well as in primary care
3. Behavioral health consultants in primary care, competent in MH/SUD disorders
4. Nurse care managers in MHN/SUD settings as well as in primary care
5. Evidence-based preventive care in all settings. Wellness programs in all settings.

A recent study to understand mental health, substance use, and health behavior activities within primary care practices recognized by the National Committee for Quality Assurance as patient-centered medical homes (PCMHs). The study showed that in PCMHs, practice organization and response to behavioral issues seem to be less well developed than other types of medical care. These results support further efforts to develop whole person care in the PCMH, with greater emphasis on access to and coordination of mental health, substance abuse, and health behavior services. Focusing primary care practices on this aspect of whole person care will benefit from program sponsors' support and rewarding better integration with behavioral health [20].

24.14 Toward a Person-Centered Addiction Treatment and Rehabilitation: Naufar Center in Qatar

Naufar's architectural, and functional design and model of care (MoC) is guided by National Health Mental Health Strategy to provide comprehensive specialized integrate 4d health care and social care pathways for people with substance misuse enabling them to recover, improve their lives and well-being and return them to their families and communities.

The MoC and its integrated care pathways are underpinned and guided by evidence-based healthcare policies and interventions benefitting from best practice provided in its hospitable physical and social environments. The proposed MoC is informed and guided by Naufar's resources, national health strategies, and best practice in UK. It is structured under headings of policy context, commissioning substance misuse services, assessment, care planning, integrated care pathways, quality criteria and improvement reviews, alongside performance monitoring and management, and treatment interventions.

Its clinical operations will be enabled by the reform of legislation related to addiction work that is being undertaken by the Joint Committee for the Review of Legislation related to Additions that was established by the Minister of Health and had produced its final report and recommendations in June 2013. Moreover, Naufar's clinical operations will be enabled by Qatar Mental Health Law which makes provisions for the treatment of people with mental disorders including those with substance misuse under voluntary and compulsory conditions. People with substance misuse are entitled to treatment including inpatient care on a voluntary basis with their rights to privacy and confidentiality fully assured [1].

The proposed MoC for Naufar shall be enhanced by the hospitality culture in tune with its strategy, values, mission, and core principles.

The hospitality culture will add value to the MoC that is also enhanced by the person-integrated diagnosis (PID). It benefits from the PLANTREE experience http://planetree.org/ and what it means to be patient-centered. Planetree's philosophy is based on a simple premise: care should be organized first and foremost around the needs of patients. To understand those needs Planetree turned to the source. Thousands of focus groups—from bedside to boardroom—with patients, long-term care residents, families and professionals caregivers across the globe have borne out their needs and desires for a more personalized, humanized, and demystified health care experience. Bringing these concepts to life requires a shift not merely in operations but fundamentally in culture. Planetree guides providers through a structured process that enables caregivers to transform the health care experience they provide. Moreover, it has used Maslow's Needs Hierarchy as a Framework for Evaluating Hospitality Houses' Resources and Services [6].

24.15 Conclusions

Substance use disorders (SUD) are among the most burdensome and stigmatizing health conditions in all communities and cultures. In this chapter, we provided an overview of SUD characteristics including characteristics of people prone to SUD and of their environment; their ethology from life history narrative. The life narrative and the multifactorial domains integral to the etiology and maintenance of substance misuse/SUD are unique to each individual and inform person-centered targets for prevention or treatment. A person-centered approach is uniquely befitting for the optimal comprehensive assessment and integrated treatment of addictions.

References

1. Abou-Saleh MT, Abdelalaim M. Mental health law in Qatar. Int Psychiatry. 2013;10:88–90.
2. American Board of Medical Specialties. Certificate statistics. 2011. Retrieved 15 May 2012 from https://shopping.ams.org.
3. Caspi A, Moffitt T, Newman D, Silva P. Behavioral observations at age 3 years predict adult psychiatric disorder. Longitudinal evidence from a birth cohort. Arch Gen Psychiatry. 1996;53:1033–9.
4. Collingwood TR, Reynolds R, Kohl HW, Smith W, Sloan S. Physical fitness effects on substance abuse risk factors and use patterns. J Drug Educ. 1991;21:73–84.
5. DiClemente CC. Motivational interviewing and the stages of change. In: Miller WR, Rollnick S, editors. Motivational interviewing: preparing people to change addictive behavior. New York: Guilford Press; 1991. p. 191–202.
6. Duncan MKW, Blugis A. Maslow's needs hierarchy as a framework for evaluating hospitality houses' resources and services. J Pediatr Nurs. 2011;26(4):325–31. doi:10.1016/j.pedn.2010.04.003.
7. Fleck JR, Fleck DT. A person-centred approach to addiction treatment. In: Cooper M, O'Hara M, Schmid PF, Bohart AC, editors. The handbook of person-centred psychotherapy and counselling. London: Palgrave Macmillan; 2011.
8. Flores P. Addiction as an attachment disorder. New York, NY: Jason Aronson; 2004.
9. Freeman HP. The history, principles, and future of patient navigation: Commentary. Semin Oncol Nurs. 2013;29(2):72–5.
10. Freeman HP, Muth BJ, Kerner JF. Expanding access to cancer screening and clinical follow up among medically underserved. Cancer Practices. 1995;3:19–30.
11. Galvin A. The teenage brain: sensitivity to rewards. Curr Dir Psychol Sci. 2013;22(2):88–93.
12. Grant JD, Scherrer JF, Lyons MJ, Tsuang M, True WR, Bucholz KK. Subjective reactions to cocaine and marijuana are associated with abuse and dependence. Addict Behav. 2005;30:1574–86.
13. Hopfer CJ, Stallings MC, Hewitt JK, Crowley TJ. Family transmission of marijuana use, abuse, and dependence. J Am Acad Child Psychiatry. 2003;42:834–41.
14. Horner M, Braxter B, Kirisci L, Tarter RE. (in press). Temperament disturbances in infancy progress to substance sue disorder 20 years later. Pers Individ Differ.
15. Horner M, Clark D, Kirisci L, Tarter RE. Modeling the association between sexual maturation, transmissible risk, and peer relationships during childhood and adolescence on development of substance use disorder in young adulthood. Am J Addict. 2013;20:1–7.
16. Hussong AM, Jones DJ, Stein GL, Baucom DH, Boeding S. An internalizing pathway to alcohol use and disorder. Psychol Addict Behav. 2011;25(3):390–404.

17. Johnson LD, O'Malley PM, Bachman JG, Schulenberg JE. Monitoring the future national results of drug use: 2012 overview, key findings on adolescent drug use. Ann Arbor: Institute for Social Research, The University of Michigan; 2014.
18. Kendler KS, Jacobson KC, Prescott CA, Neale MC. Specificity of genetic and environmental risk factors for use and abuse/dependence of cannabis cocaine hallucinogens sedatives stimulants and opiates in male twins. Am J Psychiatry. 2003;160:687–95.
19. Kendler KS, Prescott CA, Myers J, Neal MC. The structure of genetic and environment risk factors for common psychiatric and substance use disorders in men and women. Arch Gen Psychiatry. 2003;60:929–37.
20. Kessler R, Miller BF, Kelly M, et al. Mental health, substance abuse, and health behavior services in patient-centered medical homes. J Am Board Fam Med. 2014;27(5):637–44.
21. Kirisci L, Reynolds M, Tarter RE. Quick screen to detect current substance use disorder in adolescents and likelihood of disorder. Drug Alcohol Depend. 2013;128:116–22.
22. Kirisci L, Reynolds M, Tarter RE. Quick screen to detect current and future substance use disorder in adolescent females. Int J Pers Centered Med. 2013;3(4):280–5.
23. Kirisci L, Tarter RE, Vanyukov M, Martin C, Mezzich A, Brown S. Application of item response theory to quantify substance use disorder severity. Addict Behav. 2006;31:1035–49.
24. Kirisci L, Vanyukov M, Dunn M, Tarter RE. Item response theory modeling of substance use: an index based on 10 categories. Psychol Addict Behav. 2002;16:290–8.
25. Kristjansson AL, James JE, Allegrnts JP, Sigfusdottir ID, Helgason AR. Adolescent substance use, parental monitoring, and leisure-time activities: 12-year outcomes of primary prevention in Iceland. Prev Med. 2010;51:168–71.
26. Lewis JA, Dana RQ, Blevins GA. Substance abuse counseling. 4th ed. Belmont, CA: Brooks/Cole; 2011.
27. Marsden J, Eastwood B, Ali R, Burkinshaw P, Chohan G, Copello A, Burn D, Kelleher M, Mitcheson L, Taylor S, Wilson N, Whiteley C, Day E. Development of the addiction dimensions for assessment and personalised treatment (ADAPT). Drug Alcohol Depend. 2014;139:121–31.
28. Mezzich A, Tarter RE, Feske U, Kirisci L, McNamee R, Day B. Assessment of risk for substance use disorder consequent to consumption of illegal drugs: psychometric validation of the neurobehavior disinhibition trait. Psychol Addict Behav. 2007;21:508–15.
29. Miller WR, Rollnick S. Motivational interviewing: preparing people to change addictive behavior. New York: Guilford Press; 1991.
30. Miller WR, Rollnick S. Motivational interviewing: preparing people to change addictive behavior. 2nd ed. New York: Guilford Press; 2002.
31. Miller WR, Rollnick S. Ten things that motivational interviewing is not. Behav Cogn Psychother. 2009;37:129–40.
32. Miller WR, Rose GS. Toward a theory of motivational interviewing. Am Psychol. 2009;64:527–37.
33. Newlin DB, Mmiles DR, vanden Bree MB, Gupman AE, Pickens RW. Environmental transmission of DSM-IV substance use disorders in adoptive and step families. Alcohol Clin Exp Res. 2000;24(12):1785–1794.
34. Parker VA, Clark JA, Leyson J, Calhoun E, Carroll JK, Freund KM, Battaglia TA. Patient navigation: development of a protocol for describing what navigators do. Health Res Educ Trust. 2010;. doi:10.1111/j.1475=6673.2009.01079.x.
35. Prochaska JO, DiClemente CC. The transtheoretical approach: crossing the traditional boundaries of therapy. Malabar, FL: Krieger; 1984.
36. Rainey CJ, McKeown RE, Sargent RC, Valois RF. Patterns of tobacco and alcohol use among sedentary, exercising, on-athletic youth. J Sch Health. 1996;66:27–32.
37. Ridenour TA, Tarter RE, Kirisci L, Vanyukov MM. Could a continuous measure of individual transmissible risk be useful in clinical assessment of substance use disorder? Drug Alcohol Depend. 2011;119:10–7.
38. Rogers CR. On becoming a person. Boston, MA: Houghton Mifflin; 1961.

39. Salloum IM, Mezzich JE. Outlining the bases of person-centred integrative diagnosis. J Eval Clin Pract. 2011;17:354–6.
40. Tarter RE, Horner M, Ridenour T. Developmental perspective of substance use disorder etiology. In: Shaffer H, editor. Addiction syndrome handbook. Washington, DC: American Psychological Press; 2012.
41. Thombs DL. Introduction to addictive disorders. 3rd ed. New York: Guilford Press; 2006.
42. Tsuang MT, Lyons MJ, Meyer JM, et al. Co-occurrence of abuse of different drugs in men: the role of drug-specific shared vulnerabilities. Arch Gen Psychiatry. 1998;55:967–72.
43. Vanyukov M, Kirisci L, Moss H, Tarter RE, Reynolds M, Maher B, Kirillova G, Ridenour T, Clark D. Measurement of the risk for substance use disorders. Phenotypic and genetic analysis of an index of common liability. Behav Genet. 2009;39:233–44.
44. Vanyukov M, Kirisci L, Tarter RE, Simkevitz H, Kirillova G, Maher B, Clark D. Liability to substance use disorders: 2. A measurement approach. Neurosci Biobehav Rev. 2003;27:517–26.
45. Vanyukov M, Tarter RE, Kirisci L, Kirillova G, Maher B, Clark D. Liability to substance use disorders. 1. Common mechanisms and manifestations. Neurosci Biobehav Rev. 2003; 27:507–15.
46. Wagner RA, Anthony JC. Male-female differences in the risk of progression from first use to dependence upon cannabis, cocaine, and alcohol. Drug Alcohol Depend. 2007;86:191–8.
47. WHO. Preamble to the constitution of the World Health Organization as adopted by the International Health Conference, New York, 19–22 June, 1946; signed on 22 July 1946 by the representatives of 61 States and entered into force on 7 April 1948. International Heath Conference; April 7, 1948, New York.
48. Zerhouni E. The NIH roadmap. Science. 2003;302(5642):63–72.

Schizophrenia and Related Disorders 25

Wolfgang Gaebel, MD and Juergen Zielasek, MD

25.1 Concepts of Person-Centred Care in Schizophrenia

"Psychiatry is essentially about people, not (just) brains..." [53]. This conveys much of what psychiatry is about, and it is to investigate the role and function of psychiatry, of mental healthcare and all accompanying aspects of the diagnostics, therapy and care for people with schizophrenia, which is at the center stage of this chapter. Psychiatrists are holists par excellence, in that mental disorders affect the whole person and the need arises to integrate information from clinical assessments, neurobiology, socioenvironmental domains and psychological reactions of the patient to the development of a mental disorder. The major model of mental disorders is the biopsychosocial model [18], which is holistic in that it takes a multiperspective integrating several levels of analysis using empathic understanding of subjective experiences and other more objective tools to assess the presentation of mental disorders. One central aspect here is that the model may guide a "parsimonious application of medical knowledge to the needs of each patient" [8].

The publication of DSM-5 in early 2013 prompted a debate on the usefulness and validity of the "biologic" model of mental disorders, sparkled by contributions by individuals and a position statement by the British Psychological Society (http://www.theguardian.com/society/2013/may/12/psychiatrists-under-fire-mental-health). Also, the Research Domain Criteria Initiative (RDoC) of the National Institutes on Mental Health was challenged on the grounds that it overemphasized (neuro)biologic causes of mental disorders. While these arguments have been countered by the view that neither psychiatry nor the RDoC initiative rely solely on neurobiologic models of explaining mental disorders (http://www.theguardian.com/science/2013/may/12/dsm-5-conspiracy-laughable)

W. Gaebel, MD (✉) · J. Zielasek, MD
Proffessor, Department of Psychiatry and Psychotherapy, Heinrich Heine University, LVR-Klinikum Düsseldorf Bergische Landstr. 2, D-40629 Düsseldorf, Germany
e-mail: wolfgang.gaebel@uni-duesseldorf.de

J.E. Mezzich et al. (eds.), *Person Centered Psychiatry*,
DOI 10.1007/978-3-319-39724-5_25

[5, 16, 17], the question is still open how the person-centred approach of psychiatry and—for the purposes of this chapter—the underlying model of schizophrenia and related disorders can be optimized to become even more person-centred, and how such a personalized model may optimize the diagnosis and treatment of patients with schizophrenia. For the purposes of the following discussion, it is necessary to clarify that a solely neurobiology-oriented approach and a solely social or psychology-oriented approach will probably not lead to decisive improvements in the care of persons with schizophrenia. Integrated, multiperspective views taking the person affected by schizophrenia or related disorders with all his/her biological, social and psychological contexts into consideration is warranted to provide empowerment, healing and mental health for the person affected by schizophrenia.

Another conceptual issue arises and needs to be clarified: That is whether such a disease as schizophrenia (and related disorders) should be diagnosed after all. The grounds for this question arise in the observation that psychotic symptoms are frequently found in the general population, among these in many cases of people who do not develop mental disorders, and that the symptoms of psychosis are the results of childhood adversity and not due to a mental disorder at all, and can be controlled by providing coping strategies. There is now biologic evidence that childhood adversity experiences may have long-lasting impacts on individual psychosocial development including the emergence of mental disorders [4], but it seems unlikely that mental disorders can be understood solely on the basis of psychological or social adversity. Newly emerging study areas are the social neurosciences [1] and the research into gene–environment interactions [19], as examples of increasingly individualized, holistic approaches taking into consideration all putative etiopathogenetic mechanisms centering on the person and converging on common neurobiological pathomechanisms. Reductionist approaches do not seem to be promising anymore, be they purely biologic, psychologic or social. Rather, several different combinations from a multitude of genetic, life-experience or other socioenvironmental risk factors may interact to lead into a clinical picture of psychosis. As regards the notion of psychotic symptoms as parts of the normal human experience, it should be noted that such experiences are frequently associated with undetected mental disorders, situations of sleep deprivation or sensory deprivation, the influence of drugs and other substances of abuse and their withdrawal, or of a very short-term duration. In these cases, a diagnosis of schizophrenia would indeed not be warranted, however, medical diagnosis and treatment would still be warranted to detect underlying mental disorders, substance abuse or somatic disorders. Also, a significant proportion of persons of the general population who have psychotic experiences develop considerable help-seeking and distress, and fulfil the diagnostic requirements of schizophrenia, and even if no diagnosis is made, suffering may be present, as a large-scale WHO study has shown, both on the mental and the somatic level [38, 39]. These persons are in need of professional assistance and suffer from non-diagnosis and nontreatment. Efforts are therefore necessary to reduce this symptom-/disease-associated burden and will be dealt with later in the chapter. However, it would be unethical not to diagnose these persons with schizophrenia if this is warranted due to the clinical picture, simply on the ground of conceptual reasons to avoid psychiatric diagnoses. Not making a diagnosis may imply that the person may not be entitled to receive the necessary therapy or social support in the existing healthcare systems. Therefore, for the time being, it seems necessary to be able to make the diagnosis of schizophrenia. Also, the diagnosis of schizophrenia has validity as regards treatment decisions and prognostic evaluations. Whether it would be useful to abolish diagnoses of mental disorders at all as prerequisites of receiving mental health support may be discussed—of course, from an ethical point of view, even without a diagnosis, a person in need has a right to be treated and supported. This is an ethical challenge for the current healthcare systems, in which support is provided only based upon a firm expert diagnosis of a mental disorder. This situation will not be easy to resolve since most systems rely exclusively on a diagnosis of a mental disorder as a prerequisite for social or medical assistance. However, beyond such rather conceptual or academic discussions, there is an urgent need to ascertain access to mental healthcare especially for minority groups or other underprivileged groups, who may not even have access to simple healthcare services due to their social status. This part of the population is on the increase given the social unrest and ensuing migration of whole populations, and has been an issue for studies in Europe recently showing that marginalized social groups are under special pressure and lack access to mental healthcare [45, 54]. The central question for personalized psychiatry therefore is not if diagnoses are warranted, but how to close eminent mental healthcare gaps.

Schizophrenia and the related disorders like schizoaffective disorder, acute and transient psychotic disorders, and delusional disorders, are frequent, severe and cause a significant level of impairment, disability and suffering to those who are affected by these mental disorders. Schizophrenia will be the focus of this chapter, since most research in this area has been performed in schizophrenia. Beyond that, schizophrenia—for the purposes of this book chapter—may be regarded as a typical example for all mental disorders, in that there has been considerable progress in elucidating its multifaceted etiopathogenesis (which is most probably featuring interindividually different compositions of biologic, psychological and social factors), but little if any real progress on the level of individualized mental healthcare. There is a considerable gap between excellent technological breakthroughs in the characterization of the genes involved in the etiopathogenesis and the neural network disturbances underlying the symptoms of schizophrenia on the one hand, and the influence of such knowledge on everyday mental healthcare. The "bench to bedside" gap in schizophrenia appears to have a considerable size. Therefore, this chapter sets out to analyze this situation and develop suggestions for a future advancement not only for research about the brain mechanisms underlying the etiopathogenesis of schizophrenia, but also for mental healthcare research with a view to provide immediate benefits for those affected by schizophrenia and related disorders. An effort may be needed to reconcile the domains of classification criteria, the personal meaning of psychotic experiences for the individual, and the gap between neurobiological dysfunctions and patient′s subjective experiences. An optimized person-centred model of schizophrenia and related mental disorders would need to encompass these factors, relate to life experiences and individual coping strategies, and take impairments, social support and goal attainment into account (Fig. 25.1).

25.2 The Person in Schizophrenia—A Special Aspect of Schizophrenia

Schizophrenia and the related disorders are diagnosed on clinical grounds based on detecting a certain combination of clinical symptoms over a sufficient period of time and after the exclusion of somatic disorders and substance of abuse-related disorders, which may cause similar clinical pictures. There is still no gold standard accessory diagnostic instrument which may replace psychopathology, so that while the diagnostic criteria are "impersonal" in a sense that they apply to every person,

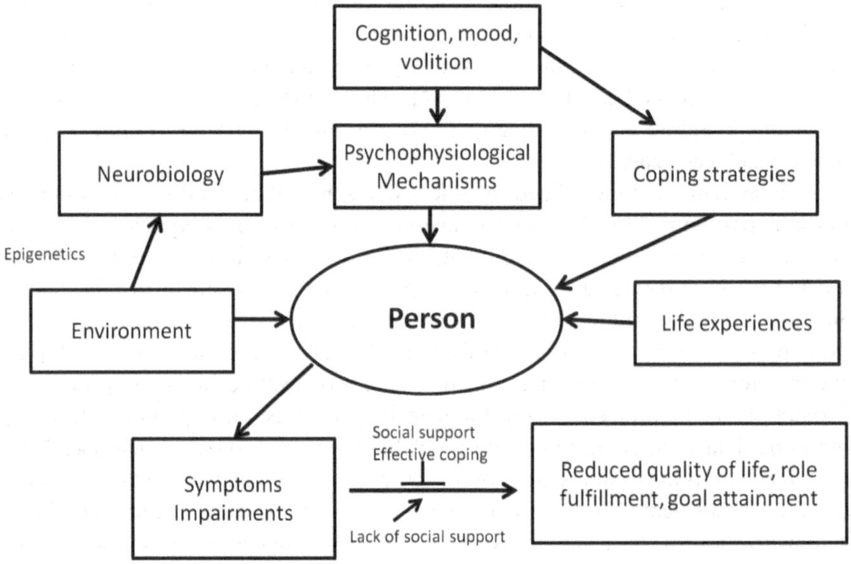

Fig. 25.1 A new person-centered model of schizophrenia and related mental disorders. The person takes centre stage and shows psychophysiologically mediated alterations of cognition, mood and volition, which are shaped by neurobiological factors, life experiences and partially alleviated by individual coping strategies. Other environmental factors may act on neurobiological pathomechanisms ("epigenetics"). The resulting symptoms and impairments may reduce quality of life, role fulfilment and goal attainment, and may lead to unfavourable outcomes which may be fostered by lack of social support and which may be alleviated by positive social support and effective coping mechanisms. Note that there are feedback loops not depicted here, for example, in that a reduced goal attainment may unfavourably affect mood, leading to vicious cycles in the process of developing mental disorders. Antipsychotic drugs and psychotherapeutic procedures are therapeutically active via neurobiologic and psychophysiological brain mechanisms most likely converging on common final pathways

they are highly personal in that they take individual experiences into account and are actually centrally based on such experiences. The diagnostic process is highly dependent on first-person accounts of subjective experiences by the person of hallucinations and/or delusions, which affect the person deeply in most cases. This implies that the person as a whole is affected by these symptoms, and the symptoms are experienced as close to the individual himself or herself, and they may have immediate meaning to the person affected. Therefore, schizophrenia has a special aspect of affecting the person in its deepest foundations, consequently leading to experiences demanding explanations, causing distress and having consequences for the person′s everyday life. Therefore, it is warranted to say that the *person* is affected in schizophrenia, not just functional systems of the brain like neurotransmitter systems or modularized, interacting networks of oscillating neural circuitry. However, the latter are conditions which may underlie the ensuing personal affection and symptoms, and therefore need to be studied if an understanding of the mechanisms of the processes leading to the hallucinatory or delusional experiences is needed. These two levels of investigation, the "person as a whole" level and the "neurobiologic" level, cannot be separated, in that they influence each other and form both a basis and a consequence of the etiopathogenetic procesess in schizophrenia and the related mental disorders. A diagnostic process in schizophrenia will therefore only be complete if it is "of the person", which means that a complete assessment including symptoms (experiences) and impairments is warranted. It needs to be "with the person" in exercising respectful and empowering partnership with a common goal of mental health. It should be "for the person", keeping in focus that it is necessary to identify the individual health aspirations of the person seeking help. There is still a considerable degree of unmet needs in patients with schizophrenia, which is only partly met by reducing the symptoms of psychosis [23, 33]. It would be necessary to optimize the diagnostic and therapeutic process towards "by the person", meaning that the person seeking help is viewed as an equal partner in a transaction involving both professional and personal aspects with joint identification of treatment needs. To advance such an approach, Salvador-Carulla and Mezzich [44] suggested to address aspects both of "ill health" and of "positive health" in this process. But there may be practical challenges and limits to these ideals in everyday clinical practice of schizophrenia mental healthcare. These include, to name some examples, on the patient side: (a) the occurrence of disorder-related overvalued ideas with lack of insight into the pathological nature; (b) challenging behaviours like threats or withdrawal; (c) suicidality; (d) nonacceptance of therapy. While these need to be addressed in proper communication, there are also challenges on the professional side. These may include—but may not be limited to—(a) nonattendance to personal beliefs or needs of the patient; (b) lack of professional knowledge; (c) lack of continuing care for the patient due to structural limitations of the mental healthcare service.

25.3 Personalized Drug Therapy

Personalized drug therapy in schizophrenia and related disorders usually implies that certain biologic markers or endophenotypes are identified which may play a role in the pharmacodynamics of the used drugs. For the antipsychotic drugs, individual dopamine-receptor blockade levels can be measured, which are associated with antipsychotic effects, but also with side effects, and there is a wide interindividual variability of these associations [15]. Also, the dopamine system is connected with other neurotransmitter systems (glutamate, serotonin, to name just two) and dopamine-receptor blockade may be a necessary, but not a sufficient action of antipsychotic drugs to control symptoms [29]. Besides, high costs, exposure to radioactive tracer substances and nonavailability of the method are barriers to the implementation of such individualized procedures. In everyday clinical practice, the selection of antipsychotic drug therapy takes a multitude of individual aspects into account and is highly personalized already [14]: parameters of the primary disorder like the disease course, the current state and the predominating symptoms, psychiatric and physical comorbidities, past treatment effects, individual patient preferences, drug availability and individual acceptability of different treatments and formulations, as well as the expected efficacy and safety of the proposed treatment. Thus, choosing an antipsychotic drug is the result of a complex and highly individualized decision making procedure involving both objective and subjective factors.

Clinical response to drug therapy as measured by psychopathological assessments is usually the response measure of choice in clinical trials assessing the efficacy of antipsychotic drugs. Increasingly, more complex "outcome" measures like "recovery" are taken into account. Model studies employing such combined approaches are available in schizophrenia and have shown that the longer-term aspect of recovery is heavily influenced by a range of factors including short-term symptomatic remission rates [47]. In a wider sense of a psychiatry of the person and its implications for schizophrenia and related disorders, this would imply that drug therapy is initiated "with the person" using strategies of shared decision making and keeping the individual´s treatment goals and values in focus. It also implies drug treatment "for the person", identifying not only health-related, but also more general aims in life with a view to integrate mental health into the context of the person´s life situation, goals and impairments. Drug therapy-related attitudes of patients with schizophrenia are predictors of treatment adherence, indicating that considering such person-related factors in patient education and information may be an important measure to increase the efficacy of antipsychotic medication [21]. Establishing a therapeutic alliance between the patient and his/her treating physician leads to drug therapy "by the person", who becomes more than a passive recipient of drugs. This then leads to drug treatment "of the person", meaning that a complete assessment of impairments including issues of quality of life, role fulfilment and social integration come into play. There are specific challenges to be expected: such assessments of treatment needs would become complex, multidimensional and time consuming. Also, such assessments may have little relevance to actual drug treatment decisions, simply because all antipsychotic drugs will have comparable side effects and excellent efficacy, with the need to find the optimal drug and dosage in each individual case. Not in all cases is it possible to integrate this into the whole life plan—simply because a person with schizophrenia may have delusion- or hallucination-driven plans, which may—from a clinical point of view—not be regarded as the person´s autonomous wish, but rather results of a disease process. Therefore, finding optimal drug regimens may always be burdened by the need to find workable compromises between the aspect of "covering every aspect of life", individual goals and the real world limitations of mental health care. Also, it may be necessary to identify and evaluate limitations of the treating physician's and the person's capacity to act ideally, and it may become prudent during the disease course to develop ways to handle such limitations rather than ignoring them.

25.4 Personalized Psychotherapy

Similar to drug therapy, psychotherapy by virtue of its nature is a personal affair in that it should benefit the patient individually and that it is heavily reliant on a personal relationship between the patient and his/her therapist. Psychoeducation has been an important aspect of forging a therapeutic alliance and is also effective in reducing rehospitalization [28], especially when combined approaches using psychoeducation and cognitive treatment are employed. A special aspect of the psychotherapy of schizophrenia is that it has long been neglected as a potentially effective therapeutic approach. In the early 2000s, increased interest in psychotherapeutic approaches emerged [3] and has accelerated with the emergence of cognitive-behavioural psychotherapies for positive and negative symptoms [31, 42]. Disputes about psychotic experiences do not negatively affect the therapeutic alliance course and applying cognitive-behavioural techniques may significantly alleviate symptom burden in patients with symptoms of psychosis [58]. Therefore, the picture of psychotic disorders as contraindications for psychotherapeutic measures is not warranted any more. Following these therapeutic successes, cognitive models of psychosis were further developed and are now increasingly based on research evidence including neurobiological studies and psychological investigations (reviewed by Sarin and Wallin [46]). In the psychoanalytic schools, there is still few research on its use for psychotic patients, but a re-emergence of interest in applying psychodynamic or psychoanalytic approaches in the care of people with schizophrenia can be observed [26, 51]. The approaches of individual understanding and highly personalized (individualized) care used in traditional psychoanalytic settings may provide interesting insights into the nature of psychotic disorders [30], but new research is necessary to prove efficacy and to show which kinds of psychoanalytic or psychodynamic approaches are best suited for which type of patient and in which disease stage. Issues of body–mind relationship and of the separation of oneself from the therapist in the patient-therapist relationship emerge. An important aspect in the sense of a more personalized approach may be the role of families, shame and guilt [36]. The studies in brief family-oriented interventions are few and a Cochrane review concluded that the size and quality of studies would need to be augmented in the future [40]. New family therapeutic approaches including culturally sensitive aspects of minority ethnicity show the feasibility of such approaches in clinical practice and some efficacy in reducing symptom loads, but would need further larger-scale trials to be generalizable [57]. Other new psychotherapeutic approaches aim at increasing the mentalizing capacities of patients with psychotic disorders, an approach designed to foster self and other understanding [10]. Person-related factors like attachment styles have been shown to be associated with the course of psychotic disorders and may provide new avenues for the psychotherapy of psychosis [32]. Another approach in psychotherapy is to deny the medical model and focus on past experiences of abuse or trauma as putative causes of hearing voices [43]. Such reductionist approaches may be superseded by the current knowledge about the social neurosciences, which integrate personal histories of adversities with neurobiological factors.

25.5 Personalized Rehabilitation Therapy

The effectiveness of individualized rehabilitation therapy for schizophrenia and related disorders has made progress in two related areas. One is research showing that cognitive therapy will improve workplace related outcomes [37], and the second is that supported employment programmes providing individualized placement and support are very effective in those countries in which traditional rehabilitation measures have not been successful. Meta-analyses show that the availability and the implementation of such effective rehabilitation programmes are the decisive factors to foster improvements of the results of workplace rehabilitation programmes for people with severe mental disorders (reviewed by [6]). In that individual life decisions like which work to chose, where to take residence and how to engage oneself in work-related or educational activities come heavily into play in rehabilitation services, these provide an area of person-centred mental healthcare for persons with schizophrenia and related disorders which deserves considerable attention. In rehabilitation medicine assessments, the comprehensive International Classification of Functions (ICF) developed by the World Health Organisation [12] provides an excellent framework for assessing and classifying not only symptoms of mental disorders, but also the kind and degree of social support, functional impairments and ensuing disabilities. The ICF approaches disorders in general from a bodily aspect, which means the psychopathological level in mental disorders, but also includes a more comprehensive perspective ("the entire health experience"), and an overarching view ("the human experience"), which considers health as part of the human condition [12]. It is mentioned here among the personalized aspects of rehabilitation, as the ICF plays a role in assessing rehabilitation needs and therapy. The ICF puts special emphasis on the person in his/her social context and the ensuing health-related issues, which play a centre role in rehabilitation medicine [13].

Beyond rehabilitation medicine, the ICF could be a first step towards holistic, person-centred diagnostic documentation of "the whole person" and his/her social relationships, their effects on mental health, and serve to identify and specify domains of putative therapeutic needs for support. A drawback is obviously the comprehensiveness of the ICF assessment, which requires much time.

25.6 Guidelines and Quality Indicators in Schizophrenia—the Inclusion of More Person-Centred Approaches

Guidelines and quality indicators are important determinants on how patients with schizophrenia are diagnosed and treated. They are constructed in elaborate structured processes, in which both scientific evidence is being considered and the views of stakeholders like patients and the families of patients with mental disorders [27]. The evidence-base is mostly a set of randomized controlled trials (RCT), and it can be assumed that what works in RCTs will also work in everyday clinical practice, as shown by previous studies [48]. A recent review showed that there is a multitude of schizophrenia guidelines available [22]. For a discussion about the role of guidelines in a personalized psychiatry of schizophrenia and related disorders, there are important associations between symptomatic remission, which usually takes centre stage in RCTs, and the levels of quality of life and subjective well-being, indicating that future outcome measures could incorporate these additional components to increase the "person-centredness" of guidelines [50]. An important aspect is, however, in which way crucial concepts like "response", "remission" or "recovery" are defined in the studies used for formulating guidelines and quality indicators. Here it is that a "psychiatry of the person" may also come into play in that it provides ideas and suggestions about the levels of understanding, insight and empowerment as additional constructs for outcome measures. Studies suggest, for example, that improving insight may improve clinical outcomes [49]. It would be necessary for a more personalized psychiatry to define its preferred clinical trial outcomes and treatment goals for the inclusion in the processes of guideline and quality indicator development. Also, measurements would be needed that assess the degree of individualization of therapies and the degree of evidence-based implementations of diagnostic and therapeutic procedures. Such scales are under development and first results show that the effects of implementing such comprehensive programs of individualization and evidence implementation may lead to only transient effects [7]. However, developing assessment tools and evaluating the efficacy of individualization and evidence-implementation programs would also necessitate a consensus between patients, psychiatrists and other stakeholders of mental healthcare in schizophrenia and related disorders to be developed about the relevant outcome measures or quality indicators. Obviously, such a process would need to lead to concrete formulations of operationalizable concepts of assessment of the "personalized" outcome measures, which would then become a part of the evidence evaluation underlying guideline and quality indicator development. Such an approach could also foster more research in this direction. An example of the complexities of such an endeavour is the discussion about the definition of the term "recovery", for which clear and internationally accepted definitions are not yet available. The diversity of definitions impedes progress in this area. Currently, the International Initiatives of Mental Health Leadership (IIMHL) is setting out to develop a consensus definition of recovery, which may serve as a model for further development in this field [52]. Trialog-based development of quality indicators and guidelines should become the rule [27].

25.7 People-Centred Systems of Mental Healthcare in Schizophrenia

Given the complexity of schizophrenia and related mental disorders, the necessary mental healthcare services are also complex ranging from prevention and early recognition over acute phase treatment to chronic phase treatment. As schizophrenia affects the whole person, mental healthcare is not limited to providing symptomatic relief, but also to provide secondary prevention, social services, rehabilitation services and support to the families and friends of those affected by schizophrenia. Aspects of comorbidity with substance-related disorders and an increased rate of somatic disorders with ensuing need for advanced somatic and general healthcare are additional factors. For example, in somatic healthcare, raising awareness for the somatic healthcare needs of patients with schizophrenia increased the rate of patients with annual medical healthcare status assessments from 20 to 58 % [56]. There is limited evidence that offering structured integrated mental health care programmes may also improve the situation of people with severe mental illnesses regarding their general somatic health [9]. Thus, there is a multi-dimensionality of potential areas of assessing and optimizing the "person-centredness" of schizophrenia health care, and there are multiple types of services and professions which need to be involved. It seems an impossible task to tackle all these issues simultaneously, but there are two major aspects concerning the nature of schizophrenia and related mental disorders, which may need to be prioritized in a future more person-centred system of mental healthcare: (A) The individual degree of medical therapy, empowerment and recovery-assistance may be very different depending on the disease course type (for example, continuous versus episodic with relapses and remissions), disease severity (for example, moderate versus severe symptoms) and the type of functional impairment (for example, need for workplace rehabilitation or housing). Schizophrenia usually affects all aspects of the person, but with time-variable degrees, and therefore comprehensiveness and flexibility of services is of high importance. (B) There is still a considerable degree of stigmatization against persons with schizophrenia and related disorders, which not only is exerted by the public, but also by mental health professionals and general medical professionals. The latter is especially concerning as studies have shown that people with schizophrenia not only have an excess mortality due to general medical conditions, but that there is also a considerable health care gap for somatic disorders in schizophrenia. To improve matters, a person-centred mental healthcare service should also implement measures to reduce the stigma of psychiatrists and the healthcare services caring for the mentally ill, since such stigmatization will reduce the acceptability of these services and have detrimental effects on the trust by users in such services [24, 25]. Therefore, people with schizophrenia pose two challenges to mental healthcare systems beyond the traditional issues, in that person-centred, needs-adapted, flexible and comprehensive mental and somatic healthcare services are necessary, which may not only lead to a need for many different kinds of mental health services, but also to the necessity of coordination of services. Therefore, structured programmes like disease management programmes may need to be developed addressing these structural and organizational challenges. As regards stigmatization, the focus should not only be on the general public, but needs to address general medical health services with a view to reduce the somatic healthcare gap and morbidity and mortality due to general medical conditions of persons with schizophrenia and related disorders. Besides these structural components, the person-centredness of services needs to be ascertained at all levels of the services, starting in the consulting room, involving the relevant mental health care organizations like hospitals (general and psychiatric), community mental health services, private practices, the families and the communities, and society as a whole, especially politicians responsible for mental health services, health insurance companies, employers and public agencies. Carrying the information about schizophrenia and the associated needs into all these circles will be a major challenge for mental health education programmes and psychiatrists, since one of the cornerstones of increasing empowerment and reducing stigmatization will be to inform those involved in the care of persons with schizophrenia about the nature of the disorder, its course types, the needs for services and how to best provide them.

New approaches for schizophrenia mental health care also warrant further investigations. For example, the Soteria approach tries to minimize drug therapy and improve empowerment, with few controlled trials so far showing that the approach shows similar results as traditional approaches [11].

25.8 Person-Centred Mental Health Education in Schizophrenia

The key aspect for providing person-centred mental health education is to address both the patient and those involved in providing or organizing mental health care for those with schizophrenia and related disorders. It would be warranted to place an emphasis on the treatment needs of people with schizophrenia, but also on the treatment options and the treatment successes possible. Psychiatrists would be experts par excellence to convey these messages to the patients, their families and their professional peers, but also to mental healthcare stakeholders like service providers, politicians and health insurance companies. This would imply new functions for psychiatrists, and would make it necessary to provide educational materials for the different target groups of such informational campaigns.

Professional psychiatric societies could become proponents of such initiatives assuring a high degree of scientific quality of such materials and campaigns. Besides this, medical schools curricula and psychiatry specialty residency programmes could include training in educational activities focused on psychoeducation, but also in anti-stigma initiatives. With a view towards strengthening person-centred approaches, a recent study showed that an educational activity including both neurobiological and social aspects of schizophrenia was effective to reduce stigmatizing attitudes of medical students [35]. Becoming proponents of person-centred mental health education in schizophrenia could provide psychiatrists with an opportunity to gain or increase trust by their patients, and could provide opportunities for joint appearences in the public with a view to destigmatize both mental disorders and the professions who care for people with mental disorders. Person-centredness would thus manifest itself on a new level, namely in the public domain breaking down barriers not only between patients and the public, but also between patients and care providers. Working together in these important educational activities could provide a new framework of empowerment and inclusion.

25.9 Person-Centred Research in Schizophrenia

Much of the research in schizophrenia has been based on group analyses. This has led to an inflation of information about genes associated with schizophrenia, brain imaging data on structural or functional alterations, and associations with social and environmental factors. While this has clearly advanced the understanding of the etiopathogenesis of schizophrenia and—by analogy mostly—of related mental disorders, these research results have had no major influence on individual diagnostic or therapeutic decisions. As it is becoming increasingly evident that there is a range of "pathways" leading into schizophrenia [55], the need arises to define the individual pathways in the individual who is affected by schizophrenia. An important step in this direction is the elucidation of the genetic risk factors, which are multiple, nonspecific and overlapping in individuals. Currently, an approach typifying sets of phenotypic and genotypic characteristics of schizophrenia patients appears promising to not only demonstrate the high degree of complexity of genotype-phenotype associations in schizophrenia, but also to allow further research based on clearly defined sets of genotype-phenotype associations [2]. It is critical to use a person-centred approach to the particular pathway from genotype to phenotype, allowing for different trajectories responsive to unique environmental, social, and therapeutic interventions. The Research Domain Criteria initiative of the National Institutes of Mental Health is conceptualizing research on such a neurobiological-individual basis, and a recent example on the pathophysiology of hallucinations from the initiative showed how this integrates constructs of auditory percepts with phenomenological experiences and individual reactions, providing a "person-centered" approach on all levels of analysis [20]. While such individualized information would be necessary to ultimately design truly individualized, pathogenetically informed therapeutic measures, it is unlikely that this ambitious goal may be reached soon. In the meantime, it is important to continue to identify the etiopathogenetic mechanisms at work in schizophrenia, but at the same time improve mental health care with a view to increase the person-centredness of the diagnostic approaches, the therapies and the mental health care services which care for people with schizophrenia. New trends reconciling (neuro)biological approaches with socioenvironmental and psychological approaches are promising to shape future research and lead to improved person-centredness of the diagnostic and therapeutic processes. These advances will also support the further development of the concepts of mental disorders in general and schizophrenia and related mental disorders more specifically [1]. Until such research has provided new breakthroughs of relevance to the concept of mental disorders, evidence-based practices fostering empowerment and recovery are available and need to be implemented (see [34], and the discussion therein). It is still difficult to identify the optimal mental health care service structures, the necessary processes and the best outcome assessment strategies. Two areas of potential research actions immediately come to mind with a view to advance in this direction and make significant progress to the best of those suffering from schizophrenia: (A) it is important to investigate the best way to educate medical doctors (not only psychiatrists, nurses, social workers and psychologists) about the nature of the person-involvement in schizophrenia with the ultimate goal to overcome stigmatizing attitudes. (B) It is important to investigate in how far awareness programmes are effective in convincing mental health politicians that persons with schizophrenia have highly different individual needs for mental health care, so that a range of services will need to be provided in each mental healthcare system. This shows that it is important to extend efficacy research beyond drug treatments, if optimized person-centred mental healthcare is to be achieved.

Ozomaro and co-workers recently described the need to go beyond physiologic markers in personalized medicine for persons with mental disorders [41]. They characterized personalized medicine in mental disorders by the major goals of predicting an individual's susceptibility to developing an illness, achieving accurate diagnosis, and optimizing the most efficient and favourable response to treatment. While all these aspects are clearly highly warranted goals, they may be extended by optimal goal fulfilment, satisfaction with life and the highest possible quality of life. This includes implementation of optimal mental healthcare services. Of note, these added goals may include a high degree of subjective estimations by the person affected by schizophrenia or a related mental disorder. But given the necessity to not only treat symptoms, but to optimize the well-being of those suffering from mental disorders to the highest possible degree, such person-centredness at the levels of diagnosis, treatment and mental healthcare may be the best road towards optimized person-centred care in schizophrenia.

25.10 Conclusions

This chapter shows that approaching schizophrenia and related disorders under person-centred perspectives has to consider several levels of analysis, ranging from the subjective experiences of a psychotic disorder to the objective assessment of psychophysiological consequences, effects of role fulfilment in life and the reaction of the social environment. This also includes questions of mental healthcare for persons with schizophrenia and how it can be optimized to yield the best possible results. Thus, two fields of action emerge for the future with a view to increase the person-centredness of schizophrenia research and health care: to obtain more information on the complex etiopathogenesis of schizophrenia and—until this is available—to optimize the person-centredness of mental healthcare for those affected by schizophrenia and related psychotic disorders.

References

1. Akdeniz C, Tost H, Meyer-Lindenberg A. The neurobiology of social environmental risk for schizophrenia: an evolving research field. Soc Psychiatry Psychiatr Epidemiol. 2014;49:507–17.
2. Arnedo J, Svrakic DM, Del Val C, Romero-Zaliz R, Hernandez-Cuervo H, Molecular Genetics of Schizophrenia Consortium, Fanous AH, Pato ME, Pato CN, de Erausquin GA, Cloninger R, Zwir I. Uncovering the hidden risk architecture of the schizophrenias: confirmation in three independent genome-wide association studies. Am J Psychiatry. 2015;172:139–53.
3. Bachmann S, Resch F, Mundt C. Psychological treatments for psychosis: history and overview. J Am Acad Psychoanal Dyn Psychiatry. 2003;31:155–76.
4. Boecker R, Holz NE, Buchmann AF, Blomeyer D, Plichta MM, Wolf I, Baumeister S, Meyer-Lindenberg A, Banaschewski T, Brandeis D, Laucht M. Impact of early life adversity on reward processing in young adults: EEG-fMRI results from a prospective study over 25 years. PLoS ONE. 2014;9(8):e104185. doi:10.1371/journal.pone.0104185.
5. Bolton D. Should mental disorders be regarded as brain disorders? 21st century mental health sciences and implications for research and training. World Psychiatry. 2013;12:24–5.
6. Bond GR, Drake RE. Predictors of competitive employment among patients with schizophrenia. Curr Opin Psychiatry. 2008;21:362–9.
7. Bond GR, Drake RE, Rapp CA, et al. Individualization and quality improvement: two new scales to complement measurement of program fidelity. Adm Policy Ment Health. 2009;36:349–57.
8. Borrell-Carrió F, Suchman AL, Epstein RM. The biopsychosocial model 25 years later: principles, practice, and scientific inquiry. Ann Fam Med. 2004;2:576–82.
9. Bradford DW, Cunningham NT, Slubicki MN, et al. An evidence synthesis of care models to improve general medical outcomes for individuals with serious mental illness: a systematic review. J Clin Psychiatry. 2013;74:e754–64. doi:10.4088/JCP.12r07666.
10. Brent BK, Holt DJ, Keshavan MS, et al. Mentalization-based treatment for psychosis: linking an attachment-based model to the psychotherapy for impaired mental state understanding in people with psychotic disorders. Isr J Psychiatry Relat Sci. 2014;51:17–24.
11. Calton T, Ferriter M, Huband N, et al. A systematic review of the Soteria paradigm for the treatment of people diagnosed with schizophrenia. Schizophr Bull. 2008;34:181–92.
12. Cieza A, Stucki G. The international classification of functioning disability and health: its development process and content validity. Eur J Phys Rehabil Med. 2008;44:303–13.

13. Cieza A, Bickenbach J, Chatterji S. The ICF as a conceptual platform to specify and discuss health and health-related concepts. Gesundheitswesen. 2008;70:e47–56. doi:10.1055/s-2008-1080933.
14. Correll CU. From receptor pharmacology to improved outcomes: individualising the selection, dosing, and switching of antipsychotics. Eur Psychiatry. 2010;25(Suppl 2):S12–21.
15. Correll CU. Mechanism of action of antipsychotic medications. J Clin Psychiatry. 2014;75(9): e23. doi:10.4088/JCP.13078tx4c.
16. Cuthbert BN. The RDoC framework: facilitating transition from ICD/DSM to dimensional approaches that integrate neuroscience and psychopathology. World Psychiatry. 2014;13:28–35.
17. Cuthbert BN, NIMH RDoC Workgroup. The RDoC framework: continuing commentary. World Psychiatry. 2014;13:196–7.
18. Engel G. The need for a new medical model: a challenge for biomedicine. Science. 1977;196:129–36.
19. European Network of National Networks studying Gene-Environment Interactions in Schizophrenia (EU-GEI), van Os J, Rutten BP et al. Identifying gene-environment interactions in schizophrenia: contemporary challenges for integrated, large-scale investigations. Schizophr Bull. 2014;40:729–736.
20. Ford JM, Morris SE, Hoffman RE et al. Studying hallucinations Within the NIMH RDoC Framework. Schizophr Bull. 2014; in press. doi:10.1093/schbul/sbu011.
21. Gaebel W, Riesbeck M, von Wilmsdorff M, et al. Drug attitude as predictor for effectiveness in first-episode schizophrenia: results of an open randomized trial (EUFEST). Eur Neuropsychopharmacol. 2010;20:310–6.
22. Gaebel W, Riesbeck M, Wobrock T. Schizophrenia guidelines across the world: a selective review and comparison. Int Rev Psychiatry. 2011;23:379–87.
23. Gaebel W, Galderisi S, Gheorghe M, et al. Unmet needs in patients with first-episode schizophrenia: a longitudinal perspective. Psychol Med. 2012;42:1461–73.
24. Gaebel W, Zäske H, Zielasek J et al. Stigmatization of psychiatrists and general practitioners: results of an international survey. Eur Arch Psychiatry Clin Neurosci. 2014a; Sep 5. [Epub ahead of print].
25. Gaebel W, Muijen M, Baumann AE. EPA guidance on building trust in mental health services. Eur Psychiatry. 2014;29:83–100.
26. Garfield DA. Psychoanalytically informed psychotherapy of psychosis: the influences of american psychoanalysis. Panel report. J Am Psychoanal Assoc. 2011;59:603–20.
27. Großimlinghaus I, Falkai P, Gaebel W, et al. Developmental process of DGPPN quality indicators]. [Article in German. Nervenarzt. 2013;84:350–65.
28. Hornung WP, Feldmann R, Klingberg S, et al. Long-term effects of a psychoeducational psychotherapeutic intervention for schizophrenic outpatients and their key-persons–results of a five-year follow-up. Eur Arch Psychiatry Clin Neurosci. 1999;249:162–7.
29. Howes OD, Egerton A, Allan V, et al. Mechanisms underlying psychosis and antipsychotic treatment response in schizophrenia: insights from PET and SPECT imaging. Curr Pharm Des. 2009;15:2550–9.
30. Kafka JS. Chestnut lodge and the psychoanalytic approach to psychosis. J Am Psychoanal Assoc. 2011;59:27–47.
31. Klingberg S, Wölwer W, Engel C, et al. Negative symptoms of schizophrenia as primary target of cognitive behavioral therapy: results of the randomized clinical TONES study. Schizophr Bull. 2011;37(Suppl 2):S98–110.
32. Korver-Nieberg N, Berry K, Meijer CJ, et al. Adult attachment and psychotic phenomenology in clinical and non-clinical samples: a systematic review. Psychol Psychother. 2014;87:127–54.
33. Landolt K, Rössler W, Burns T, et al. On the psychoanalytic treatment of a psychotic breakdown. Psychoanal Q. 2005;74:1069–99.
34. MacDonald-Wilson KM, Deegan PE, Hutchison SL, et al. Integrating personal medicine into service delivery: empowering people in recovery. Psychiatr Rehabil J. 2013;36:258–63.

35. Magliano L, Read J, Sagliocchi A, et al. Social dangerousness and incurability in schizophrenia: results of an educational intervention for medical and psychology students. Psychiatry Res. 2014;219:457–63.
36. Martindale BV. The rehabilitation of psychoanalysis and the family in psychosis: recovering from blaming. Psychiatr Danub. 2009;21(Suppl 1):51–60.
37. McGurk SR, Mueser KT, Feldman K, et al. Cognitive training for supported employment: 2–3 year outcomes of a randomized controlled trial. Am J Psychiatry. 2007;164:437–41.
38. Moreno C, Nuevo R, Chatterji S, et al. Psychotic symptoms are associated with physical health problems independently of a mental disorder diagnosis: results from the WHO World Health Survey. World Psychiatry. 2013;12:251–7.
39. Nuevo R, Van Os J, Arango C. Evidence for the early clinical relevance of hallucinatory-delusional states in the general population. Acta Psychiatr Scand. 2013;127:482–93.
40. Okpokoro U, Adams CE, Sampson S. Family intervention (brief) for schizophrenia. Cochrane Database Syst Rev 3. 2014;CD009802. doi:10.1002/14651858.CD009802.pub2.
41. Ozomaro U, Wahlestedt C, Nemeroff CB. Personalized medicine in psychiatry: problems and promises. BMC Med. 2013;11:132.
42. Rector NA, Beck AT. Cognitive behavioral therapy for schizophrenia: an empirical review. J Nerv Ment Dis. 2012;200:832–9.
43. Romme M, Morris M. The recovery process with hearing voices: accepting as well as exploring their emotional background through a supported process. Psychosis Psychol Soc Integr Appr. 2013;5:259–69.
44. Salvador-Carulla L, Mezzich JE. Person-centred medicine and mental health. Epidemiol Psychiatr Sci. 2012;21:131–7.
45. Sandhu S, Bjerre NV, Dauvrin M. Experiences with treating immigrants: a qualitative study in mental health services across 16 European countries. Soc Psychiatry Psychiatr Epidemiol. 2013;48:105–16.
46. Sarin F, Wallin L. Cognitive model and cognitive behavior therapy for schizophrenia: an overview. Nord J Psychiatry. 2014;68:145–53.
47. Schennach R, Riedel M, Obermeier M, et al. Remission and recovery and their predictors in schizophrenia spectrum disorder: results from a 1-year follow-up naturalistic trial. Psychiatr Q. 2012;83:187–207.
48. Schennach R, Meyer S, Seemüller F et al. Response trajectories in "real-world" naturalistically treated schizophrenia patients. Schizophr Res. 2012b;139:218–224.
49. Schennach R, Meyer S, Seemüller F, et al. Insight in schizophrenia-course and predictors during the acute treatment phase of patients suffering from a schizophrenia spectrum disorder. Eur Psychiatry. 2012;27:625–33.
50. Schennach-Wolff R, Jäger M, Obermeier M, et al. Quality of life and subjective well-being in schizophrenia and schizophrenia spectrum disorders: valid predictors of symptomatic response and remission? World J Biol Psychiatry. 2010;11:729–38.
51. Silver AL. Psychoanalytically informed treatment of psychosis: reflections on its U.S. history and current dilemmas. Psychoanal Rev. 2013;100:311–35.
52. Spaeth-Rublee B, Pincus HA, Silvestri F, et al. Measuring quality of mental health care: an international comparison. Int J Environ Res Public Health. 2014;11:10384–9.
53. Stanghellini G, Bolton D, Fulford WK. Person-centered psychopathology of schizophrenia: building on Karl Jaspers' understanding of patient's attitude toward his illness. Schizophr Bull. 2013;39:287–94.
54. Straßmayr C, Matanov A, Priebe S, et al. Mental health care for irregular migrants in Europe: barriers and how they are overcome. BMC Publ Health. 2012;12:367. doi:10.1186/1471-2458-12-367.
55. Sullivan PF. Puzzling over schizophrenia: schizophrenia as a pathway disease. Nat Med. 2012;18:210–1.
56. Vasudev K, Martindale BV. Physical healthcare of people with severe mental illness: everybody's business! Ment Health Fam Med. 2010;7:115–22.

57. Weisman de Mamani A, Weintraub MJ, Gurak K et al. A randomized clinical trial to test the efficacy of a family-focused, culturally informed therapy for schizophrenia. J Fam Psychol. 2014 Oct 6. [Epub ahead of print].
58. Wittorf A, Jakobi UE, Bannert KK, et al. Does the cognitive dispute of psychotic symptoms do harm to the therapeutic alliance? J Nerv Ment Dis. 2010;198:478–85.

Bipolar Disorder

26

Ihsan M. Salloum, MD, MPH and George N. Christodoulou, MD, PhD

26.1 Introduction

Bipolar disorder, a modern term that became part of the official nosology of current classification systems only in the past few decades was recognized by scholars from ancient Greece where the terms *mania* and *melancholia* appeared first [6]. Bipolar disorder, previously termed by Emil Kraepelin as manic-depressive psychosis, is a major mental disorder characterized by the occurrence of one or more lifetime manic episodes and of depressive episodes, with likelihood of regaining pre-morbid level of functioning [19].

Bipolar disorder is associated with significant clinical challenges as well as with high levels of disability, especially for younger age groups [1]. The lifetime rate of bipolar disorder is estimated about 1 % and some community estimate reported a prevalence rate up to 3.3 % [16]. Bipolar disorder, despite its relatively low frequency, is among the leading disability causes according to the World Health Organization (WHO) [41]. Bipolar disorder has one of the highest lifetime suicide risk compared to any mental or physical condition, and this risk increases when coexisting with other conditions such as substance use disorders [9, 35, 36].

I.M. Salloum, MD, MPH (✉)
Professor of Psychiatry and Behavioral Sciences, Miller School of Medicine, University of Miami, 1120 N.W. 14th Street, Rm. 1449 (LC 28), Miami, FL 33136, USA; Chair, Section on Classification, Diagnostic Assessment and Nomenclature, World Psychiatric Association, Geneva, Switzerland
e-mail: isalloum@med.miami.edu

G.N. Christodoulou, MD, PhD
Emeritus Professor of Psychiatry, University of Athens, Athens, Greece

J.E. Mezzich et al. (eds.), *Person Centered Psychiatry*,
DOI 10.1007/978-3-319-39724-5_26

Bipolar disorder often goes undetected and untreated and there is 10 years lag between the onsets of mood symptoms, typically depression, and the formulation of a bipolar disorder diagnosis [17].

Bipolar disorder is characterized by its high association with other comorbid psychiatric and physical conditions. Anxiety disorders are reportedly the most frequent psychiatric conditions among patients with bipolar disorder with reported rates ranging from 30 % to around 90 %, depending on the population studied and ascertainment methods used [11, 32]. Comorbid substance use disorders have been repeatedly reported to be very high as well. Bipolar disorder has the highest association with alcoholism and other substance use disorders (SUD) compared to any other psychiatric diagnosis with the exception of antisocial personality disorder [27]. The lifetime rates of SUD in people with bipolar disorder ranged from 40–60 % in clinical and epidemiological samples. A large epidemiological study reported that respondents with mania were 14 times more likely compared to the general population to have a drug dependence and 6 times more likely to have alcohol dependence during the previous 12-months. Additional frequent psychiatric disorders encountered in bipolar disorder patients include eating disorders, gambling and borderline personality disorders [20, 32].

The clinical course of bipolar disorder represents multiple challenges ranging from severe symptoms presentation, frequent mood episodes, higher suicide risk, higher medical comorbidities, lower functioning, lower life satisfaction and chronic disabilities for severe variants of the bipolar condition.

26.2 Challenges in the Diagnosis and Care of People with Bipolar Disorder

The Diagnostic and Statistical Manual of Mental Disorders, Fifth edition (DSM-5) [5] dedicated, for the first time, a unique chapter for bipolar and related disorders. The previous versions of the DSM [2–4] as well as International Classifications of Diseases-10th edition (ICD-10) [40] had included bipolar disorder under the rubric of mood disorders with other mood disorders such as major depressive disorders.

We will briefly discuss the diagnostic algorithm of bipolar disorder in light of the latest published revision of a major classification of mental disorders, namely the DSM-5, as conceivably it constitutes the most up-to-date nosological review of this disorder. DSM-5 places bipolar and related disorders as an independent chapter between depressive disorders and schizophrenia spectrum and other psychotic disorders. The rational for this change was stated as recognition of the place of bipolar disorder as a bridge, in terms of genetics, family history and symptomatology, between these two other major classes of disorders. Under this chapter, the three classic categories, bipolar I disorder, bipolar II disorder, and cyclothymic disorder are included in addition to substance/medications induced bipolar disorder and bipolar disorder due to another medical condition. This chapter also includes residual categories such as other specified and unspecified bipolar-related disorders [5].

The cardinal diagnostic feature of bipolar I disorder is the occurrence of one lifetime manic episode, which may precede or follow episodes of major depression or hypomania.

A manic episode is a distinct period lasting of at least one week with symptoms present every day or nearly every day, or being hospitalized during this period. Two symptoms are required during this distinct period to trigger further consideration of a manic episode. These include an abnormally and persistently elevated, expansive, or irritable mood and abnormally and persistently increased goal-directed activity or energy. Additionally, three (or four if mood is only irritable) out of seven symptoms must be present to a significant degree and represent a noticeable change in behavior. These include grandiosity or inflated self-esteem, decreased need for sleep, increased talkativeness or pressured to keep talking, racing thoughts or flights or ideas, distractibility, psychomotor activity or increased goal-directed activities, and increased activities with high potential for painful consequences. These symptoms must cause either marked impairment in functioning (social or occupational) or necessitate hospitalization to prevent harm to self or others, or for the presence of psychotic symptoms, and not due to substance/medication effects or other medical conditions.

A hypomanic episode is defined similarly to a manic episode except for the duration (at least 4 days), and absence of hospitalization with psychotic symptoms. While hypomanic episodes frequently occur, their presence is not necessary for the diagnosis of bipolar I disorder. The presence of at least one lifetime hypomanic episode and one lifetime depressive episode and the absence of a lifetime manic episode are required for the diagnosis of bipolar II disorder.

For a depressive episode, there need to be five (out of nine) symptoms present during the same 2-week period with at least one symptom being either a depressed mood or loss of interest or pleasure. Symptoms need to be present every day or nearly every day and are associated with significant impairment or distress and not attributable to physical conditions or to the effects of substances or medications. These symptoms include depressed mood, marked decreased interest or pleasure in all or most activities, significant change in weight or appetite (decrease or increase), insomnia or hypersomnia, psychomotor agitation or retardation, fatigue or loss of energy, feeling of worthlessness or excessive guilt, decreased ability to think or concentrate and indecisiveness, and recurrent thoughts of death, and the presence of suicidal symptoms (ideations, plan and/or attempts). The presence of either a manic or a depressive episode(s) are not better explained for by a schizophrenia spectrum and other psychotic disorders.

Both manic and depressive episodes are further specified in terms of severity (mild, moderate, and severe), the presence of psychotic features, and whether they are currently in partial or full remission or unspecified. Moreover, the mood episodes (manic, hypomanic and depressive) could be further characterized by using other descriptive specifiers that provide relevant information about the clinical presentation of the episode, which may have treatment implications. These further specifiers include a mood episode with either anxious distress, mixed features, rapid cycling, melancholic features, atypical features, mood-congruent and mood-incongruent psychotic features, catatonia, peripartum onset, or with seasonal pattern. Each of these clinical specifiers are further described in terms of criteria and further enrich the clinical description of the presenting episode.

Cyclothymic disorder describes a chronic disorder of at least 2 years (1 year in children and adolescents), where the criteria for an episode of major depression, mania or hypomania have never been met, however, the person had periods with hypomanic and depressive symptoms for at least half of the time and these symptoms were not absent for more than 2 months at a time. These symptoms must be accompanied by clinically significant distress and or impairment and are not explained by a schizophrenia spectrum and other psychotic disorders, and not due to substances/medications use or other physical disorders.

The Other Specified Bipolar and Related Disorders category encompass categories that causes impairment and distress but without meeting the full criteria for a specific episode. These include short-duration hypomanic (2–3 days) and major depressive episode, hypomanic episode with insufficient symptoms and major depressive episode, hypomanic episode without prior major depressive episode, and short-duration cyclothymia (less than 24 months). Finally, the Unspecified category is dedicated to presentations that do not meet the full criteria for any bipolar-related disorder or where there is insufficient information to make a specific diagnosis.

It is not surprising that, with such wide spectrum and varied clinical presentations, the recognition and treatment of bipolar disorder is typically delayed around a decade from the first onset of symptoms. DSM-5 specification of the multiple potential presenting symptoms constellation may help in enhancing the recognition of the less prototypical from of the disorder. While telltale signs and symptoms of depression or that of a typical manic episode are easily recognized, great difficulties ensues in recognizing softer manifestation of manic/hypomanic symptoms and this difficulty is magnified by the frequent presence of comorbid psychiatric and substance use disorders. Patients have difficulty recognizing the need for treatment of hypomanic/manic symptoms, which is usually not associated with subjective distress. Additionally these symptoms may also significantly impact on the patient insight into their illness, thus resulting in avoiding seeking treatment while in the hypomanic/manic phase as well as decreasing treatment adherence for those in treatment [33].

The presence of comorbid disorders, for example substance use disorders, complicate further the diagnostic recognition, as effects of many substances can induce, worsen, or masks the symptoms of bipolar disorder. The presence of comorbidity further complicates the treatment and management of bipolar disorder. Patients are usually unaware of the mutual negative effects of having multiple disorders and how each disorder may contribute to worsening of the overall condition. For example, current and past alcohol and drug use disorders increased the likelihood of switch to mania, hypomania, or mixed states in a large prospective study [24]. Furthermore, the presence of comorbid conditions may contribute to lack of response in bipolar disorder [32] and persistent residual affective symptoms, which have been linked to higher likelihood of relapse to a full affective episode [18].

Bipolar disorder, similar to other chronic medical conditions, requires an ongoing maintenance treatment, is affected by multiple comorbidities and patients usually require multiple medications to achieve stability. As with other chronic medical conditions, it presents a significant challenge in terms of preventing episode recurrences, maintaining treatment adherence and achieving long-term stability. Recovery from chronic, relapsing conditions, such as bipolar-related disorders implicate a long-term process over a continuum of care that requires the mobilization of multiple resources, including key among them the person's own resources and resiliencies. Barriers to recovery range from health system issues such as lack of integration and difficulty accessing care, to social-cultural issues such as attitudinal difficulties and stigma toward psychiatric disorders. These dynamics usually occur at multiple levels in the care for these patients, from health care provider to stakeholders, families and patients. Resistance to taking medications for bipolar disorder is a common example seen in patients, but sometime is also seen in patients' families or support network. For example, some self-help groups for addiction or alcoholism promote avoiding taking "mind & mood altering drugs" and under this rubric they misguidedly include all psychotropic medications. A practice that lead to discontinuation of much needed medication resulting in recurrence of mood episodes. Poor treatment and medication adherence is a significant challenge in bipolar disorder as well. It is unclear how much this problem has contributed to the phenomenon of polypharmacy frequently reported in patients with bipolar disorder. While many patients require more than one medication to stabilize their symptoms, the lack of effective monitoring of medication adherence and optimization of medication could not be ruled out in many patients who are prescribed additional medications to stabilize their symptoms.

26.3 Models for Diagnosis and Care for People with Bipolar Disorder

The primacy of diagnosis in the process of care is highlighted by Feinstein [15] who stated that "*Diagnostic categories provide the locations where clinicians store the observations of clinical experience*" and where "*The diagnostic taxonomy establishes the patterns according to which clinicians observe, think, remember and act*" [15]. Diagnosis is the cornerstone of the treatment plan, it guides and directs treatment intervention efforts and it frames the outcome goals. A diagnosis focused on symptoms, it directs interventions at achieving symptoms response or at best symptoms remission; a diagnosis focused on recovery, it directs interventions toward disease remission and health restoration. Contemporary psychiatric classification systems, while have at their core the diagnosis of mental disorders, have recognized the importance of an assessment that provides clinically useful information for the overall treatment of the patient. Hence, many have adopted a bio-psycho-social approach to patient assessment and have included multiaxial diagnostic schemas to organize relevant clinical information. Examples of multiaxial schemas were included in the various reiterations of the DSM system (DSM-III, DSM-III-R and DSM-IV and DSM-IV TR) of the American Psychiatric Association, the WHO ICD-10, the Chinese system [10], and the Latin-American Guide of Psychiatric Diagnosis [7] or the International Guidelines of Diagnostic

Assessment [21]. While the various multiaxial schemas include different relevant domains such as functioning, stressors and other medical conditions, the main focus of these schemas are within the ill health domains and only few included an assessment of the quality of life [21].

Traditional model of care have emphasized disease-centered approaches with primary focus on illness, acute care and on organ-system-based pathology. Secondary attention is given to preventative and health restorative efforts. Notoriously, the DSM-5 did not include a multiaxial diagnostic schema because the previously complicated algorithm included in DSM-IVTR was not widely adopted in the field. It is unclear how this change will impact on the clinical utility of the diagnostic system as a whole. A disease-centered diagnostic and intervention approach may not be sufficient to address chronic, complex diseases with high rates of comorbid conditions [28].

Bipolar disorder, a chronic and severe mental disorder, presents with all the problematics of chronic conditions, including the need for a life long illness management, the need to deal with multiple psychiatric and medical comorbidities, and the urgent need for health restoration, recovery, prevention of relapses and health maintenance. The challenges presented by bipolar disorder and other chronic conditions call for alternative models of integrated care which mobilizes the person's and their communities strengths in partnership with the health care provider with focus on long-term recovery and health restoration.

Holistic (emphasizing the importance of the whole and the interdependence of its parts), integrated concept of health have been emphasized by ancient as well as modern medical traditions (Salloum and Khazai, In Press). For example, the World Health Organization (WHO) constitution defined health as "*a state of complete physical, emotional, and social well-being and not merely the absence of disease or infirmity.*"[39].

The overreliance on disease-centered, over-specialized approach has led to artificially parceling out care, leading to fragmentation, incoordination, and decreased access to care. The interconnectedness of health problems and the exceptional burden of chronic mental health conditions, along with the crucial role of behavioral determinants of health strongly argues for dynamic care models that integrates the totality of health (including ill and positive aspects of health), with emphasis on disease prevention and health restoration. This is crucial for the long terms management for chronic severe mental disorders such bipolar disorder. Studies have shown that medical comorbidity is the most significant cause of mortality in people with mental disorders, and these disorders are less likely to receive adequate attention. High rates of comorbid physical disorders such as diabetes, cardiovascular, chronic respiratory diseases, human-immune deficiency virus (HIV) infection, hepatitis, sexually transmitted diseases (STD), tuberculosis (TB), and trauma with excess mortality have been repeatedly reported not only for bipolar disorder, but also for other chronic mental disorders such as major depression and schizophrenia. The risk of physical disorders is significantly increased in this population because of the high rates of smoking, substance abuse, obesity and sedentary lifestyle [8, 12, 26, 34]. Thus, it is not surprising that these patients have an estimated 25 years less life expectancy compared to the general population [25]. Those with comorbid substance abuse were found to be 6–8 times more likely than a non-substance abusing group, to die from injury, primarily poisoning [13].

Furthermore, the need for new approaches to care, with holistic and integrated focus stems from the disproportionate impact of psychosocial determinants on health care services [38]. Studies have repeatedly documented the overrepresentation of behavioral and life style factors among the preventable risk factor for developing chronic diseases. Furthermore, the interdependence of presenting problems is highlighted by the fact that psychosocial distress is often expressed as physical problems, and likewise, mood symptoms may develop as a consequence of chronic physical disorders [14].

26.4 The Emerging Person-Centered Integrative Diagnosis (PID) Model and Bipolar Disorder

The Person-centered Integrative Diagnosis (PID) model is an emerging approach to diagnosis and ensuing care anchored in person-centered medicine. The PID aims at putting into practice the vision of Person-centered Medicine affirming the whole person of the patient in context as the center of clinical care and health promotion at the individual and community levels [22, 30]. This model provides a conceptual approach, especially suitable for the diagnosis and care planning for complex chronic diseases, such as bipolar disorder [22, 30]. The PID is an integrated model as it considers the totality of the person's health, including both ill health and positive aspects of health and it is based on a holistic, contextual and humanistic approach to care emphasizing recovery and wellbeing. Diagnosis is also conceptualized as a process and a respectful partnership with persons seeking care, their families, care givers and other stakeholders along with health professionals.

The PID scheme, in addition of being practical and easily incorporated into the process of care, provides a dynamic and integrated multilevel assessment of the health status of the person presenting for care.

The levels of assessments include determination of the health status (positive and ill health), identification of contributors to the health status (protective and risk factors), and evaluation of the experience and values of health (illness and wellbeing).

The assessment of health status includes the assessment of ill health, such as any physical or mental disorders (using ICD-10 or ICD-10-CM conventions). This level also includes assessment of functional abilities such as personal care, occupational functioning, functioning with family, as well as social and overall functioning. Health status assessment also includes the assessment of positive aspects of health and wellbeing. Assessment of positive aspects of health and wellbeing domains is key to planning for recovery, health restoration and health preservation efforts. Support of and reliance on the strengths and resiliencies of the person seeking care will be fundamental for the process of care partnership, wellness and disease management, and functional recovery.

Aligning the domains of the health status, which would include not only the diagnosis of bipolar disorder but also all other comorbid disorders, along with functional abilities as well as the positive aspects of health and wellbeing will give the patient a road map on health as a whole, which is crucial for the process of care. This will enhance the awareness of the patient and that of the rest of the health team, on the interactions between the various comorbid conditions as well as on the most effective way to utilize strengths to optimize the recovery process.

The assessment of contributors to health status represents the second level in the PID model. Contributors to health are considered on a bio-psycho-social continuum and are divided into health promoters and health risks. A list of contributors to health has been incorporated into PID guides that include those identified in the Health Improvement Card developed by the World Health Professions Alliance [37]. Health promoters include diet, physical activity, creative activity, social involvement, stress-control, and adequate rest and sleep. Health risks include being overweight, elevated lipids, elevated glucose, high blood pressure, alcohol and tabacco use, family morbidity history, early trauma, and significant stress. A clear understanding of health promoters as well as health risks in bipolar disorder is fundamental for the long-term care of this disoder.

Assesment of the experience of health is the third level of the PID and it includes the assessment of experience and values connected to well-being and ill health. This level of assessment provides a subjective idiographic narrative of personal and cultural identity, suffering, meaning of illness and expectations (values and preferences) for health care. These subjective contributions to the process of diagnosis and care are crucial for the processes of empowerment, engagement, partnership and recovery [23, 29, 31].

26.5 Conclusions

Bipolar disorder is a chronic severe mental disorder that presents with all the challenges of chronic complex conditions including high rates of comorbidity, disability, disease burden and early mortality. Current disease-centered models of care are inadequate for the long-term care and recovery of people with these disorders. A person-centered medicine approach to care with a holistic paradigm of care and focus on health restoration and disease prevention is more likely to meet the treatment needs for this population. Person-centered integrative diagnosis is an emerging model of diagnosis and care that emphasizes holistic assessment of health using a partnership approach to diagnosis involving patients, families, caregivers, stakeholders, and health care professionals. It is a viable alternative to existing models for responding to the multiple challenges and complexities for persons with severe chronic mental health conditions such as bipolar disorder.

References

1. Alonso J, Petukhova M, Vilagut G, Chatterji S, Heeringa S, Ustun TB, Alhamzawi AO, Viana MC, Angermeyer M, Bromet E, Bruffaerts R, de Girolamo G, Florescu S, Gureje O, Haro JM, Hinkov H, Hu CY, Karam EG, Kovess V, Levinson D, Medina-Mora ME, Nakamura Y, Ormel J, Posada-Villa J, Sagar R, Scott KM, Tsang A, Williams DR, Kessler RC. Days out of role due to common physical and mental conditions: results from the WHO World Mental Health surveys. Mol Psychiatry. 2011;16:1234–46.
2. APA. Diagnostic and statistical manual of mental disorders (DSM III). 3rd ed. Washington, DC.: American Psychiatric Association; 1980.
3. APA. Diagnostic and statistical manual of mental disorders (DSM III-R). 3rd ed., revised. Washington, DC.: American Psychiatric Association; 1987.
4. APA. Diagnostic and statistical manual of mental disorders (DSM-IV). 4th ed. Washington, DC: American Psychiatric Association.
5. APA. Diagnostic and statistical manual of mental disorders (DSM-5). 5th ed. Arlington, VA: American Psychiatric Association.
6. Baldessarini RJ, Perez J, Trede K, Maggini C. History of bipolar manic-depressive disorder. In: Yildiz A, Ruiz P, Nemeroff CB, editors. The bipolar book history, neurobiology, and treatment. New York, NY: Oxford University Press; 2015.
7. Berganza CE, Mezzich JE, Jorge MR. Latin American guide for psychiatric diagnosis (GLADP). Psychopathology. 2002;35:185–90.
8. Carney CP, Jones LE. Medical comorbidity in women and men with bipolar disorders: a population-based controlled study. Psychosom Med. 2006;68:684–91.
9. Carra G, Bartoli F, Crocamo C, Brady KT, Clerici M. Attempted suicide in people with co-occurring bipolar and substance use disorders: systematic review and meta-analysis. J Affect Disord. 2014;167:125–35.
10. Chen YF. Chinese classification of mental disorders (CCMD-3): towards integration in international classification. Psychopathology. 2002;35:171–5.
11. Conway KP, Compton W, Stinson FS, Grant BF. Lifetime comorbidity of DSM-IV mood and anxiety disorders and specific drug use disorders: results from the national epidemiologic survey on alcohol and related conditions. [see comment]. J Clin Psychiatry. 2006;67:247–57.
12. De Hert M, Correll CU, Bobes J, Al E. Physical illness in patients with severe mental disorders. I. prevalence, impact of medications and disparities in health care. World Psychiatry. 2015;10:52–77.
13. Dickey B, Dembling B, Azeni H, Normand S-LT. Externally caused deaths for adults with substance use and mental disorders. J Behav Health Serv Res. 2004;31:75–85.
14. Ducat L, Rubenstein A, Philipson LH, Anderson BJ. A review of the mental health issues of diabetes conference. Diab Care. 2015;38:333–8.
15. Feinstein AR. Clinical judgment. NY: Huntington; 1967.
16. Grant B, Stinson F, Hasin D, Dawson D, Chou P, Ruan W, Huang B. Prevalence, correlates, and comorbidity of bipolar I disorder and axis I and II disorders: results from the national epidemiologic survery on alcohol and related conditions. J Clin Psychiatry. 2005;66:1205–15.
17. Hirschfeld RMA, Vornik LA. Recognition and diagnosis of bipolar disorder. J Clin Psychiatry. 2004;65(Suppl 15):5–9.
18. Judd LL, Schettler PJ, Akiskal HS, Coryell W, Leon AC, Maser JD, Solomon DA. Residual symptom recovery from major affective episodes in bipolar disorders and rapid episode relapse/recurrence. Arch Gen Psychiatry. 2008;65:386–94.
19. Kraepelin. Manic-depressive insanity and paranoia. Edinburgh, UK: Livingstone; 1921.
20. Krishnan KR. Psychiatric and medical comorbidities of bipolar disorder. Psychosom Med. 2005;67:1–8.
21. Mezzich JE. The WPA international guidelines for diagnostic assessment. World Psychiatry. 2002;1:36–9.

22. Mezzich JE, Salloum IM, Cloninger CR, Salvador-Carulla L, Kirmayer LJ, Banzato CEM, Wallcraft J, Botbol M. Person-centred integrative diagnosis: conceptual bases and structural model. Can J Psychiatry Rev Can de Psychiatrie. 2010;55:701–8.
23. Mezzich JE, Snaedal J, van Weel C, Botbol M, Salloum I. Introduction to person-centred medicine: from concepts to practice. J Eval Clin Pract. 2011;17:330–2.
24. Ostacher MJ, Perlis RH, Nierenberg AA, Calabrese J, Stange JP, Salloum I, Weiss RD, Sachs GS, Investigators S-B. Impact of substance use disorders on recovery from episodes of depression in bipolar disorder patients: prospective data from the systematic treatment enhancement program for bipolar disorder (STEP-BD). Am J Psychiatry. 2010;167:289–97.
25. Parks J, Svendsen D, Singer P, Foti ME. Morbidity and mortality in people with serious mental illness. Alexandria, VA: National Association of State Mental Health Program Directors; 2006.
26. Prieto ML, McElroy SL, Hayes SN, Sutor B, Kung S, Bobo WV, Fuentes ME, Cuellar-Barboza AB, Crow S, Osby U, Chauhan M, Westman J, Geske JR, Colby CL, Ryu E, Biernacka JM, Frye MA. Association between history of psychosis and cardiovascular disease in bipolar disorder. Bipolar Disord. 2015;17:518–27.
27. Regier DA, Farmer ME, Rae DS, Locke BZ, Keith SJ, Judd LL, Goodwin FK. Comorbidity of mental disorders with alcohol and other drug abuse: Results from the Epidemiologic Catchment Area (ECA) study. JAMA. 1990;264:2511–2518.
28. Salloum IM, Khazai L. The integration of mental health and primary care: a person-centered approach. World Med J. 2015;61(3):109–113.
29. Salloum IM, Mezzich JE. Person-centered diagnosis. Int J Integr Care. 2010;10(Suppl):e027.
30. Salloum IM, Mezzich JE. Conceptual appraisal of the person-centered integrative diagnosis model. Int J Person Centered Med. 2011;1:39–42.
31. Salloum IM, Mezzich JE. Outlining the bases of person-centred integrative diagnosis. J Eval Clin Pract. 2011;17:354–6.
32. Salloum IM, Pani L, Cooke T. Management of comorbidity in bipolar disorder. In: Yatham L, Maj M, editors. Textbook of bipolar disorder. Oxford, UK: Wiley-Blackwell; 2010.
33. Salloum IM, Ruiz P. Management of comorbid substance or alcohol abuse. In: Yildiz A, Nemeroff CB, Ruiz P editors. The bipolar book: history, neurobiology, and treatment. New York, NY: Oxford University Press; 2015.
34. Salloum IM, Williams L, Douaihy A. Diagnostic and treatment considerations: bipolar patients with comorbid substance use disorders. Psychiatr Ann. 2008;38:716–23.
35. Schaffer A, Isometsa ET, Azorin JM, Cassidy F, Goldstein T, Rihmer Z, Sinyor M, Tondo L, Moreno DH, Turecki G, Reis C, Kessing LV, Ha K, Weizman A, Beautrais A, Chou YH, Diazgranados N, Levitt AJ, Zarate C, JR A, Yatham, L. A review of factors associated with greater likelihood of suicide attempts and suicide deaths in bipolar disorder: part II of a report of the international society for bipolar disorders task force on suicide in bipolar disorder. Aust N Z J Psychiatry. 2015a.
36. Schaffer A, Isometsa ET, Tondo L, Moreno DH, Turecki G, Reis C, Cassidy F, Sinyor M, Azorin JM, Kessing LV, Ha K, Goldstein T, Weizman A, Beautrais A, Chou YH, Diazgranados N, Levitt AJ, Zarate CA, Rihmer Z, Yatham LN. International society for bipolar disorders task force on suicide: meta-analyses and meta-regression of correlates of suicide attempts and suicide deaths in bipolar disorder. Bipolar Disord. 2015;17:1–16.
37. Seyer J. Development of the health improvement card developed by the world health professions alliance. In: Medicine ICOPC, editor. The 5th Geneva conference on person-centered medicine. Geneva, Switzerland.
38. Shapiro E, Roos NP. Elderly nonusers of health care services. Their characteristics and their health outcomes. Med Care. 1985;23:247–57.
39. WHO. WHO constitution. Geneva: World Health Organization; 1946.
40. WHO. The ICD-10 classification of mental and behavioural disorders: clinical descriptions and diagnostic guidelines. Geneva: World Health Organization; 1992.
41. WHO. The World Health report 2003—shaping the future. Geneva: World Health Organization; 2003.

Depression and Anxiety Disorders

27

Megan M. Campbell, PhD and Dan J. Stein, MD

27.1 Introduction

Depression and anxiety disorders are highly prevalent across the globe [10, 11]. These conditions are associated not only with a great deal of individual suffering, but also with significant costs to society [17]. There is a clear need to understand these conditions better, to address barriers to care, and to improve treatment outcomes.

At the same time, there are important conceptual controversies. While a public health perspective has emphasized underdiagnosis and undertreatment as problematic factors that need to be addressed [12], it has been suggested that prevalence and burden of depression and anxiety disorders are overestimated [27] and that there is overmedicalization of these conditions [7]. Relatedly, from the perspective of the individual patient, the question arises of whether it is better to learn that one has a medical condition, even a brain disorder [2, 3] or whether it is better for the focus to be on one's own personal experience of the illness [5, 13] and how one can empower oneself in recovery [27].

In this chapter we will provide a conceptual framework for addressing some of these controversies. We will contrast a classical view that emphasizes depression and anxiety conditions as medical or brain disorders comprising essentialist categories, with a critical perspective that emphasizes how illness is socially constructed. We will argue that an integrative perspective to depression and anxiety

M.M. Campbell, PhD (✉)
Department of Psychiatry and Mental Health, Faculty of Health Sciences,
University of Cape Town, J-Block,
Groote Schuur Hospital Observatory, Cape Town 7935, South Africa
e-mail: mm.campbell@uct.ac.za

D.J. Stein, MD
Professor, Department of Psychiatry and Mental Health, University of Cape Town,
and MRC Unit on Anxiety and Stress Disorders, Cape Town, South Africa

J.E. Mezzich et al. (eds.), *Person Centered Psychiatry*,
DOI 10.1007/978-3-319-39724-5_27

disorders is needed. This integrative perspective emphasizes common, multi-level underlying mechanisms in depression and anxiety disorders that are influenced by sociocultural factors [9]. We argue that this perspective aligns well with a person-centred approach to psychiatry that focuses on a holistic understanding of the patient's symptomatology and illness experiences [16].

27.2 The Classicial, Critical and Integrative Perspectives

A classical perspective conceptualizes psychiatric disorders as essentialist categories, that are defined by necessary and sufficient diagnostic criteria (much as a square is defined by necessary and sufficient features). This approach has strongly influenced current nosological systems, which have in turn contributed to advances in our understanding of the psychobiology of psychiatric disorders and the development of evidence-based interventions that can be applied across diverse settings [21, 24]. From a global mental health perspective, neuropsychiatric disorders are among the most prevalent and disabling global health problems, and a significant treatment gap exists between high and middle/low income countries, but improved mental health services can address this gap [12, 23].

However, a particular limitation of this approach is that it potentially neglects more culturally specific characteristics, symptoms and categories of psychiatric illness that are influenced by context-specific and sociocultural factors, but that fall outside of recognized nosology [22, 26]. Many current diagnostic, assessment and treatment guidelines continue to be developed in western contexts. However society and culture shape illness experiences, and the application of western diagnostic categories, concepts and interventions may not necessarily take the relevant social context and key socially constructed factors into consideration [12]. In addition the classical approach arguably neglects the impact of factors like social inequality, poverty, unemployment and violence on individuals' experiences of illness [12].

In contrast, a critical perspective considers how illness is socially constructed and emphasizes the role of an individual's sociocultural context in determining the experience of a psychiatric disorder [21, 22]. It emphasizes the implicit values that individuals hold about disease, illness experiences, and expectations about treatment and recovery [5], and underscores the role of personal empowerment in recovery [9]. From this position a global mental health approach potentially downplays the value of local ways of conceptualizing, explaining and coping with mental illness, and how these can be used to empower individuals through community-based and grassroots approaches to mental health interventions [12]. Strengths of the critical approach include an emphasis on the experience and perception of suffering from psychiatric illness, and on the influence of sociocultural context and factors on the nature of psychiatric disorders [21, 22, 26].

Potential limitations to this approach include the lack of recognition of the reality of mental disorders, of sufficient emphasis on investigating their underlying psychobiological mechanisms, and of downplaying commonalities in the psychobiology of psychiatric disorders across cultures and contexts [22, 24]. Some who adopt a critical stance emphasize the social construction of all illnesses, while others focus their critique predomindantly on psychiatry, arguing that the analogy between physical and mental illness is flawed. Such foci arguably fail to capture how human language can both be fundamentally metaphoric, and yet be useful in delineating real entities, such as diseases, which are associated with human impairment and suffering [23].

An integrative perspective draws on both aspects of the classical position and the critical position. The integrative approach incorporates the view that psychiatry is a science which investigates psychobiological mechanisms, but also the perspective that subjective experience is key in psychiatry, and that human subjectivity is both embodied and embedded in particular sociocultural contexts [21, 22]. It acknowledges the complex mechanisms that underlie psychiatric disorders, and the fuzzy nature of psychiatric classification [9, 23]. While empirical epidemiological and neurobiological data provides evidence of universal psychobiological mechanisms in the pathophysiology of psychiatric disorders, psychosocial factors impact on the experience and expression of these disorders, their course and outcomes [26]. From this perspective there is significant opportunity for synergy between global mental health and neuroscience, exploring how the psychobiology and experience of mental illness plays out in different ways across the globe [23].

27.3 Person-Centred Psychiatry as an Integrative Approach

Person-centred psychiatry encourages an understanding of the patient in their totality, including both their pathology as well as positive aspects of their health [16]. This approach aims to provide treatment that extends beyond disease management into health promotion, where clinicians work collaboratively with their patients to empower them [16]. Working from a person-centred approach, an integrative diagnostic model seeks to understand and address both the symptomatology of psychiatric disorders, the social construction of illness and the patient's unique illness experience [20]. As a result, person-centred psychiatry aligns well with the integrative perspective outlined above, incorporating both the science and humanity of psychiatry. Having presented and contrasted the classical, critical and integrative perspectives, and having positioned person-centred psychiatric as an integrative approach, we now consider depression and anxiety disorders.

27.4 Depression and Anxiety

Depressive disorders are described by the Diagnostic and Statistical Manual of Mental Disorders, fifth edition (DSM-5) as characterized by "the presence of sad, empty or irritable mood, accompanied by somatic and cognitive changes that significantly affect the individual's capacity to function" [1]. Currently ranked as one of the leading causes of disability [17], depression demonstrates high prevalence globally, high risk of recurrence and high comorbidity with other mental disorders such as anxiety disorders, and chronic physical diseases such as asthma, cancer, cardiovascular disease, diabetes and hypertension [10].

The DSM-5 characterizes anxiety disorders as having "shared features of excessive fear and anxiety and related behaviour disturbances" where fear is defined as an "emotional response to real or perceived imminent threat" and anxiety as the "anticipation of future threat" [1]. Anxiety disorders are the most common mental disorders, showing a high prevalence globally [11], and high comorbidity with one another, with other mental disorders such as mood and substance use disorders, and with physical diseases such as cardiovascular disease and migraines [15]. Specific phobia and social phobia are the most commonly occurring anxiety disorders [11].

Despite the high prevalence of depression and anxiety disorders only a relatively small proportion of people with these disorders seek treatment [17]. Treatment rates are higher in more severe cases, and in high-income countries, while treatment rates are lower in middle- and low- income countries [10]. As alluded to earlier, however, a public health perspective would emphasize underdiagnosis and undertreatment [11], while others argue that estimates of prevalence and the burden of depression and anxiety disorders are misleading [27], and that there is an over-medicalization of these disorders [7]. We now discuss depression and anxiety disorders from a classical, critical and integrative perspective.

(i) A classical position—Depression and Anxiety as Essentialist Categories

From a classical position, depression and anxiety are conceptualized as medical or brain disorders and captured using essentialist diagnostic categories. Depressive disorders are mediated by the brain systems responsible for mood regulation, emotional expression, reward processing, motivation, and responses to stress [3]. The medial prefrontal cortex, amygdala, hippocampus and ventromedial parts of the basal ganglia have been identified as possible regions in the brain responsible for depressive symptoms [3]. Dysfunction in these regions may play a role in disturbances in neurotransmission, autonomic regulation, neuroendocrine responses, emotional behaviour and cognitive performance that characterize depression [3]. Antidepressant medication is the best established pharmacotherapy treatment for depression, and has shown to be efficacious, particularly in more severe cases of major depressive disorder [4].

Anxiety disorders are mediated by the medial prefrontal cortex, amygdala and hypothalamic nuclei, hippocampal formation and midbrain central grey area, which in turn have serotonergic, noradrenergic and dopaminergic inputs [2]. These regions of the brain coordinate fear responses to threat and so underpin the symptoms of anxiety disorders [2]. The relevant brain circuitry includes a defence system that responds immediately to threat, and a behavioural inhibition system that supresses behaviours that could enhance danger [2]. Selective serotonin reuptake inhibitors and serotonin–norepinephrine reuptake inhibitors act on these circuits and have demonstrated efficacy in treating most anxiety disorders [19].

Despite growing understanding of the neurobiology of depression and anxiety disorders, as well as studies demonstrating the validity of these diagnostic categories, there is also evidence that depressive and anxiety symptoms are often adaptive responses [24], that have particular value in response to various socio-cultural contexts [14]. Neurobiological changes do not map well onto diagnostic categories, and a Research Domain Criteria (RDoc) framework that focuses on broad domains cutting across a range of mental disorders may be useful in conceptualizing depression and anxiety disorders [8]. However, questions remain about the sensitivity and specificity of the RDoC framework for diagnostic practice, as well as about the clinical utility of this approach.

(ii) A critical position: Depression and Anxiety as illness experiences

From a critical position, depression and anxiety disorders are understood as socially constructed and as crucially constituted by sociocultural factors. Evidence in support of this perspective demonstrates how prevalence and symptomatology of depression and anxiety disorders vary across countries [14]. For example, somatic symptoms may be more prevalent in non-western contexts while psychological symptoms may be more typical in western contexts [6]. In addition attributions underlying depression and anxiety differ across time and place [6]. The understanding of depression and anxiety as medical disorders may be more commonly endorsed in some contexts while in others more indigenous traditional beliefs may be endorsed. In some African contexts, for example, anxiety may be more commonly associated with bewitchment and poisoning, or breaking a taboo and neglecting a ritual that leads to displeasing the ancestors [26].

Variability in prevalence rates may be a result of true differences in prevalence that exclude similar but related presentations of the same disorders [14]. However, such variability may also reflect a lack of measurement equivalence in the tools used to assess and diagnose these disorders across contexts, and challenges the validity and precision of diagnostic criteria [14]. Importantly, gender and socio-economic status or income inequality significantly influence the epidemiology of depression and anxiety disorders, with women and those of lower socio-economic status being at greater risk of developing these disorders [18].

Clearly, to neglect the influence of sociocultural factors on the expression and experience of depression and anxiety disorders is to ignore how illness is socially constructed, and the patient's unique illness experience. At the same time, to focus exclusively on this experience runs the risk of neglecting the way in which specific psychobiological mechanisms underpin these disorders and the value of pharmacotherapy and psychotherapy interventions which act on such mechanisms.

(iii) An integrative position: A person-centred approach

From an integrative position there are underlying, multi-level mechanisms involved in the pathogenesis of depression and anxiety disorders [9]. Diagnostic categories, like all human categories are socially constructed, but at the same time they reflect the operation of real proximal and distal (evolutionary) psychobiological mechanisms, and their boundaries and borders are open to rational debate. Effective treatment requires an understanding of individuals' experience of depression and anxiety, but also a knowledge of the relevant underlying mechanisms. Person-centred psychiatry offers a valuable framework to work integratively with patients presenting with depression and anxiety by drawing on this sort of understanding and knowledge [20].

First, a person-centred model focuses attention on both symptom presentation as well as the health and illness experiences of the patient [20], so promoting an integrative conceptualisation of depression and anxiety disorders. Second, the model seeks to identify positive aspects of a patient's health that support adaptive functioning, improve quality of life and are suggestive of protective factors in managing illness [20]. Depression and anxiety are typically chronic, recurring mental illnesses, and a focus on these positive health aspects may assist in identifying areas of resiliency that promote recovery. Empowerment of the patient is an important aspect of treatment that promotes recovery. Third, the model encourages a collaborative relationship between the clinician, patient, and family [20]. Both clinicians and patients hold implicit values about disease, illness experiences, and expectations about treatment and recovery [5]. Negotiation about these values, and how they relate to important aspects of illness assist in treatment considerations. For example, during the recent revision of the DSM 5, the Obsessive Compulsive-Spectrum Disorders Sub-working Group reported the value of consumer involvement during the revision process, particularly with respect to understanding issues of stigmatization [25].

27.5 Conclusions

Depression and anxiety disorders are highly prevalent, chronic, recurring conditions associated with substantial individual suffering and societal cost. However, debate surrounds the conceptualization of these disorders. A classical position often regards depression and anxiety as essentialist medical categories or brain disorders. In contrast, a critical position understands depression and anxiety as socially constructed responses and emphasizes the implicit values that individuals hold about disease, illness experiences and expectations about treatment. An integrative approach draws on both evidence-based medicine as well as values-based medicine in focusing on the underlying mechanisms involved in the pathogenesis of depression and anxiety as well as the unique illness experiences and values of the patient.

The person-centred integrative diagnosis model is arguably consistent with this integrative approach insofar as it has a focus on both symptom presentation as well as the health and illness experiences of the patient, and encourages a collaborative relationship between the clinician and patient. In this view, the patient perspective is absolutely crucial, and consumer advocacy is a key opportunity. At the same time, this perspective also emphasizes the importance of better understanding the underlying mechanisms involved in depression and anxiety disorders, so that these can be better targeted and treated.

Acknowledgments Megan Campbell is supported by a URC Postdoctoral Fellowship from the University of Cape Town. Dan Stein is supported by the Medical Research Council of South Africa.

References

1. American Psychiatric Association. The diagnostic and statistical manual of mental disorders. 5th ed (DSM 5). Arlington, Virginia: Author;2013.
2. Canteras NS, Resstel LB, Bertoglio LJ, Carobrez AP, Guimaraes FS, Stein MB, Steckler T. Neuroanatomy of anxiety. Behavioral neurobiology of anxiety and its treatment, vol. 2. New York: Springer; 2010. p. 79–97.
3. Drevets WC, Price JL, Furey ML. Brain structural and functional abnormalities in mood disorders: implications for neurocircuitry models of depression. Brain Struct Funct. 2008;213 (1–2):93–118.
4. Fournier JC, DeRubeis RJ, Hollon SD, Dimidjian S, Amsterdam JD, Shelton RC, Fawcett J. Antidepressant drug effects and depression severity: a patient-level meta-analysis. JAMA. 2010;303(1):47–53.
5. Fulford KW. The value of evidence and evidence of values: bringing together values-based and evidence-based practice in policy and service development in mental health. J Eval Clin Pract. 2011;17(5):976–87.
6. Good BJ, Kleinman AM, Tuma AH, Hillsdale MJ, Erlbaum L. Culture and anxiety: cross-cultural evidence for the patterning of anxiety disorders. Anxiety Anxiety Disord. 1985;297–323.
7. Horwitz AV, Wakefield JC. The loss of sadness: how psychiatry transformed normal sorrow into depressive disorder. Oxford, UK: Oxford University Press; 2007.
8. Insel T, Cuthbert B, Garvey M, et al. Research domain criteria (RDoC): toward a new classification framework for research on mental disorders. Am J Psychiatry. 2010;167:748–51.
9. Kendler KS. The dappled nature of causes of psychiatric illness: replacing the organic–functional/hardware–software dichotomy with empirically based pluralism. Mol Psychiatry. 2012;17(4):377–88.
10. Kessler RC, Bromet EJ. The epidemiology of depression across cultures. Annu Rev Public Health. 2013;34:119–38.
11. Kessler RC, Ruscio AM, Shear K, Wittchen HU, Stein M, Steckler T. Epidemiology of anxiety disorders. Behavioral neurobiology of anxiety and its treatment, vol. 2. New York: Springer; 2010. p. 21–36.
12. Kirmayer LJ, Pedersen D. Toward a new architecture for global mental health. Transcult Psychiatry. 2014;51(6):759–76.
13. Kleinman A. Anthropology and psychiatry. The role of culture in cross-cultural research on illness. Br J Psychiatry. 1987;151(4):447–54.
14. Lewis-Fernández R, Hinton DE, Laria AJ, Patterson EH, Hofmann SG, Craske MG, Liao B. Culture and the anxiety disorders: recommendations for DSM-V. Depression Anxiety. 2010;27(2):212–29.
15. Merikangas KR, Swanson SA, Stein MB, Steckler T. Comorbidity in anxiety disorders. Behavioral neurobiology of anxiety and its treatment, vol. 2. New York: Springer; 2010. p. 37–59.
16. Mezzich JE, Snaedal J, van Weel C, Heath I. Toward person-centered medicine: from disease to patient to person. Mount Sinai J Med. 2010;77:304–6.

17. Murray CJ, Vos T, Lozano R, Naghavi M, Flaxman AD, Michaud C, Bridgett L. Disability-adjusted life years (DALYs) for 291 diseases and injuries in 21 regions, 1990–2010: a systematic analysis for the global burden of disease study 2010. Lancet. 2013;380 (9859):2197–223.
18. Patel V. Cultural factors and international epidemiology: Depression and public health. Br Med Bull. 2001;57(1):33–45.
19. Ravindran LN, Stein MB. The pharmacologic treatment of anxiety disorders: a review of progress. J Clin Psychiatry. 2010;71(7):839–54.
20. Salloum IM, Mezzich JE. Person-centered diagnosis. Int J Integr Care. 2010;29(10) Suppl: e027.
21. Stein DJ. Philosophy and the DSM-III. Compr Psychiatry. 1991;32(5):404–15.
22. Stein DJ. Cross-cultural psychiatry and the DSM-IV. Compr Psychiatry. 1993;34(5):322–9.
23. Stein DJ. In review what is a mental disorder? a perspective from cognitive-affective science. Can J Psychiatry. 2013;58(12):656–62.
24. Stein DJ, Lund C, Nesse RM. Classification systems in psychiatry: diagnosis and global mental health in the era of DSM-5 and ICD-11. Curr Opin Psychiatry. 2013;26:493–7.
25. Stein DJ, Phillips KA. Patient advocacy and DSM-5. BMC Med. 2013;11(1):133.
26. Stein DJ, Williams DR, Stein DJ, Hollander E. Cultural and social aspects of anxiety disorders. Textbook of anxiety disorders. Washington, DC: American Psychiatric Publishing; 2002. p. 463–474.
27. Summerfield D. How scientifically valid is the knowledge base of global mental health? Br Med J. 2008;336(7651):992–4.

Eating Disorders

28

Fragiskos Gonidakis, MD, PhD and Anne-Sophie Lancien, MD

28.1 Introduction

Eating disorders (ED) is a cluster of mental disorders that affect a large number of young adults mostly in western or westernized societies. Their symptomatology ranges from the rare restrictive type of anorexia nervosa (AN) that affects mainly adolescent women to the more common binge eating disorder (BED) that has a later onset than AN and affects more men than AN and bulimia nervosa (BN) [32]. ED cause significant deterioration of the sufferer's quality of life with the most pronounced effect produced by AN. It is quite interesting that a recent review showed that the impact on the quality of life of AN sufferers persists even after weight restoration has been achieved [34]. Moreover, ED have a significant contribution to the global burden of disease attributed to mental and substance use disorders [37].

The treatment of ED has been a field of vigorous debates and extensive investigation since ED and especially AN seems to posses a unique triad among mental disorders: their mortality rate is quite high especially when they become chronic, there is no conclusive evidence that they can be treated with medication with the exception of fluoxetine for BN and possibly lisdexamfetamine and topiramate for BED and finally a high percentage of sufferers refuse to be treated even when the disorder has caused a variety of medical complications [12]. The most widely used treatment for ED is, so far, psychotherapy. For adults with AN, no specialist treatment has been shown to be superior. Cognitive behavioral therapy, enhanced

F. Gonidakis, MD, PhD (✉)
Eating Disorders Unit, 1st Psychiatric Department, Medical School, National and Kapodistrian University of Athens, Athens, Greece
e-mail: fragoni@yahoo.com

A.-S. Lancien, MD
Department of Child and Adolescent Psychiatry, Brest University Hospital, University of Western Brittany, Brest, France

J.E. Mezzich et al. (eds.), *Person Centered Psychiatry*,
DOI 10.1007/978-3-319-39724-5_28

cognitive behavioral therapy, and possibly interpersonal psychotherapy remain the most established treatments for BN and BED. Maudsley family-based therapy is the most established treatment for youth with AN and may be efficacious for youth with BN [15]. It should be noted that due to serious medical complications caused by AN symptomatology a substantial number of sufferers is hospitalized for a period of time that varies between a few weeks to 6 or more months [19, 29]. In some cases, especially for the youngest patients, a longer hospitalization may be necessary to extend the positive effect of their separation from their family. In some countries (France, Belgium, Switzerland) long-term psychiatric in-patients institutions offering study facilities are frequently used with ED patients to allow such extension without increasing their educational exclusion.

28.2 The Challenge of Treating a Patient Suffering from Eating Disorder

The implementation of a treatment plan tailored to the needs of the sufferer has not always been an easy task. Forging a solid therapeutic alliance that can lead to a successful therapeutic process and a long term remission of the ED symptomatology is not so common in everyday clinical work as it is presented in various studies on recovery from ED. Treating a person suffering from ED very often resembles a marathon with steep turns and hidden obstacles. Some of these obstacles are presented below.

28.2.1 Medical Complications

The medical complications of ED are varied and complex. They can be categorized in three groups: (a) consequences of starvation, (b) consequences of purging behaviors, and (c) consequences of binge eating [30].

Recent literature continues to reflect that multiple organ systems are frequently affected by ED and especially AN [22]. A plethora of dermatologic changes have been described, some signaling serious underlying pathophysiology, such as purpura, which indicates a bleeding diathesis. Gastrointestinal complications can be serious, including gastric dilatation and severe liver dysfunction. Acrocyanosis is common and patients with AN are at risk of various arrhythmias. Underweight patients are at high risk for osteopenia/osteoporosis. Furthermore, adolescents and children can suffer from a disruption of height growth which unfortunately cannot always be won back. Nutritional abnormalities are also common, including sodium depletion and hypovolemia, hypophosphatemia, and hypomagnesemia [22]. BN, often characterized by self-induced vomiting, is complicated by medical manifestations that affect nearly every organ system in the body [3]. Effects range from skin and dental findings to esophageal pathology, electrolyte abnormalities, cardiac arrhythmias, and in extreme cases, death [3]. In the prepubescent anorexia, a non-reversable break of the growth weight curve can be observed.

Due to the above-mentioned medical complications two issues arise. The first is that, therapy might be hindered by the constant manifestation of these complications that often require that the patient be hospitalized. Furthermore, due to these complications the therapist has to cope with the fact that for a prolonged period of time the sufferer's life will be under immediate danger. The second issue is the need for continuous medical screening and assessment of ED patients. In most of the cases the therapist has to be in close communication with the physician that is treating the sufferer. This communication raises delicate issues of confidentiality. Although both the therapist and the physician are bound by the rules concerning confidentiality, how much and which of the patient's privileged information that the therapist has access to, can be shared with her/her physician? Is the person's opinion obtained in this matter and to which extend can it be respected? The physician and the therapist have to forge a strong relation based on mutual understanding and cooperation in order to work as a team and to avoid entering a catastrophic power struggle on who carries the responsibility for the patient's well-being. The above is not rare in many cases when the patient is hospitalized in critical medical condition.

28.2.2 Mortality

AN has the highest mortality of any psychiatric disorder, estimated at 10 % occurring within 10 years of diagnosis, and is the leading cause of death in young females 15–24 years of age [26]. Death occurs due to suicide, infection, or succumbing to the effects of chronic starvation. In a recent meta-analysis, it was calculated that AN patients were 5.2 [3.7–7.5] times more likely to die prematurely from any cause, and 18.1 [11.5–28.7] times more likely to die by suicide than 15–34 year old females in the general population [17]. Mortality for BN is expectedly less, approximately one percent occurring within 10 years of diagnosis [26]. These figures could be deceiving, however, because up to 50 % of AN sufferers become bulimic somewhere during the course of their disease, but still carry the primary diagnosis of AN.

Mortality due to medical complications and high suicidality put an extremely intense strain on the therapeutic alliance and in many cases can compromise the ability of the therapist to act effectively. They can also contribute significantly to the manifestation of burnout syndrome in the therapist [11]. Furthermore, especially in severe and enduring AN patients that do not respond to treatment two ethical issues arise. The first is whether the therapist and the sufferer have the right to mutually agree to terminate therapy even when the sufferer's death is imminent and unavoidable. The second is whether the therapist has the ability to decide when to cease trying to treat the patient and to start providing palliative care. Moreover, a more delicate issue is the extent to which the sufferer's opinion can and should be taken under consideration especially when she/he is suicidal or in the verge of death.

28.2.3 Insight and Commitment to Therapy

Traditionally AN has been considered a mental disorder with poor insight specifically in the areas of the necessity for weight gain and nutritional restoration. Patients are supposed to strive to loose weight or maintain a very low body mass index (BMI) and they refuse any kind of treatment that will derive them from that. In many cases the above becomes the only life goal that the sufferer is actually dedicated to achieve. Furthermore, recent research indicates that there is possibly a group of AN sufferers where their body image beliefs are genuinely delusional [18].

Although BN and BED are not characterized by that kind of rigidity in the sufferer's beliefs around the body size and daily energy intake, the bulimic consumption of large amount of palatable food is often egosyntonic as it creates a much needed hedonic state and/or alleviates unpleasant feelings that the person is experiencing. Many sufferers report that the amount of time that the bulimic episode lasts is the only moment during their day that they have to forget all their trouble, comfort themselves, or feel free to act as they like. It goes without saying that when the above is repeated daily for years it is quite difficult for the sufferer to commit to a treatment plan that is going to reduce these highly reinforced behaviors. On certain occasions the follow-up of BN and BED patients is often difficult to maintain because of their fear to invest in a long lasting relation, due to their problem of dependence [33].

The term "food addiction" was proposed by Randolph during the mid-50s to describe: "a specific adaptation to one or more regularly consumed foods to which a person is highly sensitive, produces a common pattern of symptoms descriptively similar to those of other addictive processes" [28]. Although a substance-based addiction produced by food has not been proven so far to exist in human subjects there is consistent evidence of addictive eating behaviors [13].

Food or eating addiction, delusional beliefs around body image and nutrition, rigidity of thinking that prevents any kind of change, and self-soothing through the use of food are four factors that can weaken the person's resolve to deal with the ED that she is suffering from. Although the "stubborn" denial to follow any kind of therapeutic plan can been seen as poor insight or lack of commitment to change, fear, anxiety, or even distress are quite often the emotions that actually hinder the person's effort to overcome ED. Because of the four factors that have been mentioned these emotions can become so intense that it is impossible for the sufferer to even consider the possibility of change.

Furthermore follow-up of BN and BED patients can sometimes be quite troublesome due to the fact that a number of sufferers find difficult to commit to a long lasting therapeutic relationship.

28.2.4 Blame and Shame

Until recently, mental illness stigma research has focused primarily on conditions such as schizophrenia and depression, to the neglect of other psychological disorders. In particular, stigma towards individuals with AN has received little empirical attention [38]. AN patients are often perceived as being responsible for the onset of their illness and as having a significant amount of control over their eating disordered behaviors [38]. It has been suggested that individuals that are exposed to a biological/genetic explanation of the causes of AN tend to blame AN patients less than those exposed to a sociocultural explanation [8]. It is interesting that a study conducted by Zwickert and Rieger [38] in a sample of undergraduate students found that when compared to patients suffering from obesity or skin cancer, participants reported a significantly greater desire for social distance from the target with AN compared to targets with obesity or skin cancer, and yet attributed less blame to the target with AN.

In clinical practice it often observed that a large proportion of the sufferers and their families have been blamed or are blaming themselves for the ED symptomatology. The feeling of blame can act as the fuse for a series of misunderstandings and conflicts, thus reinforcing the vicious circle of stigmatization. The person who is blaming itself or is being blamed usually feels marginalized and reacts with more isolation and defiance. On the other hand, the family and especially the parents can react with frantic efforts to oblige the sufferer to eat and gain weight in order to avoid social stigmatization. This behavior often leads to inter-family disputes resulting in further blaming the suffer as the "black sheep" of the family whose actions destroy the family's coherence and social acceptance.

Shame has received increased attention over recent years and has been shown to be a feature of many forms of psychopathology, including ED. People with ED experience generalized shame in relation to many aspects of their self and behavior, not just shame around eating [16]. ED sufferers and especially those with bulimic and purging behaviors tend to conceal their symptoms even from their therapist as they fear that they are going to be blamed for not restraining themselves from these behaviors and subsequently be rejected as weak, degenerates, or disgusting persons. Most of them decide to live a "double" life. This "double life" has been described as a dichotomy between being active and outgoing versus performing shameful bulimic behaviors and constantly living with fear of stigmatization, and striving against exposure [27]. Concealing is well planned to avoid such fear, and to preserve dignity. Understanding the meaning of secrecy and "double life" may be crucial in a person-centered care in order to facilitate help seeking behavior and guide treatment [27].

28.2.5 Compulsory Hospitalization and Refeeding

Compulsory inpatient refeeding of patients with severe AN has caused considerable controversy. The effects of such treatment on longer term outcome are not well known [10]. In most cases the combination of severe medical complications that can endanger the sufferer's life, suicidal ideation, and denial of treatment lead to the decision for involuntary hospitalization. A recent review reported that detained patients have more severe symptoms and comorbidity and a longer duration of inpatient stay. In the short term, compulsory refeeding in AN appears to be beneficial, but the longer term effects remains uncertain. Clausen and Jones [5] reported in their review that persons that were treated involuntarily were characterized by a more severe psychiatric load. The levels of eating disorder pathology between involuntary and voluntary groups were similar and the outcome of involuntary treatment was comparable in terms of symptom reduction to that of voluntary treatment. The authors remarked that "despite inconsistent findings, the comparable levels of eating disorder pathology observed between involuntary and voluntary patient-groups together with findings of higher co-morbidity, more pre-admissions, longer duration of illness and more incidences of self-harm for involuntary patients suggest that involuntary treatment is not a reaction to the severity of eating disorder symptoms alone, but is most likely a response to the complexity of the patient's situation as a whole" [5].

Although the ethical issues concerning compulsory treatment in ED are beyond the scope of this chapter, it should be noted that until now there is no final agreement among experts on whether AN sufferers should be involuntary hospitalized. Some therapists believe that involuntary treatment is not an option, since quite often even involuntary treatment does not lead to recovery. However, others endorse this decision, in extreme cases, for lack of any other option, in order to save patients' lives [23].

Finally, it should be noted that AN usually has an onset during early (12–14 years of age) or late adolescence (16–18 years of age). These are two periods when the issue of separation/ individualization is strongly raised in young sufferers. A hospitalization in this age can, most of the times, be decided solely with the agreement of the parents without taking into account the opinion of the adolescent sufferer [1].

28.3 The Need of a Person-Centered Care for Eating Disorders

The main concept behind the term "person centered" medicine is human individuality. Each person is perceived as biologically and psychologically unique in a state of continuous transaction with the physical and social environments [36]. To treat the person is to study, understand, and respect this individuality and to use it to promote the person's psychosomatic health.

In general, the term 'person-centered medicine' can have the following meanings [14]:

(a) Medicine of the person: this is the theoretical aspect, especially the notion of person itself.
(b) Medicine for the person: this is the therapeutical aspect.
(c) Medicine by the person: this is the aspect of the medical professionals' role and self-understanding.
(d) Medicine with the person: this is the interpersonal aspect, especially the relationship between patient and doctor.

Concerning ED a person-centered approach has to take in account all the above mentioned issues that arise in the diagnosis and treatment of these specific disorders. The ED sufferer has to be put in the center of the specialists attention. Her/his ideas, wishes, narratives, explanations have to be taken under consideration and used as a guide for designing the individual's person treatment goals.

28.3.1 Diagnosis

The diagnostic process in psychiatry has always been a controversial issue. This has to do with particular features of this field: from all medical specialties, psychiatry, and psychotherapy are most intensively connected with political, historical, and social developments [14]. World Psychiatric Association created in 2005 the Institutional Program on Psychiatry for the Person (IPPP). One of the main scopes of IPPP is the development of a person-centered integrative diagnosis (PID). The concept of PID is that diagnosis can be defined as the "description of the positive and negative aspects of health, interactively, within the person's life context" [20]. Strategically, the PID model "has a bio-psycho-socio- cultural framework, articulates science and humanism, uses all pertinent descriptive tools (categories, dimensions, and narratives) in a multilevel structure, and engages clinicians, patients and families in a diagnostic partnership" [21, 31].

A person-centered diagnosis of ED has to take under consideration a number of factors beyond the symptomatology that has already been described in the existing classification systems. Family interactions, the burden of the disorder to the person and her/his family, the interplay between cultural and idiosyncratic beliefs concerning body shape, weight, and nutrition are examples of these factors. The most important factor though is the opinion and the experience of the sufferers of what, according to them, constitutes a mental disorder and what not. An illustration of the above is the threshold of the weight loss for the diagnosis of AN. This limit has been set in the classification systems according to strict medical data. What is the subjective experience of the sufferers? What is the limit of weight loss where they start to feel the negative impact of starvation on their quality of life and their ability to function according to their desire? In person-centered diagnosis the answer to the above questions would be considered a crucial contribution for setting the weight limit for the diagnosis of AN. A second example is the amount of binge episodes per week for the diagnosis of BN or BED. Again the current diagnostic criteria lack the use of the person's opinion and experience. There are cultural and family settings where the periodical impulsive consumption of large amount of food could be considered normative behavior, part of a family ritual or cultural festivity. Can we describe this as BN or BED? According to the current diagnostic criteria, under certain circumstances, yes. Furthermore, what is the number of binge episodes per week that would signal a pathological condition for the person. Two as it was in DSM-IV? One as it is in DSM-5? Even a small change in ED diagnostic criteria can have a major impact on the number of individuals that are diagnosed as suffering from an ED. It has been calculated that the implementation of the new DSM-5 criteria increased the diagnosis of AN and BN and decreased the cases of EDNOS [25].

How do we decide on these issues? According to the research data and the DSM or ICD task force expert opinion? Has the person something to say about that and what weight her/his opinion must carry in our decision on whether she/he is suffering from an ED? A person-centered diagnosis is able not only to incorporate most of these data but also to spare both the therapist and the sufferer from futile diagnostic disagreements.

28.3.2 Treatment

A person-centered approach to the treatment of ED would be tailored to suit that person's illness, situation and needs. That would involve the following:

(a) The treatment would focus on recovery for the specific person and the ED that she/he is facing.
(b) The treatment would take under consideration all the aspects of the ED: psychological, physical, behavioral, social, and interpersonal.
(c) The treatment would be adjusted to the needs and personal conditions of the person and her/his family with respect to their cultural and social beliefs system.
(d) The treatment would put the needs of the person who suffers from ED at the center of all therapeutic decisions from the beginning to the end of the whole procedure.
(e) The treatment would provide the adequate time for the person to achieve recovery and do not place arbitrary time limits based on data that are not specifically related to the individual.

To implement this kind of care for ED sufferers the mental health practitioners have to overcome the basic assumption that a person suffering from ED can not always determine what is in her/his own interest due to the symptomatology of the disorder and thereby requires a directive role from the therapist [2]. The above requires that, on a basic level, the curriculum in psychiatry and psychotherapy training would be amended to incorporate a more person-centered approach to ED treatment [4, 20].

28.3.3 Hospitalization

Most patients, even those that have voluntary admitted themselves, describe the experience of hospitalization with ambivalent words. "Terrifying, prison-like, authoritative, punitive, with too many rules that I could not dispute, holding me away from my family, I could not tolerate the loneliness" are some of the negative descriptions. "Helpful, supportive, necessarily firm, the rules helped me to focus, being separated from everything and everyone helped me a lot" are some of the positive descriptions. From the stuff point of view ED patients are usually described as "difficult" patients who "usually do not want to improve". "They lie, try to manipulate you, react badly to the slightest comment or suggestion, hide food or purge in secret, deny every help that you might want to offer to them" are some of the negative comments that stuff members make when they describe their experience in a psychiatric ward with ED patients. The question that arises is whether this kind of mutual negative feelings are a result of the ED symptomatology and its consequences or of certain therapeutic interventions that focus on weight and nutritional restoration and not on the person's needs.

The challenge in a person-centered approach is to find the balance between serving the sufferer's effort and improving her/his medical condition. A shift is needed from treating the person as a body that needs to eat more and purge less to improve its heart rate and restore it potassium levels to actively listen to what the person is experiencing, what he wants, how he feels, and try to integrate that with the fundamental obligation of the medical practitioner to preserve life. Although this might seem easy to do it is not the case in many inpatient units for ED patients around the world. It has been observed that in large mental hospitals when the staff have complete power and the patients little or no power and no successful monitoring, the practice drifts inevitably in favor of the convenience of staff and away from the patient [7].

28.3.4 Research

ED are considered as "difficult to treat" and potentially "lethal" mental disorders. This statement has led the scientists around the world to vigorously investigate different kinds of therapies. It is interesting that almost all of the published studies on the efficacy of treatment focus on the improvement of the medical condition or the amelioration of the symptomatology and specifically the symptoms that are described in the classification systems. There have been very few studies on the sufferer's satisfaction from treatment and only a handful on the factors that according to the person's opinion contributed to her/his improvement. Noordenbos [24] and De la Rie et al. [9] reported that good communication skills of the therapist, strong therapeutic alliance, and focus on ED symptoms were the factors according to the sufferer that had an impact on the positive therapeutic outcome. Similarly Swain-Campbell et al. [35] reported that the emotional bond with the therapist, trust, cooperation, and mutual commitment were the factors that the patients rated as important for their recovery. Finally, Clinton et al. [6] reported that support from their therapist and energetic participation in food and eating habits management were the two factors that patients found helpful in their treatment.

28.4 Conclusions

A quote from Copeland's [7] article on "World Federation for Mental Health perspectives on person-centered medicine" can serve as a final remark on the necessity to put the ED sufferer from a state of stigma, shame, and coercion to a state of understanding, respect, and mutual collaboration: "If we are to put the person back into medicine we must listen to what the person has to tell us about what they want. We may have knowledge of illness but we do not necessarily have knowledge, nor do we necessarily understand, what it is that an ill person wants us to do for them. They must guide us in what they want to achieve and be helped to articulate this, and we must surely listen to them".

References

1. Abbate-Daga G, Pierò A, Rigardetto R, Gandione M, Gramaglia C, Fassino S. Clinical, psychological and personality features related to age of onset of anorexia nervosa. Psychopathology. 2007;40(4):261–8.
2. Borg M, Karlsson B, Tondora J, Davidson L. Implementing person-centered care in psychiatric rehabilitation: what does this involve? Israeli J Psychiatry Relat Sci. 2009;46(2):84–93.
3. Brown CA, Mehler PS. Medical complications of self-induced vomiting. Eat Disord. 2013;21 (4):287–94.
4. Christodoulou G, Fulford B, Mezzich JE. Psychiatry for the person and its conceptual bases. Int Psychiatry. 2008;5:1–3.
5. Clausen L, Jones A. A systematic review of the frequency, duration, type and effect of involuntary treatment for people with anorexia nervosa, and an analysis of patient characteristics. J Eat Disord. 2014;2:29.
6. Clinton D, Bjorck C, Sohlberg S, Norring C. Patient satisfaction with treatment in eating disorders: cause for complacency or concern? Eur Eat Disord Rev. 2004;12:240–6.
7. Copeland J. World Federation for mental health perspectives on person-centered medicine. Int J Integr Care. 2010;10(Suppl):e009.
8. Crisafulli MA, Von Holle A, Bulik CM. Attitudes towards anorexia nervosa: the impact of framing on blame and stigma. Int J Eat Disord. 2008;41:333–9.
9. De la Rie S, Noordenbos G, Donker M, van Furth E. The quality of treatment of eating disorders: a comparison of the therapists' and the patients' perspectives. Int J Eat Disord. 2008;41:307–17.
10. Elzakkers IF, Danner UN, Hoek HW, Schmidt U, van Elburg AA. Compulsory treatment in anorexia nervosa: a review. Int J Eat Disord. 2014;47(8):845–52.
11. García de Amusquibar AM. Interdisciplinary team for the treatment of eating disorders. Eat Weight Disord. 2000;5(4):223–7.
12. Hay PJ, Claudino AM. Clinical psychopharmacology of eating disorders: a research update. Int J Neuropsychopharmacoly. 2012;15(2):209–22.
13. Hebebrand J, Albayrak O, Adan R, Antel J, Dieguez C, de Jong J, Leng G, Menzies J, Mercer JG, Murphy M, van der Plasse G, Dickson SL. "Eating addiction", rather than "food addiction", better captures addictive-like eating behavior. Neurosci Biobehav Rev. 2014;6 (47C):295–306.
14. Hoff P. Historical perspectives on person-centered medicine and psychiatry. Int J Integr Care. 2010;10(Suppl):e016.
15. Kass AE, Kolko RP, Wilfley DE. Psychological treatments for eating disorders. Curr Opin Psychiatry. 2013;26(6):549–55.

16. Keith L, Gillanders D, Simpson S. An exploration of the main sources of shame in an eating-disordered population. Clin Psychol Psychother. 2009;16(4):317–27.
17. Keshaviah A, Edkins K, Hastings ER, Krishna M, Franko DL, Herzog DB, Thomas JJ, Murray HB, Eddy KT. Re-examining premature mortality in anorexia nervosa: a meta-analysis redux. Compr Psychiatry. 2014;55:1773–84.
18. Konstantakopoulos G, Varsou E, Dikeos D, Ioannidi N, Gonidakis F, Papadimitriou G, Oulis P. Delusionality of body image beliefs in eating disorders. Psychiatry Res. 2012;200(2–3):482–8.
19. Lopez-de-Andres A, Carrasco-Garrido P, Hernández-Barrera V, Gil-de-Miguel A, Jiménez-Trujillo I, Jiménez-García R. Hospitalization trends in Spanish children and adolescents with eating disorders (1998–2007). Appetite. 2010;55(1):147–51.
20. Mezzich J. World Psychiatric Association perspectives on person-centered psychiatry and medicine. Int J Integr Care. 2010;10(Suppl):e003.
21. Mezzich JE, Salloum IM. Clinical complexity and person-centered integrative diagnosis. World Psychiatry. 2008;7(1):1–2.
22. Mitchell JE, Crow S. Medical complications of anorexia nervosa and bulimia nervosa. Curr Opin Psychiatry. 2006;19(4):438–43.
23. Mitrany E, Melamed Y. Compulsory treatment of anorexia nervosa. Israeli J Psychiatry Relat Sci. 2005;42(3):185–90.
24. Noordenbos G. Which criteria for recovery are relevant according to eating disorder patients and therapists? Eat Disord. 2011;19(5):441–51.
25. Ornstein RM, Rosen DS, Mammel KA, Callahan ST, Forman S, Jay MS, Fisher M, Rome E, Walsh BT. Distribution of eating disorders in children and adolescents using the proposed DSM-5 criteria for feeding and eating disorders. J Adolesc Health. 2013;53(2):303–5.
26. Patrick L. Eating disorders: a review of the literature with emphasis on medical complications and clinical nutrition. Altern Med Rev. 2002;7(3):184–202.
27. Pettersen G, Rosenvinge JH, Ytterhus B. The "double life" of bulimia: patients' experiences in daily life interactions. Eat Disord. 2008;16(3):204–11.
28. Randolph TG. The descriptive features of food addiction; addictive eating and drinking. Q J Stud Alcohol. 1956;17:198–224.
29. Robergeau K, Joseph J, Silber TJ. Hospitalization of children and adolescents for eating disorders in the State of New York. J Adolesc Health. 2006;39(6):806–10.
30. Rome ES, Ammerman S. Medical complications of eating disorders: an update. J Adolesc Health. 2003;33(6):418–26.
31. Salloum IM, Mezzich JE. Person-centered diagnosis. Int J Integr Care. 2010;10(Suppl):e027.
32. Smink FR, van Hoeken D, Hoek HW. Epidemiology of eating disorders: incidence, prevalence and mortality rates. Curr Psychiatry Rep. 2012;14(4):406–14.
33. Speranza M, Revah-Levy A, Giquel L, Loas G, Venisse JL, Jeammet P, Corcos M. An investigation of Goodman's addictive disorder criteria in eating disorders. Eur Eat Disord Rev. 2012;20(3):182–9.
34. Sy R, Ponton K, De Marco P, Pi S, Ishak WW. Quality of life in anorexia nervosa: a review of the literature. Eat Disord. 2013;21(3):206–22.
35. Swain-Campbell NR, Surgenor LJ, Snell DL. An analysis of consumer perspectives following contact with an eating disorders service. Aust N Z J Psychiatry. 2001;35:99–103.
36. Tarter RE, Kirisci L, Ridenour T, Bogen D. Application of person-centered medicine in addiction. Int J Person Centered Med. 2012;2(2):240–249.
37. Whiteford HA, Degenhardt L, Rehm J, Baxter AJ, Ferrari AJ, Erskine HE, Charlson FJ, Norman RE, Flaxman AD, Johns N, Burstein R, Murray CJ, Vos T. Global burden of disease attributable to mental and substance use disorders: findings from the global burden of disease study 2010. Lancet. 2013;382(9904):1575–86.
38. Zwickert K, Rieger E. Stigmatizing attitudes towards individuals with anorexia nervosa: an investigation of attribution theory. J Eat Disord. 2013;1:5.

Sexual Disorders

29

Lovorka Brajkovic, PhD, Ruben Hernandez, MD,
Felipe Navarro-Cremades, PhD, MD, Said A. Azim, MD, PhD
and Antonio Pacheco Palha, MD

29.1 Person-Centred Medicine as Framework

Person-centred medicine is a paradigmatic change within medicine, and it is dedicated to the promotion of health as a state of physical, mental, social and spiritual well-being as well as to the reduction of disease. It is founded on the articulation of science and humanism to enhance personalized understanding of illness and positive health, clinical communication, and respect for the dignity and responsibility of every person, at individual and community levels [40]. Person-centeredness is an intrinsic quality rather than an additional commodity. The following principles have been suggested for Person-centred Medicine: *wide biological, psychological, spiritual, cultural and social theoretical framework; attending to both ill health and positive health; research and education on the process and outcomes of clinical care with particular attention on communication,*

L. Brajkovic, PhD (✉)
Professor and Clinical Psychologist, Department of Psychiatry,
University Hospital Centre Zagreb, Kispaticeva 12, 10000 Zagreb, Croatia
e-mail: lovorka.brajkovic@yahoo.com

R. Hernandez, MD
Professor of Forensic Psychiatry and Medico Legal Sexology,
Universidad Central, Caracas, Venezuela

F. Navarro-Cremades, PhD, MD
Associate Professor, Faculty of Medicine, UMH, San Juan University, Alicante, Spain

S.A. Azim, MD, PhD
Professor Emeritus of Psychiatry, Cairo University, Giza, Egypt

A.P. Palha, MD
Professor of Psychiatry, Faculty of Medicine, Porto University, Porto, Portugal

J.E. Mezzich et al. (eds.), *Person Centered Psychiatry*,
DOI 10.1007/978-3-319-39724-5_29

joint understanding, and on share decision-making; respect for the autonomy, responsibility, and dignity of every person; promotion of partnership at all levels.

Furthermore, the following four essential considerations of Person-Centred Medicine are pointedly relevant for person-centred sexology: *risk and protective factors* (intrinsic and extrinsic); *illness and positive health* (vitality and resilience); *health promotion* (prevention, barriers and resources); and *health system responses to illness and health* (policies, healthcare).

Person-centred integrative diagnosis (PID) combine science and humanism to obtain a diagnosis of the person (of the totality of the person's health, both ill and positive aspects), by the person (with clinicians extending themselves as full human beings), for the person (assisting the fulfilment of the person's health aspirations and life project), and with the person (in respectful and empowering relationship with the person who consults) [39]. This model is defined by three keys: *broad informational domains* (covering ill health and positive health: health status, experience of health and contributors to health); *pluralistic descriptive procedures* (categories, dimensions and narratives) *and evaluative partnerships among clinicians, patients and families* [52].

29.2 Person-Centred Sexual Health and Sexuality

29.2.1 Sex, Sexuality and Sexual Health

Most of us are talking about sexuality, reading about sexuality, listening about someone sexuality; but a lot of this information is inaccurate and some of them are harmful. Sex is biological characteristic that define humans as female or male. Sexuality is about much more than just sex. McKinney and Sprecher [17] defined sexuality as referring to sexual behaviours, arousal and responses, as well as to sexual attitudes, desires and communication. Everyone has sexual feelings, attitudes, beliefs and experiences. However, the experience of sexuality for each of us is unique, because it was created by our own point of view. These points of view are derived from our personal convictions and beliefs which are ingrained in the culture we live, at the micro and macro social level. Therefore, it is impossible to study sexuality without taking the biological, psychosocial, cultural and religious characteristics. Sexuality includes our body (sexual and reproductive anatomy and body image), our biological sex, gender, gender identity, sexual orientation, values, attitudes, and ideals about life, love and sexual relationships as well as sexual behaviours. Sexuality is a central aspect of being human, experienced and expressed in thoughts, fantasies, desires, beliefs, attitudes, values, behaviours, practices, roles and relationships. It is influenced by the interaction of biological, psychological, social, economic, political, cultural, ethical, legal, historical, religious and spiritual factors [61].

Sexual health was defined as part of reproductive health [56], and it is a state of physical, emotional, mental and social well-being in relation to sexuality. It is not merely the absence of disease, dysfunction or infirmity. Sexual health requires a positive and respectful approach to sexuality and sexual relationships, as well as the possibility of having pleasurable and safe sexual experiences, free of coercion, discrimination and violence. For sexual health to be attained and maintained, the sexual rights of all persons must be respected, protected and fulfilled. The sexual health paradigm integrates a positive approach to sexuality with existing public health policy and practice for reducing the burdens of sexually transmitted infections, including those due to HIV [20]. Sexual health care is an essential component of overall wellness during one's developmental lifespan.

Sexual health is important throughout life, although sexual health needs vary with age. Different aspects of sexual health affect people at different times throughout their lives [36]. Until recently, sex and sexuality are commonly associated in the public domain with younger age groups, whereas sexual activities in elderly individuals are considered in many cultures to be somewhat uncommon or even strange. Some studies provided data on their sexual activity [47].

29.2.2 Sociocultural Influences

Myths about sexuality and sexual relationships are often the reason for reporting sexual dysfunction and unsatisfactory sexual relationships that is seen in clinical practice. Religious beliefs can influence sexual behaviour and how one perceives oneself as a sexual being [28]. The field of sexual health encompasses a range of issues, including STIs, STDs and reproductive tract infections (RTIs), unintended pregnancy and unsafe abortion, infertility, sexual well-being, violence related to gender and sexuality, certain aspects of mental health, the impact of physical disabilities and chronic illnesses on sexual health, female genital mutilation and so on [60]. Sexuality is considered to be an important aspect of holistic care, but that it is not routinely addressed in healthcare services. There are identified a number of personal and organizational barriers to having such discussions. Individuals' sexual health concerns are often neglected in clinical practice, although the majority of patients would prefer to have the opportunity to discuss [3]. Many people find it difficult to talk about sex; health professionals need to be aware of this and prepared to raise the subject [36].

29.3 Diagnostic Assessment and Classification

The *WPA International Guidelines for Diagnostic Assessment (IGDA)* involves four essential features: *the assessment of the psychiatric patient as a whole person*, rather than just as a carrier of disease; *the coverage of all key areas of information* (biological, psychological and social) pertinent to describing the patient's pathology, dysfunctions and problems as well as his/her positive aspects or assets; *basing the diagnostic assessment on the interactive engagement among the clinician, the patient, and his/her family*; *IGDA uses ICD-10 as a basic reference in general*, and in particular for the first three axes of its multiaxial formulation (classification of mental and general medical disorders, disabilities and contextual factors). It is very important to use culturally informed framework, both for the development of updated diagnostic models and procedures as well as for the conduction of a competent clinical evaluation of every patient [37].

The *Latin American Guide for Psychiatric Diagnosis (GLADP)* integrates the use of operational diagnostic criteria and a multiaxial system, and it includes the cultural and personalized elements of each patient. Diagnostic criteria for sexual health includes [5, 51]

1. State of sexual health (as classified in ICD-10):
   (a) sexual disorders including disease, dysfunction and sexual problems,
   (b) mental, medical and general condition related to sexual functioning of the person and the relationships as perceived by the person and by the partner,
   (c) well-being/quality of life (general, sexual and relationships)
2. Factors influencing sexual health
   (a) factors of risk and protection of sexual health
      (i) risk factors: sexual, relationship, medical and psychological, family and personal psychiatric history, including current medications, severe childhood trauma, stress, including distressing dyadic relationships,
      (ii) protective factors/promoters of sexual health: both general, and centred in the sexual and dyadic relationship, healthy diet, physical activity, personal and dyadic growth in the area of couple sexuality.
3. Experience and expectations on sexual health and a dyadic relationship.

***According to WHO ICD-10* a** sexual response is a psychosomatic process, and some types of dysfunction occur in both men and women such as lack or loss of sexual desire (including frigidity, hypoactive sexual desire disorder), sexual aversion and lack of sexual enjoyment, failure of genital response (erectile dysfunction, vaginal dryness or failure of lubrication and it includes female sexual arousal disorder, male erectile disorder, psychogenic impotence), orgasmic dysfunction, premature ejaculation, nonorganic vaginismus, nonorganic dyspareunia, excessive sexual drive, other sexual dysfunction, not caused by organic disorder or disease, unspecified sexual dysfunction, not caused by organic disorder or disease. Gender identity disorders, psychological and behavioural disorders associated with sexual development and orientation are classified as well.

DSM-5 [4] indicated that sexual dysfunctions are a heterogeneous group of disorders that are typically characterized by clinically significant disturbance in person's ability to respond sexually or to experience sexual pleasure. Sexual dysfunction includes delayed ejaculation, erectile disorder, female orgasmic disorder, female sexual interest/arousal disorder, genito-pelvic pain/penetration disorder, male hypoactive sexual desire disorder, premature (early) ejaculation, substance/medication-induced sexual dysfunction, other specified, unspecified sexual dysfunction. An individual may have several sexual dysfunctions at the same time, and in such cases, all of the dysfunctions should be diagnosed.

DSM-5 aims to avoid stigma and ensure clinical care for individuals who see and feel themselves to be different. So, it replaces the diagnostic name "gender identity disorder" with "gender dysphoria," as well as makes other important clarifications in the criteria.

The second type of sexual problems is paraphilic disorders (voyeuristsm, exhibitionism, frotteurism, sexual masochism, sexual sadism, pedophilic disorder, fetishism, transvestic disorder, as well as other specified and unspecified paraphilic disorders).

Several changes have been made to classification and criterion in DSM-5. The DSM-5 has created gender specific dysfunctions and has combined or deleted some of the previous diagnoses listed in the DSM-IV. In the DSM-5 sexual dysfunction referred to sexual pain or to a disturbance in one or more phases of the sexual response cycle; all of the DSM-5 sexual dysfunctions (except substance/medication-induced sexual dysfunction) now require a minimum duration of approximately 6 months as well as frequency of 75–100 % [4]. Genito-pelvic pain/penetration disorder is new in DSM-5, merging vaginsmus and dyspareunia in females. In DSM-5 female hypoactive desire disorder and female arousal disorder are merged into female sexual interest/arousal disorder; male orgasmic disorder is changed to delayed ejaculation; sexual aversion disorder and sexual dysfunction due to a general medical condition are absent. Male dyspareunia or male sexual pain does not appear in the sexual dysfunctions in DSM-5. DSM-5 includes lifelong versus acquired and generalized versus situational subtypes.

The WPA International Guidelines for Diagnostic Assessment suggested a comprehensive diagnostic model [27]. It includes:

1. Standardized Multiaxial formulation composed of axes
   (a) Clinical problems;
   (b) Disabilities;
   (c) Contextual Factors;
   (d) Quality of Life.

2. Personalized Idiographic Formulation:
   (a) Contextualized Clinical problems;
   (b) Patient's positive factors;
   (c) Expectations for restoration and promotion of health.

The old human response cycle from Masters and Johnson has been substituted by a six-phase cycle, which is different in men and women and it is circular pathway reinforcing model of desire, excitement, plateau, orgasm, resolution and more important, sexual satisfaction.

Hernández Serrano [27] suggested new categories for classification, advances in diagnosis and classification of sexual disorders: discronaxia—time and frequency disparity in couple; sexual post-traumatic disorders; late-onset hypogonadism; postcoital dysphoria; postcoital headache; fear of pregnancy; anaejaculation.

There are some other formulations of women's sexual dysfunction—the "three windows" approach to understanding women's sexuality [24]:

1. Current situation aspects as poor communication between partners, relationship difficulties or lack of time or privacy;
2. Individual vulnerability factors influencing the presentation of complaints, including the woman's persistently negative attitudes, a past history of sexual abuse or trauma and others;
3. Health-related factors influencing the sexual response, importantly, depression or anxiety. Included also are problems in the neural control of desire, arousal and pain perception, problems in vascular supply to the genitals, endocrine dysfunction, metabolic problems and medications.

A Comprehensive Diagnostic Formulation in Sexual health [38] is based on IGDA and includes two components

1. Standardized multiaxial formulation

    (a) Axis I Clinical Disorders (CIE-10)

        (i) Sexual Disorders
        (ii) Comorbidities

    (b) Axis II Disabilities

        (i) Areas of functioning
        (ii) Disability Scale

    (c) Axis III Contextual factors (Psychosocial problems, personal)

        (i) Problem Areas (to be specified)

            - Family/House.
            - Education/Work.
            - Economic/Legal
            - Cultural/Environmental
            - Personal

    (d) Axis IV Quality of Life

        (i) Perceived level of QoL from poor to excellent

2. Idiographic formulation

   (a) Clinical Problems and their Contextualization
   (b) Positive Factors of the Patient (Including for treatment and health promotion)
   (c) Expectations for Health Restoration and Promotion of Health.

The main purpose of the multiaxial diagnostic formulation is to inform the preparation of a comprehensive treatment plan.

29.4 Person-Centred Sexual Dysfunctions

Sexual dysfunction involves problems people experience in desiring sexual interaction, as well as physiological problems in the human sexual response cycle. Sexual dysfunctions are often accompanied by interpersonal conflict between sexual partners, and sometimes very strong feelings are associated with these problems. Both, men and women can become extremely frustrated, distressed and hostile about these difficulties. Sometimes problems are caused by biological factors and whereas in other cases they result in psychological or psychosocial adjustment problems (social, interpersonal, individual factors can contribute to a sexual dysfunction). Sexual dysfunctions affect the quality of interpersonal relationships and because of ours personal varieties we are likely to handle our own or our partner's sexual dysfunction in different ways.

The following are helpful recommendations for the clinical evaluation of men and women with sexual dysfunction [26]:

1. Attend to principles of care (patient-centred, evidence-based diagnostic and treatment and unified management); medical history; distress/interpersonal difficulty
2. Consider treatment planning for person-centred care [1]
3. Comprehensive assessment
4. Look for positive changes from illness to health and for personal and dyadic growth.

Navarro-Cremades [43] has suggested the following SAFE change model.

(i) Sensible–reasonable, rational, sage
(ii) Assumable by all who are involved: Clinician, patient, couple, environment
(iii) Feasible: Practical, achievable, and operational for clinical practice
(iv) Evaluable: Short- and long-term.

Global surveys estimate that 9–29 % of men and 16–43 % of women suffer from distressing sexual problems [2]. Overall, erectile dysfunction has been the most thoroughly studied male's dysfunction. Premature or rapid ejaculation is the most prevalent male dysfunction. Erectile dysfunction shows a systematic relationship with age, while premature/rapid ejaculation does not [18].

In women various sexual dysfunctions are associated with age and comorbid health conditions such as personal distress, depression, menopausal status, as well as the partner's sexual health [18].

29.5 Standard Procedures for Diagnosis and Treatment in Sexual Health

Flexible standards are helpful for achieving good clinical practice. A sexual history guide [3] offers health care professionals a brief, structured method for obtaining a sexual history that is person-centred and is focused on the process of the interview.

Sexual history taking may be based on three management principles:

1. Adoption of a person-centred framework.
2. Application of evidence-based medicine in a flexible manner.
3. Comprehensive approach to sexual dysfunction.

History taking should include understanding the patient's ideas, feelings, expectations and values. It should also attend to psychosocial contextual issues, sexual orientation, gender conflicts, body image concerns, sexual transmitted diseases and sexual victimization.

29.6 Sexual Dysfunctions in Men

Erectile dysfunction (ED) and premature ejaculation (PE) are the two main complaints in male sexual medicine [57]. Some antidepressants can induce erectile dysfunction, delayed ejaculation and loss of libido [23].

Erectile dysfunction [57] is defined as the persistent inability to attain and maintain an erection sufficient to permit satisfactory sexual performance. Although ED is a benign disorder, it may affect physical and psychosocial health and may have a significant impact on quality of life.

There is increasing evidence that the impact of ED extends beyond the immediate orgasmic function, to sexual desire, overall satisfaction and satisfaction with intercourse and confidence [34]. ED [19] is common among ageing men, with the prevalence ranging from 10 to 80 % depending on the populations studied and definition used to describe ED. ED is a chronic condition that exerts a negative impact on male self-esteem and nearly all life domains including interpersonal, family and business relationships [47].

Comorbidities and lifestyle factors are important contributors to the development of ED. Comorbidities such as heart disease, diabetes, dyslipidemia, hypertension and depression have been described as primary risk factors for the development of ED. Modifiable lifestyle factors, including physical activity, smoking, alcohol consumption and obesity, have been associated to ED (Glina 2013). ED is a potential warning sign of cardiovascular disease. Some drugs (i.e. antihypertensives, antidepressants, antipsychotics, antiandrogens) and some recreational drugs can contribute to erectile dysfunction.

Ejaculatory Dysfunction: Its spectrum extends from premature ejaculation (PE), through delayed ejaculation (DE), to a complete inability to ejaculate (anejaculation) and includes retrograde ejaculation [35].

Premature Ejaculation (PE) has prevalence rates of 20–30 % [57]. There are two official definitions of PE in DSM-5 and ICD-10 and they have been challenged. Definitions take into account the time to ejaculation, the inability to control or delay ejaculation, distress, and negative consequences. PE can be "lifelong" (primary) and "acquired" (secondary) [53]. The time to ejaculation may be assessed by intravaginal ejaculatory latency time (IELT).

29.6.1 Low Sexual Desire/Interest in Men [50]

It can be due to a variety of causes and can be best characterized as a syndrome rather than a disorder. LSD/I is frequent in men with ED. Prevalence average is 20 %, varying from 12.5 to 28.0 %. Risk factors for LDS are ageing, poor health, vascular disease, depression, relationships issues, low frequency of sexual relationship.

29.7 Sexual Dysfunction in Women

Women's sexual dysfunction includes reduced interest/incentives for sexual engagement, difficulties with becoming subjectively aroused and/or genitally aroused, and difficulties in triggering desire during sexual engagement. Frequently, all of these aspects are involved. Orgasmic disorder denotes sexual experiences consistently associated with high arousal and absence of orgasm. Other dysfunctions include pain and difficulty with attempted or completed intercourse or any attempts at vaginal penetration [9].

Female Orgasmic Disorder (FOD). ICD-10 specifies that the disorder impairs the patient's ability to participate in a sexual relationship in the way she would like, occurs frequently, and has been present for at least 6 months. FOD can be lifelong (primary) or acquired (secondary); generalized or situational; psychological or combined. FOD is the second most prevalent sexual disorder in women, with a high level of comorbidity with other SD, requiring a comprehensive woman-centred assessment including correlates of FOD and other relevant biopsychosocial factors, in an appropriate cultural context. FOD should not be diagnosed solely on the basis of a failure to experience orgasm during sexual intercourse in the absence of additional clitoral stimulation, as this is considered a "normal variation of sexual response" rather than a "pathological inhibition." Some risk factors should be considered: psychosocial factors, cognitive/affective factors, relationship factors, a history of childhood maltreatment (physical, psychological, or sexual abuse) or adult experiences of sexual abuse.

29.7.1 Female Sexual Arousal Disorders (FSAD)

FSAD are divided into three subtypes [22]:

1. Genital Sexual Arousal Disorder: Absent or impaired genital sexual arousal.
2. Subjective Arousal Disorder: Absence of or markedly diminished feelings of sexual arousal (sexual excitement and sexual pleasure) from any type of sexual stimulation.
3. Combined Genital and Subjective Arousal Disorder.

DSM-5 combines women's sexual desire and arousal disorders into one entity—Female Sexual Interest/Arousal Disorder. FSAD can be primary and secondary; generalized or situational.

There are some risk factors for developing FSAD

- Biological: hormonal factors
- Neurological conditions, infections, iatrogenic factors
- Psychological issues, relationship problems, partner's sexual dysfunction.
- Sexual abuse
- Cultural factors.

29.7.2 Hypoactive Sexual Desire Disorder (HSDD) [11]

DSM-5 combines women's sexual desire and arousal disorders into one entity: Female Sexual Interest/Arousal Disorder. Due to the lack of objective criteria, the importance of subjective experience and the multifactorial etiology of HSDD, it is necessary to use a diagnostic guide, using a semi-structured interview

- Biomedical factors affecting sexual desire
- Individual psychological and interpersonal factors affecting sexual desire
- Distress, relationship factors, partners sexual dysfunction.

Hypoactive sexual desire disorder is a frequently reported problem among people who visit sex therapy clinics. Emotional problems, limited sexual knowledge, low levels of sexual motivation and interpersonal problems in a relationship may be involved in this dysfunction. Some investigators have reported that low sexual desire is often symptomatic of marital adjustment problems [54]. Much attention has been given to the nature of a couple's relationship dynamics when one individual reports low sexual desire [16]. The existence of a sexual desire discrepancy between two people does not always reveal the causes or consequences of such a mismatch. Clement [16] believes that such differences in sexual desire emerge from a couple's communication and cannot be attributed specifically to one or the other person.

29.7.3 Female Genital Sexual Pain (GSP) [21]

The etiology of GSP is multifaceted and it is focusing on genital pain provoked by or exacerbated during or immediately after sexual activities in women. Currently, GSP may be classified into Genito-Pelvic Pain/Penetration Disorder and into two diagnostic entities (ICD-10 and DSM-IV RT): *dyspareunia* (persistent or recurrent pain with attempted or complete vaginal entry and/or vaginal sexual intercourse) and *vaginismus:* (persistent or recurrent difficulties to allow vaginal entry of a penis/finger/any object despite the woman's expressed wish to do so) [8].

29.8 Paraphilia, Gender Dysphoria and Hypersexuality

DSM-5 has introduced some important changes to the conceptualization of paraphilic disorders, distinguishing between paraphilias and paraphilic disorders [55, 62].

Paraphilias are defined as any intense and persistent sexual interest other than sexual interest in genital stimulation or preparatory fondling with phenotypically normal, physically mature, consenting human partners. ***Paraphilic disorders*** are paraphilias that cause distress or impairment to the individual or harm to others [55].

Gender dysphoria is a new diagnostic class in DSM-5 and it is neither a sexual dysfunction nor a paraphilia [31].

29.9 Hypersexuality

According to ICD-10, hypersexuality indicates excessive sexual drive which includes nymphomania and satyriasis. Hypersexual disorder was not included in the DSM-5. Kafka [29] proposed the diagnostic criteria for a hypersexual disorder diagnosis, describing hypersexual disorder as recurrent and intense sexual fantasies, sexual urges or sexual behaviours resulting in clinically significant personal distress or impairment in social, occupational or other important areas of functioning.

29.10 Sexual Health, Mental Disorders, Chronic Disease and Ageing

Sexual disorders associated with psychiatric illness may be related to a pre-existing primary sexual disorder, a symptom of depression and anxiety, an undesirable side effect of the psychotropic medication or because of other causes such as medical illness, substance abuse or psychosocial stressors [15]. About 40 % of females and 30 % of males suffer from sexual complaints and they are more frequent in patients with mental/mood disorders not on medications, and still more in patients on treatment with psychotropic drugs [15, 41]. It may occur with almost any medication, may be dose dependent and is fairly frequent with some psychotropic medications [6]. Iatrogenic sexual dysfunction is frequent, and treatment with psychotropic drugs such as some antidepressants and various antipsychotics is one of the most frequent causes of sexual dysfunction. Antipsychotic-induced sexual dysfunction seems to be frequent with conventional antipsychotics and others too. Pharmacological treatment of CNS disease often affects sexual functioning and it is often a reason to stop treatment prematurely [10]. Sexual disorders associated with psychiatric illness and its treatment include diminished sexual desire, arousal problems such as inhibited cognitive sexual excitement, diminished genital sensation, erectile dysfunction and failure to achieve and maintain vaginal lubrication. Orgasmic dysfunction may also occur including delayed orgasm or complete anorgasmia as well as delayed or premature ejaculation in males. The relationship between psychiatric illness and sexual disorders (SD) appears to be bidirectional.

29.10.1 Sexual Health in People with Chronic Disease and Disabilities

Regarding assessment of dysfunction in the context of chronic illness [9] the multiple factors contribute directly or indirectly to sexual dysfunction. The effects on sexual health are frequent and are rarely discussed by healthcare professionals [12, 49, 63]. The recognition that people with disabilities are sexual beings is relatively new. Historically, they have been perceived as asexual or potentially deviant. These people may experience a lack of information as well as distress and anguish around their sexual and personal relationships. They often face obstacles to maximize their sexual potential and may internalize negative societal attitudes and assumptions about their sexuality [44].

Sexual health is important to people with disabilities [49]; they have higher rates of STIs, unintended pregnancies, sexual dysfunction and sexual violence.

The development of sexual morbidity in the female cancer survivor is a multifactorial problem incorporating psychological, physiologic and sociological elements [30]. At the time of diagnosis, cancer patients may have concurrent medical illnesses, taking chronic medications that may have directly or indirectly influenced any aspect of the sexual response cycle. Sexual dysfunction encompasses a broad spectrum of issues, all of which are susceptible to insult after treatment for cancer. Sexual dysfunction affects most women treated for breast cancer, and sexual quality of life is a significant concern for breast cancer survivors [12]. All cancers can impact sexuality and intimacy and having cancer does not eliminate sexual feelings. Cancer treatments often cause sexual dysfunction, irrespective of cancer type, age, gender, culture, partnership status. Over 50 % women with breast or gynecologic cancer and 70 % men with prostate cancer report some level of sexual dysfunction (hypoactive sexual desire disorder, sexual arousal disorder, orgasmic disorder, sexual pain disorder and changes in genital sensation) [12]. Erectile dysfunction is highly prevalent in men treated for prostate cancer, about in 75 % in men treated for localized prostate cancer [14].

Sexual dysfunction is observed in many neurological disorders including its treatment [33, 48]. Sexual dysfunctions are common in patients with multiple sclerosis and it is associated with enhanced disability, pain, duration of the disease, and degree of concomitant depression and low quality of life [25, 32]. The prevalence of sexual dysfunctions is very high in men with multiple sclerosis, ranges between 64 and 91 %. First complaint is erectile dysfunction in 50 % [7]. Spinal cord injury can lead to sexual dysfunction as well (end torax region injury can affect orgasm; sacral region injury can affect ED in males and arousal in females).

Stroke has impact on individual sexual functioning, intimate relationships and sexual satisfaction, as well, as rheumatoid arthritis [63].

Sexuality is so closely identified with youthfulness, the stereotype of sexless older adults who are frail and inactive is a widely held belief. Sexuality and intimacy depends on psychological factors, health status and sexual well-being is more defined by a subjective factor, rather than objective.

Older adults who are experiencing chronic illness and are disabled find themselves devalued, denied sexual expression and excluded from meaningful relationships. Low level of testosterone and low level of oestrogen, high level of prolactin can lead to lack of sexual satisfaction.

29.11 Sex Therapy

Until the sixties, when William Masters and Virginia Johnson made a sort of revolution and, in fact created sex therapy, the dominant approach to the treatment of sexual problems was psychoanalytic [12]. Masters and Johnson were considering that identifying the cause is always less important than discovering a successful method of operationally treating the problem. Their innovation was a series of "homework" tasks such as sensory exercises designed to help couples to circumvent the usual, routine, sexual contacts within which problems grow. Later approaches, especially integrative and systemic, in many ways combine cognitive behavioural and psychodynamic approaches [12, 13].

29.12 Sexual Health Promotion, Prevention, Education and Sexual Rights

Person-centred sexual health promotion (PCSHP) include: [42].

1. General Sexual Health Promotion

   - Sexual and Reproductive Rights
   - National Policies focusing on SHP
   - Educational Considerations on SHP
   - Epidemiologic and Public Health Considerations
   - Life Cycle and Sexual Health Promotion
   - Communication and Sexual Health
   - Social, cultural and spiritual perspectives and values
   - Cultural and ethnic issues in sexual expression
   - Gender issues and diversity

2. Person-centred Sexual Health Promotion (PCSHP) in the clinical setting:

   - Ethical perspectives within the patient–doctor relationship
   - General principles of positive attitudes toward human sexuality, basic sexual information and education, basic sexual enrichment and health promotion
   - The important of active listening and relaxation training
   - Personal responsibility for self
   - Mutual cooperation with the partner.

29.12.1 Person-Centred Prevention and Education

It is important for practitioners to recognize that sexually transmitted infection (STI) risks and sexual transmitted diseases will vary from person to person and should be viewed as dynamic across the lifespan. The majority of STDs/STIs are asymptomatic and therefore go undetected, and are also underreported [58]. STDs and HIV have far-reaching public health consequences on sexual and reproductive health. A variety of prevention interventions are available to reduce the risk of acquiring STIs including risk reduction counselling, appropriate use of available prevention methods, evaluation and treatment of infected persons and their sex partners, and vaccination of persons at risk.

Parish and Rubio-Aurioles [46] and Parish and Clayton [45] proposed a comprehensive model of person-centred education which includes:

1. Attitudes: Self-awareness of own beliefs, values, attitudes, sexual behaviour;
2. Knowledge, i.e. causes of sexual dysfunction, impact of medical illness, treatment; medications, sexuality in special populations, reproductive biology, STIs/IHV, sexual abuse/violence;
3. Skills: Sexual history, general communication, integrated diagnosis.

29.12.2 Human and Sexual Rights

The World Association for Sexual Health [59] states that sexual rights embrace human rights that are already recognized in national laws, international human rights documents and other consensus statements. They include the right of all persons, free of coercion, discrimination and violence to the highest attainable standard of sexual health, including access to sexual and reproductive health care services; seeking, receiving and imparting information related to sexuality; respect for bodily integrity; choosing their own partner; deciding to be sexually active or not; consensual sexual relations; consensual marriage; deciding whether or not, and when, to have children; and pursuing a satisfying, safe and pleasurable sexual life.

The WAS Declaration of Sexual Rights [59] includes sixteen human rights pertaining to sexuality

1. Equality and non-discrimination
2. Autonomy and body integrity
3. Life, liberty and security of the person
4. The right to be free from torture and cruel, inhuman or degrading treatment or punishment
5. The right to be free from all forms of violence and coercion
6. Right to privacy
7. The right to the highest attainable standard of health, including sexual health
8. The right to enjoy the benefits of scientific progress and its application
9. The right to information
10. The right to education and right to comprehensive sexuality education
11. The right to enter, form and dissolve marriage and other similar types of relationship based on equality and full and free consent
12. The right to decide whether to have children, the number and spacing of children, and to have information and the means to do so
13. The right to freedom of thought, opinion and expression
14. The right to freedom of association and peaceful assembly
15. The right to participation in public and political life
16. The right of access to justice, remedies and redress.

29.13 Conclusions

Person-centred sexuality represents a holistic approach, considering the complex nature of human sexuality. It includes sexual health and sexual well-being (physical, psychological, social and spiritual dimensions). Person-centred sexology (PCS) is derived from models of Person-centred Medicine (PCM) and Psychiatry (PCP). PCS include key contributions from PCM and PCP to a sexological adapted Person-centred Integrative Diagnosis PID. The Comprehensive Diagnostic Formulation in Sexual Health has two components: Standardized Multiaxial Formulation and an Idiographic Formulation.

New categories and diagnostics are being proposed. Additional biopsychosocial formulations and models of sexual disorders are exposed as "three windows" and ICSM-5 steps models. Person-centred and Partnership-centered care are key for competent evaluation and treatment and include evidence-based and experienced-based contributions, looking for a positive change in sexual health.

Sexual Dysfunctions (SDs) are prevalent in both sexes. A global assessment of sexual problems and SDs should be comprehensive and person- and partner-centred. Erectile dysfunction and premature ejaculation are the most common sexual dysfunctions in men; and the main female sexual dysfunctions are female orgasmic disorder, female arousal disorders, hypoactive sexual desire disorder and female genital sexual pain. SD is a frequent problem in psychiatric patients with or without drug treatment.

Sexual health is a key issue for people with disabilities and chronic diseases such as cancer and neurological problems and ageing-related conditions. Sexual Health promotion, prevention and education are important factors to advance sexual well-being and sexual quality of life. Human and sexual rights are recognized in national and international conventions and laws and must be respected at all levels.

References

1. Adams N, Grieder DM. Treatment planning for person-centered care: shared decision making for whole health. 2nd ed. Waltham, MA: Elsevier Academic Press; 2014.
2. Althof SE, McMahon CG, Waldinger MD, Serefoglu EC, Shindel AW, Adaikan PG, Becher E, Dean J, Giuliano F, Hellstrom WJG, Giraldi A, Glina S, Incrocci L, Jannini E, McCabe M, Parish S, Rowland D, Segraves RT, Sharlip I, Torres LO. An update of the International Society of Sexual Medicine's guidelines for the diagnosis and treatment of premature ejaculation (PE). J Sex Med. 2014;11:1392–422.
3. Althof SE, Rosen RC, Perelman MA, Rubio-Aurioles E. Standard operating procedures for taking a sexual history. J Sex Med. 2013;10:26–35.
4. American Psychiatric Association. Highlights of changes from DSM-IV-TR to DSM-5. Washington, DC; 2013.
5. Asociación Psiquiátrica de América Latina (APAL). Guía Latinoamericana de Diagnóstico Psiquiátrico, Versión Revisada (GLADP-VR). Lima: APAL; 2012. Available at: http://www.apalweb.org/docs/gladpvr2012.pdf. Accessed 8 Dec 2014.
6. Balon R, Segraves RT, editors. Clinical manual of sexual disorders. Washington, DC: American Psychiatric Publishing Inc.; 2009.

7. Barbonetti A, Cavallo F, Felzani G, Francavilla S, Francavilla F. Erectile dysfunction is the main determinant of psychological distress in men with spinal cord injury. J Sex Med. 2012;9:830–6.
8. Basson R, Leiblum S, Brotto L, Derogatis L, Fourcroy J, Fugl-Meyer KS, Graziottin A, Heyman J, Laan E, Meston C, Shover L, van Lankveld JJ, Weimar Schultz W. Definitions of women's sexual dysfunction reconsidered: advocating expansion and revision. J Psychosom Obstet Gynecol. 2003;24:221–9.
9. Basson R, Wierman ME, van Lankveld J, Brotto L. Summary of the recommendations on sexual dysfunctions in women. J Sex Med. 2010;7:314–26.
10. Bijlsma EY, Chan JS, Olivier B, Veening JG, Millan MJ, Waldingerm MD, Oosting RS. Sexual side effects of serotonergic antidepressants: mediated by inhibition of serotonin on central dopamine release? Pharmacol Biochem Behav. 2014;121:88–101.
11. Bitzer J, Giraldi A, Pfaus J. A standardized diagnostic interview for hypoactive sexual desire disorder in women: standard operating procedure (SOP part 2). J Sex Med. 2013;10:50–7.
12. Brajkovic L. Sexuality and sexual health from person-oriented perspective. In: Djordjevic V, Bras M, Milicic D, editors. Person in medicine and health care—from bench to bedside to community. Zagreb: Medicinska naklada; 2012.
13. Brajkovic L, Bras M, Radic I, Djordjevic V. Sexual quality of life in women with breast cancer —croatian sample. Asia Pac J Clin Oncol. 2012;8(Suppl S3):238.
14. Chisholm KE, McCabe MP, Wootten AC, Abbott JAM. Review: psychosocial interventions addressing sexual or relationship functioning in men with prostate cancer. J Sex Med. 2012;9:1246–60.
15. Clayton AH, Balon R. The impact of mental illness and psychotropic medications on sexual functioning: the evidence and management. J Sex Med. 2009;6:1200–11.
16. Clement U. Sex in long-term relationships: a systemic approach to sexual desire problems. Arch Sex Behav. 2002;31(3):241–6.
17. DeLamater J, Hyde JS. Conceptual and theoretical issues in studying sexuality in close relationship. In: Harvey JH, Wenzel A, Sprecher S, editors. Handbook of sexuality in close relationship. New Jersey: Lawrence Erlbaum Associates Inc; 2004.
18. DeRogatis LR, Burnett AL. The epidemiology of sexual dysfunctions. J Sex Med. 2008;5:289–300.
19. Ettala OO, Syvänen KT, Korhonen PE, Kaipia AJ, Vahlberg TJ, Boström PJ, Aarnio PT. High-intensity physical activity, stable relationship, and high education level associate with decreasing risk of erectile dysfunction in 1,000 apparently healthy cardiovascular risk subjects. J Sex Med. 2014;11:2277–84.
20. Fortenbery JD. The evolving sexual health paradigm: transforming definition into sexual health. AIDS. 2013;(Suppl 1):S127–33.
21. Fugl-Meyer KS, Bohm-Starke N, Damsted Petersen C, Fugl-Meyer A, Parish S, Giraldi A. Standard operating procedures for female genital sexual pain. J Sex Med. 2013;10:83–93.
22. Giraldi A, Rellini AH, Pfaus J, Laan E. Female sexual arousal disorders. J Sex Med. 2013;10:58–73.
23. Glina S, Sharlip ID, Hellstrom WJG. Modifying risk factors to prevent and treat erectile dysfunction. J Sex Med. 2013;10:115–9.
24. Graham CA. Orgasm disorder in women. In: Binik Y, Hall KSK, editors. Principles and practice of sex therapy. 5th ed. New York: Guilford Press; 2009.
25. Gumus H, Akpinar Z, Yilmaz H. Effects of multiple sclerosis on female sexuality: a controlled study. J Sex Med. 2014;11:481–6.
26. Hatzichristou D, Rosen RC, Derogatis LR, Low WY, Meuleman EJ, Sadovsky R, Symonds T. Recommendations for the clinical evaluation of men and women with sexual dysfunction. J Sex Med. 2010;1(2):337–48.
27. Hernández Serrano R, Palha AP, Azim SA, Simonelli C, Navarro-Cremades F, Parra A. Advances in diagnosis and classification of sexual disorders. In: Salloum IM, Mezzich JE, editors. Psychiatric diagnosis: challenges and prospects. Chichester, UK: Wiley-Blackwell; 2009.

28. Kellogg Spadt S, Rosenbaum TY, Dweck A, Millheiser L, Pillai-Friedman S, Krychman M. Sexual health and religion: a primer for the sexual health clinician. J Sex Med. 2014;11:1606–19.
29. Klein V, Rettenberger M, Briken P. Self-reported indicators of hypersexuality and its correlates in a female online sample. J Sex Med. 2014;11:1974–81.
30. Krychman M, Millheiser LS. Sexual health issues in women with cancer. J Sex Med. 2013;10 (Suppl 1):5–15.
31. Lawrence AA. Gender assignment dysphoria in the DSM-5. Arch Sex Behav. 2014;43:1263–6.
32. Lew-Starowicz M, Rola R. Correlates of sexual function in male and female patients with multiple sclerosis. J Sex Med. 2014;11:2172–80.
33. Lundberg PO, Ertekin C, Ghezzi A, Swash M, Vodusek D. Neurosexology. Guidelines for neurologists. Eur J Neurol. 2001;8(Suppl 3):2–24.
34. McCabe MP, Althof SE. A systematic review of the psychosocial outcomes associated with erectile dysfunction: does the impact of erectile dysfunction extend beyond a man's inability to have sex? J Sex Med. 2014;11:347–63.
35. McMahon CG, Jannini E, Waldinger M, Rowland D. Standard operating procedures in the disorders of orgasm and ejaculation. J Sex Med. 2013;10:204–29.
36. Mercer CH. Sexual behavior. Epidemiol Sex Behav. 2014;42(6):1–3. Available from http://www.medicinejournal.co.uk/article/S1357-3039%2814%2900071-1/pdf. Accessed 15 Dec 2014.
37. Mezzich J, et al. WPA International Guidelines for Diagnostic Assessment (IGDA) project. New York; 2002. Available at: http://www.wpanet.org/uploads/Sections/Classification_Diagnostic/introduction.pdf. Accessed 3 Nov 2014.
38. Mezzich JE, Hernandez R, editors. Psychiatry and sexual health: an integrative approach. New York: Rowman & Littlefield; 2006.
39. Mezzich J, Salloum IM, Cloninger CR, Salvador-Carulla L, Kirmayer LJ, Banzato CE, Wallcraft J, Botbol M. Person-centred integrative diagnosis: conceptual bases and structural model. Can J Psychiatry. 2010;55(11):701–8.
40. Mezzich JE, Snaedal J, van Weel C, Heath I. Toward person-centered medicine: from disease to patient to person. Mt Sinai J Med. 2010;77:304–6.
41. Montejo AL, Majadas S, Rico-Villademoros F, LLorca G, de la Gándara J, Franco M, Martín-Carrasco M, Aguera L, Prieto N. Frequency of sexual dysfunction in patients with a psychotic disorder receiving antipsychotics. J Sex Med. 2010;7:3404–13.
42. Navarro-Cremades F, Hernández-Serrano R. Person-centered sexual health promotion. Presented at the World Congress of Mental Health, WMHC, 2nd–6th September. Athens; 2009.
43. Navarro-Cremades F. The change in sexology. SAFE model (El cambio en sexología. Modelo "SAFE"©). In: Actualidades en Sexología Médica, AISM. Quito, Ecuador: Editorial Fraga; 2007. p. 213–17.
44. O'Dea SM, Shuttleworth RP, Wedgwood N. Disability, doctors and sexuality: do healthcare providers influence the sexual wellbeing of people living with a neuromuscular disorder? Sex Disabil. 2012;30(2):171–85.
45. Parish SJ, Clayton AH. Sexual medicine education: review and commentary. J Sex Med. 2007;4:259–67.
46. Parish SJ, Rubio-Aurioles E. Education in sexual medicine: proceedings from the international consultation in sexual medicine. J Sex Med. 2009;7:3305–14.
47. Porst H, Burnett A, Brock G, Ghanem H, Giuliano F, Glina S, Hellstrom W, Martin-Morales A, Salonia A, Sharlip I, the ISSM Standards Committee for Sexual Medicine. SOP conservative (medical and mechanical) treatment of erectile dysfunction. J Sex Med. 2013;10:130–71.
48. Rees PM, Fowler CJ, Maas CO. Sexual function in men and women with neurological disorders. Lancet. 2007;369(9560):512–25.
49. Rowen TS. Sexual health for people with disabilities. J Sex Med. 2013;10:1667–8.

50. Rubio-Aurioles E, Bivalacqua TJ. Standard operational procedures for low sexual desire in men. J Sex Med. 2013;10:94–107.
51. Saavedra JE, Mezzich JE, Otero A, Salloum IM. The revision of the Latin American Guide for Psychiatric Diagnosis (GLADP-VR) and an initial survey on its utility and prospects. Int J Pers Cent Med. 2012;2(2):214–21.
52. Salloum IM, Mezzich JE, editors. Psychiatric diagnosis: challenges and prospects. Chichester, UK: Wiley-Blackwell; 2009.
53. Serefoglu EC, McMahon CG, Waldinger MD, Althof SE, Shindel A, Adaikan G, Becher EF, Dean J, Giuliano F, Hellstrom WJG, Giraldi A, Glina S, Incrocci L, Jannini E, McCabe M, Parish S, Rowland D, Segraves RT, Sharlip I, Torres LO. An evidence-based unified definition of lifelong and acquired premature ejaculation: report of the second International Society for Sexual Medicine Ad Hoc Committee for the definition of premature ejaculation. J Sex Med. 2014;11:1423–41.
54. Trudel G, Fortin C, Matte B. Sexual interaction and communication in couples with hypoactive sexual desire. Scand J Behav Ther. 1997;26:49–53.
55. Turner D, Schöttle D, Bradford J, Briken P. Assessment methods and management of hypersexuality and paraphilic disorders. Curr Opin Psychiatry. 2014;27(6):413–22.
56. United Nations Population Fundation UNFPA. International Conference on Population and Development—ICPD—Programme of Action. New York: United Nations Population Fund, UNFPA; 1995 Available at: http://www.unfpa.org/public/publications/pid/1973. Accessed 15 Dec 2014.
57. Wespes E, Eardley I, Giuliano F, Hatzichristou D, Hatzimouratidis K, Moncada I, Salonia AY. Guidelines of male sexual dysfunction: erectile dysfunction and premature ejaculation. Eur Assoc Urol. 2013. Available at: http://www.uroweb.org/gls/pdf/14_Male%20Sexual 20Dysfunction_LR.pdf. Accessed 10 Dec 2014.
58. Workowski K, Berman SM, Centers for Disease Control and Prevention. Sexually transmitted diseases treatment guidelines. Clin Infect Dis. 2011;53(Suppl 3):S59–63.
59. World Association for Sexual Health, WAS. 2014. Available at: http://www.worldsexology.org/wp-content/uploads/2013/08/declaration_of_sexual_rights_sep03_2014.pdf. Accessed 15 Dec 2014.
60. World Health Organization. Progress in reproductive health research, No. 67. 2004. Available at: http://www.who.int/hrp/publications/progress67.pdf. Accessed 15 Dec 2014.
61. World Health Organization. Defining sexual health. Report of a technical consultation on sexual health. Geneva: WHO; 2006. Available at: http://www.who.int/reproductivehealth/topics/gender_rights/defining_sexual_health.pdf. Accessed 15 Dec 2014.
62. Wright S. Kinky parents and child custody: the effect of the DSM-5 differentiation between the paraphilias and paraphilic disorders. Arch Sex Behav. 2014;43:1257–8.
63. Yilmaz H, Polat HAD, Yilmaz SD, Erkin G, Kucuksen S, Salli A, Ugurlu H. Evaluation of sexual dysfunction in women with rheumatoid arthritis: a controlled study. J Sex Med. 2012;9:2664–70.

Trauma: Complexity and Disruption

30

Moty Benyakar, MD, PhD, Carlos Collazo, MD
and George N. Christodoulou, MD, PhD

30.1 Introduction

Social reality filters into our clinical work without asking permission. During the last decades, mental health professionals have increased their interventions facing the needs of citizens after a natural or man-made disaster. They are increasingly facing the need to find an integrative concept that includes the interaction between biological, psychological, interpersonal, behavioral, and social reactions to disasters [1].

Today, committed professionals are beginning to pay attention to the dramatic reality that surrounds us, a reality in which violence lies in the backdrop of our daily existence. There is growing recognition that applying theoretical and clinical skills to one's social reality can no longer be viewed as an altruistic measure but, rather as

M. Benyakar, MD, PhD (✉)
Professor of Psychiatry, El Salvador Univ, Av. Del Libertador 4944, 9B,
1426 Capital Federal, Buenos Aires, Argentina; President, Iberoamerican Ecobioethics Network for Education Science and Technology, Unesco Chair in Bioethics, Paris, France; Honorary Member, World Psychiatric Association, Geneva, Switzerland; Honorary Chair, WPA Section on Disaster Psychiatry, Geneva, Switzerland
e-mail: motybenyakar@fibertel.com.ar

C. Collazo, MD
Professor of Psychiatry, El Salvador Univ, Av. Del Libertador 4944, 9B,
1426 Capital Federal, Buenos Aires, Argentina; Honorary Chair, WPA Section on Disaster Psychiatry, Geneva, Switzerland; International Fellow, American Psychiatric Association, Arlington County, VA, USA

G.N. Christodoulou, MD, PhD
Honorary Member, World Psychiatric Association, Geneva, Switzerland;
Professor of Psychiatry, Athens University, Athens, Greece; President, World Federation for Mental Health, Baltimore, ML, USA; Honorary President, Hellenic Psychiatric Association, Athens, Greece

J.E. Mezzich et al. (eds.), *Person Centered Psychiatry*,
DOI 10.1007/978-3-319-39724-5_30

an essential measure for the emotional and physical preservation of psychic stability and daily well-being.

For such purpose, it is useful to analyze the real meaning of concepts like complexity, disruption (the impact of the environment on the psyche), trauma, victim, victimization, and damaged person in order to know and understand their meaning, characteristics, similarities and differences, and the importance to include them in our clinical daily work.

Especially in disasters and daily accidents, it is important to distinguish the external factual event from the psychic process. We should perhaps reconsider the concept "traumatic situation", and analyze the characteristics of the situation and the psychic process in which trauma may or may not be the consequence of it. We must define each concept accurately. It is not a change of words; it is another way of thinking and facing the problem. In this way, we can understand different psychic reactions to external disruptive situations, letting us be more specific in our clinical approach.

It is difficult to identify and measure the type of impact that disruptive events can produce in people's psyche, as well as to evaluate responses.

Physically or psychologically affected people in these situations must be considered as "injured people" and not "victims". Labeling them as "victims," may produce chronic pathology. The term "Injured people" does not mean they suffer less; it is only used to avoid a new identity, the identity of "victims."

30.2 Complexity

> The progress of complexity has been made in spite of, with, and because of human folly.
>
> Edgar Morin

We consider that to face this new reality we should lean on the Paradigm of Complexity developed by Morin [2]. This paradigm implies a change of viewpoint of the phenomena observed, a change in the scientific method by which our present-day society is ruled, perceiving, and appreciating the real, the factual, signed by a globalized world that interconnects thoughts and phenomena, events and processes, where the physical, biological, psychological, linguistic, anthropological, social, and environmental contexts are reciprocally interdependent.

The world today moves on the basis of changing realities, with laws and rules that move step by step.

The universal problem for every citizen of the new millennium is how to get access to information, and how to acquire skills to articulate and organize that information. To perceive and conceive the context knowledge of isolated information or data is not enough. Meaning, information, and data must be placed in their context. We are faced with a complex situation and our approach should be equally comprehensive when applied to health in general and especially mental health.

Yunkap Kwankam, a world-renowned health and health consultant, explains the purpose of creating a repository of health knowledge: "There is a lot of reinvention of the wheel in eHealth. People don't know that certain things have already been done. So it is an opportunity to share more widely what is already known" [3, 4].

There is complexity and the various elements (economic, political, sociological, psychological, emotional, mythological) that compose a whole are inseparable, and there is inter-retroactive, interactive, interdependent tissue between the subject of knowledge and its context, the parts and the whole, the whole and the parts, the parts amongst themselves. Disaster situations can be one of the most paradigmatic examples of complexity.

Human complexity cannot be understood in dissociation from the elements that constitute it; all truly human development means joint development of individual autonomies, community participations, and a sense of belonging to the human species.

There is human unity. There is human diversity. Unity goes beyond the biological features of the species Homo sapiens. Diversity is more than the psychological, cultural, and social features of the human being. There is also a strictly biological diversity within human unity; there is a unity that is not only cerebral but also mental, psychological, emotional, and intellectual [5]. Moreover, the most diverse cultures and societies have common generative or organizing principles. Understanding what is human means understanding our unity in diversity.

It is possible also that there is a Cartesian separation between mind and body behind the thought of those neuroscientists who insist that the mind can be explained exclusively in terms of cerebral events, brushing aside the rest of the organism and the physical and social environment that surrounds it—and leaving outside the fact that parts from the environment are the product of the preceding actions of the organism [6].

We should also see that every human being, even a person confined in the most ordinary life, is a cosmos in himself. "He carries inner multiplicities and virtual personalities, endless imaginary characters, a polyexistence in the real and the imaginary, sleep and waking, obedience and transgression, ostensible and secret, and larval squirming in his bottomless caves and chasms. Everyone contains galaxies of dreams and fantasies, unsatisfied flights of desire and love, abysses of unhappiness, immensities of icy indifference, conflagrations of fiery stars, waves of hatred, mindlessness, flashes of lucidity, and outbursts of dementia in unity. We must conceive the unity of the multiple, the multiplicity of the one" [7].

The World Health Organization (WHO) definition of health focuses on the complete physical, mental, and social well-being of a person. This and the WHO's historical efforts to advance health make clear that health care can hardly be optimized for individual persons unless it is promoted for people in society as a whole.

The pursuit of individual wellbeing is rendered illusory in the absence of collective well-being.

Disasters are one of the clearest expressions of complexity of human beings, especially as they refer to their relationship with the environment.

30.3 Person-Centered Medicine (PCM)

We consider that when confronted with this panorama of complexity, the best-suited tool to face it, from the field of health, is the recently developed person-centered medicine (PCM) [8].

PCM is a holistic, multidisciplinary, and relational perspective aimed at promoting the highest attainable level of health, both for individuals and people collectively. PCM encompasses a wide range of concepts, tasks, technologies, and practices, which aim to place the whole person in context at the center and as the goal of clinical practice and public health. To this effect, PCM articulates science and humanism for a bio-psycho-socio-cultural understanding of health and for the undertaking of healthcare actions from individual interventions to general health policy [9].

PCM intends to study scientifically the complexity of health, including illness and disability as well as functioning, resilience, resources, wellbeing, and contributors to health. Absolutely necessary for such enterprise, considering human complexity, is a combination of philosophical, biological, psychological, social, and cultural approaches. Developmental and life course perspectives should also be considered with special attention to gender, age groups and vulnerable groups.

The director of the mHealth Competence Center, [10] believes that the key for the future does not lie on classifying people, but on personalizing medicine and patient attention. Technology can play a major role in achieving this scope.

30.4 Person-Centered Care

The twenty-first century is emerging as the century of person-centered care, and this perspective is especially compelling concerning chronic diseases, as articulated in the 2012 Geneva Declaration on person-centered care for chronic diseases [11]. Increased knowledge and scientific progress can be used for person-centered care. It is important to apply medical knowledge in person-centered care attending to the specificity and particularity of each person.

What we must emphasize now is that a person-centered approach to promotion and restoration of health is crucial to counteract the present massive epidemic of chronic diseases. People with chronic diseases cannot be effectively cared for without fully engaging them concerning their own health.

Consequently, we believe that bold new approaches to health promotion and illness intervention need to be developed and integrated in our health systems. Furthermore, the patient needs to remain at the heart of these approaches. Effective public health, clinical, medicinal, and technological procedures must be developed and implemented having the whole person at the core within a broad biological, psychological, and sociocultural framework.

Considering that healthcare is focused on the patient and that it is changing with technology, Dave de Bronckart, an ePatient, proposes that it is necessary for doctors and patients to work together "to create a new dynamic in which healthcare makes patients feel they are well looked after". One of my principles is: "If the microscope is happy but the patient isn't, have we achieved care?" [3, 4]. If the above are crucial for health care, they are even more needed in the case of disasters when the disruptive impacts are experienced by the whole community.

30.5 Disruption

"Disruptive situations" refer to actual external events that implode the psyche, violent eruptions in social environments that threaten the inner world. These changes turn a familiar surrounding into a threatening and alienated one, full of unknown, undetectable and omnipresent menaces, and may result in mental disorders. Perhaps the word "traumatic" should not be used to label an event or milieu. We prefer to say that a situation is disruptive and that one's experience of that disruptive situation may or may not be a traumatic one. The word "trauma" should be reserved for internal processes in this case, the breakdown of the articulation between affect and psychic representation [12–14]. We believe that, labeling a "Disruptive Situation" as "Traumatic Situation" can lead to an iatrogenic mistake.

An event is disruptive when it disorganizes or causes discontinuity, psychic deregulation, or disarticulation. The disorganization and what happens with it, does not correspond only to the event, it depends on the person who experiences it. Nevertheless, there are some types of events, for example, a cataclysm, accidents or critical illnesses, the death of a loved one, war, a terrorist attack, which are disruptive per se. However, this does not authorize mental health professionals to evaluate the events a priori and much less to make generalizations. The following qualities increase the chances for an event to be a disruptive one:

- To be unexpected, e.g., the explosion of a bomb, a meeting with someone important that we thought we would never see again;
- To interrupt a normal process, essential for our existence, e.g., being kidnapped or losing one's job;
- To undermine the confidence feeling in others, e.g., suffering a sexual assault or betrayal of an old friend;
- To contain innovative features, not coded or understandable according to the parameters that culture offers, as when we move to a country with customs and beliefs completely different from ours and opposite to our values;
- To be a threat to our own physical integrity, or of significant others, and
- To distort or destroy the daily habitat.

The quality and intensity of the impact will be identified after the event has occurred, observing and analyzing the reactions of every person.

At present, new expressions of human suffering, resulting from disruptive social and political environments, compel us to reexamine what we think we know. They put to test established classifications (e.g., DSM; ICD) and the ones related to disasters, stress and trauma, that not always take into account the individual and cultural elements or the peculiarities and characteristics of each event. The impact of a rape is not similar to the shock of a bomb explosion next to a group of people. It is important to consider these kinds of situations besides person-centered medicine.

It is a risk that medical classifications are based exclusively on symptoms and are oriented to the diagnosis of individual cases without incorporating social elements in an important way, as well as stress and trauma [15].

As mental health professionals, we must face a new situation that forces us not only to reconsider the understanding of how disruptive events affect the individual but, also, to develop new intervention techniques that combine inputs from many disciplines. Populations like children, pregnant women, handicapped, old persons need special intervention techniques. Different religions and cultural outlooks must also be taken in consideration [1].

30.6 Trauma

Mental health professionals frequently use the word 'trauma' to refer to a painful situation experienced by a person. They refer to the situation itself as "traumatic," failing to consider that it is the psychological aftermath of the painful situation that should be defined as trauma. We should make a distinction and characterize the different elements that are components of this complex situation: the distinctiveness of the event that comes from outside, the type of impact that the psyche suffers and the resources and lack of recourses of the person to face this complex circumstance.

Without this differentiation, which allows us to develop specific concepts for each of these elements and its characteristics, it is not possible to have an appropriate diagnosis and a treatment strategy. Without it, the word "trauma" is not capable of designating a specific phenomenon with its own characteristics differentiating it from other similar phenomena.

The concept "traumatic situation" is commonly used to refer to accidents, death of a loved one, serious disease, sudden disability, the birth of a sibling, economic breakdown, and other similar situations. It is also used to characterize disasters and catastrophes as natural cataclysms and wars or forced migrations.

A necessary step that will allow us to advance in this sense is the concept of 'disruption'. It is recommended to use the word 'disruptive' instead of "traumatic" whenever we speak about the events and the situations that take place in the external world, any event, or situation with the potential of causing reactions that change capacity for integration.

Presently, posttraumatic stress disorder (PTSD) is known as one of the most used and abused concepts in mental health and one of the most "misused" concepts. A. Shalev has reported that the co morbidity is 88.3 % in men and 79.0 % in women. There is lack of accuracy in the diagnosis of this condition.

Throughout wars and disasters, the symptomatology is diverse [16, 17]. In five different wars within the same period, there were several symptoms. Cultural and social factors lead to different reactions, such as in Malvinas' War [18], Asian Tsunami [13, 14], Athens earthquake [19]. Standardization of symptoms ignores social, economic and political impacts.

PTSD is only related to stress, missing a wide range of disorders, especially depression. This diagnostic category leaves aside the concept of "Psychic Trauma," which allows us to approach deeply the psychic processing, in the psychotherapeutic field.

The concept of "Impact by Disruption" includes a broad range of manifestations: stress, anxiety, depression, confusion, bewilderment, panic, and so on. This is important for psychopharmacological and psychotherapeutic therapies.

PTSD determines, in all cases, that the event causes psychic disorders, without considering which are its characteristics and outcome. The main problem is that the regulating authorities and medical services recognize only the diagnosis of PTSD as the psychological aftermath of the person that experienced disruptive situations, without considering the broad spectrum and the idiosyncrasy of each psychologically damaged person. One of the main dangers is that this diagnosis facilitates a process of victimization. The person often gets trapped into a self-image of victim. The psychological profile of victim includes a pervasive sense of helplessness, passivity, loss of control, pessimism, negative thinking, strong feelings of guilt, shame, self-blame, and depression. This way of thinking can lead to hopelessness and despair.

Another condition related to victimization is the long ago known and too quickly forgotten concept of "Compensation Neurosis." There has been great debate concerning the existence and meaning of compensation neurosis. It is included in the International Classification of Diseases (ICD-9 and ICD-10) but not listed in the Diagnostic and Statistical Manual of Mental Disorders, Fourth Edition, Text Revision (DSM-IV-TR). It is necessary to consider its utility as a diagnostic entity for forensic evaluations and its components as they relate to exaggeration in injury claims. It is also important to discuss how compensation neurosis differs from malingering and factitious disorder. The more modern definition of the condition is seen in the 1946 quote from Foster Kennedy that "compensation neurosis is a state of mind, born out of fear, kept alive by avarice, stimulated by lawyers, and cured by a verdict" [20].

The popularity of the diagnosis was also affected by new disease categories and diagnoses that have been introduced in the Diagnostic and Statistical Manual of Mental Disorders, Third Edition (DSM-III) and Fourth Edition (DSM-IV). Individuals who might have received a diagnosis of compensation neurosis in the past, in some cases now are erroneously subsumed into the categories of PTSD [21].

The use of "Disruptive Impacts" as a nosological entity tries to avoid victimization [15]. Its preestablished symptoms define the person in a pathological state.

In case that we diagnose a disorder, we should determine its characteristics, such as depression by disruption, anxiety by disruption, stress by disruption.

The use of "Disruptive Impacts" proposes not only a PTSD symptoms review, as we conducted in DSM-5, but also a review of the ways of using this concept in therapy and the possibilities of reconceptualizing it.

30.7 Economic Disasters

In the case of economic disasters, like the ones associated with the current economic crisis, the effects of the associated disruptive events are diverse and have been reported in detail elsewhere [22, 23]. Depression is perhaps the most frequently occurring consequence. We should, however, differentiate between depression (a psychopathological reaction) and normal sadness (an adaptive reaction) [24].

30.8 Victim and Victimization

We want to propose a specific use of the concepts of victim and victimization. Generally, both concepts are used for all the people that suffered terrorist attacks, wars, rape, and other situations that we label as "disruptive situations."

Since the start of civilization, the "victims" are needed by societies because: (1) they are used to maintain the social memory of certain events, (2) expiate the individual and social guilt, (3) relieve the distress that the presence of the evil causes while they allow to consider the evil in the "victimizer" and/or (4) retain the group identities. Often the individuals gather together for a "common reason" or "political flag." "Loving each other is having a common enemy."

In order to maintain the historical memory of disruptive events that affect individuals, community groups, or specific populations, societies need to perpetuate the event in their memory, developing special mechanisms to be able to achieve this. For example, one of the mechanisms that are used is related to those who were damaged. They are asked to tell again and again what happened, as if it could be shared and thus sooth the pain. This is one of the techniques used by some to avoid the repetition of such kinds of disruptive events.

Paradigmatic cases are the survivors of the Nazi genocide, the "living museums." Their function is to avoid the denial of what happened in the Second World War. The real victims are those who are dead, and it is a personal and social function to sustain their memories. Different articles recognize the importance of rejection of the use of the term "victims", proposing the use of the word "survivors," but not all survivors are damaged people. That is why we prefer to use the term "damaged people" to emphasize the suffering of survivors, not to diminish it.

It is important to understand that the disruptive impact in many cases changes into internal fights, disagreements, antagonism, and jealousy.

Victimization is one of the most dangerous psychological problems, product of "disruptive situations" because it encourages the development of symptomatology.

Not every person lends him/herself to the process of "victimization," but it is not easy to resist. What is needed is a vulnerable person that has been damaged, or another person that has the qualities of a leader or hero. We see the tendency to become heroes in some cases as a special vulnerability. The more this person is "victimized," the more he loses his identity and the more he acquires the identity associated with the damage. He acquires an identity according to the event and not according to his own subjective development.

The identity of a "victim" does not belong to the person. It is a social position defined in every culture or society according to the prevailing values. People cannot become victims without the interaction with society needs.

One of the functions of victimization is to strengthen the links between people of the community. This phenomenon, as old as mythology, in some cases, appears when the tendency is to develop confrontations between different groups of society. The place of the victim creates respect, and this person becomes a central symbol in the society, acquiring special rights. This sounds as a very human attitude on one hand, but on the other hand it is a way of generating secondary gains that can promote dependence and psychic pathology.

Therefore, the "victim" is not the product of the actual damage he suffered, but a product of the social process of "victimization," that involves assigning the status of "victim" to persons who have suffered damage. The damage is considered by the group as an attack on any value that the group wishes to preserve or impose.

The most frequent psychological mechanisms that take place during the process of "victimization" are projection and overidentification with the people who have suffered the type of damage that the group does not accept with impunity. By these mechanisms, the members of the group seek unconsciously to neutralize or to get rid of the guilt. We emphasize that for mental health professionals who work in the area of "disruptive situations" it is crucial to be aware of this process.

With regard to the assistance work and treatment for damaged people, especially in the mental health field, it is necessary to be aware of the risks of projection mechanisms, as well as those of overidentification induced by strong feelings of empathy.

The above apply in cases where it is very difficult to take distance from the event, and in this way the imaginary guilt is reinforced.

From the "victimized" side, the process of those who suffered damage is usually as follows: until the event, the "victimized" saw himself as a normal person who could work, love, play and have friends. From the moment that he suffered the psychic damage, these abilities are affected and he begins to suffer. From his understanding of what happened, his suffering was caused by the external world: something came from outside and harmed him. As a compensation mechanism, the "victimization" turns out to be unsuccessful.

This is not what happens in other psychological suffering, in which the person feels that the source of suffering is within oneself. The big difference with other conditions is that the damage is perceived as having been caused by the environment. Knowing that the damage came from the external world enables damaged people to claim that either one who inflicted the damage or the one who should have avoided it (a group or society in general) should repair, compensate or at least relieve their suffering.

This reaction turns on the responsibility of society, with which the imaginary guilt is associated because it is a witness of the damage. An example of this is the compensation mechanism, in which society is held responsible for all the damages suffered by its members that have been inflicted to the people that society is supposed to protect. The society should not avoid responsibility, they have to face these situations but we only stress the risks, and we propose to rethink the ways in which compensations are given.

Another aspect that we consider relevant, is to point out that when benefits, facilities, or special compensation are conferred to the injured people, society is providing them with the possibility to take advantage of the secondary gain produced by being considered as a "victim." In this way, we encourage the damaged people to crystallize themselves in that role for the rest of their lives, to fit to this definition of "victim" and leave aside the possibility of living a normal life. This is what makes the decisions about giving and accepting compensation so complex.

30.9 Injured Person and Victims

As mentioned earlier, we propose to drop the term "victim" for those who have suffered psychological damage and replace it by "injured person." The use of this term does not minimize the intensity of suffering. We consider that the word "victim" undermines the subjectivity of each person because it ignores its uniqueness and misplaces the issue in a social function to preserve collective memory.

Injured person and victim are usually used as synonyms, but it is necessary to make a subtle but vital distinction. The personal pain is what determines the condition of a damaged person, unlike the victims and victimizers that represent a social result.

There is no present or future for the victim as this person remains frozen in an unrepairable past. The victim is someone who assimilates a preestablished identity constructed by others. The present only exists for the injured people and so does the future. The injured person has a future; the victim does not have one [13].

The paradoxical and upsetting aspect is that we, mental health professionals, as part of a potentially threatened society, often become victimizers because of our own needs and the omnipotent positions in which we are often placed. The victimization tries to be a repair act of the chaotic and the unthinkable, but the emptiness increases further with it. Yet, the therapeutic role should be to help the individual face its specific condition as a person.

In summary it is appropriate to use the concept "injured person," instead of "survivor," someone who suffers injuries caused by a disaster—physical, material, psychic, or social damages. We prefer to reserve the word victim only for those who have lost their lives, for those whose retention of memory relies on the loved ones that have been affected by the victim's death.

30.10 Conclusions

Mental health professionals' responses to the needs of people after wars, disasters or daily life accidents, should be based on an understanding of the complexity of the relevant psychic reactions. It is useful to take into consideration the PCM perspective that places the whole person at the center of healthcare, and person-centered care, which is needed for healthcare and then, more importantly, to face the mental health impact of disasters.

Regarding key concepts, it is appropriate to say that a situation is "disruptive," instead of traumatic. The experience could be a traumatic one or not and "trauma" should be used when it refers to the internal processes. "Disruption" encourages researching the situations and the impact they have on each particular person. Calling an event "traumatic" a priori assumes the existence of a psychic pathology. The concept of "impact by disruption" includes many conditions, like stress, anxiety, depression, confusion, among others, and not solely PTSD.

One of the most dangerous psychological problems is victimization, because it is a way of encouraging loss of identity and development of symptomatology. A vulnerable person, leader of heroes, has been damaged. The more this person is "victimized", the more he loses his identity and the more he acquires an identity associated with the injury, the more he is "victimized." He gets an identity according to the event and not based on his own subjective development.

Therefore, we propose to drop the word "victim" to refer to those who suffered psychological damage and replace it by "injured person." It may be helpful to use the term "injured person," referring to "survivor" and the word "victim" only for those who have lost their lives.

Health professionals should take into account the specificities of each individual (person-centered approach) but also the contextual characteristics of an event, using them in an appropriate way for a proper diagnosis and treatment. A great deal of effort is needed to face a very complex situation such as the mental health impact of disasters.

References

1. Benyakar M, Collazo CR, Cohen R. Disasters: a new mental health challenge. In: Proceedings of the WPA Regional Congress, March 12–15; Athens, Greece: WPA Athens Regional and Intersectional Congress, 2005.
2. Morin E. Introduction à la pensée complexe. Paris: ESF Editeur; 1990.

3. Bau T: Interview with Yunkap Kwankam: world renowned ehealth and mhealth consultant. Retrieved from http://www.mobilehealthglobal.com/in-the-news/interviews/42/interview-with-yunkap-kwankam (2014).
4. Bau T: Epatients: Changing healthcare with technology. Retrieved from http://www.mobilehealthglobal.com/in-the-news/news/107/epatients-changing-healthcare-with-technology (2014).
5. MacLean PD. The triune brain. In: Smith FQ editor. Neurosci Second Stud Program. New York: Rockefeller University Press; 1970.
6. Damasio A. Descartes' error: emotion, reason and the human brain. New York: A Grassel/Putman Book; 1994.
7. Morin E. Les sept savoirs necessaires a l'education du future. United nations educational, scientific and cultural organization—7 place Fontenoy—75352 Paris 07 SP—France, UNESCO, 1999.
8. Mezzich JE, Snaedal J, van Weel C, Heath I. Toward person-centered medicine: from disease to patient to person. Mt Sinai J Med. 2010;77:304–6.
9. Salvador-Carulla L, Cloninger CR, Thornicroft A, Mezzich JE. 2013 Geneva declaration consultation group: background, structure and priorities of the 2013 Geneva declaration on person-centered health research. Int J Person Cent Med. 2013;3:109–13.
10. Cornet Prat J. Healthy ageing: a utopia or an opportunity for new technologies? Retrieved from http://www.mobilehealthglobal.com/in-the-news/articles/31/healthy-ageing-a-utopia-or-an-opportunity-for-new-technologies. Accessed on 06 Oct 2014.
11. International College of Person Centered Medicine. Geneva declaration on person centered care for chronic diseases. Int J Person Cent Med. 2012;2:153–4.
12. Benyakar M, Collazo CR, de Rosa E. Anxiety by disruption http://www.psiquiatria.com 2002.
13. Benyakar M, Knafo D. Disruptive: individual and collective threats. In D. Knafo, editor. Living with terror, working with trauma: a clinician's handbook. New York: Jason Aronson; 2004. p. 605.
14. Benyakar M. Five wars, five traumas: experience and insight from clinical work in Israel's trenches. In D. Knafo, editor. Living with terror, working with trauma: a clinician's handbook. New York: Jason Aronson; 2004. p. 605.
15. Lopez Ibor JJ. The psycho(patho)logy of disasters. In: Proceedings of the 12th world congress of psychiatry. Yokohama, Japan; 2002.
16. Crocq L, Doutheau C, Louville P, Cremnitter D. Psychiatrie de catastrophe. Réactions immédiates et différées, troubles séquellaires, paniques et psychopathologie collective. Encycl Med Chir Psychiatrie, 1988;37–113-D10, 8p.
17. Crocq L. Les Traumatismes Psychiques de Guerre. Paris: Edit. Odile Jacob; 1999.
18. Collazo C. Psychiatric casualties in Malvina's War. a provisional report. In: Pichot P, Berner P, Wolf R, Thau K, editors. Psychiatry: the state of the Art. New York: Plenum Press; 1985.
19. Christodoulou GN, Paparrigopoulos TJ, Soldatos CR. The experience of the Athens earthquake. In: Lopez-Ibor JJ, Christodoulou G, Maj M, Sartorius N, Okasha A, editors. Disasters and mental health, New York: Wiley, World Psychiatric Association; 2004. pp 145–50.
20. Kennedy F. The mind of the injured worker: its effects on disability periods. Compens Med. 1946;1:19–21.
21. Hall RCW, Hall RCW. Compensation neurosis. a too quickly forgotten concept? J Am Acad Psychiatry Law. 2012;40(3):390–8.
22. Christodoulou GN, Anagnostopoulos DC, Christodoulou NG, Tsipas V. The economic disaster in Europe: psychological and psychopathological consequences. Eur Psychiatry; 2013. 28 (suppl. 1, 1).

23. Christodoulou NG, Christodoulou GN. Financial crises: impact on mental health and suggested responses. Psychother Psychosom. 2013;82:279–84.
24. Christodoulou GN, Christodoulou NG. The financial crisis and its impact on mental health. Psychiatriki. 2013;24:95–8.

Personality Disorders

31

C. Robert Cloninger, MD, PhD, Dragan M. Svrakic, MD, PhD,
Nigel C. Lester, MD, Dusica Lecic-Tosevski, MD, PhD,
Nestor Koldobsky, MD and Michel Botbol, MD

31.1 Why Are Personality Disorders Important?

The assessment and treatment of personality and its disorders is a core feature of person-centered medicine (PCM) for several interrelated reasons [14]. First, recognition of the personality of another person helps to *establish an effective working alliance* because everyone likes to be known as a person with unique interests, motivation, and values, rather than being reduced to a categorical diagnosis

C.R. Cloninger, MD, PhD (✉)
Wallace Renard Professor of Psychiatry, Washington University School of Medicine,
660 South Euclid, Campus, Box 8134, St. Louis, MO 63110, USA
e-mail: clon@wustl.edu

D.M. Svrakic, MD, PhD
Professor of Psychiatry, Washington University School of Medicine, St. Louis, MO, USA
e-mail: svrakicd@wustl.edu

D. Lecic-Tosevski, MD, PhD
Professor of Psychiatry and Director, Institute of Mental Health, University of Belgrade,
Belgrade, Serbia
e-mail: dusica.lecictosevski@eunet.rs; dusica.lecictosevski@gmail.com

N. Koldobsky, MD
Professor of Psychiatry, Universidad de La Plata, La Plata, Argentina
e-mail: koldobsky@speedy.com.ar

M. Botbol, MD
Professor of Child and Adolescent Psychiatry, University Western Brittany, Brest, France
e-mail: botbolmichel@orange.fr

N.C. Lester, MD
Clinical Researcher and Instructor of Psychiatry, Washington University School of Medicine,
St. Louis, MO, USA
e-mail: lestern@wustl.edu

J.E. Mezzich et al. (eds.), *Person Centered Psychiatry*,
DOI 10.1007/978-3-319-39724-5_31

or a chief complaint about a particular organ or function. Put in a broader historical and cultural context, we see that medicine has more often adopted a whole person approach (from the Ancients to the Renaissance) and that the fragmented view of the individual is a more a recent interlude paralleling the modern industrial era.

Second, assessment of personality stimulates greater self-awareness so that people can begin to better recognize the connections between their lifestyle and their health status, thereby *promoting greater capacity for self-regulation* that will help to reduce their suffering and improve their well-being. Self-regulation, as opposed to external regulation, is the driver of sustained positive change. In order to understand and appreciate another person's health status, it is essential to know as much as possible about their personality and lifestyle behavior. Third, greater self-awareness of the impact of personality and related lifestyle activities is crucial for health promotion to prevent acute and chronic diseases from emerging before a person becomes symptomatic. Clinicians are today aware that modern medicine, so often limited to end-stage symptoms management, is increasingly recognized as an unsustainable approach to human suffering. The actual causes of most morbidity and mortality are directly related to personality and lifestyle, so greater self-regulation is essential for reducing the burden of disease and improving well-being [2, 23]. Personality disorder (PD) is the primary psychiatric illness observed in most patients with psychosocial complaints. PD is present in about one-sixth of people in the general population and in most primary care or psychiatric patients [17]. People with PDs have poor self-esteem, reduced ability to work and to love, and frequent stress responses that lead them to seek medical treatment.

In addition to generating chronic personal suffering and/or substantial social or professional consequences, PDs predispose an individual to other mental disorders, including substance abuse, mood and anxiety disorders, eating disorders, somatoform and dissociative disorders, and psychoses [19]. The complex dynamic interactions of personality are often at the root of this comorbidity that is observed across the full spectrum of psychiatric illness. Unless the underlying personality features are assessed and treated, little improvement in the comorbid disorders is likely, certainly not in a sustained way. Furthermore, PDs or extreme personality traits interfere with cooperation with prescribed treatments and outcome. Without an informed awareness of personality, the therapist runs the risk as being perceived by the patient as lacking authenticity. Consequently, effectiveness of any medical treatment is greatly impaired unless there is thorough assessment and treatment of personality and its disorders in clinical practice, as is amply demonstrated by the marked burden of chronic disease in Western societies [11, 12].

Consequently, a solid conceptual understanding and classification are critical to deal with these prevalent and chronic disorders with sensitivity and efficiency. Yet, current systems for classification of PDs have serious practical and theoretical limitations [13, 35]. The concept of PDs as sharply delineated categories, as described in the current classifications of the American Psychiatric Association and the World Health Organization, is both imprecise and clinically impractical. The categorical criteria for these disorders overlap and many individuals usually meet criteria for more than one diagnosis. In fact the most common PD diagnosis in

DSM-IV was the residual category of PD "not otherwise specified," which is used to designate cases that do not fit any one category well. Such findings raised serious questions about the validity and utility of categorical personality diagnoses.

In DSM-5 an effort was made to develop a system that could combine aspects of both dimensional and categorical features. Research has consistently shown that the boundaries between mental disorders are not sharply defined, and yet DSM persists in delineating many overlapping disorders while warning clinicians not to reify these diagnoses.

The criteria proposed by the DSM-5 working group on PD were not accepted because the APA's Scientific Review Board regarded the scientific evidence as insufficient for the major changes proposed and the APA's Clinical and Public Health Review Board regarded the criteria as too unwieldy for routine clinical use. As a result, the DSM-IV criteria for PDs were retained for official use in DSM-5, but the criteria proposed by the working group were listed as "alternative criteria" for research and clinical consideration. Reference to DSM criteria for PDs in this chapter indicates the current official criteria, which are the same in DSM-IV and DSM-5. The alternative DSM-5 criteria will also be briefly described so that the reader can appreciate the shortcomings of current criteria that the alternative criteria attempt to address, as well as how the alternative criteria are related to the more coherent approach described herein. Fortunately, scientific research allows a coherent and clinically practical approach to the assessment and treatment of personality and its disorders that transcends the limitations of current official classifications in its utility for understanding etiology, development, and treatment [7, 8, 11–13].

31.2 What Is Personality?

People differ markedly from one another in their outlook on life, in the way they interpret their experiences, and in their emotional and behavioral responses to those experiences. These differences in outlook, thoughts, emotions, and actions are what characterize an individual's personality. More generally, personality can be defined as the dynamic organization within the individual of the psychobiological systems that modulate his or her unique adaptations to a changing internal and external environment [18]. Each part of this definition is important for a clinician to appreciate. Personality is "dynamic," meaning that it is constantly changing and adapting in response to experience, rather than being a set of fixed traits. Inflexibility of personality is actually an indicator of PD. Personality is regulated by "psychobiological" systems, meaning that personality is influenced by both biological and psychological variables. Consequently treatment of PDs requires growth in psychological self-understanding and not just treatment with medications, although these can be helpful adjuncts to therapy [27]. These systems involve interactions among many internal and processes, so each person's pattern of adjustment is "unique" to them, even though they follow general rules and principles of development as complex adaptive systems [8]. Finally, to understand personality and its development we must pay attention to both the "internal" and "external" processes by which an individual interacts with and adapts to their own internal milieu and external situation. For example, when a person is under stress, they are likely to think and feel differently about themselves and other people. On the other hand, when they are calm and encouraged, they may act more maturely and happily. Everyone has personal sensitivities or "rough spots" that surface when they are under stress. Everyone has "good days" and "bad days," and this pattern of variability over time is what characterizes a person's personality. As the stressors faced in modern life grow in complexity and intensity, clinicians increasingly observe the emergence of unhealthy and maladaptive patterns in their patients.

31.3 What Is a Personality Disorder?

The diagnosis of PD requires that the patients have a maladaptive pattern of responses to personal and social stress that is stable and enduring since early adulthood, inflexible, and pervasive. These response patterns lead to chronic and pervasive impairments in their ability to work and to cooperate with others. For example, they may have problems with perfectionism or underachievement, and excessive dependency or social detachment. In addition, most patients with PD consistently have low self-esteem and handle stress poorly. The resulting subjective distress often leads them to complain about anxiety, depression, and worries about physical health. Many patients with PDs have problems with impulse control, such as being too impulsive or too rigid. They also have problems in the way they perceive and interpret themselves, other people, and events, such as cognitive deficits in empathy, tendencies to blame others, and tendencies to be suspicious of others' intentions. Lastly, these patients have difficulty in maintaining healthy lifestyle choices about their diet and personal activities, such as drinking, smoking, and exercise. Consequently, personality and its disorders influence both objective and subjective aspects of physical health. In summary, the abnormal outlook on life that is characteristic of PD leads to impairment in emotional regulation, impulse control, human relationships, cognition, and physical health.

Individuals with PD typically blame other people or external circumstances for their own physical, psychological, or social problems. Their externalizing of responsibility is a result of two characteristics of PDs to which all clinicians must be alert. First, these patients provoke strong emotional reactions from others but do not recognize the abnormality of their own attitudes, thoughts, and feelings. Second, they try to change others, instead of changing themselves. Both these features reflect an effort to reduce their distress and improve their perceived quality of life, but unfortunately in ways that actually impair their health in the long-run [8, 17],

The diagnosis of PD can be made accurately with little time or expense once their essential features are learned so that they can be recognized and understood. Recognizing the personality issues underlying somatic and psychosomatic complaints improves treatment efficiency and outcomes. Both the physician and patient need to understand that personality predisposes to objective diseases in all organ systems, and not only to functional psychosomatic complaints [28]. The impact of personality is observed at the root of many illnesses, operating through more-or less direct and indirect mechanisms.

Clinical Features of PDs: Current descriptive criteria that are diagnostic of a PD according to the American Psychiatric Association are summarized in Table 31.1.

As shown in Table 31.1, the maladaptive behavior patterns must be "stable and enduring," that is, very long term if not lifelong characteristics. The DSM criteria require that the maladaptive pattern be "of long duration and its onset can be traced back at least to adolescence or early adulthood." In practice, it can be difficult to distinguish long-term maladaptation typical of PD and chronic personality changes caused by other mental disorders (such as chronic depression) or long-term situational factors (such as financial dependency on one's spouse). Second, the maladaptive pattern must be inflexible and pervasive, that is, manifest in a wide range of personal and social contexts (i.e., at home, at work, with family, and friends), not only in isolated aspects of the person's life. Finally, there must be substantial evidence of subjective distress, impaired social and occupational function, or both. Subjective distress refers to low self-esteem and limited problem-solving skills, which often lead to anxiety, depression, and somatic complaints. The social and occupational impairments in people with PD result from their immature perspective on life, which is manifest as deficits in self-awareness and character development. More simply, individuals with PDs lack mature goals and values.

In addition to these consistent features of all PDs, there is much variation in specific styles of thinking, feeling, and relating. The Diagnostic and Statistical Manual of Mental Disorders (DSM), published by the American Psychiatric Association, distinguishes three clusters of PD (odd, dramatic, and anxious), but features of more than one cluster frequently occur in the same patient. Furthermore, each cluster is subdivided into discrete subtypes of PD (see Table 31.2), but most patients with PD have features of more than one subtype (e.g., narcissistic, histrionic, and antisocial symptoms usually occur together).

Table 31.1 Qualitative description of personality disorders

Discriminating features
A maladaptive pattern of responses to personal and social stress that is – Stable and enduring since teens – Inflexible and pervasive – Causing subjective distress and/or – Impaired work and/or social relations
Consistent features
Strong emotional reactions elicited from others (like anger or urge to rescue) Efforts to blame and change others, rather than oneself
Variable features
– Odd, eccentric – Erratic, impulsive – Anxious, fearful

Table 31.2 Qualitative clusters and subtypes of personality disorders according to the current official criteria of the American Psychiatric Association (DSM-IV, 1994 and DSM-5, 2014)

Cluster	Subtype	Discriminating features
Odd/eccentric	Schizoid	Socially indifferent
	Paranoid	Suspicious
	Schizotypal	Eccentric
Erratic/impulsive	Antisocial	Disagreeable
	Borderline	Unstable
	Histrionic	Attention-seeking
	Narcissistic	Self-centered
Anxious/fearful	Avoidant	Inhibited
	Dependent	Submissive
	Obsessive	Perfectionistic
Not otherwise specified	Passive-aggressive	Negativistic
	Depressive	Pessimistic

In contrast to the current official criteria for diagnosis of PDs in DSM-IV and DSM-5, DSM-5 also allows consideration of alternative criteria for assessment of personality functioning and pathological personality traits. The alternative assessment is comprised of three components that were developed separately and are not really coherently related to one another. The three components of the alternative assessment approach are a reduced list of specific categories, a description of healthy personality, and a list of five pathological traits like those derived by factor analysis [1], as summarized in Table 31.3.

The alternative criteria for PD in DSM-5 only consider the diagnosis of a reduced set of categories: antisocial, avoidant, borderline, narcissistic, obsessive-compulsive, and schizotypal PDs, even though there is extensive scientific support for other

Table 31.3 Alternative assessment of personality functioning and pathological traits (DSM-5, 2014)

Component of assessment	Elements to be assessed	Descriptors
Personality functioning	Functioning of self	Identity (self-esteem, sense of uniqueness with boundaries) Self-direction (rational goal-setting)
	Interpersonal functioning	Empathy Intimacy
Pathological traits	Negative affectivity	Negative emotions, like anxiety, depression, anger
	Detachment	Avoidance or withdrawal from intimate relationships
	Antagonism	Hostility, self-importance
	Disinhibition	Impulsive self-gratification
	Psychoticism	Odd or eccentric thoughts and behavior

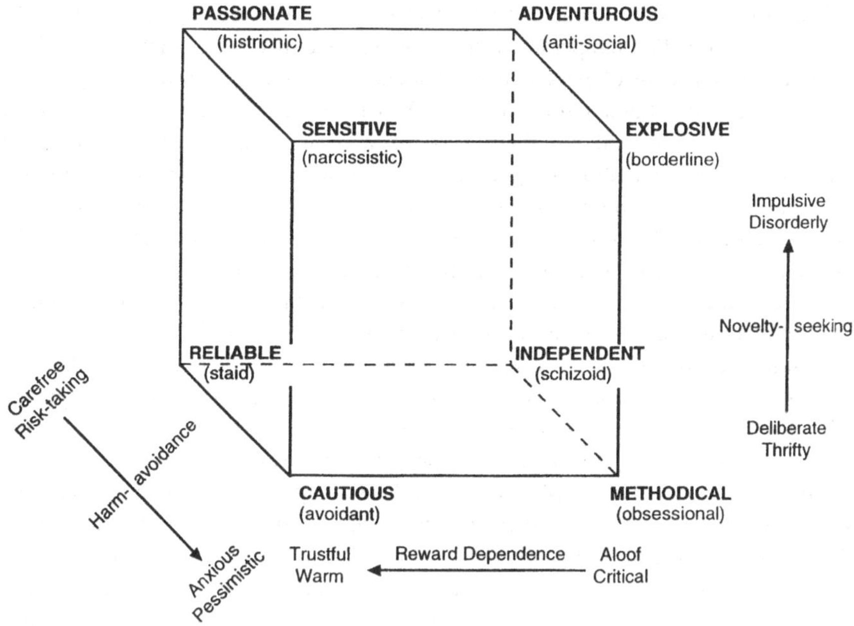

Fig. 31.1 Cube articulating personality dimensions and personality features

disorders, such as histrionic PD. Any system of profiles emerging from 3 to 7 underlying dimensions would require recognition of other syndromes, as illustrated in Fig. 31.1. However, the categories in the alternative DSM-5 approach were not systematically derived from the set of five pathological traits delineated in DSM-5, as is done in the psychobiological model of personality. Likewise, healthy personality functioning did not represent the healthy poles of the pathological personality traits. In fact, the description of healthy personality included descriptors closely related to Self-directedness and Cooperativeness. Self-directedness is not the healthy pole of negative affectivity because negative affectivity includes low self-directedness combined with high harm avoidance.

As a result of these limitations and internal inconsistencies, the alternative criteria provide an approach to diagnosis that was judged by the APA to be inadequately supported by scientific data and too unwieldy for clinical practice.

31.4 Deconstructing the Components of Personality and Its Disorders

Qualitative terms like "inflexible" and "enduring" require subjective judgments and produce little precision in the diagnosis of PD in general. Fortunately, quantifiable components of personality have been identified that allow the differential diagnosis of PDs [6, 7, 11, 12]. The features that distinguish people with any PD from those with no PD are called character traits. The features that differentiate among subtypes of PD are called temperament traits. More generally, temperament is defined as the emotional core of personality. Character is defined in terms of a person's goals, values, and human relationships. A person's character is based on their outlook on life, which allows them to regulate conflicts among the temperament dimensions. The regulation of emotional drives allows a person to accomplish meaningful goals and to maintain human relationships in accordance with his or her values and needs. Hence the harmonious integration of personality depends on the coherence of character, not on the temperament configuration.

Three dimensions of character have been distinguished: self-directedness, cooperativeness, and self-transcendence. Self-directed people are responsible, purposeful, resourceful, self-accepting, and dutiful, whereas others are blaming, aimless, helpless, vain, and insecure. Cooperative people are tolerant, empathic, helpful, compassionate, and principled, whereas uncooperative people are prejudiced, uncaring, selfish, revengeful, and opportunistic. Self-transcendent people are intuitive, idealistic, contemplative, faithful, and spiritual, whereas others are self-conscious, pragmatic, judgmental, cynical, and skeptical. Each of these aspects of character are crucial for healthy adaptation to life under current world conditions in which ego-centric behavior is threatening to produce mass extinction [11, 12].

It has been repeatedly demonstrated that poorly developed character traits, especially self-directedness, increase the risk for PD substantially [7]. Indeed, most individuals with PD have difficulty accepting responsibility, setting long-term goals, accepting their own limitations, and/or overcoming obstacles they encounter in life. Usually, but not always, they are also uncooperative, i.e., they tend to be intolerant of others, insensitive to other people's feelings, selfish, have difficulty trusting and confiding in other people, and are often hostile and revengeful when others disappoint them, but are quick to take advantage of others in an unprincipled manner when the opportunity arises.

High self-directedness is not always protective against PD. Some narcissistic and antisocial persons may appear to be highly self-directed, i.e., quite resourceful and purposeful and thus successful in pursuing their narcissistic or antisocial goals. Recent genetic research indicates that their reports of self-directedness are an expression of their egotism so their low self-acceptance serves to distinguish it from health-promoting forms of Self-directedness. Their very low cooperativeness (e.g., intolerance of others, low empathy) and low self-transcendence (e.g., lack of generosity and other virtues) may so interfere with social relations that they have a PD.

While low character traits represent the core features determining the presence or absence of PD, other quantifiable traits are used for differential diagnosis of the DSM clusters (eccentric, dramatic, anxious) and discrete subtypes of PD. The different clusters of PD are distinguished by differences in basic emotions regulated by the temperament dimensions. Four dimensions of temperament have been identified, and are labeled novelty seeking, harm avoidance, reward dependence, and persistence. Individuals high in novelty seeking are impulsive, quick-tempered, extravagant, and dislike rules, as is characteristic of antisocial, histrionic, and other erratic PDs. Individuals high in harm avoidance are anxious, fearful, shy, and fatigable, as is characteristic of avoidant and other anxious PDs. Individuals low in reward dependence are socially indifferent, aloof, cold, and independent, as is characteristic of schizoid and other odd PDs. Individuals who are high in persistence, such as some mature and some obsessional patients, are industrious and persevering, whereas those who are low in persistence are easily discouraged. Factor analyses have repeatedly supported the validity of the above three DSM clusters of PD (i.e., eccentric/odd, anxious/fearful, erratic/dramatic) except that symptoms for compulsive PD tend to load separately from other PDs thus forming a fourth cluster [25]. The fourth temperament dimension, Persistence, has been shown to correlate with symptoms for obsessive-compulsive PD.

In ICD-11 four groups of patients that correspond closely to individuals extreme in these four temperaments are being considered for simpler categorization of personality difficulties and disorders [32]. In the ICD-11 classification of personality variation, the main distinction is a severity rating of personality dysfunction ranging from no PD to personality difficulty and mild, moderate, and severe PD [31]. Personality difficulty is not a disorder but its use would allow recognition of such dysfunction as a target for intervention. The severity rating of personality dysfunction is then further qualified by description of four domain traits that describe what personality features are most prominent in the person. These four domain traits correspond to the four temperaments: negative affective traits (i.e., anxiety-prone as in high Harm Avoidance), dissocial (i.e., impulsive as in high Novelty Seeking), detached (i.e., aloof as in low-Reward Dependence), and anankastic (i.e., obsessional as in high Persistence). Peter Tyrer, the head of the ICD-11 committee on PDs, has argued that the DSM-IV criteria were unrealistic scientifically because they tried to specify sharp boundaries between categories that are better described on a continuum of severity. He has pointed out that DSM-IV criteria were also unpopular in practice for clinicians for the essentially the same reason—they had too many categories that frequently overlapped. Tyrer noted that DSM-5 has failed to address effectively either the scientific or the practical problem of many categories for PD. In fact, DSM-5 alternative criteria were rejected by the leadership of DSM-5 itself and the alternative criteria were listed for possible consideration by clinicians, but made the criteria even more unwieldly and impractical for use. He has called on psychiatrists worldwide to adopt the ICD-11 criteria in place of DSM-5 because he feels the ICD-11 approach will destigmatize the diagnosis and encourage clinical intervention by emphasizing severity of dysfunction over falsely reified categorical distinctions [31]. Fortunately, the psychobiological model of personality and its disorders is scientifically well-grounded and provides practical ways to rate the severity of PD in terms of its character dimensions and also allows specification of prominent features of personality profiles in terms of its temperament dimensions [13]. Multidimensional profiles of temperament and character have the diagnostic power that clinicians like about a categorical diagnosis and do not falsely reify the diagnosis as representing a homogeneous disease entity.

It is important to recognize that both DSM and ICD approaches to classification have serious deficiencies because they fail to describe the multidimensional structure of the normal and abnormal aspects of a person's personality in a systematic way. ICD rates severity and describes prominent traits, which is simple and practical but does not capture the information needed to guide treatment optimally. DSM-5 alternative criteria are a hybrid approach to categories and dimensions that are not really coherent because the categories cannot be derived from profiles of the dimensions.

To put these deficiencies in perspective, it is important to consider what temperament and character traits reveal about a person. Temperament traits regulate the primary emotions of fear (harm avoidance), anger (novelty seeking), and attachment/disgust (reward dependence). Often people with PD impress others as irrational and/or excessively emotional because their behavior and interactions are dominated by extreme temperament traits that are only weakly modulated by character traits. These patients have a rather limited spectrum of the elementary emotions to respond everything going on inside and around them. In contrast, mature people have a more complex emotional life including a broad spectrum of so-called secondary emotions, such as humility, compassion, empathy, equanimity, and patience. The likelihood of a well-adapted temperament and mature character is high when these complex emotions are prominent.

Character traits describe the maturity of a person's goals and values in ways that can be specified both in terms of severity and in terms of profiles that describe a person's style of mental self-government. Additional personality subtypes can each be distinguished by a unique combination of values on the temperament dimensions. These can all be assessed by mental status examination or by psychometric testing, as described elsewhere for the interested (http://psychobiology.wustl.edu). For example, borderline PD is characterized by high novelty seeking, high harm avoidance, and low-reward dependence. Antisocial personality has the same temperament profile except that harm avoidance is low. It is easy to remember the discriminating features of most PDs as the extremes of a cube with three dimensions defined by novelty seeking, harm avoidance, and reward dependence (see Fig. 31.1).

31.5 Stages in the Development of Self-awareness and Well-Being

A full assessment of personality requires consideration of a person's level of self-awareness and well-being, not just their impairments. Health and well-being are more than the absence of deviant traits. Well-being depends on a person's level of self-awareness and leads to the expression of human virtues and positive emotions that go beyond what is average in contemporary society [8].

There are three major stages of self-awareness along the path to well-being, as summarized in Table 31.4, based on extensive work by many people [8]. The absence of self-awareness occurs in severe PDs and psychoses in which there is

Table 31.4 Three stages of self-awareness on the path to well-being

Stage	Description	Psychological characteristics
0	Unaware	Immature, seeking immediate gratification ("child-like" ego-state)
1	Average adult cognition	Purposeful but egocentric able to delay gratification, but has frequent negative emotions (anxiety, anger, disgust) ("adult" ego-state)
2	Meta-cognition	Mature and allocentric aware of own subconscious thinking calm and patient, so able to supervise conflicts and relationships ("parental" ego-state, "mindfulness")
3	Contemplation	Effortless calm, impartial awareness wise, creative, and loving able to access what was previously unconscious as needed without effort or distress ("state of well-being," "soulfulness")

Adapted from [8]

little or no insightful awareness of the preverbal outlook or beliefs and interpretations that automatically lead to emotional drives and actions. Lacking self-awareness, people act on their immediate likes and dislikes, which is usually described as an immature or "child-like" ego-state.

The first stage of self-awareness is typical of most adults most of the time. Ordinary adult cognition involves a capacity to delay gratification in order to attain personal goals, but remains egocentric and defensive. Ordinary adult cognition is associated with frequent distress when attachments and desires are frustrated. Hence the average person can function well under good conditions, but may frequently experience problems under stress. At this stage of self-awareness, a person is able to make a choice to relax and let go of their negative emotions, thereby setting the stage for acceptance of reality and movement to higher stages of coherent understanding.

The second stage of self-aware consciousness is typical of adults when they operate like a "good parent." Good parents are allocentric in perspective—that is, they are "other-centered" and capable of calmly considering the perspective and needs of their children and other people in a balanced way that leads to satisfaction and harmony. This state is experienced when a person is able to observe his or her own subconscious thoughts and consider the thought processes of others in a similar way to observing his or her own thoughts. Hence the second stage is described as "meta-cognitive" awareness, mindfulness, or "mentalizing." The ability of the mind to observe itself allows for more flexibility in action by reducing dichotomous thinking and excessive emotional reactivity [21, 30, 34]. At this stage, a person is able to observe himself and others for understanding, without judging or blaming. However, in a mindful state people still experience the emotions that emerge from a dualistic perspective, so mindfulness is only moderately effective in improving well-being [8].

The third stage of self-awareness is called contemplation because it is direct perception of one's outlook—that is, the preverbal assumptions and schemas that direct one's attention and provide the frame that organize and bias our expectations, attitudes, and interpretation of events. Contemplation, which brings into consciousness what was unconscious, can be thought of as the opposite process as repression, which puts memories out of consciousness. Direct awareness of our outlook allows the enlarging of consciousness by accessing previously unconscious material, thereby letting go of wishful thinking, prejudicial biases, and the impartial questioning of basic assumptions and core beliefs about life, such as "I am helpless," "I am unlovable," or "faith is an illusion." For example, many modern psychiatrists are skeptical materialists who are not aware that their reductionist outlook is an extreme metaphysical assumption for which they have no test or adequate evidence, but which leads them to ignore considerations that are essential for well-being in themselves and their patients [11, 12, 24]. In the third stage of self-awareness people begin to become aware of such assumptions and biases of which they had previously been unconscious. The third stage of self-awareness can be described as "soulful" contemplation because in this state a person becomes aware of deep preverbal feelings that emerge spontaneously from a unitive and holistic perspective, such as hope, compassion, and reverence [8]. Contemplation is much more powerful in transforming personality than is mindfulness, which often fails to transform a person's unconscious outlook on life or to reduce feelings of hopelessness [22].

Extensive empirical work has shown that movement through these stages of development can be described and quantified in terms of steps in character development or psychosocial development, as in the work of Vaillant on Erikson's stages of ego development [33]. Such development can be visualized as a spiral of expanding height, width, and depth as a person matures or increases in coherence of personality. Likewise, the movement of thought from week to week or month to month has the same spiral form regardless of the time scale. Such "self-similarity" in form regardless of time scale is a property characteristic of complex adaptive systems, which are typical of psychosocial processes in general [8]. The clinical utility of this property is that therapists can teach people to exercise their capacity for self-awareness, moving through each of the stages of awareness just described. Their ability to do so, and the difficulties they have, reveals the way they are able to face challenges in life over longer periods of time. Cloninger [8] has developed an exercise, called the "Silence of the Mind" meditation, with explicit instructions to take people thorough each of the stages of awareness as well as they can. The first phase of this meditation results in a relaxed state in the first stage of self-awareness. The second phase facilitates entry into the second stage of self-awareness, and the third phase into the third stage of self-awareness, if the person is able to do so. Using this and a way of observing thought during mental status examination, mental health professionals can assess a person's thought and its level of coherence in a way that is constructive, easy, and precise without being judgmental [14, 19]. As the patient moves from ordinary self-awareness, through mindfulness and then contemplation, the therapist and patient can calmly discover together particular blockages in the patients' path toward well-being, and develop creative solutions to individual challenges.

31.6 Treatment

General Principles: Individuals with PD seldom think that they have a mental disorder and so seldom seek help for mental disorder unless other people (such as a spouse, a colleague, or parents) are insistent. This usually happens when maladaptive behaviors create severe marital, family, and/or career problems. In addition, individuals with PD often seek medical help when other associated mental symptoms (e.g., anxiety, depression, substance abuse) or somatic symptoms begin to bother them. Hence PCM offers the opportunity to help people with PDs to address problems that they personally care about, which is their own physical and mental well-being. Medical consultation is an important opportunity to help people with PDs to recognize the changes they need to make in order to improve their subjective well-being and their objective health. In general, patients with PD require a multifaceted treatment plan that always combines psychotherapy and pharmacotherapy.

There are three major barriers to effective treatment of PD, but, fortunately, all are preventable errors within the control of the healthcare professional. The first is the frequent loss of professional objectivity, signaled by the development of strong emotions (positive or negative) also called positive or negative counter-transference. Such inappropriate personal involvement is a red flag to reassess the treatment strategy, seek objective supervision of therapy sessions, and, if persistent, mandate referral to another psychiatrist or therapist. Frequent discussions and counseling with colleagues are useful because even strong counter-transference feelings can persist unrecognized.

The second preventable error in PD management is to believe the myth that PDs cannot be treated effectively. This myth is partly initiated by negative counter-transference of some professionals, and then sustained by a failure to consider signs showing the effectiveness of treatment. In other words, belief in the untreatability of a patient sets the stage for a self-fulfilling prophecy. However, many controlled studies indicate that even severe PDs, such as borderline or antisocial, can be effectively treated within an appropriate setting, such as a cooperative therapeutic alliance [9].

The third preventable error in PD management is to give direct advice on personal and social problems. This is counterproductive in patients with PD because they usually become dependent, non-compliant, or resentful. Occasionally, direct advice may be offered to some antisocial, narcissistic, and schizoid patients who are at low risk of developing dependency and need precise structure and direction initially. When tempted to give direct advice to patients, remember that change in personality requires more than common sense and logic. If the relationship leads to frequent advice giving, then referral to a psychiatrist or psychologist may be indicated. People change if they become self-aware and thus able to self-observe, eventually leading to recognition of their own role in chronic dissatisfaction with their health status, and with themselves and their relationships. Personal growth thus arises from new insights about oneself, the environment, and the connection between one's personality, lifestyle, and health status. Direct advice robs the patient of the opportunity to develop new insights and to learn from his or her mistakes. Although supportive psychotherapy is not recommended with PD patients, supporting their existing coping mechanisms that are mature and adaptive is always useful (e.g., joint evaluation of options and encouragement to practice skills in solving problems).

Substantial personality change, which is invariably needed people with PDs, involves an extensive reorganization of internalized concepts and coping mechanisms and thus requires precise diagnostic analysis, specific treatment strategies, and expert training. The expert treatment may include any of the several available psychotherapy approaches and is usually combined with pharmacotherapy and mind-body therapy, so optimally the treatment of PD is a prominent example of the utility of person-centered (integrative) medicine in practice. The major points relevant to integrative therapy of PDs are summarized below.

As already mentioned, individuals with PD have a peculiar capacity to elicit strong emotions from other people. They are often described as aggravating, unlikable, difficult, or bad. Alternatively, they may be seductive or dependent, and elicit inappropriate emotions or actions, such as sexual interest or the urge to rescue. Even professionals may have difficulty treating them with respectful objectivity because of a blurring of personal boundaries. Such loss of objectivity occurs because the patient's deeply felt assumptions about other people may often elicit interpersonal responses that are appropriate to the patient's assumptions. Our assumptions about ourselves and others often become self-fulfilling prophecies because of automatic mechanisms of affect transfer. If someone smiles at you, communicating appreciation, it is natural to experience feelings of social attachment and to smile back automatically. Likewise, if someone frowns, communicating anger, it is natural to feel defensive in preparation for his or her angry attack. For example, many patients with PD are suspicious and hostile about others' motives. This distrustful attitude is communicated in many verbal and non-verbal ways and often elicits disagreement or frank hostility from others. These uncooperative responses reinforce the original negative assumptions of the patient, which in turn leads to further alienation.

This vicious cycle of affect transfer can only be interrupted by professional objectivity combined with patience and compassionate respect for the patient's disability. Such objectivity arises from recognizing the overall meaning and implications of their pattern of interpersonal signals, so that their verbal and non-verbal communication takes on diagnostic and therapeutic, rather than personal, significance. In optimal therapeutic relationships, "patients" should be patiently hopeful and physicians should be compassionately realistic. Whenever professionals become aware of strong positive or negative emotions toward a patient (so-called "counter-transference" reactions), this should help to alert them to the possibility that the patient has a PD.

As many patients with PD do not recognize or admit their psychopathology they resist and resent psychiatric diagnoses and any form of mental health treatment. Accordingly, it is prudent to steadfast in a person-centered approach to health care: let the patient define his/her treatment goals and then jointly evaluate the likelihood of successful outcome until treatment goals that both patient and therapist agree upon can be identified. Initially, these goals should be as simple and concrete as possible (e.g., "to develop social skills," or "to reduce alcohol use," etc.). In many, but not all cases, successful completion of this initial phase will motivate the patient to define other, more complex treatment goals and to continue treatment.

Both primary care-takers and mental health experts need to keep in mind that there is a natural succession of stages in the treatment of patients with PDs. The four stages in the treatment of a patient with PD can be described as (1) crisis management and stabilization, (2) awakening of a positive perspective and spiritual values in life, (3) illumination, and (4) integrated intelligence [10]. Each has different goals and requires different methods. The complete care-taker should be prepared to guide people along these stages, ever ready to advance to the next stage if a person is interested and prepared to do so. In this chapter the initial stabilization and awakening phases will be discussed using an integrative medical approach that combines integrative pharmacotherapy [16, 29], mind-body therapy [3, 5, 20], and person-centered psychotherapy [14]. The more advanced phases of treatment will be considered in another chapter on psychotherapy.

Integrative treatment of PDs: The initial stage of crisis management and stabilization deals with the presenting problem and stressors in order to help the patient get into a calm enough state and a working alliance with the psychiatrist. The second stage involves elevating a person's outlook on life so that they can experience things they enjoy and value under relaxed conditions. This involves a spiritual awakening that has often been neglected in strictly cognitive-behavioral or psychodynamic approaches but without which there is little capacity for fundamental change in the quality of life. The third stage of illumination involves increases in self-awareness and capacity for contemplation that elevate a person's usual thoughts, feelings, and relationships in a wide range of conditions. The fourth stage of integration of reason and love in action allows a person to be mature and happy even under conditions that were previously stressful. Patients with PDs can pass through these stages on their own (i.e., remit spontaneously) or be guided through these stages in treatment facilitated by a scientifically designed set of physical, personal, social, cognitive, and spiritual exercises [10].

What is done in the first stage of treatment depends greatly on individual patient and his or her presenting situation. This initial stage may involve stabilization of the patient with medications if they are indicated and the patient is interested in such treatment. Medications are often helpful, but not everyone wants such treatment because they always carry some risk of side-effects and can be costly. The advantages and disadvantages must be carefully weighed to respect the patient's wishes and to help them be calm and organized enough for further growth in self-awareness. On the other hand, integrative mind-body therapy or psychotherapy requires more motivation for fundamental change than use of medication, so some people prefer to not try to develop their capacity for self-regulation and prefer to rely on more passive treatments like medication. Commitment to change requires recognition that change is possible and worthwhile. A person-centered care-taker must engage the patient by providing a range of alternative approaches to achieve what the patient values, such as relief of subjective distress (i.e., anxiety, depression, sleep problems) and enhancement of self-confidence and self-respect by accomplishing SMART (specific, measurable, achievable/assignable, realistic, time-related) goals [15].

Providing a wide range of alternative approaches to a problem gives people flexibility and hope that if one thing is too difficult or not effective, there are other pathways to well-being. Medications can be targeted to specific symptoms, particularly anxiety and mood dysregulation, aggression, emotional detachment, and magical thinking/perceptual aberrations [29]. Biofeedback for stress reduction is useful to optimize heart rate variability and other indicators of psychophysiological coherence [36]. Psychosocial interventions relying on person-centered dialog can motivate people who were not even considering change in lifestyle to improve their health related behaviors, including motivating people to improve diet, exercise regularly, and reduce stress [26]. Many mind-body and energy therapies, such as acupressure, Tai Chi, and Qi Gong, promote self-regulation, character development, and enhanced well-being [3]. Randomized controlled trials of mindfulness training promote well-being in association with increased self-directedness, cooperativeness, and self-transcendence [4]. Throughout this process, the clinician will periodically direct the patient to observe their individual progress and character development, continually building hope, and further motivating the virtuous spiral upwards.

31.7 Conclusion

In practice, a flexible person-centered care-taker must be open to what is appealing to the people they are treating and to what works regardless of their own personal preferences and theoretical biases. Such flexibility is also what facilitates the maturation and integration of personality through self-awareness, self-regulation, and beginning to consider and value the needs of others. As a deeper awareness of connectedness grows, so a sustained change in the outlook develops. Most fundamentally, a holistic approach that addresses all three aspects of a person (i.e., body, thoughts, and soul) is essential for the maturation and integration of personality in the full range of a person's life. People cannot enjoy full health without becoming aware of the interrelationships among the sexual, physical, emotional, social, cognitive, and spiritual components of their life. Accordingly, the assessment and treatment of people with PDs must address the person as a whole, rather than reducing them to an organ or a disease.

References

1. APA. Diagnostic and statistical manual (DSM-5). Washington, DC: American Psychiatric Association; 2013.
2. Balluz LS, Okoro CA, Mokdad A. Association between selected unhealthy lifestyle factors, body mass index, and chronic health conditions among individuals 50 years of age or older, by race/ethnicity. Ethn Dis. 2008;18(4):450–7.
3. Bertisch SM, Wee CC, Phillips RS, McCarthy EP. Alternative mind-body therapies used by adults with medical conditions. J Psychosom Res. 2009;66(6):511–9.
4. Campanella F, Crescentini C, Urgesi C, Fabbro F. Mindfulness-oriented meditation improves self-related character scales in healthy individuals. Compr Psychiatry. 2014;55(5):1269–78.
5. Chiesa A. Vipassana meditation: systematic review of current evidence. J Altern Complement Med. 2010;16(1):37–46.
6. Cloninger CR. A systematic method for clinical description and classification of personality variants: a proposal. Arch Gen Psychiatry. 1987;44:573–87.
7. Cloninger CR. A practical way to diagnose personality disorder: a proposal. J Pers Disord. 2000;14(2):99–108.
8. Cloninger CR. Feeling good: the science of well-being. New York: Oxford University Press; 2004.
9. Cloninger CR. Antisocial personality disorder: a review. In: Maj M, Akiskal HS, Mezzich JE, Okasha A, editors. Personality disorders: evidence and experience in psychiatry, vol. 8. London: Wiley; 2005. P. 125–9.
10. Cloninger CR. The science of well-being: an integrated approach to mental health and its disorders. World Psychiatry. 2006;5:71–6.
11. Cloninger CR. Person-centered health promotion in chronic disease. Int J Pers Cent Med. 2013;3(1):5–12.
12. Cloninger CR. What makes people healthy, happy, and fulfilled in the face of current world challenges? Mens Sana Monogr. 2013;11:16–24.
13. Cloninger CR. Validation of psychiatric classification: the psychobiological model of personality as an exemplar. In: Zachar P, Stoyanov D, Aragona M, Jablensky A, editors. Alternative perspectives on psychiatric validation: DSM ICD, RDoc, and beyond. Oxford, UK: Oxford University Press; 2015.
14. Cloninger CR, Cloninger KM. Person-centered Therapeutics. Int J Pers Cent Med. 2011;1 (1):43–52.
15. Cloninger CR, Salloum IM, Mezzich JE. The dynamic origins of positive health and wellbeing. Int J Pers Cent Med. 2012;2(2):1–9.
16. Cloninger CR, Svrakic DM. Integrative psychobiological approach to psychiatric assessment and treatment. Psychiatry. 1997;60(2):120–41.
17. Cloninger CR, Svrakic DM. Personality disorders. In: Sadock BJ, Sadock VA, Ruiz P, editors. Kaplan and Sadock's comprehensive textbook of psychiatry, vol. II. New York: Lippincott Williams & Wilkins. 2009; p. 2197–2240.
18. Cloninger CR, Svrakic DM, Przybeck TR. A psychobiological model of temperament and character. Arch Gen Psychiatry. 1993;50:975–90.
19. Cloninger CR, Zohar AH, Cloninger KM. Promotion of well-being in person-centered mental health care. Focus. 2010;8(2):165–79.
20. Fjorback LO. Mindfulness and bodily distress. Dan Med J. 2012;59(11):B4547.
21. Kuyken W, Hayes R, Barrett B, Byng R, Dalgleish T, Kessler D, Lewis G, Watkins E, Brejcha C, Cardy J, Causley A, Cowderoy S, Evans A, Gradinger F, Kaur S, Lanham P, Morant N, Richards J, Shah P, Sutton H, Vicary R, Weaver A, Wilks J, Williams M, Taylor RS, Byford S. Effectiveness and cost-effectiveness of mindfulness-based cognitive therapy compared with maintenance antidepressant treatment in the prevention of depressive relapse or recurrence (PREVENT): a randomised controlled trial. Lancet. 2015;386(9988): 63–73.

22. Linehan MM. Cognitive-behavioral treatment of borderline personality disorder. New York: Guilford Press; 1993.
23. Mokdad AH, Marks JS, Stroup DF, Gerberding JL. Actual causes of death in the United States, 2000. JAMA. 2004;291(10):1238–45.
24. Moreira-Almeida A, Santos FS, editors. Exploring frontiers of the mind-brain relationship. Mindfulness in behavioral health. New York: Springer; 2011.
25. Mulder RT, Joyce PR. Temperament and the structure of personality disorder symptoms. Psychol Med. 1997;27:99–106.
26. Nigg CR, Burbank PM, Padula C, Dufresne R, Rossi JS, Velicer WF, Laforge RG, Prochaska JO. Stages of change across ten health risk behaviors for older adults. Gerontologist. 1999;39(4):473–82.
27. Oldham JM, Gabbard GO, Goin MK, Gunderson J, Soloff P, Spiegel D, Stone M, Phillips KA. Practice guidelines for the treatment of patients with borderline personality disorder. Washington, DC: American Psychiatric Press; 2001.
28. Rosenstrom T, Jokela M, Cloninger CR, Hintsanen M, Juonala M, Raitakari O, Viikari J, Keltikangas-Jarvinen L. Associations between dimensional personality measures and preclinical atherosclerosis: the cardiovascular risk in Young Finns study. J Psychosom Res. 2012;72(5):336–43.
29. Svrakic DM, Cloninger CR. Psychobiological model of personality: guidelines for pharmacotherapy of personality disorder. Curr Psychopharmacol. 2012;2(3):190–203.
30. Teasdale JD, Moore RG, Hayhurst H, Pope M, Williams S, Segal ZV. Metacognitive awareness and prevention of relapse in depression: empirical evidence. J Consult Clin Psychol. 2002;70(2):275–87.
31. Tyrer P. Time to choose—DSM-5, ICD-11, or both? Arch Psychiatry psychother. 2014;3:5–8.
32. Tyrer P, Crawford M, Sanatinia R, Tyrer H, Cooper S, Muller-Pollard C, Christodoulou P, Zauter-Tutt M, Miloseska-Reid K, Loebenberg G, Guo B, Yang M, Wang D, Weich S. Preliminary studies of the ICD-11 classification of personality disorder in practice. Pers Ment Health. 2014;8(4):254–63.
33. Vaillant GE, Milofsky E. Natural history of male psychological health: IX. Empirical evidence for Erikson's model of the life cycle. Am J Psychiatry. 1980;137:1348–59.
34. van der Velden AM, Kuyken W, Wattar U, Crane C, Pallesen KJ, Dahlgaard J, Fjorback LO, Piet J. A systematic review of mechanisms of change in mindfulness-based cognitive therapy in the treatment of recurrent major depressive disorder. Clin Psychol Rev. 2015;37:26–39.
35. Widiger TA, Simonsen E, Sirovatka PJ, Regier DA, editors. Dimensional models of personality disorders: refining the research agenda for DSM-V. Washington, DC: American Psychiatric Association; 2006.
36. Zohar AH, Cloninger CR, McCraty R. Personality and heart rate variability: exploring pathways from personality to cardiac coherence and health. J Soc Sci. 2013;1(6):32–9.

Child and Adolescent Psychiatry 32

Michel Botbol, MD, Marco O. Bertelli, MD, PhD,
Luis Salvador-Carulla, MD, PhD, Dimitris Anagnostopoulos, MD, PhD, Angeliki Christodoulou, BSc, MA
and James Appleyard, MA, MD, FRCPCH

32.1 Introduction

More than the rest of psychiatry, Child and Adolescent Psychiatry has to deal with controversial conceptual and practical issues concerning the nature or nurture question. Neurodevelopmental processes are indeed particularly active in this stage of life. Similarly active is the influence of the environment, particularly in its relational dimension and at the earliest stage of childhood, because, as Winnicott pointed out, "'There is no such thing as an infant', meaning, of course, that whenever one finds an infant one finds maternal care, and without maternal care there would be no infant" [32]. For each of the children they have to diagnose or treat, child and adolescent psychiatrists have then to address both perspectives giving them an equal attention in spite of the inequality of the tools available to evaluate them.

M. Botbol, MD (✉)
Service Hospitalo-Universitaire de Psychiatrie Infanto Juvénile, Hôpital de Bohars, 29820 Bohars, France; Professor of Child and Adolescent Psychiatry, University of Western Brittany and Brest University Hospital, EA4686, Brest, France
e-mail: botbolmichel@orange.fr

M.O. Bertelli, MD, PhD
Research and Clinical Centre, San Sebastiano Foundation, Florence, Italy

L. Salvador-Carulla, MD, PhD
Faculty of Health Sciences, Centre for Disability Research and Policy and Mental Health Policy Unit, Brain and Mind Institute, University of Sydney, Sydney, Australia

D. Anagnostopoulos, MD, PhD
Associate Professor of Child and Adolescent Psychiatry, Department of Child and Adolescent Psychiatry, University of Athens, General Pediatric Hospital of Athens "Agia Sofia", Athens, Greece

J.E. Mezzich et al. (eds.), *Person Centered Psychiatry*,
DOI 10.1007/978-3-319-39724-5_32

Another particularity of child psychiatry, may be more than in other fields of medicine and psychiatry, is the fact that it is at the crossroad of two major concerns:

- The concern for the current child's mental health, which is a crucial dimension of his well-being and of his way to relate to the world and to himself. In this perspective, it is crucial that the approach to the child's health status integrates the specific aspects of his health manifestations and particularly the importance of development and dependency at this age. Child and Adolescent Psychiatry has then to put at its centre, aspects that are frequently considered marginal in other branches of the discipline.
- The concern for his future as the adult he will become, that is to say the protection and the development of his potentiality. In this perspective, it is important to understand that the persons presenting with symptoms of a possible illness is always experiencing not only his current heath situation but also the effect of all of their life events from perinatal period, to infancy, childhood, adolescence and adulthood, in their biological, social, psychological and spiritual dimensions.

In both perspectives, child and adolescent psychiatry and medicine have to be constantly integrative in their approach to the child and in the consideration they give to the complexity of his person. The integrative dimension of Person-Centered Psychiatry is particularly crucial to encompass the various aspects of this complexity. Child and Adolescent Psychiatry can then be seen as a good example of the usefulness of Person-Centered approaches across care settings; to the point that it can be considered that, to be efficient and close to clinical reality, child and adolescent mental heath care cannot be but person centered.

32.2 Child and Adolescent Clinical Specificities in Psychiatry

Nevertheless, the current clinical references, and particularly the leading international classification system are still quite limited in the way they consider, so far, the specificities for the child and adolescent psychiatric practice. They include only a small number of specific categories and there is a notable lack of flexibility and usability of all the categories related to personality disorder, hindering the definition of many child and adolescent mental health conditions. Moreover, in spite of the

A. Christodoulou, BSc, MA
Psychologist, Scientific Collaborator, Child and Adolescent Mental Health Unit, Department of Psychiatry, Medical School, University of Athens, Athens, Greece

J. Appleyard, MA, MD, FRCPCH
Former Consultant Pediatrician, Kent and Canterbury Hospital, Canterbury, UK; President, International College of Person Centered Medicine, London, UK

differences, these classifications are implicitly recognizing for child and adolescent psychiatry, the diagnostic process is supposed to remain strictly the same as in adult psychiatry, that is to say, based on descriptive items to type the disorders, and the use of comorbidity to correct the ill-effect of this model of the diagnostic process and to bring diagnostic categories closer to real clinical situations. These limited adaptations of the current classificatory systems to the needs of the child and adolescent psychiatric practice, contrasts with what we already have noted: the multiple specificities involved in child and adolescent psychiatry [7].

Such specificities can be considered from at least four relevant perspectives: (1) Symptomatic; (2) Developmental, (3) Environmental; and (4) Prognostic.

a. Symptomatic Specificities

In childhood and adolescence there are specific limitations in the type of externalized manifestations, as well as in the possibility to have insight-dependant symptoms. The relation between observed symptoms and underlying psychological organization are then particular in child and adolescent psychiatry. More frequently than in Adult Psychiatry a specific set of behavioral descriptive symptoms may be related to quite different underlying psychopathological organizations. Thus, at this age, consideration given to dynamic defense mechanisms and structural organizations underlying the behavioral symptoms, leads frequently to profound modification in the diagnostic evaluation and in the therapeutic indications. This perspective can lead, for example, to consider some Obsessive Compulsive Disorder (OCD) patients much closer to Schizophrenic or Narcissistic patients than it is to those suffering from other Anxiety Disorders. Although this perspective may not generally call for a change in the pharmacological prescription, the rest of the treatment strategy, so important at this age, will be more adapted to the patient specific needs when taking into account the underlying psychopathological organization rather than the sole OCD symptoms. In some cases this may lead to a therapeutic program much closer to what would be proposed to a schizophrenic patient [21] than to the one we would generally offer to other anxiety disorder patients.

Conversely, a particular psychopathological constellation may have very different symptomatic expressions. Depression in adolescence, for instance, can be expressed in very different ways: through acting out or psychotic symptoms more often than in adult psychiatry. For many authors, this should be taken into account for the pharmacological prescriptions at this age [15].

b. Developmental Specificities

Developmental considerations are of more importance in child and adolescent psychiatry than they are in adults. They are crucial to differentiate pathological symptoms and developmental conflicts, to appreciate developmental breakdowns, regressions or fixations, to recognize disharmonies on the different developmental lines, to integrate biological and environmental dimensions of development and finally to adapt therapeutic responses. Taking into account this developmental dimension allowed a team of French Child Psychiatrists to describe nearly thirty years ago a clinical condition they include in the French Classification of Child and Adolescent Mental Disorders [20] under the name of "Psychotic Disharmony"; this disorder appeared to be very similar to what Donald Cohen proposed fifteen years later under the name of Multiplex Developmental Disorders to differentiate them from other Pervasive Developmental Disorders Not Otherwise Specified (PDD-NOS) [28].

c. Environmental Specificities

There is obviously in childhood a specific dependency upon current and past environmental conditions; this implies that relational aspects have a bigger impact on the expression of mental disorders at this age. There are therefore in Child and Adolescent Psychiatry greater risks that a number of diagnostic labels might be nothing more than a psychiatric reformulation of a social impairment (e.g., the Conduct Disorders category could merely be a psychiatric formulation of Delinquency), when diagnostic labeling does not bring any added value to the social construct.

Conversely, psychopathological disorders are ignored or denied when covered by hyper adaptation to local or global social norms, even when this hyper adaptation is mainly a way to deal with underlying psychological distress (as shown in some stabilized high functioning Pervasive Developmental Disorders or in some childhood undiagnosed Obsessive Compulsive Disorders) that may be hidden to the child or the adolescent himself. It may be observed also in behavioral disorders fitting well social definitions and social responses in specific circumstances. For instance, learning difficulties at school or delinquency in educational or judicial setting have less chance to be seen as symptoms of psychological distress unless specifically addressed from a psychopathological perspective. Social norms are thus one of the main determinants of the diagnostic labeling in childhood.

Finally, in every day practice, there is a great risk in child and adolescent psychiatry that the choice between a social or a psychiatric definition of a disorder, and the assistance it will generate, would not be based as much on the disorder characteristics as it is on its social context and on the type of interaction between the child and his environment.

There is then in Child and Adolescent psychiatry a specific need to avoid diagnostic processes strictly limited to individual approaches as much as those focusing only on the adaptation to the environment; instead child psychiatry requires diagnostic processes taking into account the subjective aspects resulting from the interaction of individual and environmental dimensions. In other words, there is at this age a specific need for diagnostics to consider the psychic functioning and not to limit itself to the description of social symptoms. Moreover this approach constitutes a useful basis for multi focal approaches always required to deal with such psychopathological social expressions at this age.

d. Prognostic Specificities

Prognosis has a specific value in child and adolescent psychiatry, where the main concern is not only the current status of the disorder but its continuity into adulthood.

From this viewpoint, research data [16] shows in adolescence the lack or reliability of DSM-IV's Axis I general disorders categories alone and a significant increase in the prognostic reliability when DSM-IV's Axis II personality disorders categories are added even if they are not supposed to be used at this age. From this perspective too, child and adolescent psychiatry shows a specific need to take into account the underlying psychological functioning of the individual patient, and not to rely solely on descriptions of externalized symptomatic expressions on which current classifications base their categorical definitions.

In summary, most of the specific needs of child and adolescent psychiatry are not addressed by current classifications and diagnostic systems; the main issue is not their lack of specific categories but the diagnostic process they adopt that do not take into account what seems crucial in child and adolescent mental disorders classification: an overall evaluation of the mental functioning of the child and not only a description of his/her symptoms. To a smaller extent, this difficulty is also found in adult psychiatry, but it has more serious consequences in child and adolescent psychiatry. For instance, big differences of prevalence of Attention-Deficit Hyperactivity Disorder (ADHD) in different parts of the world can not be explained only as cultural or biological variations but rather as resulting from variations in the social use of psychiatric nosographical labeling [12].

To address these issues, classifications and diagnostic processes require conceptual modifications, such as: (a) Better integration of individual, relational and environmental dimensions; (b) Stronger references to developmental dimensions and longitudinal aspects of disorders; (c) Greater need to take into account psychic functioning and defense mechanisms to define as much the personality patterns as the process leading to the symptom.

There is then a need to introduce more complexity in the current classification systems to allow them to get closer to the clinical situations we face in child and adolescent psychiatry. The problem is that the introduction of more complexity implies necessarily more room for the psychiatrist interpretation (that is to say, for his theoretical background) while we need also to maintain common references to a universal nosographical frame.

32.3 The Impact of Early Life Experiences and Disorders on Health and Well-Being

There is now good evidence that problems in the early years of childhood may foreshadow problems in adolescence and adult life. Obviously, these problems can be of various environmental nature but can be schematically classified under two main headings: Traumatic Experiences and/or impairment of early relationships. In both cases a longitudinal approach to a patients narrative is essential in this field [14].

a. The Adverse Childhood Experience (ACE)

In a retrospective and prospective analysis in over 17,000 middle-class Americans, Lanius et al. [18] studied the effect of early traumatic life experience on later well-being, social function, health risks, disease burden, healthcare costs and life expectancy. The average starting age of the subjects was 57 years old. The study has, approximately a half century after the fact, retrospectively matched an individual's current state of health against adverse events in childhood, and then followed the cohort forward to assess the relationship of ACE Score prospectively against future doctor office visits, emergency room visits, hospitalization, pharmacy costs, and death.

The adverse reference points were grouped under the three main headings of Abuse, Household Dysfunction and Neglect. Each participant was assigned an individual ACE Score, a count of the number of categories of adverse childhood experience encountered in their first 18 years.

These are: (1) emotional abuse, (2) physical abuse, and (3) contact sexual abuse; (4) mother treated violently; (5) household member an alcoholic or drug user; (6) or in prison; (7) or chronically depressed, suicidal, mentally ill, or in psychiatric hospital; (8) the subject not being raised by both biological parents; (9) physical neglect and (10) emotional neglect.

The two Neglect categories were added part-way through the study when these began to emerge as "surprise" significant issues amongst the subjects. The scoring system took account of only one incidence in any given category, so if a subject had been raised in a household containing both an alcoholic and a drug user, this would count as one not two experiences [18].

Whenever a study participant was found to score 1 on the Adverse Childhood Experience Score, there was an 87 % probability of more such experiences. Seventeen percent of the sample tested had scores of four or above.

There is a strong relationship between ACE Score and self acknowledged chronic depression and a similar, but an even stronger, relationship between ACE Score and later suicide attempts. This relationship between ACE Score and depression is borne out by analysis of prescription rates for antidepressant medications, now 50–60 years after the fact. It appears that depression is common and has deep roots, usually going back to the developmental years of life.

The most common contemporary health risks (smoking, alcoholism, illicit drug use, obesity and high level promiscuity) are widely known to be harmful. Such unhealthy behaviors may be coping mechanisms to sooth-submerged pain and difficult to give up even though they know these things are bad for them. The higher the ACE Score the greater the likelihood of later smoking, alcoholism, intravenous drug use, etc.

The authors of the study conclude that "all told, it is clear that adverse childhood experiences have a profound, proportionate, and long-lasting effect on well-being," whether this is measured by depression or suicide attempts, by protective unconscious devices like overeating and even amnesia or by what they refer to as "self-help attempts," the use of street drugs or alcohol to modulate feelings. They say that these are misguidedly addressed solely as long-term health risks, "perhaps because we physicians are less than comfortable acknowledging the manifest short-term benefits these "health risks" offer to the patient dealing with hidden trauma." As Felitti states "it's hard to get enough of something that almost works" [14].

b. Impaired Early Relationships

Another example from developmental psychopathology demonstrates the short- and long-term effects of impaired early relationships on children's long-term development [9]. A good illustration of this phenomenon is the effect of maternal depression on infant development. Relative to control mothers, depressed mothers express less positive and more negative affect, are less attentive and engaged with their infants, and, when engaged, are more intrusive and controlling and fail to respond adaptively to their infants' emotional signals [11]. Their infants have shorter attention spans, less motivation to master tasks, elevated heart rates, elevated cortisol levels, and reduced EEG activity in the right frontal cortex, all of which correlate with the experience of negative affect in adults [11]. Longitudinal data on infants of depressed mothers indicate that elevated heart rates and cortisol can persist and may represent a functional programming of the child's autonomic set point. If true, this may explain in part that after controlling for the maternal depression status when the child was four years old, maternal depression during an infant's first year of life was predictive of the child's cognitive ability at that age [10].

Even where damage from their early years is internalized, young people and adults can become the self-destructive or depressed parents of what will become a new generation of emotionally damaged children. Untreated postnatal depression can have serious long-term consequences for the mother's ongoing relationship with her baby and for his or her mental and emotional development. Postnatal depression is thought to affect approximately 13 % of women during the early months following childbirth [22]. Yet frontline service providers, such as health visitors may only be identifying about 10 per cent of those postnatal depressed women.

Very young children need a high level of emotional responsiveness and engagement, which a severely depressed primary carer is unable to give, however much she might want to. Her baby might look well fed and clean, but might be emotionally neglected all the same. The intergenerational nature of this is underlined by the estimate that 30 to 40 per cent of abused or neglected children (versus two to three per cent of the total population) go on to abuse or neglect their own children. 56.

Reduced attention to faces of care givers, and more specifically to the eye region, may underlie traits that lead to reduced responsiveness to others distress, a lack of empathy [3].

From a stratified random sample of 213 participants drawn from a population-based sample of 1233 first-time mothers, infants' preferential faces tracking at 5 weeks and maternal sensitivity at 29 weeks were entered into a weighted linear regression as predictors of Callous Unemotional traits at 2.5 years. Controlling for a range of confounders (e.g., deprivation), lower preferential face tracking predicted higher CU traits ($p = 0.001$). Higher maternal sensitivity predicted lower CU traits in girls ($p = 0.009$), but not boys.

Physiologically as well as emotionally, infants need a stimulating, accepting environment in which they feel safe and loved. It has been said that "the greatest gift for a baby is maternal responsiveness." The more positive stimuli a baby is given, the more brain cells and synapses it will be able to develop. "The child's first relationship, the one with the mother, acts as a template that permanently moulds the individual's capacity to enter into all later emotional relationships" [26].

When this stimulus is accompanied by the type of parental attunement that fosters the development of empathy, the infant will be able to take all the needed advantages from the significant "sensitive windows" existing in the first three years of life using the brain plasticity.

The innate flexibility in sculpting the young brain has enormous survival value, because it is what enables infants to adapt to their particular environment [25].

When human infants are born they are immediately aware of and ready to be programmed by their adult carers. From our first moments of life infants are "tuned" into the facial expressions of those around them, as can be seen from the infant reflex to mimic.

At birth there are 100 billion neurons and 50 trillion synapses. By age three, the number of synapses has increased 20-fold to one thousand trillion. Because this is too large a number to be determined by genes alone, many new synapses are formed by experience [25].

The synapses are strengthened and reinforced by these experiences and the early life defines which of them live and which die. Synapses become "hard-wired," or protected, by repeated use, enabling very rapid learning via early life experience. Conversely, just as a memory will fade if it is hardly ever accessed, unused synapses wither away in what is called "pruning." This indicates that it is the nurture that infants receive based on their genetic nature that plays the lead role in creating the human personality.

Physiologically as well as emotionally, infants need then a stimulating, accepting environment in which they feel safe and loved. It has been said that "the greatest gift for a baby is maternal responsiveness." The more positive stimuli a baby is given, the more brain cells and synapses it will be able to develop. When this stimulus is accompanied by the type of parental attunement that fosters the development of empathy, the result will be a socially adapted child who is likely to be happier, healthier and more intelligent than one who has been deprived of these essentials for positive growth [1].

32.4 The Person-Centered Health Model in Intellectual Developmental Disorders

Intellectual Developmental Disorders (IDD) or Intellectual disability (ID) is one of the severe neurodevelopmental disorders, affecting both intellect and adaptive behaviors. It is a permanent condition, associated with a high comorbidity of physical and mental disorders worldwide. Consequently it is associated with high levels of care giving burden, and implies high service provision and produces high health and societal costs [5, 24]. Despite this, ID is a neglected area both in the field of general health and mental health. These challenges are more evident in Low and Middle Income Countries (LAMI).

32.4.1 Nosological and Functioning Distinctions

The case of IDD/ID is particularly challenging for multidimensional person-centered care, covering both ill health and positive health along the levels of health status [19]. In fact, there is no international consensus on whether ID is a health condition that should be classified in the International Classification of Diseases (ICD) or if it is a disability that should not be coded in the International Classification of Functioning (ICF). The fact that the international community has not reached an agreement in such a basic question and that there is an ongoing debate on its placement at the WHO Family of Classifications reflects the complexity of this construct. As a matter of fact, many national agencies follow the approach of the American Association of Intellectual and Developmental Disabilities that defines "Intellectual disability" as "a disability characterized by significant limitations both in intellectual functioning [IQ > 70] and in adaptive behavior, which covers many everyday social and practical skills. The timeframe for age of onset is defined from birth to 18 years. This has oriented the recommendations made by this group for naming and conceptualizing this condition at ICD [27, 31]. Other organizations such as the World Psychiatric Association have defined it as a group of health condition, namely developmental conditions, characterized by a significant impairment of cognitive functions, which are associated with limitations of learning, adaptive behavior and skills [23]. This definition was extended by the ICD Working Group in 2011, under the new term of "Intellectual Developmental Disorders": a group of etiologically diverse conditions that are present from birth or that arise during the developmental period, characterized by a marked impairment of cognitive functions necessary for the development of knowledge, reasoning, and symbolic representation of the level expected of one's age peers, cultural and community environment. IDD was also defined as a life span condition requiring consideration of all developmental stages and life transitions [6, 24]. Furthermore, the ICD Working Group proposed revised diagnostic criteria for ICD-11 based on an articulated model of cognitive impairment. This approach should complement measurement of IQ with assessment of specific cognitive functions and a contextualized description of consequent adaptive and learning difficulties. Within this new approach, cognitive skills should be assessed in the most comprehensive way as possible. The measurement should be done through tests, semi-structured observations, and direct clinical examination. The tests should combine measurement of IQ with that of complex aspects of executive functioning, including perceptual reasoning, processing speed, verbal comprehension, as well as specific aspects, such as attention, perception, and working memory. The evaluation should aim to identify the cognitive dysfunctions that have the greatest negative impact on the person's lifespan, not only in cognitive skills but also in terms of associated behavior, ability, adjustment, autonomy, and all other factors that rely on person-centered health [6, 24].

32.4.2 Person-Centered Medicine and Quality of Life

The current debate reflects the importance of a multifaceted approach to complex health problems and the significant contribution made by the International College of Person-Centered Medicine (ICPCM) and the International Network for Person-centered Medicine through the Person-centered Integrative Diagnostic model - PID [19], which takes into account not only the health condition and the disability but also the positive aspects defined as well-being and good functioning. IDD/ID may not be an exception in health but a prototypical example of how the holistic and comprehensive approach recommended by ICPCM is useful for understanding these complex constructs in health care.

Among person-centered approaches for persons with IDD/ID, in the last two decades Quality of Life (QoL) has increasingly gained a central place, although it is sometimes considered a concept that lacks sufficient precision to have specific usefulness in the field, and that it is more advantageous to focus on clearer concepts or simply on providing practical supports [4].

Yet, a considerable amount of substantive work has been done in the area of QoL and IDD/ID. Numerous thoughtful books, book chapters, and academic articles have been published that not only advanced our understanding of QoL, but have made ID the leading field for substantive work in QoL. It is clear from this work that achieving high quality of living is not the main purpose.

Given that QoL depends on host of individual and environmental factors that persons with IDD/ID either lack or are deprived of, the question of how we can ensure entitlement to a life of quality for people with ID who have mental health problems, is an interesting and challenging one. First it is necessary that mental health professionals value the needs and choices of people with ID, and believe that it is possible to improve their life conditions. This in turn helps them recognize the use of positive interventions that view the health—and indeed the whole life—of people with ID in more holistic and integrated ways. When mental health professionals work with people who have ID, it is helpful to consider three aspects of QoL: personal QoL, shared QoL, and family QoL. All the three are relevant in the context of care and service provision, but personal QoL is more important as ultimately it is the individual's perceptions, attitudes, values, skills and other attributes that determine how his or her life is experienced. At the same time each individual is expected to be a social being and hence shared QoL is assessed taking the social support (e.g., family, work and community) into consideration. But good QoL assessment allows for the concept to be explored at a personal level as well as at the shared level [8]. Similarly, family QoL is relevant in the context of ID for several reasons. One, families can influence and get influenced by the nature of disability in the members [29, 30]. Two, more and more families in the developed countries are living with members with disabilities as entitled by law while cultural practices or lack of residential care facilities demand the same in LAMI.

The WHO definition of QoL as a subjective construct including the self-reported assessment of both positive and negative facets of life is in agreement with the "experience" domain of the PID model of person-centered health [19]. However the

PID has a broader perspective as it highlights the importance of engagement, empathy and partnership in the clinical care process, and sustain the patients' autonomy, responsibility and dignity while advancing the recovery and promotion of well-being. To assess the domain of person's experience and values PID uses descriptive categories, dimensions, and narratives, to cultivate patient–family–clinician partnerships for achieving shared diagnostic understanding and shared commitment to care. The application of this model to the assessment of personal well-being, experiences, satisfaction and aspirations of persons with IDD faces significant challenges in persons with IDD as the self-reported assessment of these complex concepts is limited due to the cognitive and communication impairments [6].

32.4.3 Prospects for Implementation

The question of how we can ensure entitlement to a life of quality for people with ID who have mental health problems is an interesting and challenging one. Yet, the emphasis within the conceptualization of QoL on finding uniquely individual solutions to presenting problems suggests that it may be a particularly apt approach to take with this population. People with ID are characterized by lower levels of some cognitive functions, and lower potential for learning and developing logical-deductive skills. For this reason, it is not a sane goal of therapeutical interventions to attempt to provide "normal" intellectual functioning, but rather such interventions need to work within the confines of each individual's particular skills sets. Similarly, it is not a reasonable therapeutic goal to have people with IDD/ID live their lives as close as possible to people without IDD/ID, because ultimately they have to find satisfaction in those aspects of life that are important to them and that they can understand and experience. The more traditional medical approach to therapeutic interventions with people who have IDD/ID and mental health problems have tended not to consider the uniqueness of people with IDD/ID fully and have been more likely to use the general population norm as their point of reference. This has resulted in interventions that have dealt primarily with containing troublesome behaviors and helping to alleviate symptoms, rather than to address the root causes of the problems. Thus, assuming an overall QoL approach to intervention goes a long way to ensuring entitlement to a life of quality.

The conceptualization of ID should shift the traditional over-reliance on the intelligence (IQ) score in favor of the daily life expression of specific cognitive functions and the determination of the levels of severity of intellectual functioning, that was previously based on the person's IQ score, should be reached through a system that is predicated on the person's satisfaction attainment toward life.

The assessment of cognition should be aimed at identifying those dysfunctions that have the highest impact on individual behavior, skills, adaptation, autonomy, and quality of life across the life span, highlighting personal cognitive strengths and weaknesses that can be useful to understand personal functioning and to organize intervention.

Person-centeredness as a model of care provision, care individualization and lifestyle and supports was first developed in the Intellectual disability sector than in many other areas of health and social care. However, and although some agencies have actually implemented PCC over decades in the US, Australia and Europe, the claims of adherence to the PCC goals are larger than its actual application [2, 17].

As a matter of fact and in spite of the aspirations toward a PCC model, the implementation is slow due to barriers in the change in the philosophy or culture of care, power and funding structures, high levels of staff turnover and lack of training, inexperience among service management, inadequate staff supervision, and ambiguity among some stakeholders [13].

Kendrick [17] has provided an extensive review of the main 7 conditions required for such a change in the service delivery system in IDD care. The challenges related to this change include (1) Ethical Partnering With Individuals and Families and Carers; (2) A Social Inclusion/Valued Social Participation; and (3) Effective Address of People's Important Personal Needs.

Building partnerships that work requires a staff that understands ethical conduct and its aware of its absence or perversion, incorporates decision sharing, personal and organizational flexibility and demonstrates respect for persons with ID. The social inclusion/participation approach requires moving out from segregated services to fully community integration and membership, providing support for the acquisition of common social and cultural values as well as health promotion through healthy lifestyles and prevention of stigma and marginalization. The effective address of personal needs requires a monitoring system of care and support gaps, its relation to unmet needs, with an specific attention to "the essential ingredients of a good life such as employment, income, good health, a home of their own, value and respect, interesting leisure, personal growth and development, good safeguarding of vulnerabilities" [17].

To achieve these goals it is necessary to invest in the assistance to establish service user controlled entities to ensure consumer empowerment; independent personal advocacy; oversight and evaluation of services and service quality agreements directed by service users in terms of agency performance; and provide funding on the person-centered approach in education, leadership and to increase population literacy in PCC.

32.5 Conclusions

Particularly exposed to questions crucial for psychiatry in general (nature–nurture debate, dependence to relational and material context, role of subjective and psychological aspects of mental and psychic life) given the importance of developmental processes in earlier life stages, Child and Adolescent Psychiatry has to be integrative in its essence and person-centered in its practices. Whatever the etiological determinants of the mental health status of the patients they treat, psychiatric care has to be holistic, and take into consideration the person of the child and his context, implying a diagnostic process that has to go beyond the mere nosographical labeling. In this regard, the person-centered perspectives, recently developed in medicine in general and in psychiatry in particular, are particularly promising to build new paths to fulfill this ambition, promoting improvement in the current state of the art in child and adolescent psychiatry.

References

1. Appleyard J. Person centered and Integrated care across the life cycle. Int J Pers Centered Med. 2015;5:15–20.
2. Balogh R, Ouellette-Kuntz H, Bourne L, Lunsky Y, Colantonio A. Organising health care services for persons with an intellectual disability. Cochrane Database Syst Rev. 2008;4: CD007492.
3. Bedford R, Pickles A, Sharp H, Wright N, Hill J. Reduced face preference in infancy: a developmental precursor to callous-unemotional traits? Biol Psychiatry. 2014;9:22.
4. Bertelli M, Brown I. Quality of life for people with intellectual disabilities. Current Opin Psychiatry. 2006;19(5):508–13.
5. Bertelli M, Hassiotis A, Deb S, Salvador-Carulla L. New contributions of psychiatric research in the field of intellectual disability. In Christodoulou GN, Jorge M, Mezzich JE editors. Advances in psychiatry, vol 3. Athens: Beta Medical Publishers; 2009. p. 37–43.
6. Bertelli M, Salvador-Carulla L, Scuticchio D, Varrucciu N, Martinez-Leal R, Cooper SA, Simeonsson RJ, Deb S, Weber G, Jung R, Munir K, Adnams C, Akoury-Dirani L, Girimaji SC, Katz G, Kwok H, Walsh C. Moving beyond intelligence in the revision of ICD-10: specific cognitive functions in intellectual developmental disorders. World Psychiatry. 2014;13(1):93–4.
7. Botbol M, Berganza C. Specificities of diagnosis and classification in child and adolescent psychiatry In: Salloum, I Mezzich JE editors. Psychiatric diagnosis: challenges and prospects. Oxford, UK: Willey-Blackwell; 2009.
8. Brown I, Brown RI. Quality of life and disability: an approach for community practitioners. London: Jessica Kingsley Publishers; 2003.
9. Cicchetti D, Aber JL. Contextualism and developmental psychopathology. Dev Psychopathol. 1998;10(2):137–41.
10. Coghill SR, Caplan HL, Alexandra H, Robson KM, Kumar R. Impact of Maternal postnatal depression on cognitive development of young children. Brit Med J. 1986;292:1165–7.
11. Dawson, Hessel D, Frey K. Social influences on early developing biological and behavioral systems related to risk for affective disorder. Dev Psychopathol. 1994;6:759–79.
12. Diller L. Cola Coca. MacDonald's et Ritaline. Enfance et Psy. 2001;14:137–41.
13. Dowling S, Manthorpe J, Cowley S. Working on person-centred planning: from amber to green light? J Intellect Disabil Res. 2007;11(1):65–82.
14. Felitti V, Anda RF. The relationship of adverse childhood experiences to adult health, wellbeing, social function and healthcare. In: Lanius R, Vermetten E, editors. The hidden epidemic: the impact of early life Trauma on health and disease. Cambridge, UK: Cambridge University Press; 2008.
15. Jeammet PH. Les prémices de la schizophrénie. In: De Clercq M, Peuskens J, editors. Les troubles schizophréniques. Bruxelles: De Boeck Université; 2000.
16. Johnson JG, Cohen P, Skodol AE, et al. Personality disorders in adolescence and risk for major mental disorders and suicidality during adulthood. Arch Gen Psychiatry. 1999;56 (17):805–11.
17. Kendrick MJ. Getting A Good Life: The Challenges For Agency Transformation So That They Are More Person Centered. Int J Disabil Community Rehabil. 2011;11(1). http://www.ijdcr.ca Accessed 6 Feb 2015.

18. Lanius R, Vermetten E, editors. The hidden epidemic: the impact of early life Trauma on health and disease. Cambridge, UK: Cambridge University Press; 2008.
19. Mezzich JE, Salloum IM, Cloninger CR, Salvador-Carulla L, Kirmayer LJ, Banzato CE, Wallcraft J, Botbol M. Person-centred integrative diagnosis: conceptual bases and structural model. Can J Psychiatry. 2010;55(11):701–8.
20. Mises R, Quemada N, Botbol M, et al. French classification for child and adolescent mental disorders. Psychopathology. 2002;35:176–80.
21. Nechmad A, Ratzoni G, Poyurovsky M, et al. Obsessive compulsive disorder in adolescent schizophrenia patients. Am J Psychiatry. 2003;160:1002–4.
22. O'Hara MW, Swain AM. Rates and risk of postnatal depression—a meta-analysis. Int Rev Psychiatry. 1996;8:37–54.
23. Salvador-Carulla L, Bertelli M. «Mental retardation» or «intellectual disability»: time for a conceptual change. Psychopathology. 2008;41(1):10–6.
24. Salvador-Carulla L, Reed GM, Vaez-Azizi LM, Cooper SA, Martinez-Leal R, Bertelli M, Adnams C, Cooray S, Deb S, Akoury-Dirani L, Girimaji SC, Katz G, Kwok H, Luckasson R, Simeonsson R, Walsh C, Munir K, Saxena S. Intellectual developmental disorders: towards a new name, definition and framework for "mental retardation/intellectual disability" in ICD-11. World Psychiatry. 2011;10(3):175–80.
25. Shore R. Rethinking the brain: new insights into early development. New York: Families and Work Institute; 1997.
26. Stern D. The interpersonal world of the infant: a view from psychoanalysis and developmental psychology. New York: Basic Books; 1985.
27. Tassé MJ, Luckasson R, Nygren M. AAIDD proposed recommendations for ICD-11 and the condition previously known as mental retardation. Intellect Dev Disabil. 2013;51(2):127–31.
28. Tordjman S, Ferrari P, Golse B, et al. Dysharmonie psychotique et multiplex developmental disorder: histoire d'une convergence. Psychiatrie de l'enfant. 1997;2:473–504.
29. Turnbull A, Summers JA, Lee S-H, Kyzar K. Conceptualization and measurement of family outcomes associated with families of individuals with intellectual disabilities. Ment Retard Dev Disabil Res Rev. 2007;13:346–56.
30. Turnbull A, Turnbull R, Erwin E, Soodak L. Families, professionals, and exceptionality: positive outcomes through partnerships and trust. 5th ed. Upper Saddle River, NJ: Merrill/Prentice Hall; 2006.
31. Wehmeyer ML, Buntinx WH, Lachapelle Y, Luckasson RA, Schalock RL, Verdugo MA, Borthwick-Duffy S, Bradley V, Craig EM, Coulter DL, Gomez SC, Reeve A, Shogren KA, Snell ME, Spreat S, Tassé MJ, Thompson JR, Yeager MH. The intellectual disability construct and its relation to human functioning. Intellect Dev Disabil. 2008;46(4):311–8.
32. Winnicott D. The theory of the parent-infant relationship. Int J Psycho Anal. 1960;41:585–95.

Psychiatric and General Medical Comorbidity 33

Helen L. Millar, MBChB, MRCPsych and Ihsan M. Salloum, MD, MPH

33.1 Introduction

Multimorbidity, or the existence of several chronic disorders in one individual, has become a major public health concern. With the increase in prevalence of multimorbidity—the current challenges are the non-communicable diseases (NCDs)—particularly diabetes being described as a global epidemic. Health-care systems are already struggling to tackle expanding clinical workloads due to the ageing population with limited capacity and financial constraints in health-care systems worldwide. The current single disease model of delivering care is no longer sustainable given this changing climate and increasing demands for the management of multimorbidity [25].

Comorbidity is associated with high use of expensive health services leading to substantial financial burden on the individual and society. The WHO pronouncement that *Health is a state of complete physical, mental and social well-being, and not merely the absence of disease or infirmity* (World Health Organization 1948) and the global mental health strategy and the slogan emphasising that there is *no health without mental health* highlight the importance of the holistic and overall encompassing state of well-being of the individual to be described as *healthy* [28].

H.L. Millar, MBChB, MRCPsych (✉)
Consultant Psychiatrist, University of Dundee, Dundee, Scotland, UK;
Carseview Centre, 4 Tom McDonald, Dundee DD2 1NH, UK
e-mail: hlmillar1@gmail.com

I.M. Salloum, MD, MPH
Professor of Psychiatry, University of Miami School of Medicine, Miami, FL, USA;
Chair, Section on Classification, Diagnostic Assessment and Nomenclature,
World Psychiatric Association, Geneva, Switzerland

J.E. Mezzich et al. (eds.), *Person Centered Psychiatry*,
DOI 10.1007/978-3-319-39724-5_33

People suffering from long-term physical health conditions usually suffer from mental health problems and vice versa. It has been estimated that mortality in the mentally ill population is three to four times greater than in the general population and is predominantly due to cardiovascular disease with up to 30 years reduction in life expectancy [7].

33.2 Defining Comorbidity

Comorbidity, including muti-morbidity or "hyper-morbidity" has been conceptualised and defined in numerous ways over the last few decades [30]. It was originally introduced by Feinstein in 1970 to signify the coexistence of two or more diseases in the same patient [8]. This definition includes any relevant phenomena requiring clinical attention which may not be related to the index disease.

In general the term comorbidity has three meanings:

(1) Two or more coexisting but causally independent medical conditions. (2) Two or more coexisting medical conditions interdependently with each other where one medical condition is caused or otherwise related to the other condition. (3) Two or more medical conditions existing simultaneously regardless of causal relationship.

Grumbach [13] suggests that the term comorbidity should relate to the coexistence of two or more pathological conditions when one is predominant [13]. Starfield [34] suggested the term for the simultaneous presence of multiple health conditions when there is a clear index condition and other unrelated conditions [34]. Other authors have defined comorbidity as the simultaneous presence of diseases which are associated with one another through pathogenesis or more frequently than by chance in contrast to multimorbidity which refers to the presence of two or more conditions within one person without defining an index disease [14].

Goldberg [11] was first to consider that comorbidity may be better used to describe the existence of a physical condition accompanied by a mental illness [11].

Epidemiological studies have shown an increasing trend that comorbidity is a common phenomena particularly in the elderly population to the point where it has in fact been described as the norm in those over 65 years [35]. Although it is more common in this age group, it is now becoming increasingly common in the younger population, in those with mental health problems and in areas of socioeconomic deprivation and in low income countries [2].

33.3 The Burden of Physical and Mental Health Comorbidity

Non-communicable diseases (NCDs) and mental disorders constitute a large portion of the worldwide health-care burden and frequently occur together. The four primary NCDs are cardiovascular disease, Type 2 diabetes, cancers and chronic respiratory disorders [25]. Considerable progress has been made to estimate the extent to which mental disorders contribute to disease burden. Over the last 20 years, there has been a shift of disease burden, measured as Disability Adjusted Life Years (DALYs), from communicable diseases to NCDs, with neuropsychiatric disorders attributing to 28 % of the overall disease burden [28].

Importantly, studies have shown that NCDs share common risk factors namely poor diet, physical inactivity, tobacco use and harmful alcohol, exacerbated by mental health problems.

About 60 % of the excess mortality in the mentally ill population is attributed to physical health problems, predominantly cardiovascular diseases, despite an overall increased risk for completed suicide [7]. Evidence consistently demonstrates that people with long-term physical health problems are two to three times more likely to have mental health problems than the general population and overall estimates suggest that 30 % of all people with a long-term physical condition have mental health problems. Most of the evidence points to an excess in depression and anxiety disorders in this population [23].

In a Scottish cross-sectional study of 1,751,841 patients registered with 314 general medical practices, although the prevalence of multimorbidity increased substantially with age, the absolute number of people with multimorbidity was higher in those younger than 65 years of age. Of note multimorbidity occurred 10–15 years earlier in people living in the most deprived areas compared with affluent areas and socioeconomic deprivation was particularly associated with multimorbidity including mental health problems. The presence of mental health problems increased with the number of physical health problems and was more widespread in more deprived areas. It was highlighted that in the most 10 % deprived of the Scottish population, men have life expectancies 13 years shorter and women 9 years shorter that those in the most affluent 10 %. In addition, the most deprived spent twice as many years in poor health before they die than do the most affluent [2].

With multimorbidity, there is substantial increase in costs due to health service utilisation. International studies have demonstrated the financial impact of mental health comorbidity. Depression is associated with increased total medical costs for people with chronic conditions such as diabetes, asthma and congestive heart failure. Several studies have demonstrated that after controlling for the severity of the physical health condition, comorbid mental health problems are associated with 45–75 % increase in service cost [23].

In addition to the costs of medical care, comorbid mental health problems have wider economic consequences. Individuals with coexisting mental health problems are less likely to work, and productivity of those in employment is reduced. Higher levels of absenteeism are reported in those with diabetes and comorbid mental health problems than in those with diabetes alone [16].

Quality of life in this population has been examined using the health-related quality of life scores demonstrating a clear reduction in quality of life in those with coexisting mental and physical conditions [22]. Depression is highlighted as causing a reduced quality of life when coinciding with long-term physical conditions. Depression can compromise an individual's ability to cope and manage a physical health condition and therefore lead to an overall worsening of functional ability, prognosis and quality of life. This is highlighted in diabetes and depression with depression estimated at two to three times more likely in those with diabetes leading to more complications in managing the physical condition including poorer glycaemic control due to poorer compliance with pharmacotherapy and dietary/activity regime. In addition weight management becomes increasingly difficult due to poor motivation and non adherence to lifestyle interventions [9].

33.4 Links Between Mental and Physical Health: Risk Factors and Lifestyle Impact

There are a number of risk factors which contribute to comorbidity in the mentally ill population. There is increasing interest in the study of genetic factors and their contribution to the occurrence of comorbidity such as the link in genetic polymorphism affecting HTR2C and LEPR genotypes as possible predictors of weight gain and metabolic problems including diabetes mellitus. This is a rapidly developing area but practical application of this data is still a matter for future investigation [12].

Another emerging field of study is biomarker research and the possibility of identifying not only psychiatric but also somatic conditions and comorbidities that can have shared pathogenic mechanisms. A good example of this is the high comorbidity between depression and type 2 diabetes that prompted research into the effects of insulin in neurotransmission and neuroinflammation and its potential therapeutic use [1].

A landmark study by the Schizophrenia Working Group of the Psychiatric Genomics Consortium identified 108 schizophrenia-associated genetic loci providing new insights into the aetiology and associations with neurotransmission pathways supporting the hypothesised linkage between the immune system and schizophrenia and potential targets of therapeutic relevance in the field [10].

On a more practical level what is clear is that the modifiable risk factors including lifestyle and diet play a fundamental role in the well-being of the mentally ill and in determining the outcome of coexisting medical conditions.

It is well recognised that those with severe mental illness have a higher risk of obesity and therefore have shorter life spans. The extent of obesity varies with diagnosis. For example, studies have shown that those with schizophrenia have a 2.8–3.5 times increased likelihood of being obese compared to those with major depression who have an estimated 1.2–1.5 increased likelihood. Clinical research has suggested that those with a diagnosis of bipolar disorder are up to 68 % overweight or obese [7].

Obesity is associated with basic lifestyle factors such as poor diet and lack of exercise. Lifestyle is more likely to be sedentary in this population with less in the way of exercise or any physical activity due to the mental illness itself and at times due to the adverse effects of medication such as sedation. Osteoporotic changes are evident and more common with schizophrenia, schizoaffective disorders and major depression along with bipolar disorder. This can be due to the disease itself or dietary limitations in terms of Vitamin D deficiency, smoking, calcium deficiency and alcohol abuse. Antipsychotic induced hyperprolactinaemia has also been considered a further potential cause for osteoporosis but remains controversial.

Studies investigating the prevalence of cancers overall in the severely mentally ill (SMI) population have demonstrated conflicting results. The discrepancy in results may be due to the lack of screening and diagnosis in this population. For example, those with SMI are less likely to go for cancer screening. Of note there has been another hypothesis that antipsychotic medication may have an antitumour effect or that the disease itself may have a protective property. An important breakdown of cancers has found that obesity-related cancers such as endometrial, renal and bowel cancer are found more frequently in the SMI population and hence contribute to the increased premature mortality. Due to the controversial evidence for the role of prolactin in breast cancer rates, it had been assumed that exposure to prolactin raising dopamine antagonists would result in an increase in breast cancer in this population. Conflicting results have emerged and studies of the effects of typical antipsychotics showed no increased risk for breast cancer apart from a cohort described by Wang et al. [36].

Of note, diet in this population has been identified as particularly unhealthy with high levels of carbohydrate and processed foods, high levels of saturated fats and refined sugars along with low fibre. Poor dietary control can be due to a variety of factors including lack of nutritional education, poor motivation and at times lack of financial resources.

Smoking is a known risk factor for cancer, respiratory disease and circulatory disease which are all major causes for premature mortality among patients with a serious mental illness. Smoking rates amongst patients with a serious mental illness are significantly higher, estimated at around two to three times the general population and hence smoking is considered to be a major contributory factor to premature mortality in people with a serious mental illness. Oral hygiene and health in this population is poor with lack of attention to dental care. In addition medications including antipsychotics and antidepressants all cause xerostomia leading to caries, gingivitis and periodontal disease.

Sexual dysfunction in this population has received little attention with few systematic reviews in people with schizophrenia. Although there are few studies we do know that sexual dysfunction is more frequent in people with schizophrenia compared to the general population—affecting 30–80 % of women and 45–80 % of men. Dysfunction can be secondary to the disease itself but also due to physical comorbidities or adverse effects of antidepressant or antipsychotic medication with up to 70 % of those with depression describe sexual dysfunction [7].

Substance misuse including alcohol and drugs is much higher with high risk behaviour in sexual practices which also contribute to the higher risk of Hepatitis C, HIV and reduced immune function in this population. Chronic respiratory problems are increased with tuberculosis reported as particularly high in those with schizophrenia.

The most important contributor to reduced life expectancy is cardiovascular disease (CVD). The preponderance of evidence suggests that people with bipolar disorder, schizophrenia and major depression are at significantly higher risk of cardiovascular disease and mortality. The prevalence of CVD in those with schizophrenia and bipolar disorder is two- to threefold higher than the general population.

Patients with schizophrenia are three times more likely to experience sudden cardiac disease compared to the general population. QTC intervals of > 500 ms or an absolute increase of 60 ms compared to the drug free state puts a patient at significant risk of Torsade de pointes syndrome, ventricular fibrillation and sudden death. Patients on certain antipsychotic and antidepressant medications have an increased risk of QTC prolongation and are therefore at risk for these cardiac abnormalities.

The cluster of risk factors for cardiovascular disease and increased insulin resistance is described as metabolic syndrome. Although there has been increasing controversy over whether metabolic syndrome in itself is a distinct diagnosis there is a general global consensus that metabolic syndrome is characterised by central obesity with hypertension, dyslipidaemia and glucose intolerance or insulin resistance. Despite the controversy over the term there continues to be a healthy debate in the literature which will hopefully stimulate further innovative research in the area. More importantly perhaps, clinicians still appear to consider its continued use in practice as a helpful tool to quantify cardiovascular and metabolic risk in patients. Rates of metabolic syndrome have been evaluated in numerous international studies in cohorts of people with bipolar disorder and schizophrenia estimated at a prevalence of 22–30 % and 42 %, respectively [7].

With the shift to atypical antipsychotics, there has been a further advancement in pharmacotherapy for those with severe mental health problems who require long-term medication. The shift to the atypical or second generation drugs presents different challenges in terms of adverse effects profile. The older medications primarily caused movement disorders along with the physical effects of hyperprolactinaemia, i.e. galactorrhea, gynaecomastia and infertility amongst other adverse effects.

The atypical medications are a heterogeneous group of drugs, each with its own weighting of adverse effects profile in terms of cardiovascular and metabolic problems. Weight gain liability has been a concern with some of the second generation drugs.

Included in the higher risk agents for obesity are clozapine and olanzapine with intermediate risk agents risperidone and quetiapine, and asenapine, amisulpiride, ziprasidone and aripiprazole classified as lower risk agents. Mood stabilisers such as lithium and sodium valproate have also been considered as risk agents for weight gain [24, 26].

The World Health Organisation estimates that diabetes will affect more than 350 million persons worldwide by 2030 with the number doubling from the year 2000. The risk of diabetes mellitus in the SMI population is approximately two- to three-fold compared to the general population overall. Both genetic and lifestyle factors contribute to the likelihood as well as the disease itself and treatments. Overall taking into account all factors, the research suggests that those with a diagnosis of schizophrenia have an increased prevalence of diabetes of four to five times the general population with the higher rate in the older populations [5].

Some atypical medications cause an increased risk of diabetes mellitus with clozapine, olanzapine and risperidone viewed as high risk and others such as quetiapine amisulpiride and aripiprazole with no significant increase [3]. The higher individual variability in medication induced weight gain suggests that there are genetic factors at play. For example, studies have shown that HTR2C and LEPR polymorphisms are genetic predictors of weight gain. Although the results are promising this area requires further research for practical application [12].

Certain antidepressants, such as the tricyclic and SSRI groups, carry a risk of weight gain due to increased appetite and sedation. Mood stabilisers such as sodium valproate and lithium also have a propensity for weight gain [7].

33.5 Barriers to Management of Comorbidity in the Mentally Ill and Their Consequences

With the increasing fragmentation in health-care systems across the primary and secondary sectors and financial constraints the burden continues to grow. The need to coalesce research studies with clinical application and impact on early interventions with a view to improvement in outcomes requires acknowledgement and further support.

There are major challenges for the current health-care systems when an individual presents with a myriad of symptoms and at times no clear diagnosis of the index disease process in terms of either the mental or physical health condition.

There can be a number of health and social care providers as well as multiple health disciplines and agencies co-opted making it difficult to coordinate care arrangements and manage medications. It has also been noted by individuals who present with multimorbidity that despite their best motivation and intention to engage in self care it can be very difficult for them to navigate the complex health systems and just to survive and maintain both their mental and physical well-being. Time constraints for practitioners with limited budgets and ever increasing “targets” only add to the burden. Overall lack of investment in mental health-care systems has resulted in a lack of development in services to manage this population who present with complex coexisting conditions.

It is evident that people with SMI are less likely to seek care and access available services. In addition once the service has been accessed, it is also very difficult to adhere to lifestyle programmes including dietary and exercise/activity regimes.

There is considerable lack of awareness among clinicians of the importance of treating the patient as a whole and consider physical comorbid issues. At times psychiatrists feel overwhelmed with the complexity of physical comorbidities and ill equipped to manage the ongoing assessment, monitoring and medications associated with specific diseases and to treat the whole person.

Some primary care physicians feel they lack knowledge of psychotropic medications with potential adverse effects and the negative impact on a coexisting comorbid physical condition. There is still a recognised stigma for those with mental illness attending mainstream primary and secondary care services. As a result, ongoing screening and monitoring remains patchy and inconsistent within the primary care sector resulting in late diagnosis and worse prognosis.

There can also be a tendency for primary care physicians to view physical health problems as psychosomatic in this population which at times can lead to under investigation and suboptimal intervention and treatment. There is evidence that diabetic patients with mental health problems are less likely to receive standard care resulting in poorer glycaemic control. Overall studies show a delay in diagnosis with prolonged exposure to raised blood glucose levels leading to an increased risk of physical complications such as visual impairment and renal damage [7].

Hence the lack of integration in the current health systems has resulted in a lack of 'joined up' care for those presenting with mental health problems and comorbid physical conditions.

The patient with comorbid mental and physical problems often describes a very difficult journey feeling unsupported with a lack of coordination between hospital and primary care appointments leading to confusion in the organisation of polypharmacy associated with the management of complex coexisting conditions. Lifestyle changes can be very difficult to make due to poor motivation and sedation from medication leading to a reluctance to engage and actively participate in healthy lifestyle programmes. Adherence to medication can be difficult due to lack of understanding of medication, the requirement for different medications and also due to adverse effects which patients find at times unacceptable but unwilling to discuss.

As a result of the above factors, the patient with mental and physical comorbidity often faces a greater symptom burden, limited physical and psychological functioning and a reduced quality of life.

Poor coordination in care and an increased prevalence of clinical errors are reported in the care of this population as a result of the out of date single disease model of health-care delivery and complex polypharmacy.

33.6 The Way Forward

There are two main reasons why multimorbidity has become so visible. The increasing numbers in the ageing population with multimorbidity represent a major challenge and cost burden to the health-care system. Second, practitioners have great difficulty coping with the management of complex coexisting diseases in a single disease model with check lists/national guidelines provided for one presenting disease only [29].

33.7 Global Perspective

There is growing evidence to support the view that by addressing the mental health needs of those people with chronic long-term medical conditions, effective improvements will be possible in both their mental and physical well-being and their quality of life will improve. Unsurprisingly many people with mental disorders and chronic conditions do not receive the appropriate care—it is estimated that around 1–2 out of 10 in low or middle income countries has a chance of receiving treatment for their mental health condition.

The WHO Global action plan 2013–2020 for the prevention and control of non-communicable diseases outlines clearly a strategy focusing on policy development through strong national advocacy with guidance and support on implementation of programmes with monitoring and evaluation. The plan emphasises the need to promote health by reducing or preventing the exposure to risk factors such as tobacco, alcohol, drugs and other psychoactive substances, unhealthy diets, physical inactivity and unsafe sex. The focus is on building capacity to deliver an integrated, comprehensive multidisciplinary and multi sectorial approach across all programmes using ethical and evidence-based policies and practices including interventions, recommendations, standards and guidelines to reduce the occurrence of major risk factors—overall, a healthy environment to support the individual to make healthy choices [37].

The aim is to provide the appropriate governance structures with targets based on the national situation to reduce the exposure to risk factors through cost-effective and affordable interventions and monitor the progress of outcomes and the health system response. Results need to be collected on national information systems to ensure complete data to inform global analyses.

Evidence to date regarding treatment shows that clinical trials are usually designed to exclude multimorbidity and the elderly population and therefore there is less of an evidence base for the management of those with multimorbidities. Therefore, more is needed in the way of research to examine effectively a more typical population rather than a highly selected sample which is unrepresentative of the population at large. Additionally, guidelines need to include multimorbidity to help clinicians to prioritise treatments and manage the inevitable polypharmacy.

An integrated response to mental disorders and NCDs has been outlined by the WHO [38] which has been developed as a response to the fundamental connection between mental disorders and other chronic health conditions and the implications for mental health-care being integrated with general health care. The paper emphasises the challenge as not simply scaling up healthcare systems but the need for the transformation of health-care systems by implementing evidence-based approaches for integrated, effective and efficient care for those with mental disorders and other chronic disorders.

The principles include:

- Public health approach focusing on disease prevention and health promotion as well as delivery of health services
- A systems approach—including good governance, appropriate resourcing and timely information
- A whole government and multi sectorial approach

Mental disorders and other chronic diseases have common determinants and co-occur with the mental disorders at times being the precursor of a further chronic disorder with a knock on effect in terms of public, social and economic impact. For example diabetes and depression share a high disease burden, stigma and premature death along with profound effects on economic productivity and opportunities. Unfortunately when there is a comorbid mental and physical condition the levels of disability are greater than the additive effect of the two. In particular depression combined with one or more condition is associated with the worst health status overall.

Despite the increasing awareness in multimorbidity, there is an under diagnosis of comorbid conditions. Current mental health-care systems do not consider that the detection and management of chronic physical conditions falls within their remit and the converse is also true. A lot of the time this is due to lack of training and support and reportedly lack of time and pressure of workloads. This could also be due to the current prevailing model of care with heightened emphasis on specialised acute care, single disease focus.

Integration of services has to take place at various levels. At the micro level the service must be person-centred that is the service is focused and coordinated from a patient's perspective. At the meso level information systems are required within the health-care system along with professional partnerships and shared competencies, responsibilities, roles and accountability to provide a comprehensive infrastructure to deliver a continuation of health and social care from hospital into the community. At macro-level government policy, financing and shared governance is crucial.

The WHO has reviewed the chronic care model with additional roles in the community and macro-systems to improve outcomes.

At a patient level, it is crucial that the person is at the centre of the care, and not the disease model, guided by a care pathway based on a collaborative multidisciplinary model of care to deliver a comprehensive integrated package of care.

To achieve this working model of care and optimise self management support, it is crucial that health-care teams are trained in the assessment and management of comorbid conditions. This collaborative care model is an evidence-based approach to improve the management of mental disorders and comorbid chronic conditions. Key elements include the following: identification of those in need, a multidisciplinary team approach with a case manager; a clear pathway with integration across primary care and secondary care professionals, regular systematic review of caseloads, holistic care plans and electronic records with shared information to monitor treatment using validated clinical rating scales [38].

33.8 Examples of Integrated Person-Centred Collaborative Care

A recent Cochrane review has highlighted the effectiveness of this approach across a range of mental disorders including PTSD, depression and anxiety. The TEAMcare model has successfully targeted those with coexisting physical conditions such as diabetes, cardiovascular disease and hyperlipidaemia [17].

Stepped care models within primary care use a low intensity input intervention and build up a care package as required after systematic monitoring to maximise the efficiency of resources, reserving specialist complex interventions for the most complex and severe mental health problems [27].

Adequate training remains a challenge globally to deliver such integrated packages of care across mental and physical coexisting conditions. The DDD (Diabetes and Depression Dialogue) is an international collaborative effort addressing the problems related to the comorbidity of depression and diabetes. As part of its training remit the Diabetes and Depression Africa Nurse Training programme was developed out of the identified needs recognised in the Sub-Saharan area of Africa for these coexisting conditions. This programme was an example of a unique innovative educational programme about comorbidity with a practical clinical approach to enable nurses to screen, recognise and treat diabetes and depression in Sub-Saharan Africa while promoting a patient-centred collaborative approach model with early recognition and management of these comorbid conditions to improve outcomes and life expectancy in this population [21].

Locally driven health screening programmes for those with severe mental illness and coexisting physical health problems have been evolving with the plethora of guidelines and consensus statements in the field. Despite improved global awareness, consistent systematised screening and early interventions remain mostly inadequate in the majority of health-care systems. The Dundee Health Screening Clinic in Scotland was an example of an early integrated holistic multidisciplinary approach to provide health screening and lifestyle interventions for those with severe and enduring mental health problems from a highly deprived urban population—all happening 'under one roof' in a community mental health resource centre to allow easy access for the patient population [20]. The clinic was designed to address the gap in service provision for this vulnerable population by coordinating health screening and ensuring regular, structured follow-up appointments and a care pathway back to both primary care and other specialist services. The multidisciplinary screening team included a collaborative approach with medical and nursing staff, physiotherapy and occupational therapy and advice from dietetics and pharmacy on an as required basis. Staff attended training sessions to enhance knowledge of coexisting medical conditions to improve reliability and consistency of clinical measurements and investigations. This clinic scored highly on user satisfaction questionnaires and was an early example of a cost neutral (no extra staff employed) practical development addressing the needs of a highly deprived population with high levels of comorbidity and how a simple coordinated approach can be used to improve the overall well-being of this patient population [6, 15].

Comorbidity is perhaps the single area of medicine that most clearly demonstrates the inadequacy of currently prevailing models of care [31]. The above experiences of integrated care were developed in response to the recognition of the challenges posed by comorbidity and to the limitations of a care model overly focused on a specialised, single disease, acute care approach. These experiences represent a paradigm shift towards a comprehensive consideration of patients' presenting problems, emphasising care coordination and shared decision making.

Person-centred medicine is an emerging approach to care that articulates the person in context as the centre and goal for care and public health [18, 32]. This approach amplifies, makes explicit and operationalizes the consideration of the totality of the health status of the person presenting for care, including ill health as well as positive aspects of health and well-being [4, 19] including the contributors to health (ill and positive health) in a bio-psycho-social frame work. It empowers the therapeutic relationship by viewing the health-care process as a partnership between the person presenting for care, significant others and other health stakeholders and the health-care providers and it emphasises the subjective experiences of health for the protagonists of the health-care encounter. It emphasises health preservation, prevention and health restoration at the individual and community levels [18, 32]. The integrative person-centred diagnostic model operationalizes this paradigm shift into a diagnostic model articulating the integrative and dynamic interplay among the different domains of the health status and the diagnostic process [33].

33.9 Conclusions

Mental disorders and other physical health conditions frequently coexist and have much in common including causes, duration and course. There is a growing concern that there are cumulative effects related to this coexistence leading to a high burden of disease and health-care cost to the individual and society.

The problem appears to be a global phenomenon with more severe levels in low to middle income societies and also in deprived areas of high income countries. Treatment gaps are clear with a lack of integrated collaborative models of care and shortfalls in service delivery. Redesign of education and training programmes for professionals is also required to meet this challenge and contribute to effective implementation of evidence- and experience-informed collaborative holistic models of care.

Further research is needed on how best to achieve true integration in an already overburdened health-care system and how best to support health-care workers to deliver a person-centred model of care which is coordinated to meet the needs of the individual with complex physical and mental health conditions. Providing preventative and health promotional person-centred holistic seamless care, engaging the individuals and the populations involved is essential. It is the only way to address the challenge of comorbidity, to prevent and manage chronic long-term diseases, including mental disorders and achieve long-term benefits to both society and the individual in terms of improved mental and physical well-being.

References

1. Bagdy G, Juhasz G. Biomarkers for personalised treatment in psychiatric diseases. Expert Opinion; Informa Healthcare. Med Dian. 2013;7(5):417–422.
2. Barnett K, Mercer SW, Norbury M, Watt G, Wyke S, Guthrie B. Epidemiolgy of multimorbidity and implications for healthcare, research, and medical education: a cross sectional study. Lancet. 2012;380(9836):37–43. doi:10.1016/S0140-6736(12)60240-2.
3. Citrome LL, et al. Risk of treatment/emergent diabetes mellitus in patients receiving antipsychotics. Ann Pharmacother. 2007;41:1593–603.
4. Cloninger CR, Salloum IM, Mezzich JE. The dynamic origins of positive health and wellbeing. Int J Person Centered Med. 2012;2(2):179–87.
5. Danaei G, Finucane MM, Lu Y, Singh GM, Cowan MJ, Paciorek CJ, et al. National, regional, and global trends in fasting plasma glucose and diabetes prevalence since 1980: systematic analysis of health examination surveys and epidemiological studies with 370 country-years and 2.7 million participants. Lancet. 2011;378(9785):31–40.
6. Deakin B. et al. The physical health challenges in patients with severe mental illness: cardiovascular and metabolic risks. J Psychopharmacol. 2010;24(8).
7. De Hert M, et al. Physical Illness in patients with severe mental disorders II: Barriers to care, monitoring and treatment guidelines, plus recommendations at the system and individual level. World Psychiatry. 2011;10:52–77.
8. Feinstein A. The pre-therapeutic classification of co-morbidity in chronic disease. J Chronic Dis. 1970;23:455–68.
9. Fenton WS, Stover ES. Mood disorders: cardiovascular and diabetes comorbidity. Curr Opin Psychiatry. 2006;19(no4):421–7.
10. Flint J, Munafo M. Schizophrenia: genesis of a complex disease. Nature. 2014;511:412–3.
11. Goldberg D. The need for a special classification of mental disorders for general medical practice; towards ICD 11—primary care. Eur Psychiatry. 2011;26:53–6.
12. Gregoor JG, van der Weide J, Mulder W, et al. Polymorphism of the LEP- and LEPR gene and obesity in patients using antipsychotic medication. J Clin Psychopharmacol. 2009;26:21–5.
13. Grumbach K. Chronic illness, co-morbidities and the need for medical generalism. Ann Family Med. 2003;1:4–7.
14. Harrison C, et al. Examining different measures of multimorbidity, using a large prospective cross-sectional study in Australian genral practice. BMJ Open. 2014;4:e004694. doi:10.1136/bmjopen-2013-004694.
15. Heald AL, Montejo A, Millar HL, Hert M, McCrae J, Correll C. Physical health in patients with schizophrenia: current knowledge and practical recommendations. Management of physical health in patients with schizophrenia: practical recommendations. J Eur Psychiatric Assoc. 2010;25(2):S1–S46.
16. Hutter N, Schnurr A, Baumeister H. Healthcare costs in patients with diabetes and comorbid mental disorders—a systematic review. Diabetiologia. 2010;53(12):2470–9.
17. Katon WJ, et al. Multi-conditional collaborative care for chronic illnesses and depression. New Engl J. 2010;363:2611–20.
18. Mezzich JE, Salloum IM, Cloninger CR, Salvador-Carulla L, Kirmayer LJ, Banzato CEM, Wallcraft J, Botbol M. Person-centred integrative diagnosis: conceptual bases and structural model. Can J Psychiatry (Revue Canadienne de Psychiatrie). 2010;55(11):701–8.

19. Mezzich JE, Salloum IM. Comorbidity, positive health, and integration of services. In: Salloum IM, Mezzich JE, editors. Psychiatric diagnosis: challenges and prospects. Oxford, UK: Wiley-Blackwell; 2009.
20. Millar HL. The burden of multimorbidity: physical health in the severely mentally ill population. Die Psychiatrie. 2012.
21. Millar HL, Cimino L, van der Merwe AS. The dialogue on diabetes and depression African Nursing Training Programme: a collaborative training initiative to improve the recognition and management of diabetes and depression in Sub-Saharan Africa. In: Sartorius N, Maj M, Holt R, editors. Management of Comorbidity of Mental and Physical Illness. Key Issues Mental Health. Basel, Karger 2015, 179, pp 148–156.
22. Moussavi S, Chatterji S, Verdes E, Tandon A, Patel V, Ustun B. Depression, chronic diseases and decrements in health: results from the World Health Surveys. Lancet. 2007;370 (9590):851–8.
23. Naylor C, Parsonage M, McDaid D, Knapp M, Fossey M, Galea A. Long-term conditions and mental health: the cost of co-morbidities. The King's Fund for Mental Health 2012.
24. Newcomer JW. Second-generation (atypical) antipsychotics and metabolic effects. A comprehensive literature review. CNS Drugs. 2005;19:1–93.
25. Ngo VK, Rubenstein A, Ganju V, Kanellis P, Loza N, Rabadan C, Daar AS. Grand challenges: integrating mental health care into the non-communicable disease agenda. PLOS Med. 2013;10(5):e 1001443. doi:10.1371/journal.pmed.1001443.
26. Papakostas GI. The efficacy, tolerability and safety of contemporary antidepressants. J Clin Psychiatry. 2010;71:e03.
27. Patel V, et al. Effectiveness of an intervention led by lay health counsellors for depression and anxiety disorders in primary care in Goa, India (MANAS): a cluster randomised controlled trial. Lancet. 2010;376(9758):2088–95.
28. Prince M, Patel V, Shekhar S, Maj M, Maselko J, Philips MR, Rahman A, Maselko J. No heath without mental health. Lancet. 2007;370(9590):859–877. doi:10.1016/S0140-6736(07) 61238-0.
29. Salisbury C. Multimorbidity: redesigning healthcare for people who use it. Lancet. 2012;. doi:10.1016/S0140-6736(12)60482-6.
30. Salloum IM, Mezzich JE, Cordoba SE. Conceptual and methodological considerations in comorbidity. In: Salloum IM, Mezzich JE, editors. Psychiatric diagnosis: challenges and prospects. Oxford, UK: Wiley-Blackwell; 2009.
31. Salloum IM, Abou-Saleh MT, Krasnov V. Comorbidity, psychiatric diagnosis and the person-centered integrative diagnostic model. Int J Person Centered Med. 2012;2(2):168–72.
32. Salloum IM, Mezzich JE. Outlining the bases of person-centred integrative diagnosis. J Eval Clin Practice. 2011;17(2):354–6.
33. Salloum IM, Mezzich JE. Person-centered diagnosis. Int J Integr Care. 2010;10(Suppl):e027.
34. Starfield B. Thread and yarns: weaving the tapestry of co-morbidity. Ann Family Med. 2006;4:101–3.
35. Taylor A, Price K, Gill T, et al. Multimorbidity—not just an older person's issues: results from an Australian biomedical study. BMC Public Health. 2010;10:718.
36. Wang PS, et al. Dopamine antagonism and the development of breast cancer. Arch Gen Psychiatry. 2002;59:1147–54.
37. World Health Action Plan 2013–2020: Global Action Plan for the Prevention and Control of NCDs 2013-202.
38. World Health Organisation and Calouste Gulbenkian Foundation. Integrating the response to mental disorders and other chronic diseases in health care systems. Geneva: World Health Organisation; 2014.

Part V
Special Topics

Spiritualiy, Science and Person-Centred Care

34

John Cox, MD, Alison Gray, MD, Mohammed T. Abou-Saleh, MD, PhD, Roy Abraham Kallivayalil, MD, DPM, MAMS, Sam Pfeifer, MD and Alexander Moreira-Almeida, MD

34.1 Introduction

Spiritual and religious practices are important in most peoples' lives around the world. The sense that there is more to life than what we can grasp, measure and control is common. Spiritual practices and religious belief (R/S) are regarded as purveyors of culture, and understanding of these is intimately linked to the maintenance of health and the experience of illness. They cannot be ignored in any comprehensive person-centred assessment even in secular cultures. Researchers have produced over 3300 empirical studies on the connection between R/S and health. Findings show an association between R/S and health outcomes, mostly positive [31, 33]. Most patients want clinicians to address R/S, but few do [17, 35].

J. Cox, MD (✉)
Professor Emeritus, Keele University, 58 St. Stephen's Rd, Cheltenham, Gloucestershire GL513AE, UK
e-mail: john1.cox@virgin.net

A. Gray, MD
Cadbury Centre, Birmingham University, Birmingham, UK

M.T. Abou-Saleh, MD, PhD
Professor of Psychiatry, St George's School of Medicine, University of London, London, UK

R.A. Kallivayalil, MD, DPM, MAMS
Professor of Psychiatry, Pushpagiri Institute of Medical Sciences, Tiruvalla, Kerala, India

S. Pfeifer, MD
Professor of Psychotherapy and Psychiatry, Psychiatric Clinic Sonnenhalde, Riehen/Basel, Switzerland

A. Moreira-Almeida, MD
Associate Professor of Psychiatry, School of Medicine, Federal University of Juiz de Fora, Minas Gerais, Brazil

J.E. Mezzich et al. (eds.), *Person Centered Psychiatry*,
DOI 10.1007/978-3-319-39724-5_34

Since clinicians need to assess and learn how to deal with all factors that impact health, we need to deal with R/S in clinical practice, regardless of whether we are religious, antireligious or agnostic. Worldwide important health organisations have created sections on R/S and/or recommend assessing R/S in clinical practice.

34.2 Definitions of R/S in a Post-Modern World

Existential questions such as: What is true reality? Is there intelligence behind the universe? How then should I live? have been asked and answered throughout the ages. Different societies have developed their own world views, which give a coherent answer to such questions, and form the cultural basis for daily life [25]. About 84 % of the world's population self-identify is 'religiously affiliated' [53]. A further percentage of those unaffiliated would describe themselves as 'spiritual but not religious', hence for many of our patients R/S will be a significant part of their lives. In the Western democracies the secularism hypothesis—that societies inevitably become less religious as they develop [9]—has been challenged by the heightened visibility of religious groups and the recognition of the social capital found in communities of faith [16, 24].

Formerly in English, 'spiritual' referred to those who were highly committed to their religion. 'Spiritual' would not have made sense outside of a community of faith and practice. In the last 30 years 'spiritual' has become a separate category, often placed in opposition to religion. Thus spirituality is considered warm, friendly and inclusive, religion is seen as cold, hard and rule bound. Many, particularly in high-income countries, would now say that they are spiritual but not religious [15] or neither spiritual nor religious.

Multiple definitions of spirituality are found in the research literature. Some of the definitions focus on existential meaning [51]. Other definitions of spirituality are broader and include aspects of positive mental health [54]. Researchers need to be careful that any definition of spirituality does not exclude those with severe and enduring mental illness (SEMI); spiritual practices are often cited as helpful in recovery from SEMI [11].

In many definitions of spirituality aspects of positive mental health are subsumed within the definition [41], this inclusiveness is useful in clinical practice to draw attention to a significant area of life [66]. However, it makes 'spirituality' difficult to research; it is very easy to 'prove' that spirituality is good for your mental health if this is assumed in the definition of spirituality. Given these problems most researchers look at religion rather than spirituality, investigating the dimensions of religious belief, religious practice and individual spiritual experiences.

Religion refers to a collection of beliefs, practices and rituals related to the transcendent and sacred, arising out of an established tradition and from a community with common beliefs and practices. The definition of religion can be more easily operationalised for research purposes and allows for replication of research results in different populations. Most of the research on religion and health has come from North America and reflects the effect of religious involvement in a democracy where religion is highly regarded. Caution is needed when comparing results internationally, since countries vary in their tolerance of religious diversity, and the social implications of holding a minority world view differ from being in the majority; the experience of being Muslim in Cairo is different to being Muslim in Canberra. One would predict that religious adherence might have a different impact on the individual's health depending on the country studied. However, the major findings have been fairly consistent in more recent studies, throughout cultures and countries [33].

34.3 Research on Spirituality/Religion and Health

Research into the impact of religion and spirituality on health has developed and broadened over the last 20 years, with clarification of terms and approaches. Much of the research follows Evidence-Based Medicine, investigating the spiritual practices or religion as if they were a medication. A systematic review of double-blind placebo-controlled trials of the intervention would be the gold standard [49]. Clearly, it would not be practical or ethical to undertake randomised trials of religious faith and experience. When RCT are not feasible, longitudinal cohort studies can provide good quality evidence, and there are several such studies in this field [33]. Most early papers on religion and health were cross-sectional so could only demonstrate an association, being hard to define causal direction. For example, if we find that the number of currently depressed people is higher in the temple than in the general community this could mean temple attendance makes you depressed, or it could mean that people turn to their religious roots when depressed.

Religious commitment level can be established through religious activities (e.g. time spent in prayer or meditation, attendance at meetings, reading scriptures) [33]. However, simply measuring frequency of attendance at religious services and rituals conflates those who are 'true believers' and those who are 'just going along with the crowd'. We have to differentiate between those who are personally invested and committed to the religion for its own sake, and those who attend the worship place purely for social and business reasons, since the health impact may vary. This is the difference between intrinsic and extrinsic religiosities [2].

There are many scales looking at different aspects of R/S [36]. For example, Duke University Religion Index (DUREL), has 5 items, and the more comprehensive Brief Multidimensional Measure of Religiousness/Spirituality (BMMRS) has 38 items covering 11 dimensions of R/S. The WHO Quality of Life questionnaire (WHOQOL-SRPB) briefly covers spiritual, religious and personal beliefs [60].

34.4 What Do We Know About the Impact of R/S on Health in General, and Mental Health in Particular?

Much of the research and debate on religion and spirituality has come from the US, which remains a predominantly religious nation. [22]. In the US those who attend church services regularly are less likely to die in the next year than non-attenders, controlled for physical health [37]. In a large US poll, Jewish people reported the highest well-being, those with no religious adherence the lowest well-being [22].

A US study followed up over 30 years showed a correlation between attending religious services weekly, living healthier lives and being more likely to recover from depression [63]. There is a correlation between various indices of religiousness and speedier recovery from depression associated with physical illness [32]. A cohort study of over 7000 elders in the US shows that the more religious are less likely to develop depression and more likely to recover from an episode [56]. In a US longitudinal study of 114 10-year-old children those who identified that R/S were important to them had one-quarter the risk of major depression over the next 10 years. Those who had a high risk for depression, because one of their parents had experienced depression, had one-tenth the illness rate of those who did not value R/S [39]. African-Americans have one-third lower rates of depression than whites matched on demographic and health behaviours. This variance can be explained by attendance at religious services [55]. High salience of religion correlates with less prevalence of depression in Palestinian Muslim youth [5], Australian elders [50], Brazilian bipolar patients [64] and Dutch adults [38].

Several studies have shown that those who adhere strongly to a religion are at a lower risk of suicide than those with weaker or no faith. A large US case control study showed attendance at religious activities had a protective effect against suicide in a 'dose-dependent' manner [48]. A cohort study with a US nationally representative sample (n = 20,014) showed that frequent religious attendees were 68 % less likely to die by suicide over the next 16 years [30].

34.5 Religion and Psychosis

A recent review article shows a mixed picture on the interactions of religion, spirituality and schizophrenia [28], with spiritual practices being valued by patients in their recovery, but often seeming to contribute to late presentation and poor treatment concordance. US caregivers generally perceive religion as helpful to those with schizophrenia [62]. For patients with SEMI, involvement in communities of faith, when not driven by psychopathology, predicts better outcomes [7, 40, 67].

34.6 Religious Coping and Stress

At times of difficulty people commonly turn to spiritual practices for support, comfort and inspiration, e.g. Buddhist practices after the South Asian Tsunami [29]. Abrahamic practices after the 9/11 attacks in the US [58] and Japanese religions after the 2011 earthquake [46]. Religious coping is important in different physical illnesses [33]. The frequency of religious coping in a country parallels the numbers who indicate 'religion is important to me' [13]; the highest rates on this poll were in the Middle East and Asia, slightly lower in the US, with the lowest scores in Scandinavia. Moroccan Muslim religious practices were increased in 95 % of 1600 people following first cancer diagnosis [19], whereas in Demark 74.2 % of 97 patients following a myocardial infarction said they received 'no comfort whatsoever' from religion [6]. Religion helped children to cope with PTSD in Switzerland [70] and being an adolescent refugee from Bosnia Herzegovina [65].

34.7 Spiritual Experiences

Although spiritual experiences (SE) are found in the origins of most spiritual traditions and are still prevalent nowadays, this subject has received much less attention from researchers. Studies on SE can have significant clinical and theoretical implications. From the clinical perspective, SE may impact mental health and may resemble dissociative and psychotic symptoms (e.g. trances, hearing voices, visions). SE are usually not related to mental disorders and some criteria have been proposed to differentiate SE from mental disorders with religious content such as: lack of suffering, lack of social or functional impairment, compatibility with the patient's cultural background and recognition by others, absence of psychiatric comorbidities (negative or disorganisation symptoms), control over the experience, and personal growth over time [42].

The neurobiological correlates of SE and their implications for the understanding of mind–brain relationship have been examined. Trance and meditative states have revealed complex patterns of brain activation discarding more simplistic views such as the "God spot" [52]. SE such as meditation, mediumship, end of life and near death experiences, often involve altered states of consciousness, reports of anomalous experiences and of consciousness beyond the body. So, these SE may provide the empirical basis for advancing the debates regarding mind–brain relationships [43].

34.8 Mechanisms of Interaction Between Spirituality, Religion and Health

The following factors are important (after [12]):

(a) Communities of faith provide social and emotional support, particularly for those living with mental illness or learning disabilities.
(b) Religious groups provide practical and economic support.
(c) Attendance at religious meetings and services keep people physically active.
(d) Many religious and spiritual traditions teach against risk behaviours—sexual promiscuity, alcohol excess and drug usage.
(e) Religion and spirituality are positively associated with relationship stability, positive personality and psychological traits [33], purpose and meaning in life [69] and increased social capital [34].

(f) Religions generally provide a narrative of hope and eventual positive outcome. Such positive emotions and cognitions are linked to better immune, endocrine and cardiovascular functioning [33].

34.9 Negative Effect of R/S on Health and Well-Being

Religion may have negative effects on health. Specific teachings may discourage using modern medicine, e.g. the Jehovah's Witness prohibition on blood transfusion, and avoidance of psychiatric care by Scientologists [27]. Mental illness may be misidentified by religious teachers as weakness, wrongdoing or spiritual failings leading to feelings of guilt and failure. Major mental illness may be misidentified as possession by spirits, demons or *djinn*; the practices to free the person from such spirits can lead to distress and suffering, as well as delaying definitive treatment. Predatory leaders occur in all human groups, particularly those with weaker accountability structures, e.g. new religious movements. Religious fundamentalism sometimes leads to terrorist violence, however many instances of alleged religious war or terrorism actually reflects political, economic and other social conflicts [4]. Whilst many have suffered from intolerant religious groups, we would maintain that such deplorable things are considerably overwhelmed by the positive impact of the religions, in terms of personal and community quality of life, political activity and voluntary work [8].

34.10 Religion and Spirituality in Medical History

Islamic medicine flourished over 1000 years ago and was the most advanced in the world at that time. The mentally ill were cared for in the general hospital, the first of which was established in Baghdad in the ninth century followed by hospitals in Damascus, Aleppo and in Cairo [1]. The Bimaristan Al-Arghun in Aleppo is considered the most remarkable example of both Islamic architecture and the oldest hospital in the world [23]. It was converted from a princely palace into a hospital for the insane in the fourteenth century, where they were treated with humanity, music, dance and theatre performances as well as the scent of flowers, gurgling of fountains and harmonious architecture.

Ancient Indian philosophies including Upanishads are rich in their references to the theme of spirituality and health [14]. Charaka who had practiced and taught 'Ayurveda' (the 'Science of life') in ancient India had referred to positive mental health and had said absence of disease alone is not sufficient, but leading an ideal life should be the goal. Spirituality is deeply embedded in the Indian and South Asian culture, so much so, that the practice of mental health and psychiatry without understanding the strong spiritual foundations will not be ideal [61].

In Europe many hospitals were built from the Christian imperative to 'love your neighbour as yourself', and were often staffed by people with religious motivation and sustaining of their caring role. Nursing sisters were originally literally sisters of a Christian religious order—nuns, or deaconesses, including Florence Nightingale. Many American and Canadian hospitals were founded by nursing nuns [47]. In Brazil, Spiritist hospitals provide much of the inpatient mental healthcare for the poorest [57].

34.11 Implications of Faith and Spirituality for Person-Centred Medicine

All the world religions provide a metaphysical framework to develop and sustain care and compassion [3]. A failure of compassion was named in the enquiry into a recent UK hospital scandal [20]. Compassion entails thinking, feeling and will. We intellectually recognise when someone is suffering, we emotionally 'feel their pain' and we choose to act to relieve their suffering. Empathy requires self-awareness and sensitivity to others; Compassion adds in the specific desire to act to relieve suffering [26]. Basic counselling skills should be taught to all practitioners, time made available to truly care for patients, and staff be supported and cared for as well as patients, through individual and small group work [59]. Any neglect of the R/S dimension to health care provision is a degradation of those key tasks of medicine linked to care, recovery and compassion.

One model of person-centred primary health care was developed by a general practitioner in Geneva, Paul Tournier (1898–1986). Having suffered in his own life, he saw the suffering of his patients not only in the biomedical dimension but also in their personal existence. Predating psychosomatic medicine, Tournier took time to listen to his patients personal plight, encouraging them to integrate spiritual aspects in their coping with illness. This Medicine of the Person "…puts the emphasis on awareness of patients as whole persons, with places in their community and society" [68]. His approach continues to inspire physicians around the world, with annual meetings on the topic of person-centred medicine [21].

Engel's [18] Biopsychosocial model does not necessarily pay attention to aspects of life to do with values, meaning and purpose which for many people are derived from R/S. Person-centred care requires clinicians to be aware of these aspects of patients' lives.

34.12 Guidelines for Integration of R/S in Clinical Practice

While there are multiple epidemiological studies showing the relationship between R/S and health, there are fewer studies about the applications of R/S in clinical practice. Most researchers agree on the need for taking a spiritual history, where the clinician explores the importance and practical implications of R/S in patients' lives and illnesses. Patients value attention to their spiritual wellbeing.

Some general principles for integration of R/S in clinical practice follow [10, 45]:

- Open-minded approach with genuine interest and respect for patients' beliefs, values and experiences.
- Clinicians need to explore their own world view and R/S history.
- Emphasise universal values of all faiths: justice, kindness, love, compassion, forgiveness.
- The approach needs to be patient centred, not prescribing nor imposing.
- Collaborative approach exploring potential useful spiritual resources available or already developed by patients.
- Refer to religious/spiritual resources in the community.

34.13 Research Priorities and Plans

There is an urgent need for more sophisticated studies that address gaps in the available knowledge. Some possibilities include:

(a) Expand studies to a more diverse geographical and cultural base.
(b) Conduct more studies in clinical populations.
(c) Explore the impact of spiritual and spiritually integrated treatments.
(d) Investigate the mechanisms through which religious involvement and spiritual-related treatments may affect health.
(e) Study spiritual experiences, their roots, differentiation from mental disorders and implications for the understanding of mind.
(f) Develop clinical applications of the currently available epidemiological data about the interconnection between religion and health [44].

34.14 Conclusions

Research in the field of Spirituality, Religion and Person Centred Medicine is complex from a linguistic, conceptual and methodological perspective—and care must be taken to properly define and operationalize these subject areas.

Religious beliefs, spiritual practices (R/S) and existential meaning-making are pertinent to the maintenance of health, to increased longevity and to the amelioration of illness, not only in Low and Middle Income Countries (LMIC) but also in post-enlightenment High-Income countries. Our experience from Brazil, the Middle East and South Asia would confirm that the world of Spirits and their involvement with day-to-day living is taken for granted in those religious countries.

Person-Centred Care can be facilitated by sensitivity to the religious and spiritual dimensions of human life and the human search for meaning as well as by an awareness of the interconnections of body, mind and spirit.

References

1. Abou-Saleh M. Psychiatric education in the Arab world. In: Okasha A, Maj M, editors. Images of psychiatry: an Arab perspective. Cairo: Scientific Books; 2001.
2. Allport GW, Ross JM. Personal religious orientation and prejudice. J Pers Soc Psychol. 1967;5 (4):432–43.
3. Armstrong K. Twelve steps to a compassionate life. London: Bodley Head; 2011.
4. Armstrong K. Fields of blood: religion and the history of violence. New York: Knopf; 2014.
5. Barber BK. Political violence, social integration, and youth functioning: Palestinian youth from the intifada. J Community Psychol. 2001;29(3):259–80.
6. Bekke-Hansen S, Pedersen CG, Thygesen K, et al. The role of religious faith, spirituality and existential considerations among heart patients in a secular society: relation to depressive symptoms 6 months post acute coronary syndrome. J Health Psychol. 2014;19:740–53.
7. Benda BB. Factors associated with re-hospitalization among veterans in a substance abuse treatment program. Psychiatr Serv. 2002;53(9):1176–8.
8. Birdwell J, Littler M. Why those who do God do good; Faithful citizens. 2012. Demos report. http://www.demos.co.uk/publications/faithfulcitizens. Accessed 21 Dec 2014.
9. Brown CG. The death of Christian Britain: understanding secularisation 1800–2000. 2nd ed. London: Routledge; 2009.
10. Cook C. Recommendations for psychiatrists on spirituality and religion. 2013. http://www.rcpsych.ac.uk/pdf/PS03_2013.pdf. Accessed 21 Dec 2014.
11. Cornah D. The impact of spirituality on mental health: a review of the literature. London: Mental Health Foundation; 2006.
12. Cox JL, Verhagen PJ. Spirituality, religion and psychopathology: towards an integrative psychiatry. Int J Person Centered Med. 2011;1:144–7.
13. Crabtree S, Pelham B. Religion provides emotional boost to world's poor. World Gallup Poll. 2009. http://www.gallup.com/poll/116449/religion-provides-emotional-boost-world-poor.aspx. Accessed 05 Dec 2014.
14. Dasgupta SN. Philosophical essays. Calcutta: University of Calcutta Press; 1941.
15. Davie G. Religion in Britain since 1945: believing without belonging. Making contemporary Britain. London: Wiley Blackwell; 1994.
16. Eagleton T. Culture and the death of God. Yale: Yale University Press; 2014.
17. Ehman JW, Ott BB, Short TH, et al. Do patients want physicians to inquire about their spiritual or religious beliefs if they become gravely ill? Arch Intern Med 1999;159:1803–6.
18. Engel GL. The need for a new medical model: a challenge for biomedicine. Science. 1977;196:129–36.
19. Errihani IH, Mrabt IH, Boutayeb S, et al. Impact of cancer on Moslem patients in Morocco. Psycho-Oncology. 2008;17(1):98–100.
20. Francis R. The Independent Inquiry into care provided by Mid Staffordshire NHS Foundation Trust, final report. 2013. http://www.midstaffspublicinquiry.com/report. Accessed 11 Dec 2014.
21. Fulford KWM, Campbell A, Cox J. Medicine of the person: faith, science and values in health care provision. London: Jessica Kingsley; 2007.
22. Gallup poll. In U.S., very Religious Have Higher Wellbeing across All Faiths. 2012. http://www.gallup.com/poll/152732/Religious-Higher-Wellbeing-Across-Faiths.aspx. Accessed 11 Dec 2014.

23. Gorini R. Attention and care to the madness during the Islamic middle age in Syria: the example of the Bimaristan Al-Arghun from princely palace to Bimaristan. JISHIM. 2002;2:40–2.
24. Graham EL. Between a rock and a hard place. London: SCM press; 2013.
25. Gray AJ. Worldviews. Int Psychiatry. 2011;8(3):58–60.
26. Gray A, Cox J. The roots of compassion and empathy: implementing the Francis report and the search for new models of health care. Eur J Person Centered Healthc. 2015.
27. Griffith JL. Religion that heals, religion that harms: a guide for clinical practice. New York: Guilford; 2010.
28. Grover S, Davuluri T, Chakrabarti S. Religion, spirituality and schizophrenia: a review. Indian J Psychol Med. 2014;36(2):119–24.
29. Hollifield M. Symptoms and coping in Sri Lanka 20–21 months after the 2004 tsunami. Br J Psychiatry. 2008;192(1):39–44.
30. Kleinman EM, Liu RT. Prospective prediction of suicide in a nationally representative sample: religious service attendance as a protective factor. Br J Psychiatry. 2014;204:262–6. doi:10.1192/bjp.bp.113.128900.
31. Koenig HG, McCullough ME, Larson DB. Handbook of religion and health. New York: Oxford University Press; 2001.
32. Koenig H. Religion and depression in older medical inpatients. Am J Geriatr Psychiatry. 2007;15(4):282–91.
33. Koenig H, King D, Carson VB. Handbook of religion and health. 2nd ed. New York: Oxford University Press; 2012.
34. Lewis VA, Macgregor C, Putnam RD. Religion, networks, and neighborliness: the impact of religious social networks on civic engagement. Soc Sci Res. 2012;42(2):331–46.
35. Lucchetti G, Lucchetti AG, Badan-Neto AM, et al. Religiousness affects mental health, pain and quality of life in older people in an outpatient rehabilitation setting. J Rehabil Med. 2011;43:316–22.
36. Lucchetti G, Bassi RM, Lucchetti AL. Taking spiritual history in clinical practice: a systematic review of instruments. Explore. 2013;9:159–70.
37. McCullough ME, Hoyt WT, Larson DB, et al. Religious involvement and mortality: a meta-analytical review. Health Psychol. 2000;19(3):211–22. http://www.apa.org/pubs/journals/releases/hea193211.pdf. Accessed 17 Nov 2014.
38. Meertens V, Scheppers P, Tax B. Depressive symptoms in the Netherlands 1975–1996: a theoretical framework and an empirical analysis of socio-demographic characteristics, gender differences and changes over time. Sociol Health Illn. 2003;25(2):208–31.
39. Miller L, Wickramaratne P, Gameroff MJ, et al. Religiosity and major depression in adults at high risk: a ten-year prospective study. Am J Psychiatry. 2012;169(1):89–94.
40. Mohr S, Brandt PY, Borras L, et al. Toward an integration of spirituality and religiousness into the psychosocial dimension of schizophrenia. Am J Psychiatry. 2006;163(11):1952–9.
41. Moreira-Almeida A, Koenig HG. Retaining the meaning of the words religiousness and spirituality: a commentary on the WHOQOL SRPB group's "a cross-cultural study of spirituality, religion, and personal beliefs as components of quality of life" (62: 6, 2005, 1486–1497). Soc Sci Med. 2005;63:843–5.
42. Moreira-Almeida A, Cardeña E. Differential diagnosis between nonpathological psychotic and spiritual experiences and mental disorders: a contribution from Latin American studies to the ICD-11. Rev Bras Psiquiatr. 2011;33:S21–36.
43. Moreira-Almeida A. Implications of spiritual experiences to the understanding of mind–brain relationship. Asian J Psychiatr. 2013a;6(6):585–9.
44. Moreira-Almeida A. Religion and health: the more we know the more we need to know. World Psychiatry. 2013b;12(1):37–8.
45. Moreira-Almeida A, Koenig HG, Lucchetti G. Clinical implications of spirituality to mental health: review of evidence and practical guidelines. Rev Bras Psiquiatr. 2014;36(2):176–82.

46. Nakao M, Ohara C. The perspective of psychosomatic medicine on the effect of religion on the mind-body relationship in Japan. J Relig Health. 2014;53(1):46–55.
47. Nelson S. Say little, do much: nurses, nuns, and hospitals in the nineteenth century. Philadelphia: University Pennsylvania press; 2001.
48. Nisbet PA, Duberstein PR, Conwell Y, et al. The effect of participation in religious activities on suicide versus natural death in adults 50 and older. J Nerv Ment Dis. 2000;188(8):543–6.
49. OCEBM Levels of Evidence Working Group. "The Oxford Levels of Evidence 2". Oxford Centre for Evidence-Based Medicine. 2014. http://www.cebm.net/index.aspx?o=5653. Accessed 8 Nov 2014.
50. Payman V, Ryburn B. Religiousness and recovery from inpatient geriatric depression: findings from the PEJAMA study. Aust N Z J Psychiatry. 2010;44(6):560–7.
51. Pembroke NF. Appropriate spiritual care by physicians. A theological perspective. J Relig Health. 2008;47:549–59.
52. Peres JFP, Newberg A. Neuroimaging and mediumship: a promising research line. Rev Psiq Clín. 2013;40(6):225–32.
53. Pew research center's Forum on Religion & Public Life. Global Religious Landscape, December 2012. http://www.pewforum.org/2012/12/18/global-religious-landscape-exec/. Accessed 21 Dec 2014.
54. Royal College of Psychiatrists, Spirituality and Psychiatry Special Interest Group committee. Spirituality and Mental Health. 2010. http://www.rcpsych.ac.uk/mentalhealthinformation/therapies/spiritualityandmentalhealth.aspx. Accessed 11 Dec 2014.
55. Reese AM, Thorpe RJ, Bell CN, et al. The effect of religious service attendance on race differences in depression: Findings from the EHDIC-SWB study. J Urban Health Bull N Y Acad Med. 2012;89:510–8.
56. Ronneberg CR, Miller EA, Dugan E, et al. The protective effects of religiosity on depression: a 2-year prospective study. Gerontologist. 2014. doi:10.1093/geront/gnu073.
57. Schumann C, Stroppa A, Moreira-Almeida A. The contribution of faith-based health organisations to public health. Int Psychiatry. 2011;8(3):62–4.
58. Schuster MA, Stein BD, Jaycox LH, et al. A national survey of stress reactions after the september 11, 2001, terrorist attacks. N Engl J Med. 2001;345(20):1507–12.
59. Schwartz rounds, Point of care. 2014. www.Pointofcarefoundation.org.uk. Accessed 19 Nov 2014.
60. Skevington SM, Gunson KS, O'connell KA. Introducing the WHOQOL-SRPB BREF: developing a short-form instrument for assessing spiritual, religious and personal beliefs within quality of life. Qual Life Res. 2013;22(5):1073–83. doi:10.1007/s11136-012-0237-0.
61. Sharma P, Charak R, Sharma V. Contemporary perspectives on spirituality and mental health. Indian J Psychol Med. 2009;31(1):16–23.
62. Smolak A, Gearing RE, Alonzao D, et al. Social support and religion: mental health service use and treatment of schizophrenia. Community Ment Health J. 2013;49(4):444–50.
63. Strawbridge WJ, Shema SJ, Cohen RD, et al. Religious attendance increases survival by improving and maintaining good health behaviors, mental health, and social relationships. Ann Behav Med. 2001;23(1):68–74.
64. Stroppa A, Moreira-Almeida A. Religiosity, mood symptoms, and quality of life in bipolar disorder. Bipolar Disord. 2013;15:385–93.
65. Sujoldzić A, Peternel L, Kulenović T, et al. Social determinants of health—a comparative study of Bosnian adolescents in different cultural contexts. Collegium Antropologicum. 2006;30(4):703–11.
66. Swinton J, Pattison S. Moving beyond clarity: towards a thin, vague, and useful understanding of spirituality in nursing care. Nurs Philos. 2010;11:226–37.
67. Tepper L, Rogers SA, Coleman EM, et al. The prevalence of religious coping among persons with persistent mental illnesses. Psychiatr Serv. 2001;52(5):660–5.
68. Tournier P. The healing of persons. New York: Harper & Row; 1940/1983.

69. Ysseldyk R, Matheson K, Anisman H. Religiosity as identity: toward an understanding of religion from a social identity perspective. Pers Soc Psychol Rev. 2012;14(1):60–71.
70. Zehnder D, Prchal A, Vollrath M, et al. Prospective study of the effectiveness of coping in pediatric patients. Child Psychiatry Hum Dev. 2006;36(3):351.

Person-Centered Palliative Care

35

Luigi Grassi, MD, Michelle Riba, MD, Marijana Bras, MD and Paul Glare, MD

35.1 Introduction

Thanks to improvements in prevention, screening, diagnosis, and treatment, most of us no longer die suddenly, but after many months to years—or even decades—of chronic ill health caused by diseases such as cancer, end organ failures, or dementia [31]. During this time of chronic illness, we will suffer pain and other physical distress, caused by the disease directly or by its treatment which is keeping us alive but unable to cure us. We will become increasingly dependent on others for our food, water, air, and hygiene. And at some point we will have to decide—if we are still capable of deciding—if it is worth continuing with treatment. All of these problems are or will be a source of much psychological distress for us and our families.

L. Grassi, MD (✉)
Professor and Chair of Psychiatry, Program on Psycho-Oncology, University of Ferrara, Ferrara, Italy
e-mail: luigi.grassi@unife.it

M. Riba, MD
Professor, Integrated Medical and Psychiatric Services, Department of Psychiatry, University of Michigan, Ann Arbor, MI, USA; University of Michigan Comprehensive Depression Center, Ann Arbor, MI, USA; Director, Psycho-Oncology Program, University of Michigan Comprehensive Cancer Center, Ann Arbor, MI, USA

M. Bras, MD
Centre for Palliative Medicine, Medical Ethics and Communication Skills, University of Zagreb School of Medicine, 10000 Zagreb, Croatia

P. Glare, MD
Palliative Medicine Service, Division of Supportive Care and Survivorship, Department of Medicine, Memorial Sloan Kettering Cancer Center, New York, NY, USA; Department of Medicine, Weill Cornell Medical College, New York, NY, USA

J.E. Mezzich et al. (eds.), *Person Centered Psychiatry*,
DOI 10.1007/978-3-319-39724-5_35

Pain and symptom management, psychological support, advance care planning, and assistance for family and friends are important from the time of diagnosis of an eventually fatal illness [69]. However, most people do not want to die, so it is not surprising that at the beginning most of the focus is on the administration of treatments that can control the disease, even if they cannot cure it. Symptoms are often mild, the patient is relatively well and focused on disease stabilization, maintenance of well-being, and prolongation of survival. Nevertheless the treating oncologist, cardiologist, and geriatrician should be aware of these potential problems, evaluate for them and incorporate their management as part of their comprehensive treatment plan [44, 65].

Eventually, the disease progresses, the patient becomes sicker and the options for controlling it become limited or else not worth the risks and burden they cause. As the patient transitions to this point in their disease trajectory, prioritization is given to the relief of pain, other physical symptoms, psychological distress, death preparation, and anticipatory grief support for the family and friends. Unless they believe in the redemptive power of suffering [74], all patients want distressing pain, nausea and dyspnea relieved. They also need to be given information about their prognosis and the opportunity to decide how aggressive they want their treatment to be at the end-of-life.

Evaluation and management of these problems and providing this kind of help in a holistic coordinated way is called palliative care. The World Health Organization (WHO) defines palliative care as "an approach that improves the quality of life of patients and their families facing the problems associated with life-threatening illness, through the prevention and relief of suffering by means of early identification and impeccable assessment and treatment of pain and other problems, physical, psychosocial and spiritual" [64].

Palliative care can be provided by the treating physician or family physician, especially if the patient's needs are simple. This has been referred to as generalist palliative care or the palliative approach [56]. If the physician does not have the time or the skills, or the issues are complex, then a specialist palliative care team will often become involved, either in consultation or taking over the total care of the patient. Patients with limited further treatment options, a limited prognosis and for whom the focusing is on symptom control and quality rather than quantity of life are sometimes referred to as "palliative care patients."

Some aspects of palliative care, such pharmacologic and non-pharmacologic interventions for pain and symptom control, formulation of a prognosis, and the preparation of an advance care directive are largely technical, and a patient-centered approach would seem not to be mandatory to complete them successfully. However, because of the several aims that palliative care pursues (Table 35.1), such as assessing and intervening in the psychosocial and spiritual/existential issues that face a patient approaching death, and their family, the role for and the importance of a patient-centered approach clearly emerges.

This is in-line with the specific characteristics of person-centered medicine as proposed by Tournier's [71, 72] conceptualization of personalized medicine (or a 'medicine of the person'). This may be viewed as a holistic clinical approach (i.e., a

Table 35.1 Aims of palliative care (from WHO www.who.int/cancer/palliative/definition/en/)

• Provides relief from pain and other distressing symptoms
• Affirms life and regards dying as a normal process
• Intends neither to hasten or postpone death
• Integrates the *psychological and spiritual aspects of patient care*
• Offers a support system to help patients live as actively as possible until death
• Offers a support system to help the family cope during the patients illness and in their own bereavement
• Uses a team approach to address the *needs of patients and their families, including bereavement counseling*, if indicated
• Will *enhance quality of life*, and may also positively influence the course of illness
• It is applicable early in the course of illness, in conjunction with other therapies that are intended to prolong life, such as chemotherapy or radiation therapy, and includes those investigations needed to better understand and manage distressing clinical complications

basic attitude rather than a theoretical system) toward patients assuming an integration of the scientific method with psychological insights and infused with transcendental/existential awareness and the search for meaning and purpose. Historically, the approach proposed by some pioneers of holistic palliative care, such as Saunders [63] and Kübler-Ross [39], consisted of several components, which are also considered the pillars of person-centered care in medicine: (i) compassion, empathy, responsiveness to needs, values, and expressed preferences; (ii) coordination and integration; (iii) information, communication, and education; (iv) physical comfort; (v) emotional support, relieving fear and anxiety; and (vi) involvement of family and friends [24]. Thus, treatment of patients in advanced phases of medical illness can be conceived within a framework that takes all dimensions into consideration—as specifically underlined by the World Psychiatric Association and the authors proposing person-centered medicine [25, 50]—a care *of* the person (of his/her whole health, covering both illness and positive aspects), *by* the person (clinicians extending themselves as total human beings and not merely as healing technicians), *for* the person (promoting the fulfillment of the person's health, aspirations and life project, and not merely disease management) and *with* the person (working respectfully in collaboration and in an empowering manner) [51].

In this chapter, we will summarize the most significant issues related to the psychosocial dimensions of patients facing advanced phases of illness, in line with a person-centered and, by extension, family-centered, approach, which is the specific mainstream in modern palliative care [3, 6, 9].

35.2 Psychosocial Issues in Palliative Care

35.2.1 Existential and Psychosocial Needs

Patients affected by life-threatening physical illness usually present and report a series of needs within the interpersonal, psychological, and spiritual domains that often are unmet in medical settings [62]. Among the most frequent needs, [53], in a study of patients with advanced stages of cancer, indicated the following: being helped with overcoming their fears (51 %), finding hope (42 %), finding meaning in life (40 %), finding spiritual resources (39 %); having someone to talk to about finding peace of mind (43 %). Likewise, Chochinov et al. [19] found that a very high percentage of patients, also in an advanced stage of cancer, presented spiritual and interpersonal problems that needed to be taken into account, such as feeling to be a burden to others (87.1 %), feeling of not making a meaningful and/or lasting contribution in one's own life (83.7 %), not feeling worthwhile or valued (81.4 %).

Besides spiritual and existential dimensions, a huge psychosocial literature in palliative care has indicated that at least 30–40 % of ill patients with serious medical illness, present symptoms of more severe emotional distress and/or psychiatric disorders. More specifically, anxiety, depressive, and stress-related disorders (stress-related and maladjustment reactions), and delirium, are frequently reported in palliative care settings, as psychiatric conditions that need to be carefully assessed and properly treated, given the extremely negative consequences on both patients and their families [22, 75].

Other clinically significant psychosocial conditions (e.g., demoralization, health anxiety), not necessarily taken into consideration by classical nosological psychiatric systems, [30] have been reported to affect medically ill patients in an advanced stage of illness, including terminally ill patients [57]. Demoralization, in particular, has been described as a specific syndrome in palliative care settings, consisting of a triad of hopelessness, loss of meaning, and existential distress, associated with cognitive attitudes of pessimism, helplessness, sense of being trapped, personal failure, or lacking a worthwhile future; absence of drive or motivation to cope differently; a sense of social alienation or isolation and lack of support; and a fluctuation in emotional intensity. Importantly, a major depressive or other psychiatric episode is not present as the primary condition [38].

35.2.2 Communication and Relational Issues in Person-Centered Palliative Care

From this background, it is of utmost importance that physicians and palliative care teams acquire the ability to recognize, assess, and compassionately address psychosocial, existential and spiritual issues, as well as psychological disorders [2]. The model of dignity developed by Chochinov et al. [18] in palliative care represents an important example of a patient-centered approach aimed at promoting a state of physical, mental, social, and spiritual well-being, based on mutual respect for the dignity of each individual person. Dignity, as derived from the Latin nouns *decus* (ornament, distinction, honor, glory, but also worthiness for honor and esteem) and *dignitas* is "the status of human beings entitling them to respect, a status which is first and not to be taken for granted; it refers to their highest value, or to the fact that they are a presupposition for value, as they are those to whom value makes sense" [42]. According to this model, dignity of patients in the advanced stage of illness is the sum of three main dimensions: illness-related concerns (i.e., concerns related to symptoms of physical and psychological distress, functional capacity, cognitive acuity) that threaten or impinge on the individual sense of dignity; the dignity conserving perspectives and practices (i.e., continuity of the self, role preservation, maintenance of pride, hopefulness, autonomy/control, acceptance, resilience, living in the moment, seeking spiritual help, maintaining normality); and the social aspects of dignity (i.e., privacy boundaries, social support, burden to others, aftermath concerns). It is underlined that healthcare providers have a profound influence on how patients experience illness and that in medicine a main role of the physician, besides curing, is *caring* in the sense of preserving the dignity of their patients [15, 20, 32]. Upon this backdrop, Chochinov [21] has proposed an easily remembered core framework of dignity conserving care, expressed as an A, B, C, and D sequence that can guide physicians in better relating and communicating with their patients (Table 35.2). This sequence represents a roadmap to favor the maintenance of dignity (dignity conserving care) and to positively influence the experience of being a patient.

An important role to reach these aims is played by psychosocial oncology that, in-line with what a number of international guidelines recommend [35], should be part of multidisciplinary palliative care teams (MDPCTs). As Breitbart et al. [5] suggest, the specific role of the psycho-oncologist in MDPCTs is in fact to facilitate effective communication with family and medical staff, and the end-of-life discussions and decision-making among patient, family, and team; to be an advocate for patients as questions arise, favoring conflict resolution, when it is the case, between patient, family, and staff; to help to deliver culturally sensitive palliative care, with the awareness that cultural factors influence a patient and family's attitude towards death and dying; to provide support through the bereavement process, including provision of support, recognition of emotional, cognitive, physical, and behavioral features of grief, and possible complications (complicated grief) in the process; to coordinate and/or provide specific psychological interventions (see Sect. 35.3), according to his/her own training; and to help the members of the team to work through the several emotional and relational challenges that end-of-life care determine in the team members themselves. In fact, as indicated by Kutner and Kilbourn [40], physicians and health-care professionals in general must be attentive to their own needs, which include acknowledging feelings of grief and loss and pursuing healthy venues that promote adaptive coping and decrease the risk of detachment and burnout. It is confirmed that through a self-care and self-awareness plan when caring for patients with life-limiting disease, physicians may improve patient care in palliative settings [61].

As a confirmation of what has been mentioned, studies have shown that some specific attitudes and behavior on the part of physicians can be responsible for an increase of the sense of abandonment and hopelessness in patients with serious medical illness: the tendency to attend to physical aspects only, to offer advice and reassurance before the main problems have been identified, to switch the topic, to use medical jargon and to be technical and detached [29, 47]. The main series of ingredients which are considered the key communication skills in palliative care are reported in Tables 35.2 and 35.3 [1]. These are the main tools that, by favoring the promotion of reciprocal trust and consolidating the therapeutic alliance, allow the achievement of early detection and treatment of possible psychosocial problems and improves the quality of palliative care [12, 48]. A similar, yet extremely interesting framework, has been proposed by Rushton et al. [59, 60], who consider that in the clinical context, responses to the stress of the health professional–patient relationship in palliative care are thought to include four dimensions: empathy (emotional attunement), perspective taking (cognitive attunement), memory (personal experience), and moral sensitivity (ethical attunement). For the authors, if the four dimensions are highly aligned, the intensity and valence of emotional arousal will influence ethical appraisal and discernment by engaging a robust view of the ethical issues, conflicts, and possible solutions and cultivating compassionate action and resilience. On the other side, if these dimensions are not aligned, ethical appraisal

Table 35.2 ABC of dignity preserving care in a person-centered approach

A = Attitude, that is physicians' examination of their own attitudes and assumptions towards patients, including asking questions about themselves (e.g. how would I be feeling in this patient's situation? Could my attitude towards the patient be based on something to do with my own experiences, anxieties, or fears?)
B = Behavior, acknowledging that certain communication behaviors (e.g. contact, respect, sitting at a comfortable distance for conversation, at the patient's eye level when possible, small acts of kindness, like getting the patient a glass of water) enhance the trust and connection between patients and their healthcare providers
C = Compassion, referring to a deep awareness of the suffering of another coupled with the wish to relieve it, can be conveyed by any form of communication—spoken or unspoken—that shows some recognition of the human stories that accompany illness
D = Dialog as a critical element of dignity conserving care, must acknowledge personhood beyond the illness itself and recognize the emotional impact that accompanies illness. It should be also used to acquaint the healthcare provider with aspects of the patient's life that must be known to provide the best care possible

From Chochinov [21], adapted and modified

Table 35.3 Skills and abilities favoring a person-centered approach in palliative care

• Capacity to impart confidence (e.g. greeting patient with warmth, making eye contact, encouraging patient queries)
• Use of "active listening" and open questions
• Being empathetic (e.g. eliciting patient's concerns, acknowledging distress, recognizing and being sensitive to emotions)
• Providing a "human touch" (e.g. using appropriate physical contact, being attentive and present to the patient and the situation, being showing interest and compassion)
• Focusing attention to the person and asking about psychosocial and existential needs, (e.g. asking patient about his/her life, acknowledging patient's family, remembering details about patient's life from visit to visit)
• Being forthright (e.g. being honest and not withholding information, asking patient to recap conversation to ensure understanding)
• Being respectful (e.g. "actively" listening and not interrupting, taking care of the dignity of the patient)
• Being thorough (e.g. providing detailed explanations, giving instructions in writing, following up in a timely manner)

From Baile and Costantini [1], adapted and modified

and discernment will be deficient, with the risk of creating emotional dysregulation and potentially leading to personal and moral distress, self-focused behaviors, unregulated moral outrage, burnout, and secondary stress.

35.3 Intervention

Among psychosocial intervention in palliative care, several approaches have been developed and manualized over the last 20 years [43].

The majority of them, if not all, irrespective of the theoretical background, deal with the most important existential issues of human life (i.e., death and dying, freedom, isolation, meaning) (Table 35.4) and have common aims and goals (Table 35.5). It is a fact that the themes of meaning and purpose, existential approach, dignity, and spirituality are significantly overlapping [16, 70]. In all interventions, as Milstein [52] underscores, the goal is creating a "healing space," that existential and spiritually oriented interventions can serve as an experiential basis to restore a sense of order and meaning for patients and their families, improving their ability to cope and to attain a sense of wholeness, as opposite to hopelessness. Likewise, others [58] strongly recommend that, besides controlling physical symptoms, there are irrevocable elements of a person-centered approach and intervention in palliative care patients: providing a supportive presence; encouraging a life review to help the patient recognize purpose, value, and meaning; exploring guilt, remorse, forgiveness, and reconciliation; facilitating religious expression; and focusing on meditative practices.

Table 35.4 Existential issues in palliative care

• Isolation (loneliness): the existential conflict is between our awareness of absolute isolation and our wish for contacts, protection and to be part of a larger whole
• Meaning (meaninglessness): the existential conflict stems from the dilemma of being a meaning-seeking creature who is thrown into a universe that has no meaning (Why me? Why not me?)
• Freedom: the existential conflict is between freedom to choose how to live, to "create" our own world and life (confrontation with groundlessness) and the need for a structure and a ground
• Death and dying: the existential conflict is determined by the wish to live forever and the reality of death as an unavoidable fact

Table 35.5 Aims of group psychological intervention in palliative care

• Reducing anxiety, demoralization, fears
– Not to be alone with terrifying phantasies of death and nothingness
– Breaking threatening subjects into smaller, more manegeable pieces
– Making fears more tolerable (it's impossible to delete them)
• Redefining life priorities
– Define and refine life projects
– Consider time (later may be too late)
• Improving coping skills
– From passive to active coping styles
– Increasing the sense of meaning (finding hope in opening up about the meaning of life and important events of life; improving communication
– Getting one's own needs met
– Openness in group as a model for openness outside the group

Supportive-expressive group psychotherapy (SEGT) is one of the first psychosocial treatments that have been shown to be effective in advanced phases of illness [67] with building bonds (mutual support) and expressing emotions representing the two main ingredients of intervention [68]. The former ingredient stresses the fact that social and interpersonal relationships are a reservoir of instrumental assistance and coping strategies indicates against social isolation as a harbinger of death; the latter considers that since life-threatening disease are a meaningless tragedy eliciting strong emotions, openness (expressing emotions) is a way to relief and to facilitate confrontation with one's own fragility and mortality. Preliminary data reported by Spiegel et al. [66] showed that SET for metastatic cancer patients had a positive impact in improving the profile of mood states, coping, as well as physical symptoms (e.g., pain), with subsequent research also confirming these findings [13, 23].

From a perspective relying on Victor Frankel's logotherapy, Breitbart, and Poppito [10] have developed a model that has spiritual well-being and meaning at the center of the intervention (meaning-centered psychotherapy, MCT). MCT is a 7-week program that utilizes a mixture of didactics, discussion, and experiential exercises that focus on particular themes related to meaning and advanced cancer. By focusing on issues of meaning and purpose in life in the face of a limited prognosis, support and expression of emotions are also part of the intervention. This favors the discussion of existential themes in terms of patients' awareness of death and search for meaning and practitioners' promotion of personal agency and responsibility as patients face life-and-death issues. Again, data from research has shown the efficacy of MCT, particularly in its group rather than individual format, in improving spiritual well-being and a sense of meaning and reducing symptom burden and symptom-related distress [3, 5–7].

Managing Cancer and Living Meaningfully (CALM) is also a short (3–6 sessions) psychological intervention which is aimed at relieving psychosocial distress and promoting psychological growth and development. Four broad domains are covered during CALM sessions, specifically (i) symptom management and communication with health-care providers; (ii) changes in self and relations with close others; (iii) spiritual well-being or sense of meaning and purpose; and (iv) issues related to advance care planning and to end-of-life (thinking of the future, hope and mortality) [54]. Preliminary data show that CALM may be a feasible intervention to benefit patients with advanced cancer [46].

Dignity therapy (DT) [14] is a very interesting approach based on Chochinov's conceptualization of dignity, which represents the therapeutic map, guiding clinicians to find interventional strategies or insights based on each of the themes and subthemes subsumed within the dignity model. DT is based on a dialogue in which, through specific dignity-oriented questions, an opportunity is offered to terminally patients to explore aspects of life that they feel were most important or meaningful; to address issues of their personal history they most want remembered; or things that need to be said. Transcription of the tape-recorded sessions (1–2 sessions in total), are edited and returned to the patient, as a tangible product (generativity document) to be left to the family. Data from randomized trials indicate that DT is a valuable intervention in palliative care, heightening the patients' sense of dignity, increasing their sense of purpose, lessening their sense of suffering, and helping them to prepare for death and the family members for grief [17, 37].

Narrative approaches, which also have a role in palliative care, are based on the exploration of the meaning of the physical illness in the context of the patient's life trajectory, with the patients encouraged to tell their story and reflect on their perspectives on their sense of "meaning", regarding suffering and their psychological, physical, social and spiritual well-being. This type of intervention has been shown to improve anxiety and depression among cancer patients admitted to hospice, in randomized controlled trials [45].

Psychopharmacological intervention is usually integrated with psychosocial treatment, with proper drugs (e.g. antidepressants, antipsychotics) prescribed in order to treat the clinical psychiatric disorder (e.g. major depression, delirium) or to work as adjuvants (e.g. antidepressants as adjuvants in the treatment of pain) in a broader approach. We recommend readers to specific literature for more details about psychopharmacological treatment in palliative care, with the idea that, at least in cancer settings, through a 'psychopharmoncology' approach, it is possible to integrate the special components of psychological/spiritual and psychopharmacological treatment [34, 36].

As a last point to be mentioned in regards to the need to improve a person-centered approach in palliative care, health-care professionals working in the field should be also the target of intervention. With respect to this, communication skills training (CST) have been developed and applied in curricula courses [27] to improve the series of relational skills that are the key elements of caring [33, 76]. According to Larson and Yao [41], participation in CST and training courses, physicians can become more able to engage in emotional tuning with their patients both in terms of what the authors call 'surface acting' (i.e., forging empathic behaviors toward the patient, absent of consistent emotional and cognitive reactions) and 'deep acting' (i.e., generating empathy-consistent emotional and cognitive reactions before and during empathic interactions with the patient). As an example, the Project to Educate Physicians on End-of-life Care from the Institute for Ethics at the American Medical Association, was developed in the USA since 1997 and subsequently adapted to expand the scope and range of palliative care in order to include the entire spectrum of illness (e.g., oncology, emergency medicine, geriatrics, and long-term care) [28]. In the Education for Physicians on End-of-life Care (EPEC) curriculum, several areas related to doctor–patient communication (e.g., communicating bad news; depression; anxiety and delirium; withdrawing/withholding treatment; medical futility; physician-assisted suicide; psychosocial issues) are taken into consideration. The importance of CST relies also on the improvement of the clinician's ability to reflect about him/herself, about his/her relational styles and personal emotions [49], reducing the risk—as we already underlined—of developing feelings of failure, frustration, powerlessness, grief, often subsumed under the umbrella of burnout syndrome [55]. Other interventions (e.g., cognitive-behavioral interventions, mindfulness, meditation, and reflective practice intervention) have also been developed and proposed for palliative care professionals, with data showing a decrease in burnout and an increase in job satisfaction, which in turn are conducive to a more effective person-centered approach with patients and their families [73].

35.4 Conclusions

Person-centered care for patients at the end-of-life is critically important and should be provided with evidence-based techniques. There are important needs of patients, families, friends and care providers that need to be integrated into a summative process for patients, who are at the center of this care. What has emerged over the last years in the psychosocial approach to palliative care has been extremely helpful in giving the field the sense of a person-centered approach according to the philosophy of personalized medicine. Existential issues and existentially oriented interventions have particularly contributed to this approach by showing the importance for patients to explore their past, present, and future in terms of meaningful opportunities and experiences during their lifetime [4]. This has the potential to promote authentic relatedness with oneself, the world, and others and, consequently, to increase the patient's sense of dignity [8]. All these aspects are related to guidelines which consider this essential in the clinical application of palliative care: to favor patients' quality of life; their physical well-being and functioning; their psychosocial well-being and functioning; their spiritual well-being; their perception of care; and their family's well-being and functioning [31].

This is an evolving process, which also needs to be informed by cultural, gender, psychosocial concerns, as well as many other factors, and must be tailored to the specific needs of the person who should be at the center of this care. As we better understand how to provide more help regarding physical symptoms and needs, so too we need to do research to better incorporate what we understand about psychosocial issues and how best integrate this into the overall care plan.

References

1. Baile W, Costantini A. Communicating with cancer patients and their families. In: Wise T, Biondi M, Costantini A, editors. Psycho-oncology. Arlington: American Psychiatric Publishing; 2013. p. 57–90.
2. Block SD. Perspectives on care at the close of life. Psychological considerations, growth, and transcendence at the end of life: the art of the possible. JAMA. 2001;285:2898–905.
3. Breitbart W, Chochinov H, Alici Y. Palliative care. In: Levenson J, editor. APPI textbook of psychosomatic medicine. 2nd ed. Arlington, VA: American Psychiatric Publishing; 2010.
4. Breitbart W, Gibson C, Poppito SR, Berg A. Psychotherapeutic interventions at the end of life: a focus on meaning and spirituality. Can J Psychiatry. 2004;49:366–72.
5. Breitbart W, Poppito S, Rosenfeld B, Vickers AJ, Li Y, Abbey J, Olden M, Pessin H, Lichtenthal W, Sjoberg D, Cassileth BR. Pilot randomized controlled trial of individual meaning-centered psychotherapy for patients with advanced cancer. J Clin Oncol. 2012;30 (12):1304–9.
6. Breitbart W, Rosenfeld B, Gibson C, Pessin H, Poppito S, Nelson C, Tomarken A, Timm AK, Berg A, Jacobson C, Sorger B, Abbey J, Olden M. Meaning-centered group psychotherapy for patients with advanced cancer: a pilot randomized controlled trial. Psychooncology. 2010;19 (1):21–8.
7. Breitbart W, Rosenfeld B, Pessin H, Applebaum A, Kulikowski J, Lichtenthal WG.: Meaning-centered group psychotherapy: an effective intervention for improving psychological well-being in patients with advanced cancer. J Clin Oncol. 2015;33(7):749–754.
8. Breitbart W. Spirituality and meaning in supportive care: spirituality- and meaning-centered group psychotherapy interventions in advanced cancer. Support Care Cancer. 2002;10:272–80.
9. Breitbart WS, Alici Y. Psychosocial palliative care. New York: Oxford University Press; 2014.
10. Breitbart WS, Poppito SR. Individual meaning-centered psychotherapy for patients with advanced cancer: a treatment manual. New York: Oxford University Press; 2014.

11. Bretibart WS, Chochinov HM, Alici Y.: End of life care. In: Grassi L, Riba M, editors. Clinical psycho-oncology: an international perspective. New York: Wiley, 2012, pp. 249–269.
12. Bub B. The patient's lament: hidden key to effective communication: how to recognise and transform. Med Humanit. 2004;30(2):63–9.
13. Butler LD, Koopman C, Neri E, Giese-Davis J, Palesh O, Thorne-Yocam KA, Dimiceli S, Chen XH, Fobair P, Kraemer HC, Spiegel D. Effects of supportive-expressive group therapy on pain in women with metastatic breast cancer. Health Psychol. 2009;28(5):579–87.
14. Chochinov HM. Dignity therapy final words for final day. New York: Oxford University Press; 2012.
15. Chochinov HM. Dying, dignity, and new horizons in palliative end-of-life care. CA Cancer J Clin. 2006;56:84–103.
16. Chochinov HM, Cann BJ. Interventions to enhance the spiritual aspects of dying. J Palliat Med. 2005;8(Suppl 1):S103–15.
17. Chochinov HM, Hack T, Hassard T, Kristjanson LJ, McClement S, Harlos M. Dignity therapy: a novel psychotherapeutic intervention for patients near the end of life. J Clin Oncol. 2005;23(24):5520–5.
18. Chochinov HM, Hack T, McClement S, Kristjanson L, Harlos M. Dignity in the terminally ill: a developing empirical model. Soc Sci Med. 2002;54(3):433–43.
19. Chochinov HM, Krisjanson LJ, Hack TF, Hassard T, McClement S, Harlos M. Dignity in the terminally ill: revisited. J Palliat Med. 2006;9(3):666–72.
20. Chochinov HM. Dignity-conserving care–a new model for palliative care: helping the patient feel valued. JAMA. 2002;287(17):2253–60.
21. Chochinov HM. Dignity and the essence of medicine: the A, B, C, and D of dignity conserving care. BMJ. 2007;335(7612):184–7.
22. Chochinov HM. Psychiatry and terminal illness. Can J Psychiatry. 2000;45(2):143–50.
23. Classen C, Butler LD, Koopman C, Miller E, DiMiceli S, Giese-Davis J, Fobair P, Carlson RW, Kraemer HC, Spiegel D. Supportive-expressive group therapy and distress in patients with metastatic breast cancer: a randomized clinical intervention trial. Arch Gen Psychiatry. 2001;58(5):494–501.
24. Cox JL. Towards an evidence-based 'medicine of the person': the contribution of psychiatry to health care provision. J Eval Clin Pract. 2008;14:694–8.
25. Cox J, Campbell A, Fulford K. Medicine of the person: faith, science and values in healthcare provision. London: Jessica Kingsley; 2007.
26. Cox JL. Medicine of the person and personalized care: a stitch in time saves nine? J Eval Clin Pract. 2010;16(2):315–317.
27. de Haes H, Teunissen S. Communication in palliative care: a review of recent literature. Curr Opin Oncol. 2005;17(4):345–50.
28. Emanuel LL, von Gunten CF, Ferris FD.: The education for physicians on end-of-life care (EPEC) curriculum. 1999. www.epec.net.
29. Fallowfield L, Jenkins V. Communicating sad, bad, and difficult news in medicine. Lancet. 2004;363(9405):312–9.
30. Fava GA, Mangelli L, Ruini C. Assessment of psychological distress in the setting of medical disease. Psychother Psychosom. 2001;70(4):171–5.
31. Field MJ, Cassel CK, editors. Approaching death. Improving care at the end of life. Washington: Institute of Medicine, National Academy Press; 1997.
32. Grassi L. Quam bene vivas referre: curing and caring in psycho–oncology. Psycho–oncology. 2013;22(8):1679–87.
33. Grassi L, Caruso R, Costantini A. Communication with patients suffering from serious physical illness. In: Balon R, Wise TN, editors. Clinical challenges in the biopsychosocial interface: update on psychosomatics for the 21st century. Advances in psychosomatic medicine series. Basel: Karger; 2015. p. 10–23.

34. Grassi L, Caruso R, Hammelef K, Nanni MG, Riba M. Efficacy and safety of pharmacotherapy in cancer-related psychiatric disorders across the trajectory of cancer care: a review. Int Rev Psychiatry. 2014;26:44–62.
35. Grassi L, Caruso R, Nanni MG. Psycho-oncology and optimal standards of cancer care: developments, multidisciplinary team approach and international guidelines. In: Wise TN, Biondi M, Costantini A, editors. Psycho-oncology. Arlington, VA: American Psychiatric Publishing Press; 2013. p. 315–39.
36. Grassi L, Riba M, editors. Psychopharmacology in oncology and palliative care. A practical manual. Berlin: Springer; 2014.
37. Houmann LJ, Chochinov HM, Kristjanson LJ, Petersen MA, Groenvold M. A prospective evaluation of dignity therapy in advanced cancer patients admitted to palliative care. Palliat Med. 2014;28(5):448–58.
38. Kissane DW, Clarke DM, Street AF. Demoralization syndrome–a relevant psychiatric diagnosis for palliative care. J Palliat Care. 2001;17(1):12–21.
39. Kübler-Ross E. On death and dying. New York: Simon and Schuster; 1969.
40. Kutner JS, Kilbourn KM. Bereavement: addressing challenges faced by advanced cancer patients, their caregivers, and their physicians. Prim Care. 2009;36(4):825–44.
41. Larson EB, Yao X. Clinical empathy as emotional labor in the patient-physician relationship. JAMA. 2005;293(9):1100–6.
42. Lebech M.: On the problem of human dignity. A hermeneutical and phenomenological investigation. Königshausen & Neumann: Vurzberg; 2009.
43. LeMay K, Wilson KG. Treatment of existential distress in life threatening illness: a review of manualized interventions. Clin Psychol Rev. 2008;28(3):472–93.
44. Levy MH, Back A, Benedetti C, et al. NCCN clinical practice guidelines in oncology: palliative care. J Natl Compr Canc Netw. 2009;7:436–73.
45. Lloyd-Williams M, Cobb M, O'Connor C, Dunn L, Shiels C. A pilot randomised controlled trial to reduce suffering and emotional distress in patients with advanced cancer. J Affect Disord. 2013;148:141–5.
46. Lo C, Hales S, Jung J, Chiu A, Panday T, Rydall A, Nissim R, Malfitano C, Petricone-westwood D, Zimmermann C, Rodin G. Managing cancer and living meaningfully (CALM): phase 2 trial of a brief individual psychotherapy for patients with advanced cancer. Palliat Med. 2014;28(3):234–42.
47. Maguire P, Pitceathly C. Key communication skills and how to acquire them. BMJ. 2002;325 (7366):697–700.
48. Maguire P, Pitceathly C. Managing the difficult consultation. Clin Med. 2003;3(6):532–7.
49. Meier DE, Back AL, Morrison RS. The inner life of physicians and care of the seriously ill. JAMA. 2001;286(23):3007–14.
50. Mezzich JE. World Psychiatric Association perspectives on person-centered psychiatry and medicine. Int J Integ Care. 2010;10:3–7.
51. Mezzich JE. The dialogal basis of our profession: psychiatry with the person. World Psychiatry. 2007;6:129–30.
52. Milstein JM. Introducing spirituality in medical care: transition from hopelessness to wholeness. JAMA. 2008;299(20):2440–1.
53. Moadel A, Morgan C, Fatone A, Grennan J, Carter J, Laruffa G, Skummy A, Dutcher J. Seeking meaning and hope: self-reported spiritual and existential needs among an ethnically-diverse cancer patient population. Psychooncology. 1999;8(5):378–85.
54. Nissim R, Freeman E, Lo C, Zimmermann C, Gagliese L, Rydall A, Hales S, Rodin G. Managing cancer and living meaningfully (CALM): a qualitative study of a brief individual psychotherapy for individuals with advanced cancer. Palliat Med. 2012;26(5):713–21.
55. Pereira SM, Fonseca AM, Carvalho AS. Burnout in palliative care: a systematic review. Nurs Ethics. 2011;18(3):317–26.
56. Quill TE, Abernethy AP. Generalist plus specialist palliative care—creating a more sustainable model. N Engl J Med. 2013;368(13):1173–5.

57. Robinson S, Kissane DW, Brooker J, Burney S.: A review of the construct of demoralization: history, definitions, and future directions for palliative care. Am J Hosp Palliat Care. 2014. pii: 1049909114553461. [Epub ahead of print].
58. Rousseau P. Spirituality and the dying patient. J Clin Oncol. 2000;18:2000–2.
59. Rushton CH, Kaszniak AW, Halifax JS. A framework for understanding moral distress among palliative care clinicians. J Palliat Med. 2013;16(9):1074–9.
60. Rushton CH, Kaszniak AW, Halifax JS. Addressing moral distress: application of a framework to palliative care practice. J Palliat Med. 2013;16(9):1080–8.
61. Sanchez-Reilly S, Morrison LJ, Carey E, Bernacki R, O'Neill L, Kapo J, Periyakoil VS, de Thomas JL. Caring for oneself to care for others: physicians and their self-care. J Support Oncol. 2013;11(2):75–81.
62. Sanson-Fisher R, Girgis A, Boyes A, Bonevski B, Burton L, Cook P. The unmet supportive care needs of patients with cancer. Supportive care review group. Cancer. 2000;88(1):226–37.
63. Saunders C, Clark D. Cicely Saunders: selected writings 1958–2004. Oxford: Oxford University Press; 2006.
64. Sepulveda C, Marlin A, Yoshida T, et al. Palliative care: the World Health Organization's global perspective. J Pain Symptom Manage. 2002;24:91–6.
65. Smith TJ, Temin S, Alesi ER, et al. American Society of clinical oncology provisional clinical opinion: the integration of palliative care into standard oncology care. J Clin Oncol. 2012;30:880–7.
66. Spiegel D, Bloom JR, Yalom I. Group support for patients with metastatic cancer. A randomized outcome study. Arch Gen Psychiatry. 1981;38(5):527–33.
67. Spiegel D, Yalom ID. A support group for dying patients. Int J Group Psychother. 1978;28 (2):233–45.
68. Spiegel D, Classen C. Group therapy for cancer patients: a research-based handbook of psychosocial care. New York: Basic Books; 2000.
69. Temel JS, Greer JA, Muzikansky A, et al. Early palliative care for patients with metastatic non-small-cell lung cancer. N Engl J Med. 2010;363:733–42.
70. Thompson GN, Chochinov HM. Dignity-based approaches in the care of terminally ill patients. Curr Opin Support Palliat Care. 2008;2(1):49–53.
71. Tournier P.: Le personnage et la personne (English Tr. The meaning of persons). India: Harper Collins Publication; 1957.
72. Tournier P.: Médicine de la personne. (English Tr. The healing of persons). India: Harper Collins Publication; 1965.
73. Vachon MLS, Müller M. Burnout and symptoms pf stress in staff working in palliative care. In: Chochinov H, Bretibart WS, editors. Handbook of psychiatry in palliative care. 2nd ed. New York: Oxford University Press; 2009. p. 236–64.
74. Vitillo RJ. Discerning the meaning of human suffering through the discourse of Judeo-Christian scriptures and other faith teachings. J Pain Symptom Manage. 2014;48:1004–8.
75. Wilson KG, Chochinov HM, Skirko MG, Allard P, Chary S, Gagnon PR, Macmillan K, De Luca M, O'Shea F, Kuhl D, Fainsinger RL, Clinch JJ. Depression and anxiety disorders in palliative cancer care. J Pain Symptom Manage. 2007;133:118–29.
76. Zinn W. The empathic physician. Arch Intern Med. 1993;153(3):306–12.

Person-Oriented Forensic Psychiatry

36

Lana Mužinić, MD, PhD, Igor Marinić, MD, PhD
and Athanassios Douzenis, MD, MMSc

36.1 Introduction to Forensic Psychiatry Definition and Goals

Forensic psychiatry focuses on the assessment and treatment of people with a mental disorder who commit crimes and show antisocial or violent behaviors [12]. Forensic psychiatry is considered to be the branch of psychiatry in the service of the law. Forensic psychiatry deals with issues that include development and implementation of legislation relating to mental health; mental health of persons involved in court proceedings; as well as matters related to criminal law and prison systems [3].

A forensic psychiatrist has multiple roles. In criminal law, he/she assesses and diagnoses psychiatric disorders in persons who have committed a criminal offense when there is a suspicion of the existence of psychiatric disorders. The forensic psychiatrist also asseses the mental state of the examinee and gives expert opinion in court regarding questions of criminal responsibility, i.e., whether responsibility is preserved, diminished, or whether the accused is not responsible for his actions. The forensic psychiatrist also answers questions regarding the person's ability to stand trial.

L. Mužinić, MD, PhD · I. Marinić, MD, PhD
Associate Professor, Forensic Psychiatry Sub-Specialist, Department of Psychiatry, University Hospital Dubrava, Zagreb, Croatia

A. Douzenis, MD, MMSc (✉)
Associate Professor in Psychiatry, Forensic Psychiatry, Forensic Psychiatry, 2nd Psychiatry Department, «Attikon» Hospital, National and Kapodistrian University of Athens Medical School, Rimini 1, Chaidari, 124 62 Athens, Greece
e-mail: thandouz@med.uoa.gr

J.E. Mezzich et al. (eds.), *Person Centered Psychiatry*,
DOI 10.1007/978-3-319-39724-5_36

Furthermore, forensic psychiatrists offer risk/dangerousness assessments and provide recommendations for treatment. Another important function of forensic psychiatrists is the treatment and rehabilitation of mentally ill offenders, in order to reduce future crime recurrence.

Forensic psychiatrists also participate as experts in civil cases, assessing existence of psychiatric disorders, e.g., determining the presence of psychological damage after traumatic events, their intensity, and duration. Furthermore, they assess the issues of legal capacity of persons with mental disabilities; involuntary hospitalization in psychiatric institutions; as well as evaluating testamentary capacity and the capacity to decide on legal transactions.

Modern forensic psychiatry deals with various issues, including the development of new methodologies for the treatment of mental disorders, which can be implemented after the person is released from the prison system; enhancement of methods for assessment of responsibility; improvement of medicolegal understanding; as well as development and improvement of public attitudes related to mental health [3].

Forensic psychiatry differs between countries and is generally defined within the frame of the legislation in individual countries and their health systems. Nevertheless, there are several goals of forensic psychiatry that are common in different countries and their health and law systems. They include development and implementation of treatment methods for persons with psychiatric disorders who have committed criminal offenses, their rehabilitation and prevention of relapse; improvement and development of cooperation between psychiatry and the law; cooperation with other experts in the forensic area; and providing expert's opinion in the court for persons with mental disorders [22, 23].

Since forensic psychiatry acts in the common area of mental health and the law, it can be quite demanding for psychiatrists. Imperative in this area of work are cooperation and coordination among general psychiatry, forensic psychiatry, and prison psychiatry [21].

36.2 The Biopsychosocial Model in Forensic Psychiatry

Suggested by Engel's [8] the biopsychosocial model emphasized the significance of multiple factors to health, aiming to address the complexity that arises from the interaction of all three spheres of influence: biological, social, and psychological.

Engel challenged the dogmatic adherence to reductionist models of disease. He claimed that despite its successes in the physical sciences and biomedicine, analytical reductionist methods—a product of Cartesian mind–body dualism—was not adequate to address the complex needs of medical care. Engel argued that the psychosocial elements of disease are as important as the biological ones. He offered a holistic and humanistic framework for the study of disease, which focuses on how the study of interactions between biological, social, and psychic elements can aid diagnosis and treatment. Significantly, Engel's framework does not commit to one specific perspective or school [6].

The biopsychosocial model applies to all medical subspecialties including forensic psychiatry. Person-oriented psychiatry encompasses all aspects of the biopsychosocial model for the assessment and treatment of the patient as a whole person.

36.3 Person-Centered Diagnostic Process and Assessment of Dangerousness

Following the above-mentioned biopsychosocial model and dissatisfaction with prevailing reductionist models of disease and health, Psychiatry for the Person was established by the World Psychiatric Association (WPA) General Assembly in 2005 as a major institutional program following on the principles of science and humanism that informed the foundation of WPA in 1950 [10]. This institutional program aims at promoting a psychiatry of the person, for the person, by the person, and with the person [18]. This program built on the biopsychosocial model and extended it as framework for understanding both illness and positive health. It also set the goal of clinical care not only to deal with disease but to also promote health and the fulfillment of the person's life project. We believe these ideas represent a positive conceptual shift in psychiatry and, potentially, in medicine at large.

Person-centered diagnosis aims at comprehensive assessment of health status from illness to well-being, contributory risk and protecting factors, and health experience, preferences and values. It uses categories, dimensions and narratives to describe the above domains, and promotes the engagement of clinicians, patients, and families toward a collaborative diagnostic process. [19]

Assessing dangerousness specially in connection to mental disorders is an important function of the forensic psychiatrist. Forensic psychiatrists need to carefully evaluate each person and advise prison authorities and courts. In order to do this a biopsychosocial approach should be used. The risk factors for violence that need to be assessed can be divided into:

1. Patient-related risk factors: Age, sex, socioeconomic status, intelligence, education, specific psychiatric disorders, and specific neurological disorders.
2. Historical risk factors: Violence history (the strongest predictor for future violence), history of child abuse or maltreatment, employment and residential instability.
3. Environmental risk factors: Discharge earlier locations associated with violence and victimization, increased social pressures, limited social supports, and availability of substances of abuse and weapons.

The assessment of dangerousness, following psychiatry for the person principles, needs to be enriched by looking at the positive aspects of each person and not only to deficits. Social and creative skills contributing to resocialization tend to reduce the risk for violent recidivism.

36.4 Person-Centered Treatment

Forensic patients require a broad range of treatment methods, given the complexity and persistence of their mental disorders [11].

Treatment of forensic patients can be carried out in special departments of general psychiatric hospitals, in forensic hospitals, and in prisons, as well as, after prison discharge, in day hospitals and out-patient clinics.

As with other psychiatric patients, treatment of forensic patients should be person-centered using the principles of the biopsychosocial model. A careful and multidisciplinary assessment of the person should include assessment of dangerousness and risk of further criminal activity. Risk assessment of dangerousness is an important part of the care plan since one of the primary criteria of treatment success is reduction in subsequent criminal behaviors [14]. Treatment usually involves combination of psychotropic drugs, certain types of psychotherapy methods individually or in groups, as well as sociotherapeutic techniques including psychosocial rehabilitation. Therapeutic planning should be based on the specific needs and capabilities of each person [11].

The most common psychotherapeutic methods used in forensic psychiatry are psychodynamic, cognitive, and systemic [11]. It would be advisable to continue the therapy after discharge from the institution, for the purpose of remission maintenance.

Psychodynamic-oriented psychotherapy in forensic practice has a number of possible roles and activities. These include everyday clinical care as well as supervision of psychotherapists in training, psychiatrists and other staffs in the forensic setting [11].

Cognitive behavioral therapy (CBT), in individual or group form, has proven useful in forensic patients. CBT approaches can be useful in the treatment of antisocial personality behaviors and in learning to control anger, violent behavior, and alcohol and substance abuse [31].

Psychosocial interventions include education about the disorders and side effects of medication, training of social and life skills, problem-solving techniques, occupational therapy, art therapy, and music therapy. The aim of these methods is to achieve insight into criminal behavior, risk factors, and protective factors, as well as prevention of future criminal behavior and building of life projects. Gaining insight on factors underlying problematic behaviors are very difficult to achieve by individuals with antisocial personality disorder [33].

In-patient forensic psychiatric treatment may be given in a special unit because of threats to the environment. In-patient treatment is used mostly in patients with psychosis. Patients with a diagnosis of psychotic disorders may have been found to have diminished responsibility and may be the subject of assessment of risk for aggressive behavior. Patients, in forensic psychiatric hospitals often have multiple comorbidities including antisocial behavior and abuse of alcohol and other substances, with reduced insight and adherence to treatment [12].

The treatment forensic patients with schizophrenia include reduction of symptoms, increase of family, work and social functioning, improvement of quality of life, and reduction of aggressive behavior [30]. Patients with schizophrenia are often nonadherent to treatment plans and this is a significant predictor of committing new crimes. Nonadherence to treatment is a usual reason for the use of intramuscular long-acting antipsychotics with these patients [30]. Also, there is increased risk of violence in people with psychotic disorders (schizophrenia, bipolar disorder, delusional disorder) who use drugs and alcohol [9, 28].

Alcohol- and drug-addicted individuals comprise a substantial population within the prison system, which also requires carefully prepared and implemented treatment programs. Such therapeutic efforts should encompass establishing and maintaining abstinence, substitution therapy and treatment of possible physical complications of addiction. Depending on law regulations, some countries have also implemented out-patient addiction treatment programs in the context of security measures, sometimes monitored by probation systems.

Continued use of drugs and alcohol can cause severe health impairments and may lead to extremely violent behaviors and perpetration of serious crimes [25]. The time when an individual is released from a forensic institution or prison represents a time of high risk, because of increased likelihood of a drug or alcohol relapse. During that period, the person is also in danger of taking drug overdoses [26].

Therefore, addiction treatment, monitoring of abstinence as a condition of discharge or leave, as well as regular monitoring and intervening in cases where there is increased risk for these behaviors are essential components of treatment. These measures may also have a positive impact on reducing the risk of committing new criminal offenses and on successful reintegration of the offender [26]. The term dual diagnoses, which implies comorbidity of psychiatric disorders, deserves particular attention in forensic psychiatry, as people with dual diagnoses are more prone to repetition of delinquent behaviors [34].

Multilevel, multidisciplinary, evidence-based and person-centered approach to the treatment of violent offenders with psychiatric comorbidity should be a prominent concern in both in-patient and out-patient forensic settings. To obtain greater rehabilitation, family, work, and social functioning in the community, and decrease recidivism, forensic treatment should encompass individualize care using as needed psychotherapy, pharmacotherapy, and sociotherapy approaches [25].

36.5 Individualized Rehabilitation and Violence Prevention

To reduce the risk of recidivism in criminal offenses it is important to start rehabilitation as soon after admission as possible. Forensic rehabilitation can be seen as a complex process in which different components contribute to the improvement of the person. If the patient is in in-patient remission and expresses interest in out-patient care, it is a sign that the process of rehabilitation was successful and could lead to the reduction of the risk of repetition of criminal acts [14, 17].

When assessing the types of psychosocial interventions in the rehabilitation of forensic patients, it is necessary to determine the specific needs and goals of rehabilitation. Psychosocial interventions and involvement in rehabilitation programs reduce the risk of relapse [1] and thus the risk for further offenses.

Rehabilitation should be aimed at improving social skills, social awareness and change in maladaptive behaviors and coping [32]. It should be important that the person through treatment and rehabilitation gains insight into the significance of violent behavior and learns behavioral strategies that could be useful in conflictual and complex situations in life [14]. Useful psychosocial interventions and strategies are anger management, communication and general life skills training, and problem-solving in interpersonal and social relations. Furthermore, as noted above, programs should include attention to substance abuse comorbid disorders such as well as health education [14]. It is also helpful to follow the principles of rehabilitation concerning risk, criminogenic needs, and responsiveness to treatment. Rehabilitation is difficult to achieve if comorbid psychiatric disorders are not vigorously treated.

Forensic patients should actively participate in the development of a treatment plan. Programs of treatment and rehabilitation that have started in a forensic in-patient institution should continue in the community. Involvement of social services is also necessary from the beginning of the treatment process [29]. Participations of forensic patients in postdischarge out-patient follow-up reduce the risk of psychological decompensation and increase public safety [4].

Forensic assertive community treatment (FACT) represents an adjustment to assertive community treatment (ACT), which brings together a multidisciplinary team that includes psychiatrists, social workers, nurses, and counselors from various fields. The FACT model is intended for people with severe mental disorders that are involved in the forensic system [1, 5, 7, 16]. This model provides patients with medications, addiction treatment, and support services in the community. It is based on the concept that this approach can reduce repetition of offenses in persons with severe mental disorders who are prone to criminogenic activities [20]. Also, intensive case management adapted to forensic populations in different settings can be beneficial [20]. Use of assertive community treatments and intensive case management for forensic patients results in symptom improvement, decrease of relapses, reduction of hospitalizations, and lower criminal recidivism.

Gunn [13] highlighted the problem of deinstitutionalization that influenced the shift of forensic mental patients from the health care system into the justice/correctional system. The prevalence of mental disorders in prisons has increased as consequence of reduction of the number of hospital beds and increase imprisonment rates in some societies. In some parts of Western Europe, there is a recent trend toward reinstitutionalisation and increase in the number of admissions to forensic hospitals [27].

At this point we should highlight the views of Nedopil [22], who stated that cooperation between general and forensic psychiatry can lead to better prevention and that persons with mental disorders do not necessarily become offenders or victims of crime. Furthermore, this cooperation can also lead to protection of younger people who are at risk of exhibiting antisocial behavior. Closer integration of forensic psychiatry into regular health care systems as well as intensive exchanges of knowledge and skills between forensic and general psychiatrists may be helpful.

36.6 Human Rights, Ethics, and Legal Principles in Person-Oriented Forensic Psychiatry

When working with mentally ill offenders it is important to respect their human rights and to follow ethical principles in their treatment, according to the laws of individual countries and international conventions. The observance of such laws is supervised by different institutions. Forensic psychiatrists must be experts in both psychiatry and in laws that relate to ethical care [35]. This means that a forensic psychiatrist must be familiar with the ethical principles of psychiatry in general and of forensic psychiatry specifically.

Forensic psychiatrists often face intricate situations. Specifically, one segment of their work relates to the role of witness expert and another to clinical care in a doctor–patient relationship [2]. Because of inherent conflicts, it is not recommended that a psychiatrist who has treated a patient take part in the person's trial as a psychiatric expert.

The European Court of Human Rights is responsible in this part of the world for the preservation of human rights of involuntarily committed psychiatric patients [24]. In forensic psychiatry, particular ethical dilemmas may occur concerning mechanical restrictions, isolation of patients, administration of treatment without consent, and research with forensic patients. Therefore, there is a continuing need for observance of ethical principles as well as development of refined ethical experience in the treatment of forensic patients [12].

Knoll [15] has identified four principles that forensic psychiatrist should comply with, and these are respect for the person, honesty, justice, and social responsibility. Also he pointed out that forensic psychiatrists should not ever distort information and should always be aware of the possibilities and limitations of psychiatric science. The need of continued professional development for forensic psychiatrists cannot be underestimated.

36.7 Conclusions

Forensic psychiatry, as other specialties of psychiatry and medicine, must be person-oriented, especially because forensic patients have a special legal position that puts them in an intricate position. They should receive good quality psychiatric care in special conditions of deprivation of freedom. Given the need to protect the community from potential recidivism, the mental health system should provide forensic patients necessary treatment, to be in frequent contact with them to detect early signs of relapse, and offer long term treatment in the community. Therefore, proper rehabilitation is crucial to achieve better social functioning and prevention of clinical relapse and criminal recurrence. Comprehensive person-centered diagnosis, continuous evaluation of dangerousness, treatment and rehabilitation efforts must be individually targeted, i.e., according to the patient's needs and biological, psychological, and social characteristics and the causes of disorder and violence. Therapy approaches should be selected according to the characteristics and needs of the individual.

Person-centered psychiatry should inform the further development of forensic psychiatry and provide the framework for comprehensive assessment of the individual's needs and treatment planning. Forensic psychiatrists should be leading well trained and experienced psychiatric teams, with access to appropriate resources for health restoration and promotion and the diminution of potentials for dangerousness and recidivism.

References

1. Adams C. Psychosocial interventions for schizophrenia. Effective Health Care. 2000;6(3):1–7.
2. Appelbaum PS. A theory of ethics for forensic psychiatry. J Am Acad Psychiatry Law. 1997;25(3):233–47. Retrieved from http://www.ncbi.nlm.nih.gov/pubmed/9323651.
3. Arboleda-Flórez J. Forensic psychiatry: contemporary scope, challenges and controversies. World Psychiatry. 2006;5(2):87–91.
4. Butz M, Mokros A, Osterheider M. Specific outpatient treatment for forensic patients after release. Psychiatr Prax. 2013;40(1):36–42.
5. Weinstein LC, Henwood BF, Cody JW, Jordan M, Lelar R. Transforming assertive community treatment into an integrated care system: the role of nursing and primary care partnerships. J Am Psychiatr Nurses Assoc. 2011;17(1):64–71. doi:10.1177/1078390310394656.
6. Douzenis A, Seretis D. Descriptive and predictive validity of somatic attributions in patients with somatoform disorders: a systematic review of quantitative research. J Psychosom Res. 2013;75(3):199–210. doi:10.1016/j.jpsychores.2013.05.005.
7. Dixon L. Assertive community treatment: twenty-five years of gold. Psychiatr Serv. 2000;51(6):759–65. Retrieved from http://www.ncbi.nlm.nih.gov/pubmed/10828107.
8. Engel GL. From biomedical to biopsychosocial: being scientific in the human domain. Families Syst Health. 1996;14:425–33.
9. Fazel S, Långström N, Hjern A, Grann M, Lichtenstein P. Schizophrenia, substance abuse, and violent crime. JAMA. 2009;301(19):2016–23. doi:10.1001/jama.2009.675.
10. Garrabe J, Hoff P. Historical views on psychiatry for the person. Int J Person Centered Med. 2011;1:125–7.
11. McGauley G, Humphrey M. Contribution of forensic psychotherapy to the care of forensic patients. Adv Psychiatr Treat. 2003;9:117–24.
12. Gordon H, Lindqvist P. Forensic psychiatry in Europe. Psychiatr Bull. 2007;31(11):421–4. doi:10.1192/pb.bp.107.014803.
13. Gunn J. Future directions for treatment in forensic psychiatry. Br J Psychiatry J Ment Sci. 2000;176:332–8. Retrieved from http://www.ncbi.nlm.nih.gov/pubmed/10827880.

14. Jeglic EL, Maile C, Calkins-Mercado C. Treatment of offender populations: implications for risk management and community reintegration. In: Gideon L, Sung H, editors. Rethinking corrections: rehabilitation, reentry, and reintegration. Thousand Oaks: Sage Publications Inc; 2011. p. 37–70.
15. Knoll JL. Ethics in forensic psychiatry. In: Simon RI, Gold LH, editors. Textbook of forensic psychiatry. 2nd ed. Washington, DC, London: The American Psychiatric Publishing; 2010.
16. Lamberti JS, Weisman R, Faden DI. Forensic assertive community treatment: preventing incarceration of adults with severe mental illness. Psychiatr Serv. 2004;55(11):1285–93. doi:10.1176/appi.ps.55.11.1285.
17. Lindqvist P, Skipworth J. Evidence-based rehabilitation in forensic psychiatry. Br J Psychiatry J Ment Sci. 2000;176:320–3. Retrieved from http://www.ncbi.nlm.nih.gov/pubmed/10827878.
18. Mezzich JE. Psychiatry for the person: articulating medicine's science and humanism. World Psychiatry. 2007;6(2):1–3.
19. Mezzich JE, Salloum IM, Cloninger CR, Salvador-Carulla L, Kirmayer L, Banzato CE, Wallcraft J, Botbol M. Person-centered integrative diagnosis: conceptual bases and structural model. Can J Psychiatry. 2010;55:701–8.
20. Morrissey J, Meyer P, Cuddeback G. Extending Assertive Community Treatment to criminal justice settings: origins, current evidence, and future directions. Community Ment Health J. 2007;43(5):527–44. doi:10.1007/s10597-007-9092-9.
21. Nakatani Y. Treatment of offenders with mental disorders: focusing on prison psychiatry. Seishin Shinkeigaku Zasshi = Psychiatria et Neurologia Japonica. 2011;113(5):458–67. Retrieved from http://www.ncbi.nlm.nih.gov/pubmed/21706853.
22. Nedopil N. The role of forensic psychiatry in mental health systems in Europe. Crim Behav Ment Health CBMH. 2009;19(4):224–34. doi:10.1002/cbm.719.
23. Nedopil N, Gunn J, Thomson L. Teaching forensic psychiatry in Europe. Crim Behav Ment Health CBMH. 2012;22(4):238–46. doi:10.1002/cbm.1845.
24. Niveau G, Materi J. Psychiatric commitment: over 50 years of case law from the European Court of Human Rights. Eur Psychiatry J Assoc Eur Psychiatrists. 2006;21(7):427–35. doi:10.1016/j.eurpsy.2006.04.004.
25. Palijan TZ, Muzinić L, Radeljak S. Psychiatric comorbidity in forensic psychiatry. Psychiatr Danubina. 2009;21(3):429–36. Retrieved from http://www.ncbi.nlm.nih.gov/pubmed/19794370.
26. Pickard H, Fazel S. Substance abuse as a risk factor for violence in mental illness: some implications for forensic psychiatric practice and clinical ethics. Curr Opin Psychiatry. 2013;26(4):349–54. doi:10.1097/YCO.0b013e328361e798.
27. Priebe S, Badesconyi A, Fioritti A, Hansson L, Kilian R, Torres-Gonzales F, Wiersma D. Reinstitutionalisation in mental health care: comparison of data on service provision from six European countries. BMJ (Clinical Research Ed.). 2005;330(7483):123–6. doi:10.1136/bmj.38296.611215.AE.
28. Putkonen H. Schizophrenia and comorbid substance abuse substantially increases risks of violent crime. Evid Based Ment Health. 2010;13(1):31. doi:10.1136/ebmh.13.1.31.
29. Sauter J, Voss T, Dahle K-P. Effectiveness of aftercare treatment after release from prison: a first evaluation of the forensic therapeutic outpatient clinic for serious violent and sexual offenders in Berlin. Der Nervenarzt. 2014. doi:10.1007/s00115-014-4185-5.
30. Stompe T, Schanda H. Psychopharmocotherapy of schizophrenia in forensic and general psychiatry. Neuropsychiatrie : Klinik, Diagnostik, Therapie Und Rehabilitation : Organ Der Gesellschaft Österreichischer Nervenärzte Und Psychiater. 2011;25(2):75–84. Retrieved from http://www.ncbi.nlm.nih.gov/pubmed/21672506.
31. Tafrate RC, Mitchell D, editors. Forensic CBT: a handbook for clinical practice. Chichester: Wiley-Blackwell; 2013.
32. Timmerman IGH, Emmelkamp PMG. The effects of cognitive-behavioral treatment for forensic inpatients. Int J Offender Ther Comp Criminol. 2005;49(5):590–606. doi:10.1177/0306624X05277661.

33. Tsopelas C, Tsetsou S, Ntounas P, Douzenis A. Female perpetrators of sexual abuse of minors: what are the consequences for the victim. Int J Law Psychiatry. 2012;35(4):305–10. doi:10.1016/j.ijlp.2012.04.003.
34. Van Horn JE, Eisenberg MJ, Van Kuik S, Van Kinderen GM. Psychopathology and recidivism among violent offenders with a dual diagnosis. A comparison with other subgroups of violent offenders. Tijdschrift Voor Psychiatrie. 2012;54(6):497–507. Retrieved from http://www.ncbi.nlm.nih.gov/pubmed/22753182.
35. Vukota L, Mužinić L. Person oriented/centred medicine in prisons. In: Đorđević V, Braš M, Miličić D, editors. Person in Medicine and Healthcare: From Bench to Bedside to Community. Zagreb: Medicinska naklada; 2012. p. 479–93.

People-Centred Organization of Psychiatric Services

37

Roy Abraham Kallivayalil, MD, DPM, MAMS
and Varghese P. Punnoose, MD

37.1 Introduction

The provision of mental health services remains highly inadequate in most parts of the world. Treatment gap is sometimes as high as 90 % and more pronounced in low and middle-income countries [19]. Even when the services are available the potential beneficiaries are not gaining full access to them due to several reasons. The main roadblock seems to be related to the organizational aspects of mental health care delivery [18].

The traditional organization of mental health care is centred around hospitals which are specialized for treating mental illness. This hospital centred system has the advantage of operational feasibility from the point of view of health administrators. The fact that this system is very efficient in providing services for serious mental disorders in acute stage need to be acknowledged. But looking from the consumer side this system is unfriendly and insufficient in several ways. Unfriendly in the sense that it is not very sensitive to the user needs and insufficient in the sense that it does not capture the broad range of mental health problems nor provide adequate attention to health promotion. There is a neglect of the needs of real people [14]. Similarly, neither does it address the promotional aspects of mental health nor it prioritizes prevention. These proven deficiencies in the conventional hospital-based system clearly call for a more person-centred and broad system of

R.A. Kallivayalil, MD, DPM, MAMS (✉)
Vice-Principal, Professor and Head, Dept of Psychiatry,
Pushpagiri Institute of Medical Sciences, Thiruvalla, Kerala, India
e-mail: roykalli@gmail.com

V.P. Punnoose, MD
Professor of Psychiatry, Government Medical College Kottayam, Kottayam, Kerala, India

J.E. Mezzich et al. (eds.), *Person Centered Psychiatry*,
DOI 10.1007/978-3-319-39724-5_37

psychiatric services. Needless to say that the services within the hospital should be reorganized to be more people-centred. Collaborative extension of person-centred approach to general medicine [11], and integrating mental health in general health and public health may be a useful step in filling up the deficiencies in health care delivery systems and making it more person-centred [7, 13].

Greater participation by patients in healthcare decision-making has been the trend in high-income countries which are facing the problems of ageing of population and a shift in focus from acute care to chronic care [17]. This stems from the notions that citizens as responsible consumers must become co-producers of their care and less dependent on paternalistic models of health care [15]. The concept of person-centred practice which evolved in general primary care is expected to become influential in mental health care delivery in primary and specialist settings in the near future [18].

37.2 The Person-Centred Approach in Psychiatry

Recent movements emphasizing recovery and resilience place patients as active participants in the treatment process. The fundamental assumption of the recovery movement in mental health is the principle of "people first" and this places person-centred care planning for individuals with serious mental illness at its core [3].

In the field of mental health care 'person-centeredness' is generally understood as a holistic approach with an attitude of respect for the individual and his or her unique experience and needs [5]. The World Psychiatric Association Institutional Program on Psychiatry for the Persons (IPPP) affirms the whole person of the patient in context as the centre and goal of clinical care [10]. IPPP emphasizes the person's involvement as user and citizen in creating policy, plan and delivery of services.

Person-centred care has recently been emphasized in psychiatric rehabilitation as well [2]. This new approach in rehabilitation of the chronic mentally ill opens up hopes of moving beyond the rhetoric of recovery to concrete practices. Partnership in decision-making in person-centred approach may reorient rehabilitation from patienthood to personhood. Similarly, the family's role in person-centred care has been analyzed in a focussed manner [1].

37.3 Models and Guidelines

Models based on person-centred approaches have started to emerge. Recovery-oriented behavioural health care and community health of Yale University School of Medicine is one such model. This model focuses on culturally responsive person-centred care for psychosis in urban mental health system. Illness management and recovery, facilitated person-centred planning and community inclusion programmes are the components of this programme [16].

Recently, the influential mental health care provider organization, NICE, has given recommendations on "improving the experience of people who use adult NHS mental health services" [12]. NICE guideline makes some quality statements with hopes that people using mental health services, and their carers feel optimistic that care will be effective and they are treated with empathy, dignity and respect. Quality statements also hope for easy accessibility to mental health services when people need it. Care from a single, multidisciplinary community team, familiar to patients and with whom they have a continuous relationship is expected. Patients are actively involved in shared decision-making and supported in self-management. The views of service users are used to monitor performance of services. Patients are informed about the assessment process, their diagnosis and treatments options, and receive emotional support for any sensitive issues. People using mental health services jointly develop a care plan with mental health and social care professionals. Those who may be at risk of crisis are offered a crisis support and a comprehensive assessment, undertaken by a professional competent in crisis working. People in hospital for mental health care have daily one-to-one contact with mental healthcare professionals known to the service user and regularly see other members of the multidisciplinary mental healthcare team. People receiving in-patient care can access meaningful and culturally appropriate activities 7 days a week, not restricted to the convenience of day duty staff in the regular working hours. Control and restraint, and compulsory treatment including rapid tranquillisation, will be used competently, safely and only as a last resort with minimum force. People using mental health services feel less stigmatized in the community and health service system, including within mental health services.

The spirit of people centeredness in the delivery of psychiatric services is reflected in the quality statements in the guidelines. The guidelines aim to promote person-centred care that takes into account service users' needs, preferences and strengths. It is expected that by practising these guidelines people who use mental health services get the opportunity to make informed decisions about their care and treatment, in partnership with their health and social care practitioners.

However, the person-centred approach in psychiatric care is not without reservations. Practitioners might have apprehensions whether allowing people with mental illness to make their own decisions increases the liability of the care giving professional. Its applicability in acute settings, labour intensive and time-consuming nature, not having sufficient evidence base, conflicts between patients choice and clinical wisdom are some of the other concerns [16].

The NICE Guidelines suggests that people-centred approach in organization of psychiatric services should ensure the following:

1. Care and support across all points on the care pathway.
2. Access to care.
3. Comprehensive assessment.
4. Community care.
5. Access to interventions in crisis.

6. Hospital care.
7. Discharge and transfer of care.
8. Assessment and treatment under legal provisions.

37.4 Organizing Services Based on the Person-Centred Approach

The above models of care are based on the situation in the western world. Though they are very well based on the principles of person-centred approach, their feasibility in the less-developed and resource-limited settings may be limited. So each country needs to evolve its own model of person-centred delivery of mental health care services.

In middle and low-income countries, several hurdles like lack of human resources, low priority of mental health in health policy and budgeting, limitations of infrastructure, poor awareness about mental disorders and stigma and discrimination are to be tackled in organization of person-centred care for persons with psychiatric disorders. These issues need to be kept in mind when the western models are adapted to middle- and low-income countries.

The services for the mentally ill should be organized with "person first" principle at every point in the pathway of care starting from assessment to rehabilitation.

1. Person-Centredness in Assessment.
2. Person-Centredness in Hospital Care.
3. Person-Centredness in Family and Community Care.
4. Person-Centredness in Rehabilitation.

37.5 Person-Centred Assessment

When people are referred to mental health services a face-to-face appointment with a professional within the shortest time should be ensured. Patient's preference regarding the place and choice of services should be given due consideration. Transparency should be ensured by providing the name and professional designation of the person who will assess them. The process of assessment should be explained using plain language.

The assessment should take place in a warm, empathic, dignified and professional manner. The patient has to be explained that the assessment will cover all aspects of their experiences and life and the basic approach is that of shared decision-making. Although they can be accompanied by a family member or carer, it is preferable to see the person alone for some of the assessment. They should be told that they can refuse permission for any other member of staff, such as a student, to be present. Limitations of confidentiality should be disclosed.

When carrying out an assessment ensure there is enough time for the patient to describe and discuss their problems. Explain the use and meaning of any clinical terms used. Give information about different treatment options, including drug and psychological treatments, and their side effects, to promote discussion and shared understanding.

If the patient is unhappy about the assessment and diagnosis, give them time to discuss this and offer them the opportunity for a second opinion. Waiting periods should be minimized. Ensure that waiting rooms are comfortable and have areas of privacy.

37.6 Person-Centred Hospital Care

In the event of admission to a hospital, the person should be received in an atmosphere of hope and optimism. Ensure that he feels safe and address any concerns about safety. Give adequate information to the patients, and their families or carers about the hospital and the ward in which they will stay, treatments, activities and services available, rules of the ward (including substance misuse policy), service users' rights, responsibilities and freedom to move around the ward and outside and visiting arrangements. Undertake shared decision-making whenever possible. Service users in hospital should be offered daily one-to-one sessions with a healthcare professional known to the service user and regular one-to-one sessions with their consultant.

The overall coordination and management of care should ideally take place at a regular multidisciplinary meeting led by the consultant and team manager with full access to the service user's treatment records. The advocates of those who are treated under legal provisions should be encouraged to be in contact with the treatment team through the manager.

Health and social care providers should ensure that service users in hospital have access to the pharmacological, psychological and psychosocial treatments recommended in standard guidelines provided by competent health or social care professionals. Control and restraint, and compulsory treatment including rapid tranquillisation, should be used as a last resort, only after all means of negotiation and persuasion have been tried, and only by healthcare professionals trained and competent to do this. Document the reasons for such actions.

When a patient is subject to control and restraint, or receives compulsory treatment including rapid tranquillisation use minimum force, make sure the service user is physically safe, try to involve healthcare professionals whom the service user trusts and explain reasons for the episode of compulsory treatment to the patient and involved family members or carers. Offer to discuss episodes of compulsory treatment with there at the time of discharge and do so in a calm and simple manner.

Psychological and psychosocial treatments may be provided by health and social care professionals who work with the service user in the community. Those receiving community care before hospital admission should be routinely visited while in hospital by the health and social care professionals responsible for their community care.

Ensure that service users in hospital have access to a wide range of meaningful and culturally appropriate occupations and activities. Patients should be permitted to access Internet and telephone during their stay in hospital.

Discharge should be discussed and planned carefully beforehand with the patient and care giver in family. Assess the service user's financial and home situation, including housing, before they are discharged from in-patient care. Agree discharge plans with the patient and include contingency plans in the event of problems arising after discharge. Ensure that a 24-h helpline is available to service users so that they can discuss any problems arising after discharge. Give service users clear information about all possible support options available to them after discharge or transfer of care.

37.7 Person-Centred Care in Family and Community

37.7.1 Involving Families

As a general principle, the involvement of family should be encouraged. However, providers should discuss with the person using mental health services if and how they want their family or carers to be involved in their care. As the involvement of families and carers can be quite complex, staff should receive training in the skills needed to negotiate and work with families and carers, and also in managing issues relating to information sharing and confidentiality. Service users may be ambivalent or negative towards their family for many different reasons, including as a result of the mental health problem or as a result of prior experience of violence or abuse. The more tolerant and stable family system in less-developed countries are potential assets for ensuring person-centred care.

37.7.2 Avoiding Stigma and Promoting Social Inclusion

The professionals caring for the patient should be respectful of and sensitive to his gender, sexual orientation, socioeconomic status, age, cultural, ethnic and religious backgrounds. They should have competence in assessment skills and using explanatory models of illness for people from different cultural, ethnic, religious or other diverse backgrounds. They should work with local authorities and all other local organizations with an interest in mental health (including social services, other hospitals, voluntary, organizations, local press and media groups, and local employer organizations) to develop a strategy to combat the stigma in the community and even inside the health care system. The success of involvement of community gate keepers in community-based programmes like suicide prevention gives optimism for the effectiveness of such interventions in other aspects of mental health [8].

37.8 Person-Centred Rehabilitation

The principle of "*nothing about us, without us*" accepted in the planning and management of physical disabilities should be adapted in mental health care as well. Develop rehabilitation plans jointly with the recovering patient, and include activities that promote social inclusion such as education, employment, volunteering and leisure activities. Health and social care providers should consider employing service users to be involved in training teams of health and social care professionals and supporting staff (such as receptionists, administrators, secretaries and housekeeping staff) in 'person-centred care'. Recovering patients themselves should be provided with training and supervision to undertake this role. Support service users to develop strategies, including risk- and self-management plans, to promote and maintain independence and self-efficacy, wherever possible. Incorporate these strategies into the care plan.

For people who may be at risk of crisis, a crisis plan should be developed by the service user and their care coordinator, which should be respected and implemented, and incorporated into the care plan.

37.9 Challenges Ahead

There are many foreseeable hurdles for the implementation of these changes in reorganizing psychiatric services [4, 6]. These include

1. Resistance to change from the existing system itself: The existing organization of mental health care delivery is designed to suit the convenience of the providers. Feasibility issues may come up as roadblocks if sufficient planning and preparations are not undertaken. It is very important to impart training programmes for the professionals in the service with an objective to reorient them to a person-centred approach. Person-centred approach should be incorporated into the curricula of mental health professionals.
2. Difficulties of service users and families to adapt to a system which requires more active involvement from their part: The service utilizers and their family members (especially in the non-western world) are used to the paternalistic care being provided by the existing system. Changing over from this passive recipient mode to the actively involved and responsible mode is likely to create difficulties.
3. Limitations of resources and funding: The changeover to the person-centred services may require employment of more manpower and development of more infrastructures. This calls for more investment and budget allocation for mental health services. This factor can be an important hurdle which needs to be tackled especially in resource limited countries.

37.10 Conclusions

Psychiatry has slowly started embracing a person-centred approach which is a holistic approach with an attitude of respect for the individual and his or her unique experience and needs as a patient. Mental health care delivery needs to be reorganized in a way which is sensitive to the needs of the users. Integrating mental health in primary care and general health care can make mental health care more affordable and feasible in most parts of the world. Models like the NICE guidelines [12] have essentially captured the spirit of person-centeredness in the organization of mental health services. Though these guidelines are drawn upon the system in a western world setting, other countries including the low- and middle-income countries can adapt this model for initiating effective person-centred organization of mental health services. This may serve as a model upon which innovations can be tried keeping with resource limitations. A simple model of person-centeredness at four levels—assessment, hospital care, family and community care, and rehabilitation is introduced and briefly described. Associations of mental health professionals may contribute to and catalyze the organization of person-centred mental health services in each country in a manner that suits its social, cultural and economic realities. They should be incorporated into the national health policy of each nation.

References

1. Boise L, White DJ. Family's role in person centred care: practice considerations. Psychosoc Nurs Ment Health Serv. 2004;42(5):12–20.
2. Borg M, Karlsson B, Tandora J, Davidson LM. Reorientation from patienthood to personhood. Negotiation and partnership in decision making. Israel J Psychiatry Relat Sci. 2009;46(2):84–93.
3. Deegan PE. The independent living movement and people with psychiatric disabilities: taking back control over our own lives. Psychosoc Rehab J. 1992;15:3–19.
4. Deuchar N. Review of "Freeth R (2007): humanizing psychiatry and mental health care: the challenge of the person-centred approach. Oxford: Radcliffe Publishing". Br J Psychiatry. 2008;193:262.
5. Freeth R. Humanising psychiatry and mental health care: the challenge of the person-centred approach. Oxford: Radcliffe Publishing; 2007.
6. Gask L, Coventry P. Person-centred mental health care: the challenge of implementation. Epidemiol Psychiatr Sci. 2012;2:139–44.
7. Herrman H, Saxena S, Moodie R. Promoting mental health: concepts, emerging evidence, practice. Geneva: World Health Organization; 2005.
8. Kallivayalil RA, Punnoose VP. Suicide prevention: a handbook for community gate keepers. Kottayam: National Alliance for Mental Health Kottayam; 2009.
9. Kallivayalil RA, Punnoose VP. Person centred medicine and primary health care: academic perspectives. Int J Pers Cent Med. 2011;1(3):433–4.
10. Mezzich JE. Psychiatry for the person: articulating medicine's science and humanism. World Psychiatry. 2007;6(2):65–7.
11. Mezzich JE. WPA perspectives on person-centered psychiatry and medicine. Int J Integr Care. 2010;10.

12. NICE. Common mental health disorders: identification and pathways to care. Clinical guideline 123. London: National Institute for Health and Clinical Excellence; 2011.
13. Rutz W. Social psychiatry and public mental health: present situation and future objective. Time for rethinking and renaissance? Acta Psychiatr Scand. 2006;113(suppl 429):95–100.
14. Sharfstein SS. Presidential address: advocacy for our patients and our profession. Am J Psychiatry. 2005;162:2045–7.
15. Thompson AGH. The meaning of patient involvement and participation in health care consultations: a taxonomy. Soc Sci Med. 2007;64:1297–310.
16. Tondora J, Miler R, Davidson L. The top ten concerns about person-centred care planning in mental health system. Int J Pers Cent Med. 2012;2:410–20.
17. Wagner EH, Austin BT, Von Korff M. Organizing care for patients with chronic illness. Milbank Q. 1996;74:511–44.
18. World Health Organization. People centred healthcare: a policy framework. Manila: World Health Organization Regional Office for the Western Pacific; 2007.
19. World Health Organization. World Mental Health Atlas 2011. Geneva: World Health Organization; 2011.

Evaluation of Person-Centered Health Services

38

Levent Kirisci, PhD, Jeanine M. Hayes, RN, MSL
and Juan E. Mezzich, MD, MA, MS, PhD

38.1 Introduction

Economics Nobel laureate, Stiglitz [11] has stated that "What you measure affects what you do. If you don't measure the right thing, you don't do the right thing." Furthermore, concerning his field of economics, he pointed out that assessment tools should incorporate a broader concern for human welfare, not just economic growth. *Mutatis mutandis* concerning the health field, one could argue that evaluation should not be restricted to diseases and their management but also cover positive health and well-being.

Along these lines, person-centered care seems to be emerging as the most important matrix for health care evaluation. Although traditionally health care evaluations have relied solely on the concept of patient satisfaction to evaluate the care of a person's experience in a health care setting, serious doubts have been expressed about the validity of the this concept. Satisfaction is unable to encompass the range of feelings, values, and experiences of a person using a health care

L. Kirisci, PhD (✉)
Professor, Department of Pharmaceutical Sciences, University of Pittsburgh School of Pharmacy, 3520 Forbes Avenue, Suite 203, Parkvale Annex, Pittsburgh, PA 15213, USA
e-mail: levent@pitt.edu

J.M. Hayes, RN, MSL
Psychiatric Nurse and Master of Science in Health Law, Pittsburgh, PA, USA

J.E. Mezzich, MD, MA, MS, PhD
Former President, World Psychiatric Association, Geneva, Switzerland;
Professor of Psychiatry, Icahn School of Medicine at Mount Sinai, New York, NY, USA;
Editor in Chief, International Journal of Person Centered Medicine, New York, NY, USA;
Secretary General, International College of Person Centered Medicine, New York, NY, USA

J.E. Mezzich et al. (eds.), *Person Centered Psychiatry*,
DOI 10.1007/978-3-319-39724-5_38

system. Additionally, many health care workers believe that they already provide person-centered care, but there is usually little evidence that this is the case. Such care is rarely monitored or measured in a way that reflects the key elements of person-centeredness.

In response to this situation, a review of the literature was conducted specifically on person-centered evaluation of health services. The methods and results of this effort are then summarized.

Presented next in a concise manner is work of the International College of Person-Centered Medicine toward the systematic conceptualization of person-centered medicine and health care, the development of a prototype person-centered care index, the analysis of its metric features, and its initial validation.

38.2 Literature Review for Evaluation of Person-Centered Care in Health Services

The intended review of the literature on evaluation of person-centered care in health services was conducted using Medline or Index Medicus from the US National Library of Medicine. The period of review was 1946 (onset of Medline) to July 2015.

38.2.1 Selection of Articles

A systematic search of Medline used the key words "evaluation" or "assessment" or "measurement" as applied to "person-centered" or "patient-centered" "health services". This led to the identification of 792 articles. A more focused selection of articles was guided by the following question: Which articles are relevant for scaling methods evaluating conceptual elements of person and people-centered health care systems?

Of the 792 articles reviewed, 28 articles were potentially relevant from which 9 final relevant articles described instruments or assessment tools to measure person-centered care in different health care settings and patient populations. Relevant articles described tools that were questionnaires completed by the person receiving health care with the exception of articles describing questionnaires completed by health care staff (P-CAT and POPAC).

Of the nine articles, two articles described a questionnaire (P-CIS) developed and assessed person-centered care on patients discharged from general medical, surgical, and otolaryngology wards and a recently discharged frail, older adult population (indices of personalization, empowerment, information, approachability and availability of staff, respectfulness, and miscellaneous); two articles described a questionnaire (CCCQ) evaluating the client-centeredness of professional home nursing care from a client's perspective (questions generated from formulation and consensus of client expectations and underlying values-equality, partnership, and interdependence); two articles describing a health care staff self-report assessment scale (P-CAT) aiming to measure the extent to which staff in aged care facilities rate their care as being patient-centered (questions generated from three subscales: extent of personalizing care, amount of organizational support, and degree of environmental accessibility); one article evaluating the reliability and validity of Patient-Centered Medical Home survey (CAHPS-PCMH) developed to enable evaluation of patient care experiences in sites of care at different stages of implementation of the medical home model of care delivery (indices related to questions regarding access to health care, communication with providers, courteous and helpful office staff, shared decision-making about medicine, self-management support, attention to mental health issues, and care coordination); and lastly, two articles describing the development of an instrument (POPAC), a staff-report questionnaire to assess person-centered care of older people with cognitive impairment in acute care (items generated by nursing best practice with older people experiencing cognitive impairment in acute care settings and staff attitude toward older people).

38.2.2 Literature Review Results

The results of this literature review are summarized in Table 38.1. For each of the analyzed nine articles, the paper's authors, year of publication, and abbreviated title are presented first. The second column indicates the general content area of the study at hand. The third summarizes the main results. The last column outlines the key ideas emerging from the paper.

38.2.3 Literature Review Conclusions

The review revealed that person-centered health services represent a complex domain that tends to be multidimensional. There were no articles in this database search that were found to present a standardized, validated, scale for use across health care facilities and clinical populations. Most of the instruments presented were developed within the framework of institutions working with a particular type of population or in a particular care setting. About half of the articles reviewed dealt with instruments aimed to older populations in specific settings. The need for generic instruments is quite apparent given the importance of comparative studies across settings, systems, and populations.

Table 38.1 Tabulated literature review on evaluation of person-centered health services

Authorship, year/abbreviated paper title	General content area	Main results	Key ideas
Hays et al., 2014 [6] Evaluating the Psychometric Properties of the CAHPS Patient-Centered Medical Home Survey.	Study to evaluate the reliability and validity of Consumer Assessment Of Health Care Providers and Systems (CAHPS) Patient-Centered Medical Home (PCMH) survey. Survey was developed to enable evaluation of patient care experiences. Survey content contains elements related to access to health care (5 items); communication with providers (6 items); courteous and helpful office staff (2 items); shared decision making about medicine (3 items); self-management support (2 items); attention to mental health issues (3 items); and care coordination (4 items).	The study provided further support for the reliability and validity of the CAHPS PCMH survey, but refinement of the self-management support and shared decision-making about medicines scale is needed. Further refinement of these scales to improve reliability and to distinguish shared decision making from communication with providers is recommended.	Patient experience measure and evaluation of health care in medical homes using 5 elements related to person-centered care, access of health services, and coordination of services.
De Witt et al. 2006 [2]. Development of the client-centered care questionnaire.	The CCCQ is a 15 item Dutch questionnaire (total score range 15–75) aimed at evaluating the client-centeredness of professional home nursing care from a client perspective. To develop the CCCQ, researchers first conducted a qualitative 2 phase study into client perspective of home nursing care. Items were formulated that closely	Study results suggested that clients perceive their care as client-centered when they feel recognized and respected by their caregivers. Based on these outcomes, 15 items were formulated; Item 1–10 covered the concept conduct by caregivers and item 11–15 covered the perception of autonomy. Clients tended to be	Development of a 15- item self-report questionnaire to evaluate client-centeredness in a home health setting with clients that had chronic diseases.

(continued)

Table 38.1 (continued)

Authorship, year/abbreviated paper title	General content area	Main results	Key ideas
	followed the aspects clients mentioned were central to client-centered home care.	most critical about their say in the practical arrangements and organization of care. Internal consistency was high (Cronbach's alpha = 0.94). Principal components analysis and internal consistency analysis show strong internal consistency of the items. All items had strong factor loadings on one dimension.	
Muntinga et al., 2014 [8]. Measurement properties of the Client-Centered Care Questionnaire (CCCQ) in a population of frail, older adults.	Data from a 2-year clinical trial was collected to evaluated client-centeredness of home care services by frail, older adults using the Client-Centered Care Questionnaire (CCCQ) to test the factor structure, reliability, content validity and acceptability of the CCCQ in this population.	The researchers concluded that the CCCQ's reliability parameters were acceptable, however, were cautious to make a definitive statement regarding the instrument's construct validity. The respondents often answered "don't know/no opinion" to the CCCQ questions which could be indicative a high respondent burden, caused by the theoretical nature of the construct client-centeredness (which causes items to be abstract) and by the fact that in home care practice, older clients, especially those which have chronic conditions or with complex care needs, often with multiple caregivers. Based on these findings, the authors concluded that the	Testing an existing instrument, the CCCQ, in a population of frail, older people in the Netherlands.

(continued)

Table 38.1 (continued)

Authorship, year/abbreviated paper title	General content area	Main results	Key ideas
		CCCQ may not be the most feasible instrument to use in assessing client-centeredness in older, chronically ill people.	
Edvardsson et al., 2010 [4]. Development and initial testing of the Person-centered Care Assessment Tool.	Development and initial testing of a self-report assessment scale (P-CAT), which measured the extent to which long term staff rate their residential-care settings to be person-centered. A preliminary 39 item tool was generated through the process of review of research literature, expert panel consultations, and research interviews with staff working in long-term aged care facilities (n = 37), people with early onset dementia (n = 11) and family members (n = 19). The P-CAT was distributed to a sample of Australian aged care staff (n = 220) and subjected to item analysis and reduction.	Exploratory factor analysis resulted in a three-factor solution: extent of personalizing care, amount of organizational support, and degree of environmental accessibility Psychometric evaluation of the final 13-item tool was conducted using statistical estimates of validity and reliability. Internal consistency was satisfactory except for subscale 3 (Cronbach's α = 0.31). Test-retest was also found to be satisfactory. The authors suggested that the dimensionality and internal consistency of the scale needed further investigation.	Development and initial testing of the P-CAT, a self-report assessment scale by long-term aged care staff as to rating their settings to be person-centered.
Sjogren et al., 2012 [10]. Psychometric evaluation of the Swedish version of the Person-Centered Care Assessment Tool (P-CAT).	A study which evaluated the psychometric properties of the Swedish version of the Person-Centered Care Assessment Tool (P-CAT), an instrument aiming to measure the extent to	The authors discussed that although the findings of the study indicated a two-factor dimensionality of the P-CAT which included the person and the environment, it did not	Psychometric evaluation of the Swedish version of the Person-Centered Care Assessment Tool.

(continued)

Table 38.1 (continued)

Authorship, year/abbreviated paper title	General content area	Main results	Key ideas
	which staff in aged care facilities rate the care provided as being person-centered. A cross-sectional sample of 1465 staff from 195 residential care units for older people in Sweden participated in the study.	capture the dimension of person-environment fit. Confirmatory factor analysis, parallel analysis and exploratory factor analysis supported the construct validity of a two-factor solution. Reliability and homogeneity were satisfactory for the whole P-CAT (Cronbach's $\alpha = 0.75$). Questions remained regarding the endorsement frequency of some items and the underlying construct of the scale. On the basis of this study, the authors recommended using a two-scale/two-factor structure when using the Swedish version of the P-CAT.	
Coyle and Williams, 2001 [1] Valuing people as individuals: development of an instrument through a survey of person-centeredness in secondary care.	A cross-sectional survey involving 97 inpatients from medical, surgical and otolaryngology units who completed a questionnaire developed from a qualitative study containing items on dehumanization, objectification, disempowerment, and devaluation in these health care settings.	The research suggested that patients' identity was threatened by experiences perceived as dehumanizing, objectifying, disempowering and devaluing in the health care setting. The concept of "patient identity threat" showed the extent to which people felt valued (or not) as individuals. Problems highlighted around	Development and initial testing of questionnaire developed measuring the client experience of "personal identity threat" in clinical care settings.

(continued)

Table 38.1 (continued)

Authorship, year/abbreviated paper title	General content area	Main results	Key ideas
		power/control, involvement in care, and approachability/availability of staff. Additionally, findings of the research suggested that women were more at risk than men of threats to identity in these health care settings.	
Davis et al., 2008 [3] Measuring person-centered care in a sub-acute health care setting.	A study in which a 20 item Patient-Centered Inpatient Scale (P-CIS) developed by Coyle and Williams [1] was studied to determine its utility with a frail older Australian population. A random sample of 144 clients recently discharged from a sub-acute setting were sent a 20 item questionnaire and asked to respond. Core statements related to five specific dimensions (personalization, empowerment, information, approachability/availability and respect) are included in the P-CIS. Scoring for the P-CIS is based on positive responses to the statements.	Core statements for each of the P-CIS dimensions were examined against the various dimensions of person-centeredness. Results for the pilot study showed the overall Person-Centered Care Score was 0.68 which the researchers described as revealing a fundamental core of person-centeredness in the approach to care. Personalization and respect dimensions were the main strengths of person-centered care in the health care setting in which was P-CIS was studied, with personalization scoring 0.75 and respect scoring 0.77. Empowerment and information dimensions scored 0.58 and	An existing instrument, the Patent-Centered Inpatient Scale was studied in a population of frail older persons.

(continued)

Table 38.1 (continued)

Authorship, year/abbreviated paper title	General content area	Main results	Key ideas
		approachability/availability scored the lowest at 0.43.	
Edvardsson et al., 2013 [5] The person-centered care of older people with cognitive impairment in acute care scale (POPAC).	The POPAC is a 15- item scale which aims to measure staff perceptions of person-centered care in older adults with cognitive impairment in acute care clinical settings. The scale consists of 3 subscales, "using cognitive assessment and care interventions", "using evidence and cognitive expertise" and "individualized care". Development of the scale was based on an Australian sample of acute care nursing staff (n = 212).	The POPAC was reported to have satisfactory psychometric properties with an overall Cronbach's alpha of 0.87 and subscales Cronbach's alpha values of 0.74, 0.79, and 0.78. The three subscales explained 53% of the total variance in the original factor model. The content and construct validity of the POPAC was reported as satisfactory.	An instrument to measure staff perceptions of person-centered care in older adults.
Nilsson et al., 2013 [9]. Measuring levels of person-centeredness in acute care of older people with cognitive impairment: evaluation of the POPAC scale.	The POPAC (Person-Centered Care of Older People with Cognitive Impairment in Acute Care Scale) was translated from the English version to Swedish to evaluate its psychometric properties in a sample of acute hospital staff.	The results indicated that the Swedish version POPAC provides a tentatively construct-valid and reliable contribution in measuring the extent to which acute inpatient hospital services have processes and procedures that can facilitate person-centered care in older patients with cognitive impairment. However, questions remain regarding the dimensionality of POPAC.	Psychometric evaluation of the Swedish version of the Person-Centered version of the Person-Centered Care of Older People with Cognitive Impairment in Acute Care Services Scale.

38.3 Development, Metric Analysis, and Initial Validation of a Person-Centered Care Index

The International College of Person-centered Medicine (ICPCM) has conducted a project with support of the World Health Organization toward the systematic conceptualization and delineation of person- and people-centered medicine and health care and the construction and initial validation of procedures to measure progress in these directions. A technical report [7] outlining these evolving studies have been presented at recent ICPCM Geneva Conferences on Person-Centered Medicine. A full report in an academic paper will be published elsewhere.

More specifically, the objectives of the overall study are the following:

1. Exploration of the conceptual bases of person- and people-centered health care.
2. Development of a prototype procedure, a Person-centered Care Index, to assess progress in person- and people-centered care based on suitable scaling of the key factors identified under the previous objective.
3. Exploration of the metric characteristics of the Person-centered Care Index.
4. Preliminary validation of the Person-centered Care Index in terms of its content or face validity and its applicability to available health systems as well as in terms of its reliability.

The phases of the overall study corresponding to the above-listed objectives will be presented next in a summarized manner.

38.4 Exploration of the Conceptual Bases of Person- and People-Centered Health Care

This initial phase of the study was conducted with the involvement of two international panels. A Core Workgroup was composed of 17 experts from the Americas, Europe, Africa, Asia, and Oceania, including physicians from multiple specialties as well as nursing and social work representatives and patient and family representatives. Work with them was conducted through teleconferences. A broader Consultation Group included 56 international experts from across the world, including physicians and other health professionals and scholars. They responded to questions by email.

The first step of this phase was a Systematic Literature Review. The literature review was aimed at exploring the bases of person- and people-centered health care as reflected in the literature. It involved two parts. The first one was based on papers presented at the 2008, 2009, and 2010 Geneva Conferences on Person-centered Medicine and others from the archives of the International Network for Person-Centered Medicine as well as those identified by members of the Core Workgroup. The second one involved a systematic search of Pub Med using as key words "person-centered medicine, person-centered health care, person-centered clinical communication, diagnostic and treatment shared decision making, and person- and people-centered health systems." The review was conducted by a research associate under the supervision of the study director, with input and guidance from the Core Workgroup. A tabulated summary of the literature review containing authors and year, paper title, general content area, main results, and key ideas, as well as other details of the literature review will be included in an academic paper to be published elsewhere.

The second step of the initial phase involved the Elucidation, Rating, and Delineation of Literature-based Features of Person-centeredness. Upon reviewing the tabulated summary of the literature review, the Core Workgroup identified a set of key domains relevant to person- and people-centeredness in health systems. This set included first a subset of 14 domains related to "Personal Health and Care" and a second one of 7 domains related to "Public Health and Services Organization." More specifically, the first subset seemed to refer to person-centeredness and the second to people-centeredness. The domains elucidated from the literature were organized into a form to facilitate its presentation to and handling by the Consultation Group. The form also included space at the end for additional domains to be possibly identified by Consultation Group members. These individuals were asked to rate the importance (high, medium, low) for person-centeredness of each of the presented domains, and to identify and delineate within each domain crucial elements characterizing person- and people-centered care.

38.5 Development of a Prototype Person-Centered Care Index

On the basis of the above-mentioned responses from the Consultation Group, the Core Workgroup drafted a Person-centered Care Index (PCI). It includes 33 items nested under eight broad categories, as follows: 1. Ethical Commitment, 2. Cultural Sensitivity, 3. Holistic Approach, 4. Relational Focus, 5. Individualized Care, 6. Common Ground for Diagnosis and Care, 7. People-centered Systems of Care, and 8. Person-centered Education and Research. The rating instructions are called for marking the level of presence of each indicator in a given health system using a 4-point scale: not present, moderately present, substantially present, and highly present. Along with some adjustments in wording, the anchor points of the rating scale were reformulated in terms of the frequency of the presence of each of the instrument's items. The PCI also calls for computing a global average score by adding the partial scores and dividing the result by the number of items actually rated. Finally, the PCI offers space at the end for narrative evaluative comments. Table 38.2 presents all broad categories and individual items and the rating scale of the PCI.

Table 38.2 Person-centered Care INDEX (PCI)

No	Indicators	Never	Occasionally	Frequently	Always
1. Ethical commitment					
1.1	The dignity of every person involved (patients, family, clinicians) is honored	1	2	3	4
1.2	Patient's rights are respected	1	2	3	4
1.3	Patient's autonomy is supported	1	2	3	4
1.4	Patient's empowerment is advanced	1	2	3	4
1.5	The fulfillment of the patient's life project (purpose in life) is enabled and encouraged	1	2	3	4
1.6	The patient's personal values, choices, and needs are understood and respected	1	2	3	4
2. Cultural sensitivity					
2.1	The patient's ethnic identity and cultural values are recognized	1	2	3	4
2.2	The patient's language and communication needs and preferences are actively considered	1	2	3	4
2.3	The patient's gender and sexual preferences are acknowledged and respected	1	2	3	4
2.4	The patient's spiritual needs are factored in	1	2	3	4
3. Holistic scope					
3.1	The biological, psychological, social, cultural, and spiritual factors of health inform understanding and care	1	2	3	4
3.2	Both ill-health (health problems, disabilities) and positive health or well-being (functioning, resilience, strengths, resources, and quality of life) are focus of attention	1	2	3	4
4. Relational focus					
4.1	Clinicians, patients and families work in partnership	1	2	3	4
4.2	Empathy in clinical communication is emphasized	1	2	3	4
4.3	Interpersonal trust is fostered throughout the care process	1	2	3	4
5. Individualized care					
5.1	The patient's individuality and unique qualities inform care	1	2	3	4
5.2	The patient's historical and social context are factored in	1	2	3	4
5.3	The patient's personal growth and development are promoted	1	2	3	4

(continued)

Table 38.2 (continued)

No	Indicators	Never	Occasionally	Frequently	Always
6. Common ground for diagnosis and care					
6.1	Diagnosis of health status, experience, and contributory factors involve shared understanding	1	2	3	4
6.2	Diagnosis is worked out taking into account the whole person	1	2	3	4
6.3	Care plan decisions are made collaboratively	1	2	3	4
7. People-centered systems of care					
7.1	The health and rights of all people in the community are advocated and promoted	1	2	3	4
7.2	The community participates in the planning of health services	1	2	3	4
7.3	Collaboration across disciplines and programs is promoted at all levels of service organization	1	2	3	4
7.4	Personalized services are aimed at attaining high quality and excellence	1	2	3	4
7.5	Health services are responsive to specific community needs and expectations	1	2	3	4
7.6	Health services are integrated and coordinated around patients' needs	1	2	3	4
7.7	Services emphasize people-centered primary care	1	2	3	4
7.8	Services ensure continuity of care	1	2	3	4
7.9	Services are informed by person-centered international perspectives and developments	1	2	3	4
8. Person-centered education and research					
8.1	The health system promotes person-centered public education	1	2	3	4
8.2	The health system promotes person-centered health professional training	1	2	3	4
8.3	The health system promotes person-centered clinical research	1	2	3	4
Global average score					
Additional evaluative comments:					

This instrument is being developed by the International College of Person-centered Medicine. Please rate the following person-centered care indicators in terms of the frequency of their presence in a given health system. The term "patient" here refers to a person who experiences health problems and/or uses health services, whose personhood transcends these roles and circumstances. To obtain a global average PCI score, please add the partial scores and divide this by the number of items actually rated.

38.6 Exploration of the Metric Characteristics of the Person-Centered Care Index

On the basis of exercises with the PCI completed by the members of the broad Consultation Group, data on the internal structure of the PCI was obtained. The initial database encompassed the ratings made by each of the raters on each of the items of the PCI. A first analysis of the correlational matrix of items versus items yielded a tight internal correlational structure for the PCI expressed as a very high Cronbach alpha of 0.95.

The factorial structure of the PCI scale was studied through a principal component factor analysis of its broad categories. The first eigenvalue was 5.49 and explained 69 % of the variance. The factor loadings on the first factor were 0.87 for Ethical Commitment, 0.55 for Cultural Sensitivity, 0.90 for Holistic Approach, 0.80 for Relational Focus, 0.93 for Individualized Care, 0.91 for Common Ground for Diagnosis and Care, 0.79 for People-centered Systems of Care, and 0.82 for Person-centered Education and Research. The second eigenvalue was 1.04 and explained only 13 % of the total variance. These results indicate that the PCI has a unidimensional factor structure. Also noteworthy is that all the PCI broad categories loaded substantially on the first factor, a factor that therefore could be labeled as "person-centered health care."

An additional analysis of the items versus items correlational matrix, led to the exploration of the correlation of each of the broad categories with the PCI global score. The correlations ranged from substantial to high. The correlations with PCI global score were 0.86 for Ethical Commitment, 0.62 for Cultural Sensitivity, 0.85 for Holistic Scope, 0.73 for Relational Focus, 0.81 for Individualized Care, 0.87 for Common Ground for Diagnosis and Care, 0.82 for People-centered Systems of Care, and 0.78 for Person-centered Education and Research.

A further analysis of the items versus items correlational matrix involved the exploration of subsets of variables that correlated linearly in a substantial manner with the PCI global score. A stepwise linear regression analysis was conducted to determine the best subset of broad categories to predict the PCI global score. Individualized care was the first category entered into the model and explained 83 % of the variance. People-centered systems of care contributed an additional 9 % of the variance and, on the next step, person-centered education and research explained 4 % of the variance beyond the contributions of the first two categories entered.

Another stepwise linear regression analysis was conducted to determine the best subset of the 33 PCI items in predicting through a linear model the PCI global score. The best subset of items to predict the PCI global average score that were entered into the model were "5.3. The patient's personal growth and development are promoted", "7.7. Services emphasize people-centered primary care", "1.6. The patient's personal values, choices, and needs are understood and respected", "1.5. The fulfillment of the patient's life project (purpose in life) is enabled and encouraged", "7.2. The community participates in the planning of health services", and "1.3. The patient's autonomy is supported". Their corresponding standardized beta coefficients in the linear model were 0.27, 0.27, 0.27, 0.25, 0.12, and 0.12. They were all significant at a p 0.001 level.

38.7 Preliminary Validation of the Person-Centered Care Index

The validation component of the overall study has been conducted in two parts. The first one took place within the framework of interactions with the broad Consultation Group. The second one was carried out in three difference sites: California (USA), London (UK), and Lucknow (India).

38.7.1 Content Validity Assessed Through Consultation Group Ratings

The members of the Consultation Group were asked to rate six aspects of the content validity or acceptability of the PCI using a 4-point scale (none, moderate, substantial, and high) to rate the degree to which content validity was fulfilled. It was found that all six content validity aspects received quite positive ratings in terms of the combined percentage of the top two scale points (substantial and high), as follows: Broad categories being suitable and clear: 92 %; subcategories or individual items being suitable and clear: 84 %; the global score being a useful indicator of total person-centered care: 74 %; the four-point rating scale being suitable and clear: 84 %; the space for additional evaluative comments being valuable: 79 %; and the whole PCI being valuable: 87 %.

The Consultation Group members were also asked to conduct an exercise to study the applicability of the PCI to a health system (national, city, or other) available to each of them. A wide diversity of ratings were found across the four levels of presence, which suggested the suitability of the PCI to cover a broad range of person-centeredness. On each of the eight broad categories of person-centeredness, the ratings of the available health systems tended to focus between moderately present and substantially present person-centeredness.

Finally, the Consultation Group members were asked to evaluate their PCI application exercise just mentioned above in terms of two validation aspects. One, ease of completion of the PCI was rated as 96 % combining the top two positive ratings (substantial and high levels of satisfaction). The other, suitability of the PCI to describe person-centeredness of the rated health system obtained a 76 % combining the top two positive suitability levels.

38.7.2 Content Validity Assessed with a Group of Mental Health Service Users in London, UK

This exercise was conducted with seven mental health service users by a colleague of this paper's authors, researcher Jan Wallcraft from the University of Birmingham. First, the participants were asked to evaluate with a 4-point scale the acceptability of the PCI on six aspects of content validity. The ratings obtained in terms of the combined percentage of the top two scale points (substantial and high), were as follows: Broad categories being suitable and clear: 80 %; subcategories or individual items being suitable and clear: 80 %; the global score being a useful indicator of total person-centered care: 60 %; the four-point rating scale being suitable and clear: 100 %; the space for additional evaluative comments being valuable: 100 %; and the whole PCI being valuable: 80 %. The participants were also asked to evaluate a health system of their choice with the PCI, and then were asked to evaluate the PCI on the basis of their preceding experience. By combining the top two rating options on a 4-point scale, ease of completion attained 60 % and suitability to describe person-centeredness attained also 60 %.

38.7.3 Inter-rater Reliability in the Evaluation of Mental Health Facilities in California, USA

Five mental health services in Santa Cruz County, California, USA were evaluated with the PCI by two independent raters, under the supervision of our colleague Dr. Neal Adams. Services and raters were randomly chosen from a larger number of services and raters. A two way random model was used to compute intraclass correlation coefficients (ICCs) as indices of inter-rater reliability. The ICC for the overall PCI was 0.89, which is quite high. The ICCs for specific broad categories and items of the PCI was rather variable, probably because the small number of cases involved.

38.7.4 Inter-rater Reliability in the Evaluation of Four Medical Services by Medical Residents in Lucknow, India

Under the supervision of our colleagues Prof. J.K. Trivedi and Dr. Sujit Kar, a group of 20 psychiatric medical residents became familiar with the PCI and applied it in groups of convenience to four different medical services: psychiatry, neurology, internal medicine, and trauma. A two-way random model was used to compute intraclass correlation coefficients (ICCs) as inter-rater reliability indices with facilities and raters assumed to represent random effects. The ICC for the PCI Global Average Score for the rating of psychiatry and neurology services was 0.89, for the psychiatry and trauma services it was 0.99, and for the psychiatry, neurology, and internal medicine services the ICC was 0.86. Most of the ICCs for PCI broad categories were quite high. In fact for 85 % of them the corresponding ICC was 0.75 or higher.

38.8 Conclusions

The review of the literature on evaluation of person-centered health services revealed a number of efforts in this field. Most of them were developed for quite specific populations and settings such as services for older people. No instrument for the generic evaluation of person-centered health care across populations and settings was apparent.

The recent work of the International College of Person-Centered Medicine to study the systematic conceptualization of person-centered medicine and heath care and the development of instruments for evaluating person-centered health care has been quite productive. A valuable profile of key concepts for person-centered medicine and health care has been elucidated and a prototype person-centered care index has been developed. Its preliminary validation in terms of applicability, ease of use, content validity, and inter-rater reliability suggests its value for the generic assessment of person-centered health care across settings and populations. At the same time, further evaluation of the instrument with larger samples across settings and populations is warranted.

References

1. Coyle J, Williams B. Valuing people as individuals: development of an instrument through a survey of person-centeredness in secondary care. J Adv Nurs. 2001;36:450–5.
2. De Witte L, School T, Proot I. Development of the client-centered care questionnaire. J Adv Nurs. 2006;56:62–8.
3. Davis S, Byers S, Walsh F. Measuring person-centred care in a sub-acute health care setting. Aust Health Rev. 2008;32(3):496–504.
4. Edvardsson D, Fetherstonhaugh D, Nay R, Gibson S. Development and initial testing of the Person-Centered Care Assessment Tool (P-CAT). Int Psychogeriatr. 2010;22:101–8.
5. Edvardsson D, Nilsson A, Fetherstonhaugh D, Nay R, Crowe S. The person-centered care of older people with cognitive impairment in acute care scale (POPAC). J Nurs Manage. 2013;21:79–86.
6. Hays RD, Berman LJ, Kanter MH, Hugh M, Oglensby RR, Kim CY, Cui M, Brown J. Evaluating the psychometric properties of the CAHPS patient-centered medical home survey. Clin Ther. 2014;36(5):689–96.
7. Mezzich JE, Kirisci L, Salloum IM. Towards developing measures to assess progress towards person- and people-centered care. Technical report. New York: International College of Person Centered Medicine; 2015.
8. Muntinga ME, Mokkink LB, Knol DL, Nijpels G, Jansen APD. Measurement properties of the Client-centered Care Questionnaire (CCCQ): factor structure, reliability and validity of a questionnaire to assess self-reported client-centeredness of home care services in a population of frail, older people. Qual Life Res. 2014;23:2063–72.

9. Nilsson A, Lindkvist M, Rasmussen BH, Edvardsson D. Measuring levels of person-centeredness in acute care of older people with cognitive impairment: evaluation of the POPAC scale. BMC Health Serv Res. 2013;13:327.
10. Sjogren K, Lindkvist M, Sandman PO, Zingmark K, Edvardsson D. Psychometric evaluation of the Swedish version of the Person-Centered Care Assessment Tool (PCAT). Int Psychogeriatr. 2012;24:406–15.
11. Stiglitz J. On assessment tools. New York Times, 23 Sept 2009.

Person-Centered Psychiatric Education 39

Rodrigo Ramalho, MD, PhD, Roger Montenegro, MD, Veljko Djordjevic, MD, PhD, Marijana Braš, MD, PhD and Nikos Christodoulou, MBBS, MSc, PhD, MRCPsych

39.1 Introduction

> What the educator does in teaching is to make it possible for the students to become themselves.
>
> *Paulo Freire*

To understand education as a unidirectional transference of knowledge is to dismiss the human substance involved in the process. Education is an interactional process, dialogical in nature, and transformative in essence. Acknowledging this interactive, dialogical, and transformative nature of education is the first step

R. Ramalho, MD, PhD (✉)
Centre for Addiction Research (CFAR) and Department of Social and Community Health, School of Population Health, University of Auckland, Private Bag 92019, Victoria Street West, Auckland 1142, New Zealand
e-mail: rram417@aucklanduni.ac.nz

R. Montenegro, MD
President, Fundacion Contener, Buenos Aires, Argentina; Former Secretary of Education, World Psychiatric Association, Geneva, Switzerland; Former Director, Institute of Post Graduate Education, Association of Argentinean Psychiatrists, Buenos Aires, Argentina

V. Djordjevic, MD, PhD · M. Braš, MD, PhD
Professor, Department of Psychological Medicine, Clinical Hospital Centre Zagreb and School of Medicine, University of Zagreb, Zagreb, Croatia

N. Christodoulou, MBBS, MSc, PhD, MRCPsych
Consultant Liaison Psychiatrist and Honorary Assistant Professor in Psychiatry, University of Nottingham, Nottingham, UK

J.E. Mezzich et al. (eds.), *Person Centered Psychiatry*,
DOI 10.1007/978-3-319-39724-5_39

towards a person-centered education. Disregarding these qualities does not exclude them from the learning process, but rather shapes them in directions that could prove opposite to the goals of the educational enterprise. This is particularly relevant when related to medical education and the continuing professional development of psychiatrists and other physicians. Health professionals feel called to their professions by an inner desire to care for others. Educators should allow and encourage this personal aspiration to flourish *by means* of the educational process, rather than *despite of it*.

In medical education, an authoritarian and unidirectional interaction that disables the learners' voices has a transformative effect that, mirroring the learning experience, promotes a paternalistic and exclusionary health care. In other words, a reductionist approach to education generates a reductionist approach to health care. A person-centered psychiatric practice requires a person-centered psychiatric education (PCPE), as one is not possible without the other. The distinctive characteristic of a person-centered approach to psychiatric education is the acknowledgment that people constitute the core substance of the educational process. This approach does not overlook the importance of knowledge and continuous professional development, neither it ignores the fundamental roles of research, new technologies, and the use of the best evidence in practice. But, what distinguishes PCPE is its focus on the person, a focus that, in the words of Paulo Freire, demands educators "to come from speaking *to* into speaking *with*" the students [25, p. 180]. It is on this distinctive concern that this chapter focuses its content.

First, an overview is presented of the foundational elements of a person-centered medical education, as introduced in the Zagreb Declaration on Person-Centered Health Professional Education [4] and further expanded by Appleyard et al. [1]. Then, key features and strategies of PCPE are introduced in relation to medical students, psychiatrist trainees, and trained psychiatrists. The main goal is not to present an exhaustive description of all possible methods that educators can use to provide PCPE, but rather to provide a sense of what lies underneath this educational approach. It is hoped that this will allow readers to implement the approach by creating, adapting, or expanding specific strategies that can be integrated into the local contextual realities of their educational and professional environments.

39.2 Overview of Person-Centered Medical Education

As stated by Appleyard et al. [1], person-centered clinical practice enables preventing, promoting, curing, and rehabilitating simultaneously, which in return increases the efficiency of care and health systems. Several authors have highlighted the importance of a clinical practice that, grounded on ethics and human rights, focuses on the person and the person's life context, well-being, and life projects, rather than on the disease [10, 14, 31, 37, 45]. But for person-centered health care to be possible, person-centered education of health professionals is indispensable.

Person-centered medical education should start at the undergraduate level and continue throughout the physician's professional life. This educational approach moves away from education as unilateral transfer of knowledge to a framework of dialogical participation and experiential learning [3, 4]. This is very important, as learning person-centered principles is more connected to the interactive nature of the educational process than to the cognitive acquisition of information [13]. An environment of dialogical interaction where learners are engaged as individuals with specific backgrounds and motivations, promotes the development of critical thinking and an active search for meaning and understanding [34, 47]. In other words, person-centered education makes learning a transformative experience grounded in positive and supportive relationships.

Medical schools should be optimised for the support of this person-centered education. Such optimization process should include complementing biomedical sciences with social sciences, medical ethics, humanities and theology, as well as systems of knowledge about the whole person [13, 18, 33]. At the same time, medical schools should recognise the importance of engaging with patients and patients' families as equal partners in the health professionals' education [54]. Engaging with patients and their families as educators is a valuable educational resource that further promotes a deeper appreciation of the patient as a person [51, 55, 61].

Medical schools offering person-centered education cannot neglect the diversity of their student bodies and the general population they serve. This implies widening the access to medical schools to all social groups, and the development of an educational process that is not alienated from these social groups [21, 57]. If necessary, changes on the policies of selection of students and educators should be made to ensure person-centered education [4]. These changes need to take into account that not only students should be suited for the goals and responsibilities required of health professionals, but also that educators should be equally suited for their educational responsibilities [1].

Person-centered medical education should enable health professionals to develop interventions regarding prevention and health promotion that are guided by person-centered principles [12]. That is, interventions that are focused on enhancing the well-being of all members of the population while showing a profound respect for cultural diversity. In addition, person-centered medical education prepares health professionals to acknowledge and comprehend the influence of social and cultural factors on health, and to address them in health care [1, 4].

39.3 Person-Centered Psychiatric Education for Medical Students

PCPE aims to provide medical students with the knowledge, skills and attitudes necessary to offer person-centered psychiatric care. In line with the principles of person-centered health care, learners should be at the core of person-centered education [52]. The PCPE of medical students should provide them first hand experience of what is like to participate in a person-centered approach, while acquiring the knowledge and dexterities indispensable for person-centered psychiatric care. Therefore, students should be engaged as persons with unique characteristics, potentialities, and needs, within an environment of experiential learning, positive relationships, and dialogical participation [5, 8, 19].

Medical schools should do their best to provide and support person-centered education, which requires a multidisciplinary team. An education that relies on a multidisciplinary effort promotes the skills and attitudes necessary to work as part of a person-centered care team [2, 24]. In this regard, medical schools should formalise the study of social sciences and humanities, and actively introduce them as having the same value than the biomedical sciences [1, 2, 32, 33]. In medical schools that are grounded in person-centered principles, the PCPE of medical students will be part of a coordinated effort. Thus, the person-centered principles will be continuously reinforced by the whole learning process. However, if medical schools were not engaged with person-centered principles as a whole, the PCPE of medical students should introduce them to these principles, as well as to the value of teamwork and of systems of knowledge different from conventional biomedical approaches.

Introducing medical students to person-centered principles, teamwork, and the knowledge necessary for person-centered psychiatric care demands educators to become role models. The educators' attitudes are of formative importance for the students' development of person-centered attitudes. Students' engagement with non-person-centered role models is an obstacle for their development of person-centeredness [5]. If possible, medical students' person-centered education should be designed to offer them mentorship, enhancing their strengths and talents while addressing their needs whenever necessary [7, 13, 27]. Web-based technologies could complement face-to-face interactions, providing a resourceful learning environment that could foster follow up communication [41]. Medical students should have a direct experience of an interaction that is tailored to address their unique characteristics, potentialities, and needs, as this type of interaction is the basis of a person-centered psychiatric care.

Person-centered health care requires the ability to engage in dialogical communication with patients and patients' families. This communication should be committed to address patients' specific characteristics, strengths, and needs, while having a deep respect for their perspectives [39]. Thus, teaching communication skills must be considered crucial in the education of medical students [7, 44]. There are several ways in which education on communication skills can be introduced to medical students, e.g. role plays [36] or communication sessions [50]. In any case, building up a relationship with the patient should always be at the core of the learning experience [7]. This is key for medical students to develop an awareness about the essential role of communicating with patients as persons in clinical practice [26, 44].

The PCPE of medical students should include patients and patients' families as equal partners in the educational process. Recognising the patients' voices, perspectives, and experiences as educational resources will help medical students to develop person-centeredness [54], and it could have therapeutic benefits for psychiatric patients [58]. If necessary, the use of settings different from standard educational institutions as learning environments could be a valuable tool for the person-centered education of medical students [2, 23, 27]. At the same time, students themselves should also be considered equal partners in their PCPE, and they should have an active role in their own learning experience. This learning process should prepare medical students for the continuous process of acquiring and transferring knowledge that is involved in being a physician [3].

The PCPE of medical students focuses on helping students to develop the attitudes necessary to practice person-centered care. However, neither knowledge nor skills are disregarded in the educational process. PCPE should not only provide both theoretical and practical psychiatric education to medical students, but it should also encourage them to do research. As mentioned in the 2013 Geneva Declaration on Person-centered Health Research [49], person-centered health needs more person-centered research, and medical students could assist in meeting these needs. Additionally, students should also be encouraged to attend conferences, symposia, workshops, and lectures that could further benefit their person-centered learning experience, and whenever possible, they should be motivated to conduct and present their own research.

Finally, person-centered psychiatric practice emphasises the importance of considering the persons' value and dignity at the core of public health policies [37, 38], and the PCPE of medical students should help them to learn that person-centered care also involves public health actions. Working towards the patients' well-being requires addressing social determinants of health [2], and the education of medical students should encourage them to become involved in the design, implementation, and evaluation of health policies [4]. Medical students should be able to see that the relevance of focusing on persons' well-being goes beyond medicine and health and it reaches other social sectors, including government goals and policies [56].

39.4 Person-Centered Psychiatric Education for Psychiatrist Trainees and Trained Psychiatrists

Mirroring the PCPE of medical students, the PCPE of psychiatrist trainees has the trainees as its main focus. A person-centered education focuses on the whole person, as well as the learning environment [60]. The PCPE of psychiatrist trainees should take place within a framework of positive relationships, where trainees' needs, expectations, skills, and talents are addressed, helping them to develop both personally and professionally. At the same time, the PCPE of trained psychiatrists, as part of their continuing professional development, should also be framed in a positive environment where they are the focus. This will help them to experience person-centeredness, while enabling them to develop, maintain, or enhance a person-centered approach in their practice.

A person-centered educational style is particularly relevant for psychiatrist trainees, whom, unlike medical students, may be able to immediately implement this approach during their daily clinical practices. Trainees' education must provide them with the knowledge, skills, and attitudes necessary to offer, from the beginning of their professional careers, what Mezzich [37] refers to as a 'psychiatry for the person'. Educators should be mindful that although imparted knowledge has a valuable impact on the trainees' professional practice, the educators' behaviours and attitudes have a deep and long-lasting formative effect on them [59]. Trainees should have positive role models who are invested in their doctor-patient relationships [30]. Whenever educators engage with patients, they should provide trainees with professional models they will be able to mirror in their professional careers, as no textbook or chalk and talk class will be able to replace the opportunity to observe, experience, and then internalise a person-centered approach.

Developing effective communication skills is indispensable to provide person-centered care, and teaching communication skills through role modelling is also key in the PCPE of psychiatrist trainees. Trainees' education should include the development of person-centered interviewing skills that enable trainees to communicate with patients as persons [46], and patients could have an important role teaching these skills [29]. Moreover, trainees should also learn to share the decision-making process regarding treatment with their patients, as this would further help them to address the patients' specific needs [20]. Educators should not only offer trainees with professional behaviours to imitate whenever they approach a patient, but they should also engage with trainees in the same way they expect them to engage with patients. The PCPE of psychiatrist trainees should always be a constant exercise of dialogical interaction, where trainees are acknowledged as persons with specific characteristics, potentialities, and needs.

PCPE is also very important for trained psychiatrists as part of their continuing professional development. Focusing on the persons' uniqueness, potentialities, and needs should also be a key component of trained psychiatrists' PCPE. The PCPE of trained psychiatrists should also be done via mentoring relationships that provide both mentor and mentee the possibility to learn and grow from each other's knowledge and experience [42]. A person-centered education can also be implemented through programmes aiming to promote reflective and person-centered practice that may or may not be followed by an on-going mentoring [19]. However, regardless of the delivery method, trained psychiatrists' PCPE should always try to be an interactive and dialogical experience, as learning person-centered principles has to do more with the interactive nature of the educational process than with the transference of theoretical knowledge [13]. That is, whether it is for medical students, psychiatrist trainees, or trained psychiatrists' continuing professional development, PCPE should always aim to be a highly personal and transformative experience.

When talking about educators, other members of the health care team should also be acknowledged as active participants in psychiatrists' education. The PCPE of psychiatrist trainees should allow them to experience the continuum of health promotion, prevention, treatment, rehabilitation, and palliative care in their educational process, and this can only be done by means of a multidisciplinary approach. In this regard, educators serving as role models, showing respect for the knowledge and skills that all members of the health care team provide, are of utmost importance [24]. In addition, ensuring collaborative care should also be part of trained psychiatrists' continuing professional development. Psychiatrists' continuing professional development should integrate interprofessional programmes that help them to better understand their roles within a care team, promoting respect and positive attitudes towards all members of the team [9].

Besides fellow health professionals, patients should also be considered equal partners in the psychiatrists' education [35]. The PCPE of trainees should consider the patients' involvement beyond one-off and isolated events, and include the patients' voices throughout the programme [54]. Although there might be several issues that need to be considered when implementing this approach [16, 22], it will nevertheless be highly significant in assisting psychiatrist trainees to regard patients as persons and not merely as disease carriers. Patients should also be part of the psychiatrists' continuing professional development, for example through direct participation as educators or through patient directed research [17, 35]. In other words, if PCPE is to promote a partnership with patients in care, it should also promote this partnership in the psychiatrists' education throughout their professional careers.

During their education, psychiatrist trainees should also have the opportunity to provide PCPE. Psychiatrist trainees should be involved in the PCPE of medical students, and developing a departmental manual that they could use as a toolkit might be helpful in this regard [53]. Encouraging trainees to be role models for medical students will help them to notice that attitudes are as important as, and perhaps more than, knowledge and skills when it comes to helping others to learn person-centered care [59], and it will also help them to solidify their own person-centered approach styles. Moreover, while developing their own styles, psychiatrist trainees should also offer a person-centered role model to their peers, for example, during liaison consultations. This should also be extended to trained psychiatrists within the health system. In both cases, role modelling fellow health professionals requires trained psychiatrists and psychiatrist trainees to have a person-centered approach to patients, patients' families, and their peers.

The PCPE of psychiatrist trainees should also provide them with the chance to learn how to care for themselves. Caring for others should not be accompanied by a disregard of the carer [8]. Residency years have a great impact on the personal and professional lives of physicians, and they should be encouraged to engage with these years reflectively [6, 43]. This need to care for the carer also includes trained psychiatrists working in both educational settings and the health system. Both trainees and trained psychiatrists should develop a space where they can share their own experiences of caring for others. Furthermore, all members of the educational team should be invited to participate in this space. Psychiatrists working in the health system should also try to create these spaces of sharing in their working environments, as peer support should be presented as a normal feature of caring for others [28].

Framing the psychiatrists and psychiatrist trainees' learning process in an environment of caring and reflective practice should further guide their actions to a macro level [8], as caring for the value and dignity of the person involves public health actions [11, 38]. This requires medical educators to promote not only person-centered approaches, but also cultural competence [48]. Psychiatrists should be able to extend the relevance of a person-centered approach beyond medical care and into social activities, research, and government policies [56]. A person-centered approach to care allows an understanding of the patient in context, enabling the possibility to see the impact of socioeconomic, cultural, and environmental factors on the person's health and well-being [2]. Furthermore, the PCPE of psychiatrists, whether it is during training years or as part of continuing professional development, should include building knowledge and awareness of social determinants of health, and it should also encourage them to become actively involved in shaping health policies. Educators should promote policies that help health professionals to obtain and enhance the knowledge, skills, and attitudes necessary to provide person-centered care [15].

In summary, the PCPE of psychiatrists and psychiatrist trainees is supported by the same principles that guide the PCPE of medical students. However, as professionals who are already involved in the process of providing health care, psychiatrists and psychiatrist trainees should align their clinical practice to the person-centered principles they are acquiring, developing, or enhancing in their educational process. This aspiration demands from educators and learners alike to ground their interactions with patients, patients' families, other members of the educational and care team, and each other in the co-construction of a medicine of the person, for the person, by the person, and with the person [40].

39.5 Conclusions

PCPE is an interactional process, dialogical in nature, and transformative in essence. In parallel to the person-centered care it promotes, PCPE regards learners as the core substance of the educational process. Therefore, it requires educators to engage with learners as individuals with unique characteristics, potentialities, and needs, and most importantly, to be committed to be role models. PCPE of medical students, psychiatrist trainees, and trained psychiatrists aims to be a transformative experience that allows learners to observe, experience, internalise, develop, and enhance person-centeredness. It is a process that both advocates and enables a person-centered approach to psychiatry and mental health.

Acknowledgments The authors would like to acknowledge the invaluable contribution of Professor Bulent Coskun in the development of this chapter.

References

1. Appleyard J, Ghebrehiwet T, Mezzich J. Development and implications of the Zagreb declaration on person-centered health professional education. Int J Person Centered Med. 2014;4(1):8–13.
2. Balzarini F. Perspectives from collaborating major medical and health organizations: international federation of medical students' association (IFMSA). Int J Person Centered Med. 2012;2(1):144–5.
3. Baron D, Coskun B. Psychiatrist educators. In Gask L, Coskun B, Baron D, editors. Teaching psychiatry: putting theory into practice. Chichester, West Sussex, UK: Wiley; 2011. p. 247–259.
4. Board of the International College of Person Centered Medicine (ICPCM). Zagreb declaration on person centered health professional education. Croatian Med J. 2014;55(1):81–2.
5. Bombeke K, Symons L, Debaene L, De Winter B, Schol S, Van Royen P. Help, I'm losing patient-centredness! Experiences of medical students and their teachers. Med Educ. 2010;44 (7):662–73.
6. Brady DW, Corbie-Smith G, Branch WT. "What's important to you?": the use of narratives to promote self-reflection and to understand the experiences of medical residents. Ann Intern Med. 2002;137(3):220–3.
7. Brajkovic L. The CEPAMET approach to teaching communication skills to medical students. Int J Person Centered Med. 2015;4(3):167–72.
8. Branch WT Jr. The ethics of caring and medical education. Acad Med. 2000;75(2):127–32.
9. Chan AK, Wood V. Preparing tomorrow's health care providers for interprofessional collaborative patient-centred practice today. UBC Med J. 2010;1(2):22–4.
10. Christodoulou GN. Moral theories and medicine for the person. Int J Integr Care. 2010;10 (Suppl.):48–49.
11. Christodoulou GN, Christodoulou N. Mental health promotion: concept and practice. Int J Person Centered Med. 2012;2(1):24–8.
12. Christodoulou N, Ramalho R. Changement de paradigme d'une médecine préventive centrée sur la maladie à une médecine préventive centrée sur la personne. In: Kipman SD, editor. Médecine de la personne: Un manifeste collectif qui s' adresse aux médecins, soignants, malades et décideurs (ou ceux qui se pensent tels). Paris: Doin; 2012. p. 47–54.
13. Christodoulou N, Ramalho R, Larsson M, Karpenko O. Person-centred medicine and professional development. Int J Person Centered Med. 2011;1(3):581–4.
14. Cloninger CR, Abou-Saleh MT, Mrazek DA, Möller HJ. Biological perspectives on psychiatry for the person. Int J Person Centered Med. 2011;1(1):137–9.
15. Epstein RM, Fiscella K, Lesser CS, Stange KC. Why the nation needs a policy push on patient-centered health care. Health Aff. 2010;29(8):1489–95.
16. Fadden G, Shooter M, Holsgrove G. Involving carers and service users in the training of psychiatrists. Psychiatr Bull. 2005;29(7):270–4.
17. Faulkner A, Thomas P. User-led research and evidence-based medicine. Br J Psychiatry. 2002;180(1):1–3.
18. Gayvoronskaya E. Eastern European considerations on the person with the disease at the center of teaching. Int J Person Centered Med. 2012;2(1):33–7.
19. Gee SB, Scott-Multani ME. Walking in another's shoes: encouraging person-centred care for people living with dementia in New Zealand. World Fed Occup Therapists Bull. 2014;70 (1):13–5.
20. Goss C, Moretti F, Mazzi MA, Del Piccolo L, Rimondini M, Zimmermann C. Involving patients in decisions during psychiatric consultations. Br J Psychiatry. 2008;193(5):416–21.
21. Greenhalgh T, Seyan K, Boynton P. "Not a university type": focus group study of social class, ethnic, and sex differences in school pupils' perceptions about medical school. BMJ. 2004;328 (7455):1541–7.

22. Haeney O, Moholkar R, Taylor N, Harrison T. Service user involvement in psychiatric training: a practical perspective. Psychiatr Bull. 2007;31(8):312–4.
23. Henschen BL, Garcia P, Jacobson B, Ryan ER, Woods DM, Wayne DB, Evans DB. The patient centered medical home as curricular model: perceived impact of the "education-centered medical home". J Gen Intern Med. 2013;28(8):1105–9.
24. Herbert CP. Changing the culture: interprofessional education for collaborative patient-centred practice in Canada. J Interprof Care. 2005;19(suppl. 1):1–4.
25. Horton M, Freire P. We make the road by walking: conversations on education and social change. Philadelphia: Temple University Press; 1990.
26. Hovey RB, Apelian N. Is our incapacity for conversation a serious barrier to person centred medicine? Int J Person Centered Med. 2014;4(1):52–9.
27. Howe A. Patient-centred medicine through student-centred teaching: a student perspective on the key impacts of community-based learning in undergraduate medical education. Med Educ. 2001;35(7):666–72.
28. Hu YY, Fix ML, Hevelone ND, Lipsitz SR, Greenberg CC, Weissman JS, Shapiro J. Physicians' needs in coping with emotional stressors: the case for peer support. Arch Surg. 2012;147(3):212–7.
29. Ikkos G. Engaging patients as teachers of clinical interview skills. Psychiatr Bull. 2003;27 (8):312–5.
30. Jochemsen-van der Leeuw HR, van Dijk N, van Etten-Jamaludin FS, Wieringa-de Waard M. The attributes of the clinical trainer as a role model: a systematic review. Acad Med. 2013;88 (1):26–34.
31. Kallivayalil RA, Kumar PS. Education in person-centered medicine: Indian perspectives. Int J Person Centered Med. 2012;2(2):155–8.
32. Karle H. World federation for medical education perspectives on person-centered medicine. Int J Integr Care. 2010;10:14–7.
33. Kruithof R, Kaduru CC. International federation of medical students association: views on person-centered medicine. Int J Person Centered Med. 2011;1(1):90–1.
34. Lévesque M, Hovey R, Bedos C. Advancing patient-centered care through transformative educational leadership: a critical review of health care professional preparation for patient-centered care. J Healthc Leadersh. 2013;5:35–46.
35. Livingston G, Cooper C. User and carer involvement in mental health training. Adv Psychiatr Treat. 2004;10(2):85–92.
36. Luttenberger K, Graessel E, Simon C, Donath C. From board to bedside-training the communication competences of medical students with role plays. BMC Med Educ. 2014;14 (1):135–45.
37. Mezzich JE. Psychiatry for the person: articulating medicine's science and humanism. World Psychiatry. 2007;6(2):65–7.
38. Mezzich JE. World Psychiatric Association perspectives on person-centered psychiatry and medicine. Int J Integr Care. 2009;10(suppl.):e003.
39. Mezzich JE. Building person-centered medicine through dialogue and partnerships: perspective from the international network for person-centered medicine. Int J Person Centered Med. 2011;1(1):10–3.
40. Mezzich JE, Snaedal J, van Weel C, Heath I. Toward person-centered medicine: from disease to patient to person. Mount Sinai J Med. 2010;77:304–6.
41. Motschnig-Pitrik R, Standl B. Person-centered technology enhanced learning: dimensions of added value. Comput Hum Behav. 2013;29(2):401–9.
42. Paice E, Heard S, Moss F. How important are role models in making good doctors? BMJ: Br Med J. 2002;325(7366):707–10.
43. Plack MM, Greenberg L. The reflective practitioner: reaching for excellence in practice. Pediatrics. 2005;116(6):1546–52.
44. Ramalho R. Doctor-patient relationship. New perspectives. Anales de la Facultad de Ciencias Medicas (Asuncion). 2008;41(1–2):82–5.

45. Ramalho R. Psychiatry and mental health. Anales de la Facultad de Ciencias Medicas (Asuncion). 2009;42(1):55–8.
46. Rimondini M, Del Piccolo L, Goss C, Mazzi M, Paccaloni M, Zimmermann C. Communication skills in psychiatry residents—how do they handle patient concerns? An application of sequence analysis to interviews with simulated patients. Psychother Psychosom. 2006;75(3):161–9.
47. Rogers CR. Freedom to learn for the 80's. Columbus: Ohio, Charles E Merrill Publishing Company; 1983.
48. Saha S, Beach MC, Cooper LA. Patient centeredness, cultural competence and healthcare quality. J Natl Med Assoc. 2008;100(11):1275–85.
49. Salvador-Carulla L, Cloninger CR, Thornicroft A, Mezzich JE. Background, structure and priorities of the 2013 Geneva declaration on person-centered health research. Int J Person Centered Med. 2013;3(2):109–13.
50. Shield RR, Tong I, Tomas M, Besdine RW. Teaching communication and compassionate care skills: an innovative curriculum for pre-clerkship medical students. Med Teach. 2011;33(8): e408–16.
51. Spencer J, Blackmore D, Heard S, McCrorie P, McHaffie D, Scherpbier A, Gupta TS, Singh K, Southgate L. Patient-oriented learning: a review of the role of the patient in the education of medical students. Med Educ. 2000;34(10):851–7.
52. Stewart M, Weston WW, McWhinney IR, McWilliam CL, Freeman TR. Patient-centred medicine: transforming the clinical method. 2nd ed. Oxford, UK: Radcliffe Medical Press Limited; 2003.
53. Swainson J, Marsh M, Tibbo PG. Psychiatric residents as teachers: development and evaluation of a teaching manual. Acad Psychiatry. 2010;34(4):305–9.
54. Towle A, Bainbridge L, Godolphin W, Katz A, Kline C, Lown B, Madularu I, Solomon P, Thistlethwaite J. Active patient involvement in the education of health professionals. Med Educ. 2010;44:64–74.
55. Turner P, Sheldon F, Coles C, Mountford B, Hillier R, Radway P, Wee B. Listening to and learning from the family carer's story: an innovative approach in interprofessional education. J Interprof Care. 2000;14(4):387–95.
56. Wagner P, Perales A, Armas R, Codas O, de los Santos R, Elio-Calvo D, Mendoza-Vega J, Arce M, Calderón JL, Llosa L, Saavedra J, Ugarte O, Vildózola H, Mezzich JE. Latin American bases and perspectives on person centered medicine and health. Int J Person Centered Med. 2014;4(4):220–227.
57. Walsh K. Medical education: a new pedagogy of the oppressed? Med Teach. 2013;36(2):175–6.
58. Walters K, Buszewicz M, Russell J, Humphrey C. Teaching as therapy: cross sectional and qualitative evaluation of patients' experiences of undergraduate psychiatry teaching in the community. BMJ. 2003;326(7392):740–6.
59. Wear D, Skillicorn J. Hidden in plain sight: the formal, informal, and hidden curricula of a psychiatry clerkship. Acad Med. 2009;84(4):451–8.
60. Weston WW, Brown JB. The learner-centered method of medical education. In: Stewart M, Weston WW, McWhinney IR, McWilliam CL, Freeman TR, editors. Patient-centred medicine: transforming the clinical method. 2nd ed. Oxford, UK: Radcliffe Medical Press Limited; 2003.
61. Wykurz G, Kelly D. Developing the role of patients as teachers: literature review. BMJ. 2002;325(7368):818–21.

Person-Centered Psychiatric and Mental Health Research

40

Luis Salvador-Carulla, MD, PhD, Arnstein Finset, PhD
and Alberto Perales-Cabrera, MD, DMedSc

40.1 Introduction

The crucial role of research and of building the broader possible bases of solid evidence for PCM had been recognized early on by the International College of Person Centered Medicine (ICPCM). In 2012, and in consonance with priorities of other sponsoring organizations, such as the WHO, the ICPCM decided it was timely to dedicate the 2013 Geneva conference to this topic. The aim of this chapter is to describe the development of the 2013 Geneva Declaration on Person-centered Health Research and to provide additional information on the research priority areas identified during this iterative process in mental health.

In summary, ICPCM recognized Person-Centered Medicine and Person-Centered Health care (PCH) as a complex construct which articulates science and humanism for a bio-psycho-socio-cultural understanding of health and for the undertaking of

L. Salvador-Carulla, MD, PhD (✉)
Centre for Disability Research and Policy, Faculty of Health Sciences, and Mental Health Policy Unit, Brain and Mind Centre, University of Sydney, 75 East St Lidcombe, NSW 2141, Australia
e-mail: luis.salvador-carulla@sydney.edu.au

A. Finset, PhD
Professor, Department of Behavioral Sciences in Medicine, Institute of Basic Medical Sciences, Faculty of Medicine, University of Oslo, Oslo, Norway
e-mail: arnstein.finset@medisin.uio.no

A. Perales-Cabrera, MD, DMedSc
Professor, Department of Psychiatry and Institute of Ethics in Health, Faculty of Medicine, Universidad Nacional Mayor de San Marcos, Lima, Peru; Honorary Member, Academia Nacional de Medicina, Lima, Peru
e-mail: perales.alberto@gmail.com

J.E. Mezzich et al. (eds.), *Person Centered Psychiatry*,
DOI 10.1007/978-3-319-39724-5_40

health care actions from individual interventions to people's health to general health policy, guided by the ethical principle of respect for the autonomy, dignity, and responsibility of each person. Due to its inherent characteristics PCH demands a complexity approach to its study and analysis.

PCH involves complex structures, functions, and high-dimensional interactions among multiple factors, where the meaning of the measurements becomes crucial for proper interpretation, and where phenomena are very difficult to model under classical approaches. The complexity and nonlinearity of PCH [28] has major implications to data analysis, too often based on techniques and procedures designed for linear phenomena, which should not be applied to systems characterized by nonlinearity, self-organization and constant change, fragmented but highly interconnected, history-dependent, and counterintuitive. In order to analyze and to understand complex systems, prior expert knowledge should be incorporated into the analysis itself. Generalizing classical data analysis methods to be guided by prior expert knowledge permits a better modeling of these phenomena and improves the quality of the results. Taking the prior expert knowledge into account is not necessarily related to a loss of scientific rigor, since, from the beginnings of the artificial Intelligence developments in the mid 1950s, there are strictly rigorous frameworks, based on logical paradigms, to handle expert knowledge in a formal and automatized manner. As an example, the 'Expert-based Collaborative Analysis' (EbCA) [9] completes classical data analysis with prior expert knowledge as a mean to extract relevant knowledge in complex health domains and shows how explicit and tacit or implicit expert knowledge are critical to guide the scientific analysis of very complex decisional problems such as those found in health system research.

Framing analysis is the first step of the EbCA process and other methods that incorporate prior expert knowledge in the analysis of complex phenomena. Until very recently health research has paid very little attention to framing tools which have been regarded as irrelevant or as 'evidence' within the classical Evidence-based Medicine framework [29].

40.2 Main Domains to Develop a PHC Research Roadmap in Mental Health

The main areas of research focus identified at the 2013 Declaration include: Conceptual, terminological, and ontological issues; research to enhance the empirical evidence of PCM main components such as PCH informed clinical communication; PCH-based diagnostic models; person-centered care (PCC) and interventions; and people-centered care (PCC), research on training and curriculum development. Dissemination and implementation of PCH knowledge-base is integral to Person-centered Health Research and shall engage currently available scientific and translational dissemination tools including eHealth. All these areas apply to current challenges and research needs in the mental health sector.

1. **Conceptual, Terminological, and Ontological Issues**: The development of a knowledge-base and the generation of evidence that can be transferred and applied in different settings requires common conceptual frameworks, terms, and taxonomy. For example it is relevant to provide a 'synset' (set of synonyms and semantically related terms) [30] of the key concepts in this field and the conceptual map or the formal relationship across these terms to enhance scientific communication. Under the umbrella term of 'Person-Centered Health' it is necessary to set up the definitions and boundaries of "Person-Centered Medicine," "Person-Centered Care," "Person-Centered Planning," "People-Centered Care," and also the links with "Personalised Medicine" [27]. It is also important to set up an internationally agreed glossary of terms and consensus-based guides to develop research that can be effectively compared across settings, territories, and cultures. Finally the relationship of PCH and the partnership approach in medicine [19] should be established with other fields of collaborative health such as integrative medicine, integrated care, chronic care, bridging, and knowledge transfer. A comprehensive approach should encourage analysis from different perspectives including philosophy of science, biological, psychological, social, and cultural approaches. International comparison should be encouraged [20].
2. **Evidence on the Main Components of PCH and its Implications for Mental Health**: It is important to generate more evidence on the different domains of PCH taking into account the complexity approach [32]. These domains include illness and wellness, disability and functioning, resilience and resources, plus experiences of health and contributors to health, and well-being in PCH [18]. In particular, the development of well-being can be characterized in terms of the nonlinear dynamic interaction among plasticity, virtue, and functioning as the "motor of well-being" [4, 5]. Within this context the experiences of health such as suffering, meaning and understanding of illness, contentment, fulfillment, and flourishing constitute a core element of PCH that deserve special attention. Developmental and life course perspectives should also be studied within the context of PCH (e.g., mental capital approach) [1] with special attention to gender and age groups (children and elderly population) and to other vulnerable groups [17, 24]. The standardization of international assessment procedures and instruments of the main components of PCH should be encouraged [4]. Finally, a translational approach should be adopted in the integrative study of these domains linking person-centered research to genomics, neurosciences and epigenetics, as well as, to social, environmental, economics, and policy research [3].
3. **Clinical Communication in Mental Health**: The doctor–patient relationship constitutes a key element of PCH. This relationship represents the fundamental matrix for the whole of care. It should encompass empathic listening, comprehensive diagnosis beyond symptom checklists, appreciation for symbolic meaning, nonverbal communication, engagement, and information exchange and transfer. The doctor–patient relationship represents at its best a therapeutic partnership advancing the process and outcome of care.

Del Piccolo and colleagues have investigated doctor–patient communication in psychiatric consultations in Italy, using the Verona Coding Definitions of Emotional Sequences (VR-CoDES) [7]. The VR-CoDES makes a distinction between cues or hints to underlying emotions and concerns, which are explicit expressions of negative emotions. They found that cues were more frequent among female patients across most diagnostic categories, while concerns were more frequent among patients with mood disorders. When responding to cues and concerns, psychiatrists often provided space to further disclosure, but referred explicitly to the affective dimension of patients' expression only when the psychiatrist him- or her-self had initiated the patient's cue or concern. In a subsequent study, they found that a vague hint or cue could be elaborated into a more explicit concern if the psychiatrist actively had provided room for further disclosure [7].

A majority of patients with mental health problems are treated in general practice. In a study of the attitudes and learning needs of general practitioners (GPs) regarding mental health issues in general practice. Based on the results of previous study that found that a majority of GPs was interested in training in mental health and in communication skills to promote patient coping; Stensrud et al. developed and tested a training program for GPs based on six specific skills in emotional and cognitive domains and related to individual coping. Three of the skills were "explorative": (i) be sensitive to and explore patients′ hints, concerns and emotions; (ii) explore the patient's perspective and understanding; and (iii) assess the patient's resources and strengths. The other three were "therapeutic skills" elaborating on patients' responses to the explorations: (iv) be explicitly empathic to emotional content; (v) provide insight into possible cause–effect relations of the problem; and (vi) promote empowerment by focusing on resources, strengths, and coping strategies. Skills exploring emotions, cognitions and resources, and the skills aimed to promote coping, increased significantly after training [31]. In any case more research is needed to understand patient's problems and concerns; to establish the therapeutic alliance by acknowledging and responding to patient's emotion, and to inform and involve patients and their families in the decision-making process [6].

Within this context, topics that require special attention are integrative/translational research in PCH communication, shared decision making [33], the impact of health information technologies, and the roles of patients and health professionals in relation to empowerment and new models of care [25, 26]. International guidelines for person-centered research on clinical communication are emerging [16].

4. **PCH Diagnostic Models and Mental Health**: This includes the development, validation, and comparison of the usability of PCH diagnostic models, guides and assessment instruments. For example, the Person-centered Integrative Diagnosis (PID) model [18] not only identifies and classifies illnesses, disabilities, and related problems but also assesses positive health [5]. It also includes a comprehensive evaluation of biological, psychological, and social contextual factors contributing to health. This model is also unique as it includes

a narrative component to complement each domain considered. It further includes in a narrative format domains on the experience of and values relevant to ill and positive health. The PID intends to serve as effective informational base for understanding the clinical situation and planning for care collaboratively among clinicians, patients, and families [18, 25, 26]. Other models, while not as comprehensive and balanced on including the totality of health as the PID include the "pragmatic model" which describes the behaviors shown by persons with mental disorders as the base for diagnosis and intervention in mental health [16]. Other contextualized models also include the International Classification of Primary Care (ICPC-2). This classification system allows for simple linkage between reason for encounter, diagnosis, and intervention, taking into account the complex relationship between biological, psychological, mental, and social problems and their temporal variations [2, 8].

5. **Person-centered Care and Interventions in Mental Health**: The International Alliance of Patients' Organizations have defined five principles of patient-centered healthcare: Respect, choice and empowerment, patient involvement in health policy, access and support, and information [10]. A better understanding of individual PCC and interventions for health promotion, prevention, treatment, and rehabilitation is required, including aspects related to empowerment of patients and their families, and care issues such as usability, efficacy and effectiveness, efficiency, appropriateness, equity, parity, and quality of interventions following the PCH care models [21]. These developments should be framed in the context of the new International Classification of Health Interventions (ICHI) [22]. The international standardization of instruments for assessing the different facets of PCC and the development of indicators of individual interventions on PCC deserve special attention. Furthermore, PCH research calls for patient active partnership and engagement in the research endeavor from identifying priority areas and research questions to study design and choice of meaningful outcomes to dissemination of results and practical implementation of research findings.
6. **People-centered Care**: More research is needed on indicators of PCC [10] as well as on health system analysis and policy that are conducive for PCC and planning at all levels of care (community, regional, country, and international levels) [19]. Particular topics that should be mentioned are patient involvement in health policy, links between PCC and integrated care to develop and to implement person-centered integrated care systems, PCC in vulnerable population groups, and use of new methods of system analysis in PCC.
7. **Research in Training and Curriculum Development** is also required, as training and education are key contributors to the development and implementation of PCH. The 2006 World Health Report documented the severe shortages of health professionals around the globe and their poor fit to health service delivery needs, including training on person-centredness, as well as limitations in opportunities for health professional students of different disciplines to learn together and interact adequately during their training [11, 12]. The Buenos Aires Declaration on Humanism and Science in Latin America for

Person Centered Medicine, included important recommendation on methods and instruments for "promoting a person-centered health professional education founded on both ethical and scientific bases" [13]. Traditionally, medical schools have emphasized, almost exclusively, scientific training of undergraduate students neglecting aspects of their emotional maturity as a person. Medical students pass a minimum of six years assimilating the technological and scientific teachings that provide them with the necessary skills for professional practice; however, during that period, the university has not wondered what happens to these potential leaders with regard to their psychological, spiritual, and moral growth for becoming better persons. As an example, a survey made in 2010 on medical students (n = 601) of a Peruvian public university gave, within other results, the following life-prevalences: suicidal attempts, 4 %; homicidal ideation, 12.9 % and indicators of antisocial behavior, 19.2 % [23]. Such worrisome results, indicates that student´s mental health should be assessed and their personal development should be an outstanding commitment of our medical education systems.

8. **eTools for Person Centered Mental Health**: These tools may include internet-based informational platform and substructures to support PCH activities and research, such as workgroup efforts and inter-institutional and scholarly collaboration [14, 15], and specific apps.

40.3 Conclusions

There is a need for more PCH research and for the incorporation of the PCH approach into mental health research and medical education. The ICPCM has recognized this need in a series of documents, mainly in the 2013 Geneva Declaration on Person Centered Health Research. Major areas of development are conceptual, terminological, and ontological issues; evidence on the main components of PCM and its implications for mental health; clinical communication in mental health; PCM diagnostic models in mental health; PCC and interventions in mental health; PCC; research in training and curriculum development; and the development of eTools for person-centered mental health.

References

1. Beddington J, Cooper CL, Field J, Goswami U, Huppert FA, Jenkins R, Jones HS, Kirkwood TB, Sahakian BJ, Thomas SM. The mental wealth of nations. Nature.2008;455 (7216):1057–60.
2. Boot CR, Meijman FJ. Classifying health questions asked by the public using the ICPC-2 classification and a taxonomy of generic clinical questions: an empirical exploration of the feasibility. Health Commun. 2010;25(2):175–81.
3. Cloninger CR, Abou-Saleh M, Mrazek DA, Moller HJ. Biological perspective on psychiatry for the person. Int J Person-centered Med. 2011;1(1):135–7.

4. Cloninger CR, Cloninger KM. Development of instruments and evaluative procedures for contributions to health and illness. Int J Person-centered Med. 2011;1(3):446–55.
5. Cloninger CR, Salloum IM, Mezzich JE. The dynamic origins of positive health and wellbeing. Int J Person-centered Med. 2012;2(2):179–87.
6. Del Piccolo L, Goss C. People-centred care: new research needs and methods in doctor-patient communication. Challenges in mental health. Epidemiol Psychiatr Sci. 2012;21(2):145–9.
7. Del Piccolo L, Mazzi MA, Goss C, Rimondini M, Zimmermann C. How emotions emerge and are dealt with in first diagnostic consultations in psychiatry. Patient Educ Couns. 2012;88:29–35.
8. Gask L, Klinkman M, Fortes S, Dowrick C. Capturing complexity: the case for a new classification system for mental disorders in primary care. Eur Psychiatry. 2008;23(7):469–76.
9. Gibert K, Garcia-Alonso C, Salvador-Carulla L. Integrating clinicians, knowledge and data: expert-based cooperative analysis in healthcare decision support. Health Res Policy Syst. 2010;8:28.
10. International Alliance of Patients' Organizations (IAPO). Patient-centred healthcare indicators review; 2012. IAPO, London, viewed 17 Jan 2016. www.patientsorganizations.org.
11. International College of Person-centered Medicine (ICPCM). Geneva declaration on person-centered care for chronic diseases. Int J Person-Centered Med. 2012;2(2):153–4.
12. International College of Person Centered Medicine (ICPCM). Geneva declaration on person centered health research. Int J Person Centered Med. 2013;3:106–7.
13. International College of Person Centered Medicine (ICPCM). The 2014 Buenos Aires declaration on humanism and science in Latin America for person centered medicine. Int J Person Centered Med. 2014;4:217–8.
14. Kirisci L, Reynolds M, Vanyukov M, Ridenour T, Hayes J, Mezzich JE. Developing an institutional information base and bibliographical clearinghouse. Int J Person Centered Med. 2011;1:109–12.
15. Kovacevic A, Dehghan A, Filannino M, Keane JA, Nenadic G. Combining rules and machine learning for extraction of temporal expressions and events from clinical narratives. J Am Med Inform Assoc. 2013;20(5):859–66.
16. Ladd PD, Churchill AM. Person-centered diagnosis and treatment in mental health. A model for empowering clients. London: Jessica Kingsley Publ.,: 2012.
17. Lüthi H, Geyh S, Baumberger ME, Dokladal P, Scheuringer M, Mäder M, Cieza A. The individual experience of functioning and disability in Switzerland—patient perspective and person-centeredness in spinal cord injury. Spinal Cord. 2011;49(12):1173–81.
18. Mezzich JE, Salloum IM, Cloninger CR, Salvador-Carulla L, Kirmayer LJ, Banzato CE, Wallcraft J, Botbol M. Person-centred integrative diagnosis: conceptual bases and structural model. Can J Psychiatry. 2010;55(11):701–8.
19. Mezzich JE, Snaedal J, van Weel C, Botbol M, Salloum I, van Lerberghe W. Articulating person-centered medicine and people-centered public health: a report from the fourth geneva conference. World Med J. 2011;57:171–4.
20. Nolte E, Knai C, Mckee M. Managing chronic conditions experience in eight countries. World Health Organization, European Regional Office, on behalf of the European Observatory on Health Systems and Policies, Geneva;2008.
21. Olsson LE, Jakobsson UNG E, Swedberg K, Ekman I. Efficacy of person-centred care as an intervention in controlled trials - a systematic review. J Clin Nurs. 2013;22(3–4):456–65.
22. Paviot BT, Madden R, Moskal L, Zaiss A, Bousquet C, Kumar A, Lewalle P, Rodrigues JM. Development of a new international classification of health interventions based on an ontology framework. Stud Health Technol Inform. 2011;169:749–53.
23. Perales A, Alarcón J, Sánchez E, Arcaya M, Cortez E, Parhuana A, Caballero J, Carrera R, Torres H. Conducta suicida en estudiantes de medicina de una universidad nacional peruana. En Violencia y Trauma en el Perú. Desafíos y Respuestas. In Bustamante I, Rivera M, Matos L, editors. Programa Trauma y Salud Global. Lima: UPCH, McGill University; 2013. p. 105–13.
24. Raudonis BM, Daniel K. Frailty: an indication for palliative care. Geriatr Nurs. 2010;31 (5):379–84.

25. Salloum IM, Mezzich JE. Person-centered diagnosis. Int J Integr Care. 2010;10(suppl. e027).
26. Salloum IM, Mezzich JE. Conceptual appraisal of the person-centered integrative diagnosis model. Int J Person Centered Med. 2011;1(1):39–42.
27. Salvador-Carulla L, Mezzich JE. Person-centred medicine and mental health. Epidemiol Psychiatric Sci. 2012;21(2):131–7.
28. Salvador-Carulla L, Garcia-Alonso C, Gibert K, Vazquez-Bourgon J. Incorporating local information and prior expert knowledge to evidence-informed mental health system research. In: Thornicroft G, Ruggeri M, Goldberg D, editors. Improving mental health care: the global challenge. Chichester: Willey; 2013. p. 209–28.
29. Salvador-Carulla L, Fernandez A, Madden R, Lukersmith S, Colagiuri R, Torkfar G, Sturmberg J. Framing of scientific knowledge as a new category of health care research. J Eval Crit Pract. 2014;20(6):1045–55.
30. Sanchez D, Batet M, Valls A, et al. Ontology-driven web-based semantic similarity. J Intell Inf Syst. 2010;35:383–413.
31. Stensrud TL, Gulbrandsen P, Mjaaland TA, Skretting S, Finset A. Improving communication in general practice when mental health issues appear: piloting a set of six evidence based skills. Patient Educ Couns. 2014;95:69–75.
32. Sturmberg JP. Caring for people with chronic disease: is 'muddling through' the best way to handle the multiple complexities? J Eval Clin Pract. 2012;18(6):1220–5.
33. Van Dulmen S, Humphris G, EIDE H. Towards a guideline for person-centered research in clinical communication: lessons learned from three countries. Int J Person Centered Med. 2012;2:58–63.

Index

Note: Page numbers followed by *f* and *t* indicate figures and tables respectively.

J.E. Mezzich et al. (eds.), *Person Centered Psychiatry*,
DOI 10.1007/978-3-319-39724-5